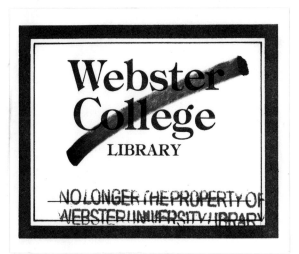

INTEGRATED MEDICINE

INTEGRATED MEDICINE

VOLUME II
OF A COMPANION
TO THE LIFE SCIENCES

Edited By

STACEY B. DAY, M.D., Ph.D., D.Sc.

*Retired Professor, Sloan Kettering Division, Cornell University
Medical College, New York; Consultant and Member,
Board of Directors, American Institute of Stress; Consultant
Communications and Medical Education, Division of Surgery,
St. Barnabas Hospital, Bronx, New York.*

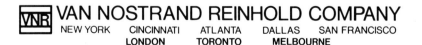
VAN NOSTRAND REINHOLD COMPANY
NEW YORK   CINCINNATI   ATLANTA   DALLAS   SAN FRANCISCO
LONDON   TORONTO   MELBOURNE

Van Nostrand Reinhold Company Regional Offices:
New York Cincinnati Atlanta Dallas San Francisco

Van Nostrand Reinhold Company International Offices:
London Toronto Melbourne

Library of Congress Catalog Card Number: 78-8300
ISBN: 0-442-25163-7

Manufactured in the United States of America

Published by Van Nostrand Reinhold Company
135 West 50th Street, New York, N.Y. 10020

Published simultaneously in Canada by Van Nostrand Reinhold Ltd.

15 14 13 12 11 10 9 8 7 6 5 4 3 2 1

Library of Congress Cataloging in Publication Data

Main entry under title:

Integrated Medicine, Vol. II of A companion to the life sciences

   Includes index.
   1. Life sciences. I. Day, Stacey B.
[DNLM: 1. Biology. 2. Science. 3. Behavioral
sciences. 4. Medicine. QH307.2 C737]
QH307.2.C65   574   78-8300
ISBN 0-442-22010-3 (v.1)
ISBN 0-442-25163-7 (v.2) Integrated Medicine

Preface

Notwithstanding the extraordinary increase in knowledge over the last three decades, there appears to be a marked lack of responsiveness to understand *what* this knowledge portends, and *how it may best be managed* for the good of society generally. It is a paradox of the teaching profession that while researching presumed new knowledge, it either fails or is reluctant to recognize that hand in hand with change must come new perspective in comprehension of the knowledge process and its potential to change existing boundaries or limits. Reasonably it is held that education is a goal of teaching institutions and must remain so, but few medical educational systems are concerned with change in society; neither do they evaluate the critical truth that management—or handling—of knowledge information must keep apace of the process of discovery. It is precisely to this area of medical knowledge—the management and strategies of handling health knowledge power (management of knowledge)—that we have addressed ourselves over the last 12 years.

Clinical and basic research knowledge accrue so rapidly that few investigators are able to keep abreast of their own unique fields. Furthermore, what might be called the *form* of knowledge changes. New problems are posed.

In the relatively brief span of 25 years, broad scientific advance has moved to molecular levels. Experimental philosophy must provide a context for change of educational prospect as well as process of change in the onward passage of knowledge toward improving scholarship. During this time, we have engaged methodologies relating procedure and governance via interdisciplinary learning.

The concept of the first volume of *A Companion to the Life Sciences* was to encourage search for a timely strategy which can cope with rapid increase in knowledge, in multiple disciplines, widely dispersed, yet presentable in a synthesis acceptable on a broad general educational front, as far as is possible within the dimensions of the fields under review. The present volume continues these efforts. Widely integrated medical knowledge is presented here.

It is hoped that comprehensive attention to the text will suggest that we have now arrived at a point when the interdisciplinary approach is fully accepted. Those at the cutting edge of these efforts have long recognized that knowledge is a power source, and dynamics of synthesis of new information must be integrated into as wide a sphere of daily life as is possible. *Science* and *technology* are words that sit comfortably on the heads of citizens as well as of students and professors. The next front in the medical field must be to establish a synthesis between health communications/health education and biosocial development and biopsychosocial health. This direction, I submit, will serve creative policies of human resources, basic human needs, justice rather than ethics, quality of life and of the biosphere, cultural diversity and transcultural tolerance, and many other forms of social growth. Good health is not only good clinical health but also good social health. The choice of papers in this integrated medical volume emphasizes this. Although social health is not yet as structured as clinical medicine, it must be considered of equal importance.

The basis of the editorial conviction is the faith that integrated views on medicine are needed; that we have moved, in our societies, from strictly clinical or curative philosophy of disease to augmented understanding of the social foundation of illness. Health care, as a dominant force in the decade ahead, must include teaching of the social process of problems as well as the treatment of pathophysiologic anatomy of disease per se. Aspects of both medical viewpoints are included in this volume.

STACEY B. DAY, M.D., PH.D., D.SC.
Retired Professor, Sloan-Kettering Division,
Cornell University Medical College, New York

Contents

III DISEASES OF THE BLOOD VESSELS

IV CURRENT CLINICAL MANAGEMENT

I
PHYSIOLOGICAL AND MOLECULAR PERSPECTIVES RELEVANT TO CLINICAL PROBLEMS

Introduction

EVERETT V. SUGARBAKER, M. D.
University of Miami
Miami, Florida

The fields of clinical medicine at large interrelate with the ever expanding body of knowledge in other health sciences, as well as with an even broader perimeter of multiple and increasingly specialized disciplines included loosely under the heading "Life Sciences." The volume of data/knowledge being generated in each life science specialty is virtually exploding, and increasingly specialized journals, specialty associations and meetings, and so on continue to proliferate. And, indeed, the need for more intense intraspecialty communication is real. Many new and highly specialized scientific observations need to be refined, replicated, and their relevance to life science determined, with these specialty review mechanisms fulfilling this requirement. On the other hand, this real need for highly specialized communication has perhaps too often created a series of discrete islands of knowledge. The scientists so isolated and pressured by constraints of time, and so forth, frequently do not or cannot interrelate with other specialists in related disciplines; and, of equal importance, very limited interaction with the broader spectrum of the life sciences occurs.

From the viewpoint of the educator our islands of specialization can create an impasse for the trainee in the life sciences. It is difficult to integrate specialty data meaningfully. One of the most difficult educational challenges with allotted curriculum time and space is to balance the amount of relevant specialty data with meaningful and useful generalizing concepts. The new scientific trainees often crave guidance in their desire to sift the irrelevant data from the important. They also frequently find a synthesis or an overview of a subject even if its central tenets must be eventually discarded in light of even newer knowledge— a useful point of reference. Our problem of specialty islands, therefore, not only impairs the mutually desired progress of the life sciences as a whole, but greatly complicates our educational process and burdens both educator and trainee.

This problem of islands of specialization and their potentially harmful effect on the life sciences has received national attention, with such truisms as "improved technology transfer" and "interdisciplinary programs" as general expressions of the desire to improve intercommunication among disciplines. Many

3

mechanisms to effect this goal of improved interaction are currently being in-vestigated on many levels. One approach that could be of real benefit is being explored in this series of *Companion* volumes. Why not ask the specialists themselves, many of whom are also experienced educators and widely read scientists, to sift their own specialty for its most relevant data and present in verbal and graphic form a state-of-the-art overview? Thus the authors of these volumes were charged:

> The goal for this contribution is that it should be an authoritative state-of-the art overview definitively selecting the most important facts in your area. As you write be cognizant of the fact that it should have a multi-disciplinary appeal to those who would not be expected to read your specialty literature.

References were severely curtailed to encourage forthright statements and avoid bibliographic elections of a given viewpoint. Likewise space was severely limited in the confidence that the knowledgeable specialists/contributors could under these constraints meaningfully characterize the core concepts of their chosen areas of specialization.

Thus, specialists generally acclaimed in their field of endeavor and with ex-perience in education were chosen to participate. Since Volume II is dominantly centered about clinical problems, areas of recent major scientific or clinical advance not included in other volumes of this series are described. Clearly space limitations demand that this selection of topics be somewhat arbitrary. Included in this volume are recent but established advances in disease pathophysiology and nutrition, restorative and replacement surgery, cardiac and peripheral blood vessel disease, the cancer problem, biomethods as applied to clinical medicine, and environmental considerations in clinical and infectious disease.

In summary, the *Companion* concept is viewed as one of the several possible methods for effectively bridging the islands of knowledge that have developed as a natural result of increasing specialization. The thrust of this approach is to request that recognized scientist-educators assume some of the responsibility for intercommunication themselves, and additionally channel these efforts into a concise yet meaningful format. If other scientists and trainees can better interrelate to other specialties or new areas of interest because of this mecha-nism, the objectives of this volume will be well on the way to fulfillment.

The Thymus and Its Functions

OSIAS STUTMAN
Memorial Sloan-Kettering Cancer Center
New York, New York

The 1971 edition of the *Oxford English Dictionary* still defines the thymus as "a glandular body of obscure function (one of the so-called 'ductless glands')" *Webster's New Collegiate Dictionary* (1973) goes one step further and defines the thymus as "a glandular structure . . . that is held to function esp. in the development of the body's immune system." In the calf and lamb the thymus is the neck sweetbread of the butchers, a gourmet's delicacy. However, dictionaries cannot be considered as authoritative sources on biological matters. Although there are still unresolved questions concerning mechanisms of thymus action, there is total agreement that such a "glandular body" has a critical role in regulating the development and maintenance of a major part of the immune system in animals and man. For the chronologers, the first clear observations of the role of the thymus on the regulation of immune functions in mammals were published in 1961.

The notion that there are two broad categories of immune responses—humoral and cellular—although simplistic in its inception, has been extremely useful for the study of lymphoid physiology. Humoral immunity is mediated by antibodies present in the serum, whereas cellular immunity is mediated directly by lymphoid cells. Both systems, although showing extensive interaction with each other at a functional level, are independent from each other for their development. The thymus regulates the production of the lymphocytes involved in cellular or cell-mediated immunity. The development of the antibody-producing cells which operate in humoral immunity is independent of the thymus, and in mammals probably regulated by special microenvironments in the marrow or the sites for early hemopoiesis such as liver in the embryo. In birds, the development of the humoral immunity system is regulated by a specific organ called the bursa of Fabricius. Based on this "dichotomy" the cell-mediated system has been termed "thymus-dependent," and its effector cells are globally described as "T cells." The cells composing the humoral immunity system, which is thymus-independent for its development, have been termed "B cells." Humoral immunity includes responses such as antibody production, immediate hypersensitivity, allergic reactions, and bactericidal reactions to various microorganisms. On the other hand, cellular immunity includes delayed hypersensitivity reactions, rejection of foreign tissue grafts, immunity to intracellular parasites, and immunity to some viral infections. In experimental models, humoral immunity can be transferred to naive animals with serum, whereas cellular immunity can be transferred passively only with the appropriate immune cells. With this brief introduction, we will discuss the functions of the thymus and the functions of T cells.

FUNCTIONS OF THE THYMUS

The process of blood cell formation, including formation of T lymphocytes, is called hemopoiesis. The fact that all the lymphoid cells of the blood and tissues have finite life spans but are constantly replenished and maintained at defined numbers, argues that there must be a mechanism for such cell renewal. This type of renewal system also applies to the other blood cells such as red cells, leukocytes, monocytes, and so on. A general statement about hemopoiesis is that it is the consequence of complex events that include especially the interaction between hemopoietic stem cells, which give rise to committed precursor cells for the different lineages, under the influence of local microenvironments. This general statement applies also to the thymus and the formation of T cells. In fact, one of the functions of the thymus is to provide the local microenvironment that is necessary for hemopoietic precurosrs to become irreversibly committed to differentiation along the T lineage.

During the early studies using neonatal thymectomy in mice, it was observed that the immunological defects produced by the procedure could be restored by the grafting of a thymus. When the phenomenon was analyzed in further detail, it was determined that the competent T cells in the restored animals were derived from the host and not from the thymus donor. These results were interpreted as indicative of two possible mechanisms of action: (1) the traffic of hemopoietic cells of host origin through the thymus, with subsequent export, and (2) some form of indirect mechanism on the host mediated by humoral factor(s). Further studies demonstrated that both mechanisms are indeed operative, with the intrathymic step being a necessary but not sufficient event for the generation of T cells with defined immune functions, usually termed immunologically competent cells.

Our present knowledge of T cell development can be summarized as follows: (1) traffic of hemopoietic stem cells to the thymus; (2) the intrathymic stage, which includes expansion of the population and irreversible commitment to the T lineage, mediated by cell contact with the thymic stroma (which is a reticulo-epithelial framework derived from the 4th and/or 5th pharingeal pouches in mammals) as well as by local effects of the thymic humoral factors (or "thymic hormones"); and (3) export of postthymic precursor cells, which will give rise in the peripheral lymphoid tissues to the immunologically competent T cells under further influence of the secreted humoral thymic factors (such factors have been defined in serum as well as in thymic extracts and probably represent a family of related peptides that can drive T cell differentiation). The exported population is further expanded in the periphery by the thymic factors as well as by influence of the local microenvironments and most probably also antigenic stimulation. In summary, T cells are derived by the special processing within the thymus of precursor cells of hemopoietic origin, which are exported to the periphery and are further expanded into the different functional sets of T cells. Recent evidence has suggested that the intrathymic step may also be critical not only for the development of the lineage but for the definition of the immunological repertoire of the differentiated cells. For example, the T cell precursors may be selected intrathymically for capacity to react with modification of self antigens as well as non-self antigens, while cells with self reactivity would be deleted. Thus, the intrathymic step also defines the possible range of specificities of the T cells.

Although the magnitude of the two differentiative events discussed—thymus traffic and peripheral maturation—may be different at different ages (i.e., thymus export being more apparent early in life and a decline of thymic factors production with advanced age), both mechanisms are indeed operative during the whole life span of the individual. The concept of "thymic involution" is erroneous and a consequence of two phenomena: (1) the average size of the thymus (i.e., the relation of thymus weight to whole body weight) is larger during early life and smaller late in life, and (2) the thymus is exquisitely sensitive to "accidental involution" which is mediated by adrenal corticosteroids, so that any acute or chronic stress will produce marked thymus involution. As a matter of fact, the older literature contains spurious descriptions of "hypertrophy" of the thymus in adults who had committed suicide. However, these findings merely indicated that such adults had their normal thymus which was detected at autopsy as a consequence of the sudden death. In summary, although the adult thymus may be smaller than the thymus in the infant, it is readily detectable in the normal individual. From experimental as well as clinical studies it is apparent that the two main functions described for the thymus as regulator of the peripheral T cell pool are operative throughout life.

FUNCTIONS OF T CELLS

Although T cells are thymus-dependent for their development, the functionally mature T cells are independent from the thymus for their function, i.e., T cells will function in vivo or in vitro in the absence of the thymus or its humoral factors. Although morphologically T cells are quite homogeneous and are represented by the classic small lymphocyte, they have a degree of heterogeneity based on function. Several major T cell categories can be defined (based on functional studies, surface markers, life span, recirculating capacity, and so on (1): helper T cells, cells that are capable of helping B cells in the antibody response to certain antigens (the T cells do not produce antibody by themselves but they are required for the optimal antibody response of the B cell, most probably as cells that deliver the appropriate signal to the B cells); (2) killer or cytotoxic T cells, cells capable of specifically attaching and destroying foreign cells, virus-infected cells, parasites, and so forth (helper T cells are also needed for the generation as well as amplification of the T killer response); (3) suppressor T cells, a complex population whose main function is to regulate immunological responses of both T and B effector cells; and (4) a less-defined group of regulatory or precursor (or "early") T cells that interact with the above ones for the optimal expression of defined T cell responses (this population also includes the postthymic precursor cell discussed above, which is the precursor cell exported by the thymus and can give rise to T cells of the different functional subsets). In summary, this is a rather complex set of interacting populations with effector as well as regulatory functions, which can affect all stages of humoral as well as cellular immunity.

SUMMARY

The thymus plays a critical role in the development and regulation of the lymphoid system. The role is exerted via the action of special cell interactions and thymic humoral factors, at both intrathymic and extrathymic locations, on hemopoietic precursors, which give rise to immunologically competent T cells with defined effector and regulatory functions.

References (Books)

Golub, E. S. *The Cellular Basis of the Immune Response.* Sunderland, Massachusetts: Sinauer Assoc., 1977.
Greaves, M. F., Owen, J. J. T., and Raff, M. C. *T and B Lymphocytes: Origins, Properties and Roles in Immune Responses.* Amsterdam: Excerpta Medica, 1974.
Loor, F., and Roelants, G. E. *B and T Cells in Immune Recognition.* London: Wiley, 1977.
Moller, G. Acquisition of the T Cell Repertoire, *Immunological* Reviews, Vol. 42. Copenhagen: Munksgaard, 1978.
Stutman, O. *T Cells,* Contemporary Topics in Immunobiology, Vol. 7. New York: Plenum Press, 1977.

On Cellular Immunity and the Biological Role of the Major Transplantation Antigens

ROLF M. ZINKERNAGEL
Scripps Clinic And Research Institute,
La Jolla, California

For quite some time medical scientists have known that lymphocytes that are processed by the thymus (T cells) are critically involved in life-saving immunity against intracellular parasites, such as viruses or facultative intracellular bacteria. In addition, T cells participate in graft rejection, the response to an invention of modern medicine. These apparently quite different phenomena are actually opposite sides of the same coin. That is, T cells' reactivity against infected cells expressing foreign antigens induced by the intracellular parasites is identical to that against foreign cells expressing foreign transplantation antigens. In fact, T cells' ability to recognize and kill virus-infected cells is specific not only for the infectious agent, but also for the host's own transplantation antigens. This fact implies a very important biological role for major transplantation antigens.

Our understanding of the major transplantation antigens' functions, particularly polymorphism, is fragmentary. Evidence suggests that these antigens play a major role in cellular communication and interaction between the members of the mobile, immunological police force of the vertebrate host—the lymphocytes—not only from one lymphocyte to others but from lymphocytes to the rest of the somatic cells. Investigation of these questions may reveal answers about structure, function, and activation of T cells' receptors as well as lead to a better understanding of virus-induced immunopathology and the empirical association between the major histocompatibility gene complex (MHC) and certain disease susceptibilities.

MAJOR TRANSPLANTATION ANTIGENS AND IMMUNITY TO VIRUS

Double specificity for both self-MHC and foreign antigenic determinants is a quality of all T cell functions examined so far in the mouse and has been confirmed in other species such as humans, rats, guinea pigs, and chickens. Although all T cell functions of mice are restricted by the hosts' MHC, as explained below, we shall examine only one class of T cells: virus-specific cytotoxic T cells. These virus-immune T lymphocytes are called cytotoxic because they can destroy virus-infected cells grown in tissue culture. One measures T cell-mediated cell destruction in vitro by using a radioactive substance to label the infected cells, which when destroyed, release this label in measureable amounts.

The crucial experiment in this work involved infecting mice of three different strains—A, B, and C—with lymphocyte choriomeningitis virus (LCMV). About 7 to 10 days after mice were injected with LCMV and developed systemic infection, cytotoxic T cells specifically reactive to the infecting virus were found in the animals' blood, spleens, and lymph nodes. When these immune T cells from strain A mice infected with LCMV were tested for the capacity to destroy LCMV-infected target cells, only cells from the same strain—strain A—were destroyed; the LCMV-infected cells from the unrelated strains B and C remained intact. Subsequent studies revealed that the genetic information enabling virus-immune T cells to destroy infected target cells, and only from the appropriate animal strain, is located in the MHC*—the part of the germ line that also codes for major transplantation antigens involved in graft rejection.

Various T cell subsets, each with its own distinct function, express specificity for different MHC antigens. Cytotoxic T cells are predominantly restricted to interacting with cells that express the MHC specificities H-2K and D in the mouse or HLA-A, B in humans, whereas noncytotoxic T cells interact only with cells that express H-2I. These noncytotoxic T cells act as helper cells for antibody-producing cells (B cells), activation of macrophages, or production of delayed-type hypersensitivity immune responses. In terms of the structural conformation that provides this MHC restriction over the diverse activities of T cells, it is still not clear whether T cells express two recognition sites, one for the foreign antigen plus one for self-MHC, or whether T cells possess only one recognition site that is specific for a complex antigen formed between the foreign antigen and self antigen.

What is the biological relevance of this cytotoxic phenomenon we have observed in vitro; that is, how does it relate to immunologic responses to viruses?

---

*The major histocompatibility gene complex of mice (H-2), located on the 17th chromosome, is about 0.5 recombination units (centimorgans) long, which approximates the length of the genome of *E. coli*. This gene complex is subdivided into K, I, S, and D regions. K and D regions correspond to the human A and B regions of HLA and code for serologically defined major transplantation antigens present on all cells of an individual; the I region, in humans the D region, codes for Ia antigens expressed on certain subsets of lymphocytes and for immune response genes regulating antibody response; the S region codes for complement factors and other serum proteins. The allele coded for by H-2 or by one of the regions (K, I, D) is usually noted in lower case letters added in superscript (e.g., H-2^k mice express K^k, I^k, D^k antigens.

And why this double specificity of T cells? One possible teleological and mechanistic explanation is based on the assumption that intracellular parasites, such as viruses and certain bacteria, were major selective forces in shaping the immune system during evolution.

Although cytolytic T cell phenomena have been studied for many years, and the role of these lymphocytes in graft rejection is well recognized, the wider significance is unclear. In experiments done with cultured cells, virus-immune splenic T cells that destroy infected cells in vitro are the same group of cells that protect mice against virus infection in vivo. The cells involved in this protection are predominantly T lymphocytes. Newer experiments now reveal that the protection so afforded requires H-2 compatibility at the K and D loci between immune T cells and recipient mice, and lack of such compatibility or compatibility at the I region alone obviates a protective effect. Furthermore, the kinetics with which cytotoxic activity is generated in vitro and the development of T cells' protective capacity in vivo, are virtually identical. Thus, identification of cellular characteristics, kinetics, and H-2 restriction specificities all suggest that the cytotoxic effector T cell assessed in vitro and the antiviral effector T cell tested in vivo are probably the same. But, because T cell-mediated responses to viruses kill infected host cells, the protective immune response can become "autoaggressive." These findings are important for understanding the concepts of viral immunity and immunopathology.

How can host cell destruction act antivirally? After virus absorbs onto and penetrates a cell, its genetic information is integrated into the host cell's genetic replication machinery. Eventually, virus components reassemble, and mature virus is released by budding or by cell decay. Considering these mechanisms, immune cytolysis must take place reasonably quickly after infection if the host is to be protected. Indeed, maximum protection can be expected if the target cell is killed and removed during the "eclipse" phase of the virus, that is, after the viral antigens are expressed on the cell surface but before new viral progeny assemble. Some protection can still be provided once assembly of new viral progeny is in progress, but steadily diminishes. With all new viruses assembled, the cytolytic T cell ceases to be protective. It is important to emphasize that cytotoxic T cells are certainly not the sole defense mechanism of higher vertebrates. Various humoral and cellular mechanisms, such as complement, antibody, antibody-dependent cell-mediated cytotoxicity, lymphotoxins and lymphokines, interferon, natural killer cells, and activated macrophages, simultaneously act together to protect the host.

Because viruses as a class of infectious agents may infect all host cells, although with differential preference (called tropism), any self antigen that might be involved in the lysis of uninfected cells must be expressed on all cells. The serologically defined major transplantation antigens, that is the products of K, D (or A, B), seem to fulfill this requirement excellently; they are expressed on all cells and are receptors for lytic signals that are delivered in an immunologically specific fashion.

In contrast to viruses, intracellular bacteria or fungi do not undergo an eclipse phase (therefore cell lysis cannot eliminate the parasites), nor can they infect all cells. Because the parasites must be phagocytized to become intracellular, their antigens probably associate only with cell membranes of phagocytes. Bacterial parasites are most effectively destroyed by intracellular digestion. The self-cell-surface markers involved (a) are expressed on phagocytic cells (e.g., macrophages), and (b) function as receptors for *nonlytic* but digestive enzyme-activating signals. The I region coded antigens expressed by certain macrophages seem to comply with this requirement. Similarly, I structures on bone marrow-derived B cells, the antibody-producing cells, may serve as receptors for specific B cell differentiation signals. In this situation, T cells may trigger immunoglobulin (Ig) synthesis or switch the class of Ig produced from IgM to IgG in an antigen-specific way. Therefore, under the assumption that during evolution infectious diseases exerted major selective pressures to form cellular immunity and its association with MHC products, major transplantation antigens may be viewed as an array of receptors for cell-specific differentiation or lytic signals that are triggered by antigen-specific T cells.

How and when the apparent intimate relationship between MHC products and T cell–mediated immunity developed are undetermined. Possibly the MHC-coded interaction system evolved out of a system for recognizing differentiation signals, to become the immune-recognition system. Alternatively, molecules that regulate differentiation and some genetic material of some endogenous viruses may be related if not identical. For example, endogenous viruses may have inserted genetic material into cells' genomes as a means of accelerating evolution dramatically, and, in such a mechanism, recognition of the presence or absence of insertion appears to be vital. Therefore, one could theorize that the immune system evolved around this primitive surveillance mechanism, in which H–2 antigens functioned either as virus receptors or as viral products. This reasoning could explain the efficiency of T cells in recognizing cell surface alterations caused by *acute* viruses, which are similar to endogenous viruses, but differ significantly in that they cannot insert themselves into the germ line. Inert antigens are handled accordingly by a similar but modified pathway.

This view could explain tumor growth as resulting from an imbalance among many possible factors influencing endogenous virus self-recognition, and immunologic recognition, with two specific consequences. First, since oncogenic viruses use the same pathways as endogenous viruses, the intruding virus may not be detected by the recognition system. Uncontrolled cellular proliferation could follow because of the viruses' intrinsic capacity to regulate the proliferative mechanism. Alternatively, oncogenic viruses may cause uncontrolled proliferation of the recognizing lymphocyte population. Tumors of nonlymphoreticular origin may well be of the first type, and tumors of the lymphoreticular cell type more of the second kind.

The foregoing mechanistic explanation and the hypothesis that endogenous viruses are intimately involved in the evolution of the immune system are pure speculations, which one expects to contain readily apparent contradictions. Yet these theories offer a starting point for explaining the preoccupation of the immune system with MHC antigens, the functional association of viruses with MHC antigens, and the special relationships between the immune system and endogenous and tumor-associated viruses.

IMMUNE RESPONSIVENESS AND MHC

The first hint of the biological relevance of the MHC in cell-mediated immunity came from research on inbred strains of mice that were the same in all respects except MHC type. These mice, differing only at the MHC, differed in their capacity to respond to certain antigens. This phenomenon is also true for the response to viruses. For example, mice bearing the MHC type $H-2^k$ (K^k D^k) generate strong T cell responses against vaccinia virus restricted to $H-2K^k$, but virtually no response restricted to $H-2D^k$; the response against LCMV is strong for D^k, but only weak for K^k. Two other interesting features common to both T cells' restriction specificity and capacity to respond are the facts that a particular T cell can express only one of the various K, I, or D restriction specificities, and that, if the restriction specificity expressed is linked to nonresponsiveness, then responsiveness is not expressed even though the genes for responsiveness are present in the genome. For example, in the heterozygote F_1 offspring from a mating between a mouse that does respond immunologically to a given virus (responder) and a mouse that does not (nonresponder), T cells specific for the MHC of the nonresponder parent never become responsive, whereas T cells restricted to the MHC of the responder parent do respond. Consequently, the restriction specificity of T cells and their capacity to respond to an antigen seem to be intimately linked. That these two qualities are regulated or coded by identical genes is only a vague speculation, but nevertheless an attractive possibility.

THE ROLE OF THE THYMUS IN SELECTING T CELLS' RESTRICTION SPECIFICITY AND RESPONSIVENESS

About 17 years ago research showed that the thymus was critically involved in T cell maturation and differentiation. Now we know that T cells, in fact, acquire the capacity to recognize self-MHC in the thymus. An important experiment in arriving at this conclusion was the following: Heterozygote F_1 offspring from an $H-2^a$ parent and an $H-2^b$ parent of mouse strains that have no thymuses and, therefore, no functional T cells received fetal thymus grafts taken from homozygous $H-2^a$ donors. Some weeks later these thymically reconstituted mice were infected with virus and soon produced virus-specific cytotoxic T cells that could only destroy infected target cells of $H-2^a$ but not of $H-2^b$ origin, and vice versa. Thus, the MHC type of the thymus seems to dictate the restriction specificity of maturing T cells; whether this occurs via selection or another mechanism is unclear.

Interestingly, as stated earlier, the restriction specificity selected by the thymic MHC automatically determines the capacity of T cells to respond to antigen. Thus, if the thymus's MHC expresses an H-2K, I, or D type that does not generate a response to a particular antigen, then T cells from that thymus, and the animal that houses them, are both automatically unresponsive to that antigen. T cells' specificity for self-MHC is therefore "learned" or "selected," and this process also determines responsiveness. These findings have important implications not only for understanding T cell recognition but also for attempting to reconstitute patients who lack either a thymus or lymphohemopoietic stem cells. An experimental example is mice without thymuses or T cells. Even though such mice were transplanted with MHC-incompatible thymuses, they failed to generate a great number of immune-competent T cells, the reason probably being that T cells cannot fully mature if the specificity for self-MHC learned in the thymus does not match the MHC encountered on lymphocytes or somatic cells. In applying this finding to patients, the reconstitution of immunological defects might improve if the MHC of lymphohemopoietic stem cells, thymus, and other somatic cells are tested and matched for at least one of the HLA A or B and D regions of the MHC.

WHY IS T CELLS' RECOGNITION OF SELF-MHC SO FLEXIBLE AND ADAPTIVE AND WHY ARE MAJOR TRANSPLANTATION ANTIGENS POLYMORPHIC?

Polymorphism of a genetically determined trait is exemplified by the MHC which apparently codes only a small number of cell surface structures, although these structures differ markedly from individual to individual. The polymorphism of H-2 or HLA antigens could be allelic, with the germ line of the individual containing a single gene to code just one of the possible alleles, or could be regulatory, with the germ line containing genes for all possible allelic structures but allowing expression of only one. Strikingly, the most polymorphic systems known in biology are those of major transplantation antigens coded by the MHC, which also control responsiveness of T cell–mediated immunity *and* of immunoglobulin (Ig) allotypes involved in regulating the responsiveness of antibodies.

The studies of immune responsiveness of mice to virus, assessed as the potential to generate K- or D-restricted cytotoxic virus-specific T cells, show that immune protection depends on which H-2 allele a host expresses. For example, mice of the H-2^k MHC type that are infected with LCMV generate a good T cell response restricted to H-$2D^k$ but markedly less to K^k plus LCMV. In contrast, the same mice infected with vaccinia virus, a pox virus, generate strong cytotoxic activity against K^k plus vaccinia, but virtually none with specificity for D^k plus vaccinia. Because LCMV and pox virus are among the most prevalent natural pathogens of mice, this difference in responsiveness is as interesting as the finding that all inbred strains of mice known have strong K- or D-restricted responses to these viruses. The frequent finding of specific immune response defects suggests that the number of possible antigenic determinants on viruses recognized by T cells must be rather limited. Although the reason is unknown, these findings may suggest a substantial difference between the receptor repertoires of T and B cells.

The profound regulatory role of the MHC in immune responsiveness, and its link with the restriction specificity of T cells, suggests a direct relationship between the polymorphism of MHC, the immune response, and the survival of some animals in the face of infectious disease. The apparently great selective pressure exerted by infectious agents, particularly viruses, may in fact have helped to shape the MHC's polymorphism during evolution. Although this view is attractive, it is by no means generally accepted, and MHC polymorphism has also been interpreted to represent an "accident" of nature.

To illustrate, if mice as a species possessed only one cell surface structure H-$2D^k$ to receive lytic messages transmitted by T cells immune to LCMV, for example, then these mice could not generate T cells with specific immunity for pox virus. Obviously, the species would then be in great jeopardy at the first outbreak of mouse pox. Even though the murine immune system could handle LCMV very efficiently with that one restricting MHC product, the other equally common virus would destroy the species.

A twofold purpose is served by the duplication of MHC genes and the polymorphism of the cell surface structures that receive the immunologically specific signal: Duplication and polymorphism (a) diminish the chances of viruses or other infectious agents to escape immune surveillance, and (b) severely limit the incidence of low response or unresponsiveness, or restrict it to homozygous individuals. The probability that each individual will express different self markers is further enhanced by duplication of the gene system coding for these markers; examples are K, D in mice and A, B in humans. These proposals fit either single *or* dual receptor models for immune interaction by T cells and are compatible with the hypothesis that immune response genes are expressed at the levels of T cell recognition *or* of antigen presentation by B cells or macrophages. Besides these theoretical implications, the evidence and speculations discussed may provide a better understanding of the clinical and empirical finding that some diseases or susceptibilities to disease may be linked to certain MHC types in humans.

IMMUNOPATHOLOGY AND THE ASSOCIATION
OF MHC AND DISEASE SUSCEPTIBILITY

The clinical outcome of an infection is determined by the effectiveness of T cells in destroying infected cells and thereby preventing viral spread. The intrinsic implication is that the balance of beneficial versus harmful effects of cellular immunity depends on such factors as: cytopathogenicity of the virus, rapidity of its spread, its organ and/or cell tropism, and its antigenicity as well as the host's immunocompetence and immune response phenotype.

Two sets of virus infections, in man and in mice, illustrate these concepts. Infection by pox virus in humans and ectromelia virus in mice is highly cytopathic but is overcome by cell-mediated immunity, as documented by the facts that T cell–deficient children often develop general vaccinoses upon pox vaccination and T cell–deficient mice infected with mouse pox rapidly die. Hepatitis virus in humans and LCMV in mice seem to elicit the other extreme of immune response to infection. The viruses are *not* particularly cytopathic, and immunodeficient hosts do *not* die of the infection. Therefore, in the immunologically competent hosts infected with these nondestructive viruses, any associated tissue damage is caused by the host's T cell response rather than by the virus per se. In these cases, disease develops when (1) the tissue-damaging effect or cytopathogenicity of the infectious agent and/or the destructive effects of the immune response outweight immunoprotection, and (2) susceptibility to disease outweighs resistance. Because the quality of a host's immune responsiveness is determined by the restriction specificity of its T cells, resistance to disease versus susceptibility to disease is influenced by MHC-linked immune response genes.

Since the susceptibility of mice to tumor induction was first related to the MHC almost 20 years ago, an ever increasing number of diseases have been categorized as appearing in patients with particular HLA types. For example, arthropathies often occur in patients with the HLA-BW27 antigen; other diseases have been observed in patients who lack a certain HLA antigen. However, resistance to infectious disease also occurs nonimmunologically or nonspecifically, often not visibly linked with the MHC. Therefore, the comments that follow refer only to intracellular parasites and their relationship to T cell–mediated immunity.

In a simplified concept of the relationship between cellular immunity and disease, one may divide susceptibility to disease into four main categories: High immunologic responsiveness results in relatively *increased* resistance to infections by cytopathogenic agents, but may *decrease* resistance to poorly cytopathogenic agents, since the latter tend to spread widely and, therefore, cause extensive T cell-mediated autoaggression. In contrast, *low responsiveness* results in relatively *increased* susceptibility to infections by acute cytopathogenic agents, and therefore, has probably been eliminated by selective pressure during evolution, but could *decrease* the susceptibility to virus-induced autoaggressive disease.

For some time chronic infectious disease, particularly viral infections, has been the suspected cause of so-called autoimmune disease. This term may in fact be inaccurate, since these immune processes could be directed against foreign cell surface determinants induced by infectious agents. Susceptibility to acute viral infections influences survival of the species dramatically, since acute viral infections can kill the afflicted before reproduction, and natural selection would tend to eliminate these low or nonresponders. However, most associations between disease and MHC relate to chronic autoaggressive or autoimmune disorders rather than acute infections. Of course, the autoaggressive diseases may be acute, such as fulminant autoaggressive hepatitis, but more commonly tend to be slow processes that end life after the reproductive years. Therefore, with autoaggressive-type diseases the host's responder status is not subject to great selective pressures, and positive MHC-disease associations may become manifest.

CONCLUSION

Research on the multiple relationships between MHC and T cell immunity makes the MHC one of the best understood gene regions of higher vertebrates. Although our knowledge of this subject is far from complete, particularly with respect to the regulatory roles of MHC genes, biochemists have analyzed some of the gene products in detail. The aspects of immunology discussed here represent one of the few areas in which recognized gene products have been traced in relatively well-studied differentiation processes such as T cell maturation and function in precise cellular communication. We still do not know the structure of the T cell receptor(s) nor its relationship to antibodies. The thymus and all regulatory phenomena of the immune system remain so complex as to escape simple experimental analysis. Still, the unfolding science of immunology and cell biology of lymphocytes are certain to reveal much that is applicable to understanding the pathogenesis of human disease and improving related medical practice.

References

(References for more detailed information containing pertinent references to original papers.)

Transplantation Review **19**, 1974.
Transplantation Review **29**, 1976.
Immunological Reviews **42**, 1978.
Bodmer, W., *Nature* **237**: 139, 1972.
Paul, W. and Benacerraf, B., *Science,* **195**: 1293, 1977.
Dausser, J. and Svejgard, A., eds. *HLA-disease,* 1977.
Zinkernagel, R. M. and Doherty, P. C. MHC-restricted cytotoxic T cells: Studies on the biological role of polymarphic major transplantation antigens determining T cell restriction-specificity, function and responsiveness. *Adv. Immunal.* **27**: 52–142, 1979.

Pathways of B-Cell Development

DANIEL LEVITT
MAX D. COOPER
The Cellular Immunobiology Unit of the Tumor Institute,
Departments of Pediatrics and Microbiology, and
The Comprehensive Cancer Center,
University of Alabama in Birmingham
Birmingham, Alabama

Cellular differentiation implies a process advancing in time, involving a multitude of phenomena and factors that interact to achieve a defined goal. This process involves (1) precursor populations of multipotent cells capable of differentiating along several developmental pathways, (2) eventual commitment of stem cell progeny to specific cell lineages, determined by both environmental stimuli and genetic potential, (3) expression of features characteristic for the specialized cells of each pathway, and (4) stable expression of the specialized cell phenotypes.

Nowhere has the spectrum of cell specialization evolved to such a complex degree as in the developing lymphoid system. Unlike most differentiated cell types, which are limited to the production of less than a hundred specialized molecules, lymphocytes create products that have greater than a million distinct binding specificities and are involved in a diverse spectrum of interactions rivaled only by the central nervous system. In this article, we will describe the development of B cells as a model of programmed cellular differentiation. The consistent and orderly progression of these cells through a unidirectional and irreversible series of transformations to sequentially specialized cell types will be emphasized.

A B cell can be functionally defined as a cell whose ultimate purpose is to produce antibody molecules. As will be seen, there are multiple changes that a B cell undergoes during its journey to become an efficient antibody-producing "factory," and the regulatory events controlling most of these steps are still uncertain. It is possible, however, to integrate the available information to give a meaningful description of a B cell's life history.

B lymphocytes, as well as all other formed elements of the blood, are ultimately derived from hemopoietic stem cells (Figure 1). Adoptive transfer of bone marrow cells to lethally irradiated mice is followed by formation of colonies of cells in the recipient's spleen. Transfer of cells in one spleen colony (void of lymphocytes) to a second lethally irradiated mouse will reconstitute all hematopoietic elements of the second animal. Because each of the splenic colonies is derived from a single cell, it can be assumed that a common stem cell exists for all hematopoietic elements. This concept is supported by information obtained from the cells of a women heterozygous for the X-linked enzyme glucose-6-phosphate dehydrogenase (G-6-PD). Her cells were examined to determine their clonal diversity because of an underproduction of red cells. As the Lyon hypothesis would predict, random inactivation of her X-chromosomes

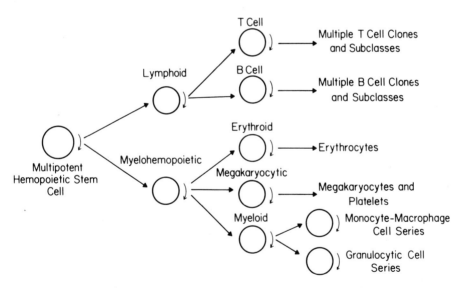

FIG. 1. Commitment of stem cells to different pathways of differentiation. Reproduced from Cooper, M. D., Kearney, J. F., and Lawton, A. R., III. The life history of antibody producing B cells. In *Birth Defects. Proceedings of the Fifth International Conference, Montreal 21-27 August 1977*, J. W. Littlefield and J. de Grouchy, eds. Amsterdam-Oxford: Excerpta Medica, 1978. With permission of the publisher.

in skin fibroblasts allowed expression of both A and B isoenzymes. Only *one* isoenzyme was demonstrable in her blood cells. The data imply inactivation of one specific X-chromosome in a hemopoietic stem cell which served as the progenitor for all of her blood cell types.

The mechanism by which hemopoietic stem cells give rise to progeny cells that are still capable of self-renewal yet have more restricted potentials for differentiation is still poorly understood. Evidence supporting the idea that one of these branch points leads to a lymphoid stem cell that differs from myeloid-erythroid-megakaryocyte precursors (see Figure 1) was obtained from analysis of cells from women heterozygous for the G–6–PD isoenzymes who had an overproduction of red cells (polycythemia vera). While only one isoenzyme was detectable in their red cells, myeloid cells, and platelets, lymphocytes in these patients expressed equal amounts of A and B G–6–PD isoenzymes.

In contrast, adoptive transfer of bone marrow cells with specific chromosomal aberrations (marked cells) to lethally irradiated mice reconstituted either all hematopoietic cells or only T cells. Sole development of B and T cells by the marked population was not demonstrated. In vitro systems generating B lymphocytes from stem cells are not available as yet, thereby complicating direct examinations of generation of these cells.

It has become increasingly evident that an important factor instigating cellular transformations during specific stages of differentiation is a cell's microenvironment. Studies of environmental influences in cell development date back to the pioneering research of Spemann and Mangold on the amphibian blastula and gastrula. These investigators and their colleagues convincingly demonstrated that the ultimate fate of a cell in an organism was determined by its position during a specific period of the developmental continuum. Cells could be translocated from one area of the blastula to another and subsequently develop according to the program of their neighbor cells. The concept of positional fating (or fate-mapping) can also be extended to developing *Drosophila* imaginal discs and the chick limb.

In the lymphoid system, the idea of environmental determination of lymphocyte development was strongly supported by the discovery of the avian bursa of Fabricius as the site of B lymphocyte commitment and the thymus as the equivalent organ for T lymphocyte specialization. Prevention of B cell development by embryonic removal of the bursa suggests that it is the only environment in the chicken in which B cells begin their development. Experiments using bursal cells with distinct chromosomal markers reveal that B cell progenitors migrate or "home" specifically to the bursa and no other organs. These cells, after acquiring phenotypic characteristics of B cells, then seed other lymphoid organs, e.g., bone marrow and spleen. Thus, the primacy of the bursa as the generative microenvironment for antibody-producing cells in birds seems to be irrefutable.

A great deal of evidence suggests that fetal liver is an early and major site of B cell generation in mammals. Recent evidence indicates that cells having the capacity for developing into B cells under laboratory culture conditions are present in mouse placental tissue even earlier than in fetal liver. Circulating stem cells of uncertain origin find the proper microenvironment for hematopoiesis in the fetal liver. It is unclear when and where actual commitment to the B cell lineage becomes irreversible during embryogenesis, but there is clear evidence that this decision can be supported by the fetal liver. In the adult, the bone marrow serves as the primary source of lymphoid stem cells. Fetal liver cells or adult bone marrow injected into lethally irradiated mice will migrate to bone marrow and completely reconstitute the host's hematopoietic system, including antibody-producing cells. When murine fetal liver at a stage prior to the appearance of B lymphocytes is placed into tissue culture, antibody-forming cells develop in a reproducible, orderly fashion.

LIFE HISTORY OF B CELLS

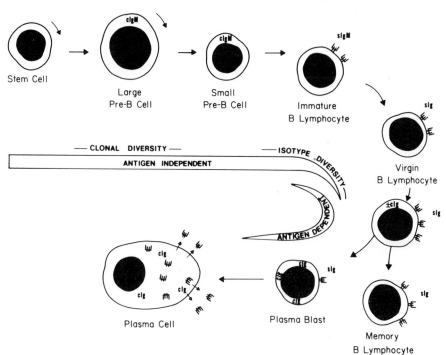

FIG. 2. Developmental pathway of B cell differentiation. (Reproduced from Lawton, A. R., Kearney, J. F., and Cooper, M. D. Immunoglobulin diversity: Regulation of expression of immunoglobulin genes during primary development of B cells. In *Biological Regulation and Development,* Vol. II, R. F. Goldberger, ed. New York: Plenum Publishing Corporation, 1978. With permission of the publisher.)

Ontogenetic analysis of B cell development has permitted the description of cells with varying phenotypic expression (Figure 2). The earliest recognizable cell in the lymphoid line is termed the precursor B or pre-B cell. These cells have been found in the liver as early as the eighth week of human gestation. They are large mononuclear cells, most of which are synthesizing DNA, and their direct progeny are small, nondividing cells. Both large and small pre-B cells contain cytoplasmic immunoglobulin M (IgM) molecules (Figure 3) in small quantities, but no surface IgM detectable by immunofluorescent staining. Using other methods, studies performed on mouse fetal liver cells prior to the appearance of cells with stainable surface IgM (sIgM) suggest that pre-B cells may possess small quantities of IgM on their surface which has a rapid turnover rate. It may be more important to note that pre-B cells almost surely lack functional immuno-globulin receptors; it has not been possible to affect their development in either a positive or negative fashion by exposure to antibodies or antigens known to modify behavior of sIg$^+$ B lymphocytes.

Pre-B cells also lack several other surface markers commonly associated with more mature B lymphocytes, including receptors for the Fc portion of IgG and receptors for complement. They may (humans) or may not (mice) express the major histocompatibility locus product Ia antigen, which is of great importance in cell–cell interactions necessary for immune responses.

Immunofluorescent studies of mammalian B cell ontogeny, injection of radio-actively labled fetal liver and bone marrow cells into lethally irradiated mice, and examination of cultured fetal liver all support the proposal that B lympho-

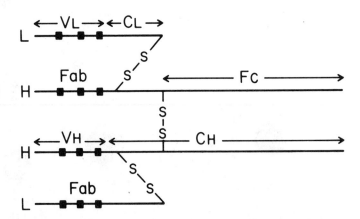

FIG. 3. Schematic representation of an immunoglobulin molecule. L: light chain (kappa or lambda). H: heavy chain (μ, δ, γ, α, or ϵ). V_L: variable region of light chains. V_H: variable region of heavy chains. C_L: constant region of light chains. C_H: constant region of heavy chains. Fab: antigen combining fragment. Fc: heavy chain constant region (after protease digestion of molecule). ■: complementarity or antigen combining sites of variable regions.

cytes bearing membrane-bound immunoglobulin are derived directly from pre-B cells. In birds, the earliest detectable cells of B lineage in the bursa possess both cytoplasmic and surface immunoglobulin molecules. Treatment of immature or mature B lymphocytes from birds or mammals with divalent antibody against light or heavy chain (Figure 3) determinants of IgM removes surface immunoglobulin via an energy-dependent mechanism leading to movement of cross-linked sIg to one pole of the cell ("capping") and endocytosis of capped material. Early B cells fail to re-express surface IgM, whereas mature B cells re-exhibit surface immunoglobulin within 12 to 24 hours after removal. This modulation of "young" B lymphocytes occurs with anti-μ concentrations several-fold less than necessary for mature cell modulation. Moreover, administration of anti-IgM to mice during the immediate postnatal period can severely diminish subsequent development of B lymphocytes and plasma cells producing all immunoglobulin classes or isotypes. This phenomenon can also be demonstrated in chick embryos injected with anti-μ in ovo, but not after hatching.

Such studies strongly suggest a functional differentiation between early B lymphocytes (immature) and late B lymphocytes (mature). Further support for this concept can be gleaned from investigations of tolerance* induction in fetal versus adult B cells. Tolerance of fetal and neonatal B cells can be induced by exposure to multivalent antigens in the absence of T lymphocytes sensitized to the antigen. When such T cells are present, a normal antibody response can be generated. Adult B cells cannot be made tolerant in a similar manner except for a small population of cells residing in the bone marrow, which generates young B cells throughout life.

Generation of isotype diversity† is a primary feature of B lymphocyte differentiation. Recent data suggest that switching from expression of one antibody class to another proceeds in an orderly, programmed manner. In all vertebrate systems examined, IgM is always the first immunoglobulin synthesized during development (8 to 9 weeks in humans, 12 days in chickens, 16 days in mouse). Removal of μ-bearing B cells from embryonic or neonatal tissue by physical or immunochemical methods eliminates or severely reduces the expression of all other antibody classes. It can be concluded, then, that B cells possessing surface IgM stand as the immediate progenitors of all antibody-producing cells. Cells bearing other immunoglobulin classes appear at approximately 10 weeks in humans and around birth in the mouse. Co-expression of IgM with each isotype early in B cell differentiation is an invariable rule (Figure 4). In mice and

Studies performed in our laboratory were supported by grants CA 16673 and CA 13148 awarded by the National Cancer Institute, DHEW, USPHS.
*Immune tolerance is the lack of response of lymphocytes when stimulated by an antigen to which they had been previously exposed.
†Isotype is defined as a specific class of antibody molecule determined by the type of heavy chains, i.e., IgM, IgG, IgA, IgD, or IgE.

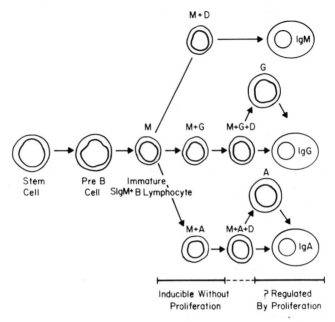

FIG. 4. Development of isotype diversity. Note sequential expression and co-expression of multiple isotypes of B lymphocytes. (Reproduced from Lawton, A. R., Kearney, J. F., and Cooper, M. D. Immunoglobulin diversity: Regulation of expression of immunoglobulin genes during primary development of B cells. In *Biological Regulation and Development*, Vol. II, R. F. Goldberger, ed. New York: Plenum Publishing Corporation, 1978. With permission of the publisher.)

humans, IgG can be detected on the surface of a subpopulation of B lymphocytes prior to the appearance of sIgA-bearing cells. IgD expression during ontogeny occurs slightly after IgG and IgA, and again is found on lymphocytes also exhibiting IgM on their surface. For a transient period during development, virtually all sIgG- and sIgA-positive B lymphocytes also bear sIgM and sIgD, so that these subpopulations of B cells express three isotypes, i.e., IgM, IgD, and either IgA or IgG. After birth, and probably as a result of antigen stimulation, many sIgG$^+$ and sIgA$^+$B cells bear only one of these classes of surface immunoglobulin molecules. These mature subpopulations of cells, like the majority of B lymphocytes which possess IgM and IgD on the cell membrane, probably function as immediate precursors to cells that synthesize antibodies in large quantities (plasma cells; see Figure 2). Normal plasma cells produce only one class of antibody. This pattern of isotype diversification at the level of the B lymphocyte surface appears to be both antigen- and T cell–independent, since germ-free and congenitally athymic (nude) mice, as well as germ-free chickens, share identical sequences of cell surface antibody development with normal animals. Thus the initial generation of antibody class diversity occurs in selective microenvironments and follows an orderly, consistent pattern of expression with temporal stabilization of the differentiated cell phenotypes.

Similar ontogenic patterns of gene expression also occur in developing erythrocytes and connective tissue cells. As differentiation proceeds, the characteristics of several distinctive specialized macromolecules (globin, collagen, proteoglycans) change in a reproducible manner. The simultaneous appearance of more than one type of globin chain or collagen molecule in progeny of a single cell has also been demonstrated.

We have not yet approached the problem of how antibody specificity is created. Immunoglobulin reactivity with specific antigens is determined by the amino acid structure of the variable (V) region, with antigen binding sites appearing as hypervariable areas (Figure 4-3). Both heavy and light chains contain distinct V regions; their combination and folding provide the unique structural differences between antibody molecules. Estimates of the complexity of the antibody repertoire range from 10^5 to 10^7 specific molecules. Generation of this diversity must be intimately coupled with ontogenic events regulating B lymphocyte development.

Two basic theories, with multiple variations, have attempted to explain how such an incredible array of proteins might have arisen. The germ-line hypothesis predicts that all specificities of the repertoire are encoded by germ cell genes. Evolutionary forces are determinant in selecting the ultimate spectrum of antibody diversity. Thus, for 10^5 distinct pairs of V regions, cells would require approximately 350 distinct V_L genes and 350 distinct V_H genes. These approximations assume, of course, that shuffling among various V_H and V_L molecules occurs normally, and that any V_H specificity can combine with all V_L specificities. Recent estimates of V region gene frequency using nucleic acid hybridization techniques and DNA sequencing suggest that such numbers of genes could exist in mammalian cells. If the recently described J (joining) genes for V and C genes provide for further diversity among antibody molecules, the complexity of the immunoglobulin repertoire can be expanded even further.

The somatic mutation theory holds that diversity arises via programmed mutations of a small number of V region genes in lymphoid precursor cells following a consistent, reproducible pattern. This concept requires the existence of hypermutable sequences in stem cell genes and/or specific mutator proteins (enzymes) that recognize the variable region genes of heavy and light chains in developing B cells, altering the genome to allow production of any antibody molecule in the repertoire. No such enzymes or regions of nuclear DNA have been described, and it remains doubtful whether such a mechanism could account for most antibody diversity. Recent modifications of the germ-line and somatic mutation theory would permit reasonable, known mutation frequencies to provide for generation of a limited degree of antibody diversity in cells containing 100 to 200 distinct V_L and V_H genes.

If lymphoid stem cells contain all or most of the genetic material necessary for a complete antibody response, when and how might clonal commitment to a distinct antibody specificity occur? Evidence obtained from both embryonic chickens and mice suggests that cells capable of binding a variety of antigens appear in an orderly sequence during development; exposure to a particular exogenous immunogen is not necessary to elicit cells producing antibodies. In fetal mice, spleen cells producing anti-hapten antibody of a specific clonotype (idiotype)* can be initially detected during distinct periods of development in both germ-free and normal mice. These studies support the concept that generation of antibody diversity begins well before birth, precedes exposure to environmental stimuli, and follows an orderly, programmed pathway. External signals appear not to be required to instruct a B cell precursor to become committed to production of a specific antibody.

Information dealing with the precise stage of B cell development where antibody commitment occurs is meager. Studies of humans with the disease multiple myeloma reveal synthesis of antibody molecules with the particular myeloma idiotype by cells that appear to be pre-B in phenotype. These data would indicate that in certain malignancies, a number of B lymphocyte precursors are already committed to the formation of immunoglobulins with one specificity. Since occasional normal pre-B cells have been observed to express idiotypic determinants, the antigen-independent expression of antibody specificity seems quite likely.

It was proposed almost 15 years ago that variable and constant region genes were physically separated in the germ cell genome; during B cell differentiation, these loci were then joined prior to antibody synthesis. Such a model seemed to be unique for immunoglobulin formation. Recent studies using DNA complementary to λ light chain messenger RNA annealed to restriction endonuclease fragments of either embryonic or myeloma DNA reveal that V_L and C_L genes appear on distinct cleavage pieces in embryonic DNA. These genes are then joined and can be recognized on the same fragments of the myeloma genome. Sequence analyses of cloned V genes from myeloma cells support the concept that families of V_L genes exist, and only one member of a family is joined to a C_L gene during differentiation. Such information buttresses the proposal for at least two genes joining to direct synthesis of one polypeptide chain of an antibody molecule.

As stated earlier, B cells can express more than one surface immunoglobulin class at the same time during development. Cells bearing surface IgM are the

---

*Idiotype or clonotype defines the antibody molecules synthesized by a single antibody-producing cell and possessing uniqueness in the variable region of the molecule.

precursors for lymphocytes producing all other isotypes. In cells producing two different antibody classes, the variable regions of both classes are identical. How might sequential formation of immunoglobulin isotypes with identical specificities occur in the same cell? One postulated mechanism would involve integration of a single V_H gene with distinct C_H genes in a temporally ordered fashion (Figure 5). This process could be regulated by linear arrangement of C_H genes on a particular chromosome and looping-out/excision of C_H genes either after expression by the cell or prior to transcription of other C_H loci. Recent information employing myeloma cells producing different immunoglobulin classes and subclasses supports the preceding model.

Abnormal development of the lymphoid system in humans has provided significant information regarding possible regulatory mechanisms of cellular differentiation. Defects of development at every step of the B cell lineage (Figure 2) have been recognized. Lymphoid stem cell deficiencies are suggested in patients with severe combined immunodeficiency (SCID) who lack both B and T cells. A maturation arrest of B lymphocytes at the pre-B level was recently described in X-linked agammaglobulinemia (Bruton's disease); other agammaglobulinemic patients possess B lymphocytes that are unable to further differentiate to plasma cells.

In summary, B lymphocyte development shares many features common to other specialized cells yet possesses characteristics that distinguish it from virtually all other differentiating systems. Stem cell origin of B cells is common to all other vertebrate tissues and most invertebrate systems. Restriction of developmental potential by a precise microenvironment has been exemplified by

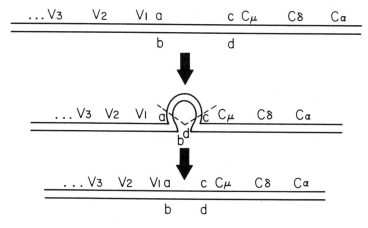

FIG. 5. Loop-excision model for variable-constant gene integration. A single chromosome is shown. A segment of DNA, separating V and C genes, is excised, bringing a gene for a specific V region closer to one of a small number of C region genes.

specific epithelial–mesenchymal interactions in numerous organs, including hematopoietic cells. For instance, combination of limb-bud mesenchyme with any nonspecific epithelium prohibits formation of limb tissue or structure. Similar results are obtained with heterospecific combinations of liver and thyroid epithelium and mesoderm.

The migration of lymphoid stem cells to specific inductive microenvironments also occurs with neural crest and germ cells. The "homing" signals for these cells remain a mystery, but the patterns of migration are so precise that exact mechanisms of recognition are required.

Sequential activation (or de-repression) of the genome to allow production of large quantities of specialized macromolecules is the hallmark of the differentiated state. Numerous theories on regulation of these events have appeared during the past ten years. Most developing systems need account for the synthesis of very few "luxury" molecules (i.e., globin by erythrocytes, actin and myosin by myocytes, certain hormones by endocrine cells, proteoglycan and collagen by chondrocytes). Collectively, B lymphocytes can potentially produce upwards of 10^7 distinct molecules. Each antibody will share certain regions with other immunoglobulins (C_L, C_H), yet still contain a distinctiveness that permits its recognition by both biochemical and immunochemical techniques. Determining how these individual molecules are chosen for synthesis among a group of similar molecules is an awesome task.

We have not mentioned the role of hormonal influences or second messengers during development, but they are clearly of major significance in determining developmental fates of several different cells (T cells, erythrocytes, mammary tissues, limb tissue). There exists little information about such regulator molecules in early B cell development; most factors characterized seem to influence terminal differentiation of B lymphocytes into plasma cells. It would not be surprising to find specific extrinsic signals that influence B cells during their progression toward specific antibody production.

ACKNOWLEDGEMENT

We are grateful for the help of Mrs. Summer King in typing and editing this manuscript, and Mrs. Susie Gray in preparing the figures.

References

Cooper, M. D., and Lawton, A. R. The development of the immune system. *Sci. Am. 231*: 58–72, 1974.
Cooper, M. D., Kearney, J. F., Lydyard, P. M., Grossi, C. E., and Lawton, A. R. Studies of generation of B-cell diversity in mouse, man, and chicken. *Cold Spring Harbor Symp. Quant. Biol. 41*: 139–145, 1977.

Klinman, N. R., Sigal, N. H., Metcalf, E. S., Pierce, S. K., and Gearhart, P. J. The interplay of evolution and environment in B-cell diversification. *Cold Soring Harbor Symp. Quant. Biol. 41*: 165–173, 1977.

Melchers, F. Immunoglobulin synthesis and mitogen reactivity: Markers for B lymphocyte differentiation. In *Development of Host Defenses,* M. D. Cooper and D. H. Dayton, eds. New York: Raven Press, 1977, pp. 11–29.

Katz, D. H., ed. *Lymphocyte Differentiation, Recognition and Regulation.* New York: Academic Press, 1977.

Experimental Approaches to Study of Transplantation Immunology

C. B. CARPENTER, M. D.
Department of Medicine
Peter Bent Brigham Hospital
Harvard Medical School
Boston, Massachusetts
Investigator, Howard Hughes
Medical Institute

When living cells are transplanted from one individual to another, they are subjected to an increasingly hostile environment as the recipient's immune system is stimulated to reject the foreign tissue. Only if the donor and recipient are syngeneic, that is, identical for all tissue antigens, will there be no rejection response. In man, only identical twins are syngeneic. Transplantation of vital organs, such as kidneys, hearts, liver, or bone marrow, has already reached a point of clinical application, supported by the empiric application of nonspecific chemical and biological immune suppressive agents. In experimental animals, skin grafting, also of considerable potential in clinical practice, has been the primary tool for experimental study of the antigens provoking rejection. More recently, direct study of organ transplantation has been possible in rats because the necessary microvascular surgery is possible in animals of this size, and a variety of defined genetic stocks have become available. Information about the genes determining transplantation antigens in mice is known in much greater detail, but vascularized organ transplantation in such small animals has been difficult to accomplish in all but a few studies. Transplantation among non-syngeneic members of the same species is denoted by the prefix "allo-," as in the terms allograft or allogeneic. Inbred strains of mice and rats have been of immense value in determining the nature of allograft rejection, and of the positive and negative controls that can be exerted on the complex allogeneic response.

HISTOCOMPATIBILITY ANTIGENS OF THE MAJOR HISTOCOMPATIBILITY COMPLEX (MHC)

Central to consideration of allograft rejection is the nature of the antigens responsible for stimulation of the immune response to transplanted tissue. In every mammalian species studied so far, vigorous rejection of tissue grafts is promoted by "strong" antigens which are the gene products of a relatively restricted area of a single chromosome (e.g., H-2 in mice, chromosone no. 17; HLA in man, short arm of chromosome no. 6; RTI in rats) (Table 1).[1,2] The region of the major histocompatibility gene complex (MHC) is also known to contain immune response genes (Ir) and some of the genes for synthesis or structural variation of certain complement components. Hence, the biological significance of the MHC goes far beyond its role in transplantation phenomena, most of which are artifacts of modern surgery. Nevertheless, MHC antigens are defined by study of transplantation phenomena; and whether one's interest is in promotion of unresponsiveness to transplants for clinical purposes, or in definition and biological role of MHC gene products in the immune response in general, allotransplantation in animal models is the necessary reference point for assessment of MHC alleles.

Pregnancy is a form of allograft, and maternal immunization to antigens of the fetus usually occurs. Nature, therefore, performs successful allografts with ease in the special environment of the uterine cavity. Understanding of the physical and immunological barriers leading to successful parturition is still meager, and must in the future be integrated with other knowledge gained in studies of transplantation phenomena.

The reasons that MHC gene products serve as potent transplantation antigens are not precisely known; however, they may in part elicit strong allogeneic immune responses because these glycoproteins are prominently displayed on cell surfaces. Of greater importance is the concept that allogeneic MHC antigens are recognized as "altered self," eliciting a vigorous immune response because the recipient immune system recognizes the allogeneic antigen as a variant of its own MHC structure, the variation normally being the association of environmental (viral or bacterial) antigen with self MHC antigen. The evidence for the role of the MHC in normal immune responses is reviewed in detail elsewhere

TABLE 1. Characteristics of Gene Products of the MHC

Antigen	Structure	Tissue	Identification Technique	NOMENCLATURE			Function
				Mouse (H-2)	Rat (RTI)	Human (HLA)	
Class I	β_2-microgulin plus heavy chain	Virtually all cells except human red blood cells	Serology	D, K	Ag–B (A region)	A, B, C	Targets for effector antibodies and killer cells
Class II	α-chain plus β-chain	Absent on platelets, T cells, red blood cells	Mixed lymphocyte response (MLR) and serology (Ia)	I (LAD, Ia)	MLR/Ia (B region)	D, DR (Ia)	Key role in initiation of immune response (Ir genes)

(Chapters 12 and 16). It is important to understand, however, that the fundamental physiology of the alloimmune response in the dual context of rejection of transplanted tissue and in modulation of the immune response to environmental pathogens, and possibly also to unique tumor antigens, is the same.

NON-MHC ANTIGENS

Before reviewing some of the information being obtained from study of experimental models of transplantation, a brief word about "minor" transplantation antigens is in order. In simplest terms, any structural difference between members of a species may be recognized as a foreign antigen, and an immune response can be made to it. Animals, including humans, matched for the MHC antigens will still reject tissue grafts of all types, but with much less vigor. Multiple minor antigenic differences can be additive; for example, rejection of skin grafts across an MHC barrier will be within 7 to 10 days, whereas minor differences (encompassing any number of chromosomal differences) may survive over a range of 12 to 150 days. The sum total of all non-MHC antigenic strength is equivalent to that induced by the MHC alone, as far as skin grafts are concerned[3]. It is currently assumed, though not strictly proved, that whereas major MHC antigens are cell surface structures that are functional components of the normal immune response, minor antigens represent allotypes of structures that may serve a variety of physiologic functions in cell economy. In man the major red cell blood group antigens (A and B) also serve as potent transplantation antigens, particularly in organ transplantation wherein vascular injury develops very rapidly when naturally occurring anti-A or anti-B antibodies contact the endothelium of grafts mismatched for these antigens. Although not MHC antigens, the ABH system functions as a "strong" barrier to transplantation. Comparable systems have not been defined as yet in animal models. Rat antigens of the Ag-F(pta) system, restricted to peripheral T lymphocytes, and genetically linked to genes for albinism, are potent immunogens in eliciting antibody responses, but appear to play a minor role in graft rejection. Rejection of tissue bearing MHC antigens produces quantities of recognizable effector molecules, either as immunoglobulins, or as antigen-specific cytotoxic cells, commonly called "killer T cells." In contrast, although rejection of tissue bearing only minor incompatibilities does occur, it is generally much more difficult to detect specific antibodies and effector cells as a result of immunization to a large number of weak antigens. This is another way of emphasizing the relative immunogenicity of a small number of MHC antigens, a point of practical value when one studies the latter, since the measurable responses to completely allogeneic (major plus minor) cells are almost always directed to the MHC. At the same time, there is a disadvantage in study of minor systems because of the difficulties inherent in raising reagents for their detection. The situation with cytotoxic "killer" cells is, in fact, not quite the same as for antibody production, since it has been appreciated that there is genetic restriction by MHC antigens of cell-mediated killing directed to minor antigens. In simplest terms, killer cells with specificity to minor antigens will not injure target cells bearing those antigens unless MHC anrigens of attacking and target cells are identical. Such genetic restriction does not apply to antibody-induced cytotoxicity.

It is of considerable interest that the difference in strength between MHC and minor antigens is more exaggerated with vascularized organ grafts than with skin grafts. Some examples are shown in Table 2 of prolonged survival (> 300 days) of kidney allografts between strains of rats matched for major portions of the MHC, while skin grafts are rejected in 7 to 13 days. It is apparent then that the effector mechanisms triggered by minor histocompatibility differences are more important for skin graft rejection than for the vascularized organ graft. The presentation of alloantigen is most important in this regard, and more important than the total antigen content of a tissue. If a heart, for example, is implanted as bits of tissue, rather than via connections to the major blood vessels by micro-surgery, it will be rejected as rapidly as a skin graft from the same donor.

NATURE OF THE REJECTION PROCESS

Detailed study of the components of rejection in a vascularized organ graft model has shed considerable light upon the effector mechanisms in rejection and upon the apparent discrepancies in the role of MHC antigens in skin (or bone marrow, which is similarly susceptible to rejection by minor histocompatibility differences) and kidney or heart graft rejection[4]. If A and B represent inbred rat strains differing for the MHC, when kidneys from inbred donor strains of the $(A \times B)F_1$ genotype are transplanted to A or B parental genotype recipients ($A/B \rightarrow A/A$, e.g.), progressive renal failure develops between days 4-5 post transplantation, with total cessation of function by days 7-8. At this time the organ is seen upon pathological examination to be heavily infiltrated with

TABLE 2. Differential Survival of Skin and Kidney Allografts in MHC-Compatible Rat Strains*

Donor	Recipient	Skin (days)	Kidney (days)
LEW	F344	10–12	46– > 500
F344	LEW	7–10	89– > 300
LEW	AS	12	> 300
AS	LEW	13	> 300

*Inbred stains, all of the $RT1^{\varrho}$ ($Ag-B^1$) genotype

mononuclear cells, and also to have necrotic lesions of major blood vessels and glomeruli. When MHC-matched, but minor-antigen-different strains are employed, only minimal cellular infiltration develops, and the kidneys function for long periods. The key to understanding this difference comes from comparative studies in a model of immunological manipulation called enhancement, in which indefinite graft prolongation is achieved in the A/B → A/A situation when immune IgG from an A anti-B alloantiserum is given intravenously to the A/A recipient at the time of transplantation. Instead of promoting a more accelerated rejection response, such passive transfer of anti-donor IgG prevents the recipient's own IgG, but not IgM, antibody response to MHC antigens, and results in the absence of the vascular lesions mentioned above, lesions that contain IgG and complement[4]. In contrast, the degree of cellular infiltration is not reduced, even though the grafts maintain reasonable function for prolonged periods. The cellular infiltration is a reflection of killer T cell activity, as shown by direct recovery of infiltrating cells from rejecting grafts of heart and kidney[5]. Clearly an important effector mechanism in skin graft and bone marrow rejection, the role of cell-mediated responses in the actual destruction of an organ allograft appears to be less critical than antibody (usually IgG)-mediated assault upon MHC antigens expressed in the vasculature. Clinical experience shows also that the most important factor in the rejection of renal allografts is humoral immunity leading to vasculitis[4].

With regard to the nature of the cellular infiltrate in rejecting organ allografts, recovery of viable monodisperse cells from rejecting and rejected rat tissues has established the presence of T lymphocytes having "killer" activity against donor MHC antigens, and also of B lymphocytes, macrophages, and K cells (mediators of antibody-dependent cell-mediated cytotoxicity)[5]. When tissues are treated with acidic buffers, immunoglobulins fixed to tissue are eluted into the fluid phase. These can then be studied for their class and specificity. When this is done with rejecting rat organs, donor-specific immunoglobulins are recovered; these antibodies are not present in enhanced and vasculitis-free grafts. Hence, the vascularized organ graft, in comparison to skin in the same animal model, has been extremely valuable in the analysis of those effector mechanisms that are operative in rejection. Immunopathological similarities to clinical transplant biopsies are in fact quite striking.

There is increasing application of in vitro tissue culture techniques for isolation and study of components of the immune system. The mixed lymphocyte response (MLR) in vitro is a measure of allogeneic incompatibility for a locus, or loci, of the MHC, which is closely associated with, if not identical to, genes coding for Class II Ia antigens (Table 1). The degree of lymphocyte proliferation, measured by assessing DNA synthetic rates in clones of responding T cells (mostly helper T cells having receptors for alloantigens), is an in vitro model for the early recognition of Ia-related structures on donor tissue. One can also discern the evolution in vitro of killer T cells directed to Class I (β_2-microglobulin-containing) antigens, or closely related structures, maturing as a result of the helper T cell effect upon those cytotoxic precursor cells having receptors for the alloantigens in question. Further, the establishment of immunological memory can be studied by restimulation of cultures that have gone through this wave of clonal proliferation and differentiation. The secondary response of primed cells in vitro is markedly accelerated when the appropriate antigen is introduced. These systems are now being exploited for study of suppressor T cells and other factors that many modulate the immune response to alloantigens. Although less work has been done with alloantibody-producing cells in vitro, mainly for technical reasons, approaches to in vitro study of antibody production are under development. This is an important area because of the role of antibodies in organ transplantation. Helper and suppressor T cell activation is also known to modulate the maturation of the IgG response, and this needs study at the cellular level.

ENHANCEMENT

The phenomenon of *passive graft enhancement* by administration of anti-donor immune serum has been mentioned above. Data thus far explain this effect as a blockade of the IgG humoral antibody response to those donor MHC antigens recognized by the antiserum used. Further, a number of studies have shown that antigens of the rat I region (RTl-B) and mouse H-2I region are more important immunogens than the classical β_2-microglobulin containing (RTl-A) antigens (H-2D/K in mouse). The precise mechanism of this anti-immunogenic effect of antibody is unknown. Its action is not entirely upon the humoral response, as there is some delay in appearance, though no suppression, of cytotoxic "killer" T cells in the spleens of passively enhanced animals. These alterations in immune response might be explicable in terms of alteration of the T cell-B cell collaboration necessary for full development of an IgG and killer cell response. Whether this occurs by interference with T helper cells, or by activation of T suppressor cells, has yet to be worked out (see Chapter 12). The enhanced state is immunologically specific to donor strain MHC antigens. *Active enhancement* may occur when the recipient strain has been actively immunized with donor cells, usually blood or lymphoid tissue, at some interval prior to organ engraftment. Present evidence in the rat model suggests an activation of a T cell population capable of suppressing the normal alloimmune effector response. Thymocytes from actively enhanced, graft-bearing rats can transfer a state of donor-specific unresponsiveness to an untreated recipient syngeneic to the thymus donor.[6] Models such as these should provide important data relevant to current clinical interest on the role of blood transfusions or other antigenic preparations in preconditioning potential graft recipients to a state of enhancement.

TOLERANCE

The distinction between enhancement and the type of specific unresponsiveness classically called tolerance is less clear than formerly believed. Specific unresponsiveness means that reactivity to antigens other than those used for tolerance induction is unimpaired, and is, of course, the ideal goal of transplantation research. The classic example of specific unresponsiveness to transplantation antigens is that of *neonatal tolerance,* in which immunization of newborn animals with allogeneic lymphoid cells results in development of specific tolerance to tissue grafts from the same donor strain[7]. Inbred mice and rats have been particularly valuable for such experiments. Such a state of tolerance develops because the immunologically immature newborn does not reject the inoculum, and a state of chimerism develops in which the animal has lymphoid cells of the donor strain circulating along with its own. Maintenance of the chimeric state is essential for persistence of specific unresponsiveness. Graft versus host reactions (GVH) do occur if the immunocompetent inoculum encounters alloantigens in the host. Animal models have been particularly valuable in studies on the genetic requirements for, and control of, GVH. Injection of histoincompatible lymphoid cells into mature animals does not result in tolerance, but in various degrees of immunity. However, a number of manipulations designed to decrease immunologic responsiveness of the mature host have yielded some success. In particular, successful bone marrow engraftment following drug or X-ray therapy also results in establishment of a chimeric state, and in such hosts other tissues from the same donor strain may then be transplanted. Recent studies on the nature of unresponsiveness after establishment of chimerism show that true tolerance, in the sense of a deletion of reactive clones, is probably never established. Rather, an active immune process, sometimes transferable with lymphoid cells to syngeneic recipients, seems more likely, and has focused attention upon the phenomena of enhancement and suppressor-modulator cell activity as underlying states of unresponsiveness.

Another phenomenon that may be operative in specific unresponsiveness, and which has been discerned in inbred rat, mouse, and guinea pig models, is that of anti-idiotype autoimmunity, in which an animal's auto-antibody response to the specific idiotypes of its anti-donor response serves to block the continuation of that response[8]. The variable region of a specific antibody, or of the cellular receptor that recognizes antigen, has a closely associated configuration that can be recognized as antigenic. Hence, after clonal expansion of cells and production of large amounts of antibodies to a given set of alloantigens, the animal is confronted with such quantities of an idiotype that it may be induced to make an autoimmune response to it. Experimentally this can be induced by hyperimmunization, and such animals can then be shown to be specifically unresponsive to tissue grafts from the appropriate donor strain. Practical application of this approach awaits further study. In particular, further understanding of how unresponsiveness is induced in relation to donor Class I or Class II MHC antigens, and whether there is a state of clonal deletion of suppressor cell activation, is needed.

CONCLUSIONS

Animal models of transplantation will grow in importance as the components of the immune system are better characterized and their interactions understood. Important developments from animal experimentation that have already contributed to our present level of understanding include the identification of lymphocyte subsets (e.g., Ly markers in the mouse) in relation to specific functions, the preliminary definition of I-region analogues and lymphocyte subset markers in rats in which organ grafting is possible, the appreciation that the MHC has an important role in immunobiology of which transplantation is only a special case, and recognition that specific unresponsiveness can be induced by a number of active processes involving altered regulation of the cellular and humoral immune systems. Although in vivo experimentation is considerably more complex than isolated in vitro systems, even when genetically defined strains of animals are employed, further study relating in vitro findings to in vivo events in allograft systems promises to provide a great deal of important knowledge regarding transplantation immunity, some of which will certainly be of value in clinical areas.

References

1. Snell, G. D., Dausset, J., and Nathenson, S. *Histocompatibility*. New York: Academic Press, 1976.
2. Götz, D., ed. *The Major Histocompatibility System in Man and Animals*. Springer-Verlag: Berlin, 1977.
3. Graff, R. J. Minor histocompatibility genes and their antigens. *Transplant. Proc.* **10**: 701-705, 1978.
4. Carpenter, C. B., d'Apice, A. J. F., and Abbas, A. K. The role of antibodies in the rejection and enhancement of organ allografts. *Adv. Immunol.* 22: 1-65, 1976.
5. Strom, T. B., Tilney, N. L., Paradysz, J. M., Bancewicz, J., and Carpenter, C. B. Cellular components of allograft rejection: Identity, specificity, and cytotoxic function of cells infiltrating acutely rejecting allografts. *J. Immunol. 118*: 2020-2026, 1977.
6. Hendry, W. S., Tilney, N. L., Baldwin, W. M. III., Grave, M. J., Milford, E., Strom, T. B., and Carpenter, C. B.: Transfer of unresponsiveness to organ allografts by thymocytes: Specific unresponsiveness by thymocytic transfer. *J. Exp. Med.* 149: 1042-1055, 1979.

7. Brent, L., Brooks, C. G., Medawar, P. B., and Simpson, E. Transplantation tolerance. *Br. Med. Bull. 32*: 101–106, 1976.

8. Andersson, L. C., Aguet, M., Wight, E., Andersson, R., Binz, H., and Wigzell, H. Induction of specific immune unresponsiveness using purified mixed leukocyte culture-activated T lymphoblasts as autoimmunogen. I. Demonstration of general validity as to species and histocompatibility barriers. *J. Exp. Med. 146*: 1124–1137, 1977.

Composition and Dynamics of Lipids in Cellular Membranes and Serum Lipoproteins

MICHAEL INBAR
Weizmann Institute of Science, Rehovot, Israel
Institut de Cancerologie et d'Immunogenetique, Villejuif, France
Harvard Medical School, Boston, Massachusetts

The involvement of lipids in specific protein reactions regulating normal and abnormal cell growth and differentiation has been much debated since the introduction of the concept of "fluid" structural organization of biological complexes. Throughout the past several years, it has become increasingly obvious that cellular membranes and serum lipoproteins are highly dynamic, specialized structures containing proteins and lipids. The dynamic structural organization of such complexes is now widely accepted and, in some cases, even well documented. However, the general term "fluidity," which is commonly employed in this respect, is actually complex and covers different properties of such a complex. The most prominent of these are: (a) the degree of lateral and rotational mobilities of protein receptors and (b) the degree of viscosity of the lipid core. These dynamic features of cellular membranes and serum lipoproteins, which to some extent are interrelated, are now believed to play a major role in control mechanisms regulating specific biological reactions. Moreover, since by definition all specific protein receptors are embedded to some extent in a lipid domain, the dynamic nature of the lipid region, which is determined by its composition, may determine to a large extent functional activities of proteins that are embedded in it.

During the last decade, with the improvement of physical techniques such as electron spin resonance, nuclear magnetic resonance, and fluorescence, dynamic parameters of lipid layers have been studied extensively, mostly with liposomes as model systems. These studies have established that three main characteristics determine the physical state of a lipid complex. The most prominent of these is the relative amount of cholesterol in the system. At a constant temperature an increase in the molar ratio of cholesterol to phospholipids in cellular membranes and an increase in the ratio of cholesterol to phospholipids and triglycerides in serum lipoproteins will cause an increase in the rigidity of the system. The two other characteristics are the relative amount of the different phospholipids and the degree of saturation of the fatty acids in the system. The main conclusion obtained from experiments with model system was that an increase in the fluidity of a lipid complex can be obtained by: (a) a decrease in the ratio of cholesterol to phospholipids or cholesterol to phospholipids and triglycerides, (b) a decrease in the ratio of sphingomyeline to phosphatidylcholine, and (c) a decrease in the ratio of saturated to nonsaturated fatty acids. Some of these results are illustrated in Table 1.

Based on results obtained with model systems, dynamic parameters of lipids both in membranes of lymphoid cells and in serum lipoproteins were quantitatively analyzed. These recent results have shown that the fluidity in the surface membrane lipid core of malignant leukemic lymphoblasts is much higher than that of normal lymphocytes (Table 2). This difference in dynamics between normal and malignant lymphocytes originates from a significant reduction in the molar ratio of cholesterol to phospholipids in the surface membrane of the leukemic cells as compared to plasma membranes isolated from normal lymphocytes (Table 3). Moreover, since the cholesterol deficiency in acute lymphoblastic leukemia (ALL) is greater than in chronic lymphatic leukemia (CLL), the degree of lipid fluidity is higher in ALL as compared to CLL cells. These results have established a clear correlation between fluidity and lipid composition of normal and leukemic lymphoid membranes.

Moreover, introduction of exogenous cholesterol into the surface membrane of intact leukemic cells can be performed by incubation of cells with lecithin/

TABLE 1. Lipid Fluidity in Artificial Liposomes of Different Lipid Composition*

Composition of Liposomes	Lipid Fluidity at 25°C
Phosphatidylcholine	15.55
Sphingomyeline	0.57
Phosphatidylcholine/cholesterol (M/M)	2.07
Phosphatidylcholine + 10% stearic acid	4.51
Phosphatidylcholine/cholesterol + 10% linoleic acid	96.45

*From C. Rosenfeld et al., in *Recent Results in Cancer Research,* in press.

TABLE 2. Fluidity of Membrane Lipids in Normal Lymphocytes
and Leukemic Lymphoblasts*

Cells	Origin	Fluidity of Cellular Membranes at 25°C
Normal lymphocytes	T-cells	2.64
	B-cells	2.77
	Null-cells	2.70
Leukemic lymphoblasts	T-ALL	5.29
	Null-ALL	4.79

*From S. Yanovich et al., *Cancer Research*, 38: 4654, 1978.

TABLE 3. Molar Ratio of Cholesterol to Phospholipids in Plasma Membranes
Isolated from Normal Lymphocytes and Leukemic Lymphoblasts*

Membrane Origin	Cholesterol/Phospholipids (M/M)
Normal lymphocyte membranes	0.67
Leukemic lymphocyte membranes	0.39

*From M. Petitou et al., *Proceedings of the National Academy of Science* 75: 2306, 1978.

cholesterol liposomes, such a treatment resulting in a decrease in membrane fluidity to a value characteristic of untreated normal lymphocytes. On the other hand, extraction of native cholesterol from the surface membrane of intact normal lymphocytes can be performed by incubation of cells with lecithin liposomes, such a treatment resulting in an increase in membrane fluidity to a value similar to that found in untreated leukemic lymphocytes. The changes induced in vitro in the molar ratio of cholesterol to phospholipids and in its corresponding fluidity are practically reversible for both types of cells in both directions, and, in principle, the treated cells can assume any of the characteristics between the lower and upper fluidity limits presented by untreated normal and leukemic lymphocytes, respectively.

Concomitant with these changes in composition and dynamics of cellular membranes, the degree of fluidity of lipids in the blood serum of leukemic patients in clinical relapse in markedly increased as compared to blood serum obtained from normal donors and leukemic patients in complete clinical remission (Table 4). A complete biochemical analysis of serum lipids has shown that the increased fluidity of serum lipids in leukemic patients in relapse is associated with a significant reduction in the ratio of cholesterol to phospholipids and triglycerides as compared to sera with low fluidity obtained from normal donors

TABLE 4.   Fluidity of Serum Lipid Complexes in
Normal Donors and Leukemic Patients*

Serum Origin	Lipid Fluidity of Serum at $25°C$
Normal donors	1.63
Leukemic patients in relapse	3.50
Leukemia patients in remission	1.86

*From M. Petitou et al., *Proceedings of the National Academy of Sciences 75:* 2306, 1978.

or leukemic patients in remission. Moreover, a complete lipid analysis of purified serum lipoproteins has shown that the decrease in the total ratio of cholesterol to phospholipids and triglycerides is due to (a) a significant increase in triglycerides in the very-low-density lipoprotein fraction and, more important, to (b) a marked decrease in cholesterol in the low-density lipoprotein fraction.

The facile exchange in vitro of cholesterol between artificial liposomes and lymphoid cells indicates that similar translocations of cholesterol can also occur in vivo, between cellular membranes and serum lipoproteins. Direct experimental evidence for this assumption was obtained from the experiment where leukemic and normal lymphocytes were incubated in vitro in normal and leukemic sera, respectively. A significant decrease in fluidity of cellular membranes was obtained following incubation of leukemic lymphocytes with high fluidity with normal serum with low fluidity, whereas a marked increase in fluidity of cellular membranes was obtained following incubation of normal lymphocytes with low fluidity with leukemic serum with high fluidity, suggesting cholesterol translocations (a) from normal serum to leukemic lymphocytes and (b) from normal lymphocytes to leukemic serum. This suggestion was further supported by the experiment indicating direct cholesterol translocation from low-density lipoproteins isolated from serum of normal donors to leukemic lymphocytes (Table 5). Indeed, it is well established that most cholesterol exchange processes between serum lipids and cells in the blood circulation resulted from efficient interactions between cellular membranes and the low-density lipoprotein complex and its cholesterol reservoir.

By virtue of controlling the fluidity of the cell surface membrane, the level of cholesterol may play a major role in determining biological activities of specific membrane protein receptors in the cell surface of both normal and leukemic lymphocytes. Since by definition all cellular membrane receptors are embedded to some extent in the surface membrane lipid bilayer, changes in the dynamic behavior of the lipid region induced by changes in the relative amount of cholesterol may turn on and off specific biological signals and reactions on the cell surface. This hypothesis is supported by the following recent observa-

TABLE 5. Decreased Fluidity of Leukemic Lymphocytes upon Incubation in
Low-Density Lipoproteins Isolated from Normal Donors*

Incubation Medium	Lipid Fluidity of Cellular Membranes at 25°C
Phosphate-buffered saline	4.85
Normal low-density lipoproteins	2.65

*See also M. Inbar et al. *Cancer Research 37:* 3037, 1977; and M. Petitou, *Proceedings of the National Academy of Sciences 75:* 2306, 1978.

tions: (a) Malignant lymphoma cells from mice that have accumulated cholesterol up to the level found in mouse normal lymphocytes show a marked decrease
in their tumoriginicity. (b) On the other hand, mitogenic stimulation of normal
lymphocytes is associated with a marked increase in membrane fluidity, and
cholesterol-deficient normal lymphocytes are more susceptible to activation by
plant lectins than native lymphocytes. (c) Serum stimulation of contact-inhibited
mouse fibroblasts showed a significant increase in membrane fluidity, and the
highest fluidity was found to be associated with the S-phase of the cell cycle
as compared to G_0 or G_1 phases. (d) Dynamics and composition of membrane
lipids isolated from both normal and regenerating liver cells have shown a
marked increase in membrane fluidity and a significant decrease in the ratio of
cholesterol to phospholipids in membranes isolated from regenerating cells as
compared to normal rat liver cells. (e) A direct correlation between dynamics of
serum lipids and specificity and crossreactivity of HLA antigens was reported. (f)
An increase in serum lipid fluidity was observed during spontaneous development of mammary tumors in C3H mice. (g) The amount of membrane cholesterol was found to determine directly the rate of uridine transport in normal and
leukemic lymphocytes. (h) Dynamics and composition of membrane lipids
were found to be directly associated with lymphocyte–target cell interactions
and with specific binding of Epstein-Barr Virus to lymphoid cells.

Although not much is known about the distribution pattern of lipids in the
cell surface membrane, it was suggested that composition and dynamics of
membrane lipids may act on two distinct levels in determining biological activities of normal and malignant cells: (a) on the molecular level, by determining the
amplitude of specific biochemical signals that depend on the degree of lateral or
rotational mobilities of specific protein receptor sites embedded in the lipid
core; and (b) on a cellular level, by creating a gross tensile force over the cell
periphery that will act as a mechanical barrier in cell growth, differentiation,
and proliferation processes. The outline given above strongly suggests that exchange of lipids between cellular membranes and serum lipoproteins can be
utilized by different biological mechanisms to regulate processes that are as-

sociated with normal and abnormal cell growth. As was suggested for cholesterol and leukemia, in normally regulated cases, where the molar ratio of cholesterol to phospholipids in the cell surface membrane of normal lymphocytes and the molar ratio of cholesterol to phospholipids and triglycerides in serum lipoproteins are within the normal range, the rate of cholesterol exchange can preserve and regulate a normal degree of membrane fluidity which will determine the appropriate normal expression of surface antigens, and controlled growth and differentiation. However, when the ratio of cholesterol to phospholipids and the ratio of cholesterol to phospholipids and triglycerides in leukemic cells and leukemic serum, respectively, are below the normal range, the rates of cholesterol exchange and accumulation in the cell surface membrane can decrease to a critical level where the membrane fluidity will retain an increased value that is characteristic of malignant leukemic cells.

The above mechanism suggested for leukemia can be of a more general nature. Genetic defects in the rates of cellular lipid biosynthesis or in the rates of serum lipid biosynthesis, as well as nutrition or metabolic defects, may induce alterations in lipid composition that will change the degree of fluidity of protein-lipid complexes.

Such changes may be part of a general control mechanism in determination and regulation of various physiological functions of cells because by definition all cellular membranes of each individual organ in the body are in direct contact with serum lipoprotein complexes. Therefore, our basic working hypothesis is that exchange of lipids between different lipid–protein complexes may introduce a new approach to elucidate the molecular basis of specific biochemical signals that are associated with turning on and off specific biological functions of cells.

References

Berke, G., Tzur, R., and Inbar, M., *J. Immunol. 120*: 1278-1384, 1978.

Inbar, M., and Shinitzky, M. *Proc. Nat. Acad. Sci. USA 71*: 4229-4231, 1974.

Inbar, M., Yuli, I., and Raz, A. *Exp. Cell Res. 105:* 325-335, 1977.

Petitou, M., Tuy, F., Rosenfeld, C., Mishal, Z., Paintrand, M., Jasmin, C., Mathe, G., and Inbar, M. *Proc. Nat. Acad. Sci. USA 75*: 2306-2310, 1978.

Shinitzky, M., and Inbar, M. *J. Mol. Biol. 85*: 603-615, 1974.

Van-Blitterswijk, W. J., Emmelot, R., Hilkmann, H. A. M. Oomenmeulemans, E. P. M., and Inbar, M. *Biochim. Biophys. Acta 467*: 309-320, 1977.

Lymphokines: Mediators of Delayed Hypersensitivity

ROSS E. ROCKLIN, M.D.
Chief, Allergy Division
Department of Medicine
Tufts–New England Medical Center

Delayed hypersensitivity plays an important role in a number of host responses to foreign antigens, including the rejection of organ transplants, the expression of tuberculin-type skin reactions, certain autoimmune diseases, and host defense against cancer and such microorganisms as viruses, fungi, protozoa, and bacteria. The peripheral manifestation of delayed hypersensitivity is the tuberculin-type skin reaction, and the central manifestations are those of host defense.

A delayed hypersensitivity skin reaction evolves slowly, often taking days to develop. This sets it apart from anaphylactic reactions, which occur within minutes, and Arthus-type reactions (lesions produced by antigen–antibody complexes), which evolve over a period of hours. The antigens that provoke delayed reactions are usually protein or conjugated molecules containing protein. Once the eliciting antigen in or on the skin is destroyed, the process ceases.

A delayed hypersensitivity reaction begins with the perivenous accumulation of sensitized lymphocytes and other mononuclear cells. These infiltrative lesions enlarge and multiply with time, and there is cellular invasion and destruction of tissue elements. It is now quite clear from the accumulation of experimental evidence that most, if not all, of the cells participating in the delayed hypersensitivity reaction come from the bloodstream and that they are capable of tissue destruction. How these infiltrating cells are attracted to the site of the lesion, how they are kept there, and what influences their behavior is the subject of this presentation.

When sensitized lymphocytes interact in vitro with antigen, they release a variety of protein factors which have profound effects on cells involved in these reactions. A list of these factors is given in Table 1. It may be seen that these substances have profound effects on macrophages, other lymphocytes, neutrophils, basophils, and eosinophils.

The first of the lymphokines described was that of the macrophage migration inhibitory factor (MIF). This substance was shown to retard the random movement of macrophages in vitro. There is also a chemotactic factor, which selectively attracts macrophages. In addition, there is a macrophage activating factor,

TABLE 1.   Lymphokines

Mediators affecting macrophages	Migration inhibitory factor (MIF)
	Macrophage activating factor (indistinguishable from MIF)
	Macrophage aggregation factor (MAF) (?same as MIF)
	Factor causing disappearance of macrophage from peritoneum (?same as MIF)
	Chemotactic factor for macrophages
	Antigen-dependent MIF
Mediators affecting neutrophils	Chemotactic factor
	Leukocyte inhibitory factor (LIF)
Mediators affecting lymphocytes	Mitogenic factors
	Antibody-enhancing factors
	Antibody-suppressing factors
	Chemotactic factor
Mediators affecting eosinophils	Chemotactic factor (requires antigen–antibody complexes)
	Migration stimulation factor
Mediators affecting basophils	Chemotactic augmentation factor
	Histamine Releasing Factor
Mediators affecting other cells	Cytotoxic factors–lymphotoxin
	Growth inhibitory factors (clonal inhibitory factor, proliferation inhibitory factor)
	Osteoclast activating factor (OAF)
	Procoagulant activity
	Interferon

which alters the stickiness of this cell and increases its metabolism, phagocytosis, bactericidal activity, and tumoricidal activity.

Lymphocytes are affected by several lymphokines. One factor, a mitogenic factor, causes lymphocytes to nonspecifically increase their DNA synthesis and undergo cell division. Other factors cause B lymphocytes or plasma cells to be activated and increase their synthesis of immunoglobulin or antibody. On the other hand, certain factors inhibit the production of immunoglobulin synthesis by B cells. There is also a chemotactic factor, which causes lymphocytes to direct their movement toward the chemotactic stimulant.

The migration of neutrophils is affected by two factors. One factor, termed leukocyte inhibitory factor or LIF, selectively retards the random movement of neutrophils. This factor may be analagous to MIF on macrophages and is also thought to increase the metabolism and phagocytic activity of these cells. Neutrophils are also selectively attracted by a chemotactic factor. The directed movement of eosinophils and basophils are also affected by chemotactic factors produced from lymphocytes.

These lymphokines have effects on a variety of other target cells. For example, there is a family of molecules called the cytotoxins that includes substances that are capable of bringing about lysis of susceptible target cells or can inhibit the growth of these cells. There is an osteoclast activating factor capable of activating osteoclasts in bone and bringing about its resorption. Lymphocytes also produce molecules that have interferon-like activity. They are also thought to produce a procoagulant-like activity, which has been identified as being tissue factor.

The various cell types involved in the production of lymphokines have recently been clarified. It has been shown that thymus-derived or T lymphocytes, which are the mediators of delayed hypersensitivity, produce all of the factors that have been described. In addition, bone marrow–derived or B lymphocytes also have a capacity to elaborate these factors with the appropriate immunologic stimulus. This means that under certain circumstances B lymphocytes would be able to initiate a delayed-type reaction, perhaps in the absence of T cells. It should be noted, however, that unless the host possesses immunocompetent T cells, then no lymphokine production is noted by either cell type. In addition, macrophages or monocytes are important for the initiation of certain T cell reactions and, therefore, lymphokine production as well.

The interaction between the lymphocytes producing lymphokines and their target cells can be modulated by a number of agents. It has been shown, for example, that lymphocytes must be alive and able to metabolize in order for these substances to be produced. Inhibitors of protein synthesis prevent lymphokine production and in addition the response of the target cell to the lymphokine, if present. Agents that affect microtubule and microfilament function also inhibit lymphokine production. Corticosteroids do not appear to affect lymphokine production but do affect the response of the target cell to the preformed substance. Drugs that raise intracellular levels of cyclic nucleotides also have a profound effect on lymphokine production and the response of the target cell to the mediator as well.

While lymphokines were originally described as in vitro phenomena, more recent experiments have been directed toward elucidating their in vivo effects. For example, the injection of lymphokines into the skin of normal animals provokes the development of an accelerated delayed-type hypersensitivity reaction at that site. This reaction begins after several hours and peaks by eight hours. Histologically, it mimics the classical tuberculin-type reaction. If lymphokines are injected intravenously or intraperitoneally into animals, one finds that the blood monocyte level or the numbers of macrophages in the peritoneum decrease. These changes are thought to reflect the increased stickiness of the cells with their margination or adherence to surfaces. If an immunologic reaction is induced in a host, then one can detect the presence of lymphokines circulating in the blood of these animals. Furthermore, there have been some reports of lymphokine-like activity in patients with abnormalities in their cellular-immune system or in the synovial fluid of patients who have rheumatoid arthritis.

These in vitro observations permit a fairly complete interpretation of what happens at the site of a local delayed hypersensitivity reaction. A circulating sensitized lymphocyte(s) reacts with antigen and releases several of its products, the first of which might be chemotactic factors that selectively attract inflammatory cells, particularly monocytes, to the site of reaction. The monocytic cells stick to the endothelium either because of their increased stickiness or because the endothelium has been damaged, and ultimately pass through the vessel wall. Once these cells arrive at the site of the lesion, they are held there by the migration inhibitory factor. Their function as phagocytic elements becomes enhanced by the macrophage activating factor. The initially small lesion is amplified by products such as the mitogenic factor, which nonspecifically activates other lymphocytes in the milieu so that these cells may, in turn, produce more factors. This process may be modified by enzymes extruded by the various phagocytic leukocytes that are capable of breaking down the lymphokines. In addition, when the supply of antigen is exhausted, the lack of a further stimulus to drive the reaction will result in a diminution in the inflammatory process. Substances such as the interferon-like molecules or the cytotoxic factors will be able to destroy the invader, be it a virus as in the former instance or a tumor cell in the latter.

The use of in vitro lymphokine production to detect circulating sensitized lymphocytes has been employed in a variety of clinical circumstances. These instances have included an evaluation of delayed hypersensitivity in patients who have defects in this arm of the immune response such as those with sarcoidosis, Hodgkin's disease, chronic mucocutaneous candidiasis, and certain collagen-vascular diseases. One can also detect lymphocytes sensitized to tissue antigens in patients who have autoimmune diseases such as idiopathic polyneuritis, glomerulonephritis, multiple sclerosis, and thyroiditis. Sensitivity to certain drugs has been detected with the use of these techniques. Investigators have also been able to demonstrate the presence in patients of lymphocytes sensitized to a variety of tumor antigens. A few examples will be given.

In patients with impaired cellular immunity, several patterns of reactivity have been observed. An analysis of their reactivity has been carried out by use of the delayed skin test reaction, and in vitro by the production of migration inhibitory factor and lymphocyte proliferation. Three groups of patients could be discerned. The first group included those who were positive with respect to all three of the parameters being studied, so that within the limits of the studies one could say that they had normal delayed hypersensitivity mechanisms, and those who were negative or completely anergic (unresponsive) to all three. The second group had negative delayed skin tests and negative MIF assays but had positive lymphocyte proliferation. Third, a small group of patients were negative on skin testing, so that by conventional criteria they were anergic, but had positive MIF assays and lymphocyte proliferation. Therefore, by in vitro criteria, they could be assumed to have sensitized lymphocytes. Perhaps they were not making the right lymphokine, or perhaps they had a defect in their monocytes, or in their microvasculature or their clotting mechanisms. The possibilities remain myriad, but a significant beginning has been made in dissociating the various parts of the hypersensitivity reaction.

Another approach has been the study of patients with glomerulonephritis. The question asked was whether or not these patients had sensitized lymphocytes using glomerular basement membrane as an antigen in vitro. The MIF test in response to glomerular basement membrane antigen was positive in 6 of 14 instances. By means of fluorescent microscopy, it was found that 7 of the 8 patients incapable of making MIF had either the immune complex type of disease or no fluorescence. Those patients who produced MIF had linear deposits in their glomeruli, indicating that they had antibody directed against the glomerular basement membrane. These experiments point to the utility of lymphokine assays as a means of determining the presence or absence of sensitized lymphocytes and perhaps of differentiating between the roles of sensitive cells and humoral antibodies in the pathogenetic situations where both appear to be present.

It should be stressed that clinical applications of our knowledge of lymphokines are still remote, but the possibilities are considerable. It would be of interest to determine whether tumor antigens are capable of inciting cellular hypersensitivity, and our ability to detect MIF or chemotactic factors or cytotoxic factors could well provide useful information on this problem. Nor can the possibility be excluded that breakdown in host tumor defenses might involve a specific failure in the production of one or more lymphokines.

Similarly, the shortcomings of the present means of immunosuppression are, for the most part, results of our inability to narrow the effects down to just the desired one. Here again, the dissection of the cellular defense mechanism being sought through understanding of lymphokines might afford a solution. Another possibility is the speculation that in situations where cellular hypersensitivity is a pathologic mechanism, that mechanism could be thwarted by inhibiting the production of one of the factors while leaving all other aspects of host defense mechanism intact. It is hoped that the study of these molecules will eventually lead to a situation in which the immune response can be manipulated to the benefit of man.

Granulocyte and Monocyte-Macrophage Production—Studies with in Vitro Colony-Forming Cells

Ross D. Brown
Kevin A. Rickard
Haematology Department
Royal Prince Alfred Hospital
Sydney, Australia

Hemopoiesis is a cellular process occurring primarily in the bone marrow and involving an orderly progression of both proliferation and differentiation from the earliest stem cell through various progenitor cell pools to the mature blood cells. The concentration of the different types of mature blood cells in the peripheral blood is relatively constant under normal conditions, and yet the bone marrow can increase the output of one or more of these hemopoietic cell types in response to increased demand. Our knowledge of the factors involved in the control of hemopoietic proliferation and differentiation, although still far from complete, has increased greatly in recent years. The introduction of in vivo and in vitro cloning techniques into experimental hematology has led to a greater understanding of hemopoietic precursor cells and the mechanisms involved with the regulation of hemopoiesis.

HEMOPOIETIC STEM CELLS

In animals, hemopoietic pluripotential stem cells can be assayed in vivo by their ability to generate colonies in the spleen of heavily irradiated syngeneic recipients after bone marrow transplantation. It has been demonstrated that each of these colonies, containing erythroid, myeloid, and megakaryocytic elements, arises from a single cell which has been referred to as the multipotential stem cell or spleen colony-forming unit (CFU-S). The CFU-S has proved the "stemness" of its character by its capacity for extensive self-regeneration, migration throughout the body to repopulate hemopoietic organs, and the production of specific progenitor cells for each blood cell series.

There is now substantial evidence to indicate that the pluripotential stem cell feeds into a unipotent or committed stem cell compartment for each of the three major blood cell series. A morphologically unrecognizable compartment of the megakaryocytic series actively synthesizing DNA and differentiating into the megakaryoblast was described in 1965 by Ebbe and Stohlman. In the following year, Morse and Stohlman demonstrated the presence of a committed erythroid stem cell compartment for the erythroid series by studying the differential effect of vincristine on erythropoietin-stimulated red cell precursors as compared with platelet precursors. Later, Rickard and Stohlman utilized a murine model for granulopoiesis to demonstrate that the cell responsible for colony formation in agar was a stem cell committed to granulopoiesis (Stohlman et al., 1973).

Although all the committed stem cell compartments are actively involved in cellular proliferation, and their progeny may also be committed stem cells, they are not entirely self-sustaining. In times of increased demand for differentiated cells, the pluripotential stem cell, which is normally in a G_0 or resting state, can enter the cell cycle and release cells into the committed stem cell compartments. However, under normal conditions the committed stem cell compartments have the capacity for proliferation and amplification in response to humoral regulation and thus demand very little from the pluripotential stem cell compartment. An increase in demand for one cell type may cause a slight decrease in production of other cell types. Thus, the various hemopoietic elements may be forced into a "stem cell competition" situation.

IN VITRO COLONY-FORMING CELLS

The phenomenon of colony growth in semisolid agar by hemopoietic cells was first discovered by two groups independently. Bradley and Metcalf in Melbourne and Pluznik and Sachs in Rehovot demonstrated that discrete cellular colonies developed when bone marrow or spleen cells were cultured in nutrient agar. These colonies consisted of granulocytic and mononuclear cells, but would only form if a specific colony stimulating factor for granulocytes and macrophages (GM-CSF) was present in the cultures (Metcalf and Moore, 1971).

In 1970 Robinson and Pike adapted this technique to culture granulocytic and mononuclear colonies from human bone marrow. In the ensuing years, agar cultures and other support matrix like methylcellulose and plasma clots have been utilized to grow colonies containing erythrocytes, megakaryocytes, plasma cells, B lymphocytes, T lymphocytes, and bone marrow stromal cells. Thus, cloning techniques are now available for all major hemopoietic subpopulations (Metcalf, 1977). However, there is still no in vitro cloning technique that can assay the multipotential stem cell. These semisolid culture systems can determine the concentration of various hemopoietic progenitor cells, kinetic and biophysical characteristics of these cells, and the response to specific hemopoietic regulatory factors. As most of the experimental studies using semisolid cloning cultures have involved the granulocyte/macrophage colony-forming cell (GM-CFC), the remainder of this chapter will be concerned only with studies of GM-

CFC cultures. However, the principles emerging from these studies are generally applicable to other cell systems.

IN VITRO COLONY FORMATION BY GM-CFC

Cells forming granulocytic and/or macrophage colonies (GM-CFC) in vitro have been demonstrated in the seven-day-old yolk-sac of mice. By the tenth day of gestation, GM-CFC's can be detected in the developing fetal liver, and by days 13-14 gestation the number of fetal liver GM-CFC's reaches a maximum level. As the bone marrow and spleen develop on days 16-18 gestation, CM-CFC's appear in these organs. Liver GM-CFC's can reappear in this organ if damage occurs to other hemopoietic organs (Metcalf, 1977). In the normal adult mouse, GM-CFC's occur only in the bone marrow (about one in every 10^3 nucleated cells), spleen, and blood (about one in every 10^5 nucleated cells). In man, GM-CFC normally occur at lower concentrations (about one in every 5×10^3 nucleated bone marrow cells and one in every 5×10^5 peripheral blood leukocytes). GM-CFC have been demonstrated to be sensitive to many different stimuli, both in vitro and in vivo. In response to demand for new granulocytes, caused by irradiation, bacteremia, or endotoxemia, a marked increase in serum GM-CSF levels precedes a wave of granulopoiesis in which increased numbers of recognizable granulocytic precursor cells enter DNA synthesis.

The size of in vitro colonies varies considerably. Clones containing more than 50 cells have been called colonies, whereas smaller clones (less than 50 cells) have been called clusters. The pattern of granulocyte-macrophage differentiation varies with culture conditions and the source of the specific stimulating factor (GM-CSF). It appears that granulocytic colonies transform into macrophage colonies toward the end of the culture period. Although eosinophilic colonies develop in agar cultures, there is some disagreement between reports as to the incidence of eosinophilic colonies. Differences in the source of GM-CSF are probably the cause of these apparent discrepancies.

RELATIONSHIP BETWEEN CFU-S AND GM-CFC

It was suggested soon after the introduction of the in vitro culture technique that the cell responsible for colony formation in vitro was possibly identical to the in vivo spleen colony-forming unit. However, it is now realized that the GM-CFC and CFU-S are different cellular entities. At any particular time less than 5% of CFU-S in the normal animal are synthesizing DNA, whereas between 30 and 50% of GM-CFC are in DNA synthesis. Thus, while the GM-CFC are predominantly in cycle, CFU-S are predominantly in G_0 —a resting state. Murine CFU-S and GM-CFC have been separated physically on the basis of size by velocity sedimentation, density by centrifugation in discontinuous albumin gradients, and active adherence on glass-bead columns. It has been shown that there is a differential effect by vinblastine on the survival of CFU-S and GM-CFC, and there is an increased growth potential of GM-CFC in fetal liver. GM-CFC are increased in the shielded limb of leg-shielded mice, and CFU-S are decreased in W^v/W^v and W/W^v mice and genetically determined anemia. Further studies have indicated that GM-CFC are the progeny of CFU-S, and in vitro cluster-forming cells are the progeny of GM-CFC (Metcalf and Moore, 1971).

COLONY STIMULATING FACTOR FOR
GRANULOCYTES AND MACROPHAGES
(GM-CSF)

As mentioned earlier, the formation of colonies of granulocytes and macrophages in vitro is entirely dependent on the presence of a specific stimulating factor in each culture. GM-CSF can be bioassayed in cultures of marrow cells at concentrations as low as 10^{-11} M. There is a sigmoid dose–response curve between GM-CSF concentrations and the number of colonies developing.

The purification and characterization of GM-CSF has proved to be a difficult problem because of the low concentration of GM-CSF in most potential sources, the apparent heterogeneity of the GM-CSF molecule (not only between different species, but also from the same species), and the instability of the activity of the GM-CSF molecule.

GM-CSF has been extracted from a wide range of tissues and extracellular fluids in many species. However, there appears to be a wide heterogeneity in the molecular size, antigenicity, and functional activity of GM-CSF from these sources (Metcalf, 1977).

The active material in human placental conditioned medium which will stimulate human marrow cells has a molecular weight of 30,000 daltons. Active GM-CSF extracted from human leukocytes has been reported by one group of workers to have a molecular weight of 1,300 daltons, while another group reports three types of GM-CSF with molecular weights of 93,000, 36,500, and 14,700 daltons. The GM-CSF from human urine has been reported to be a glycoprotein with a molecular weight of 45,000 daltons.

Despite these apparently conflicting data, the specific biological activity of all forms of GM-CSF is to stimulate granulocyte/macrophage production. When other agents like endotoxin and cyclic AMP stimulate granulopoiesis in vivo or in vitro, this response is apparently mediated by the stimulation of GM-CSF production and/or release, which subsequently stimulates GM-CFC proliferation.

Although in vitro studies suggest that GM-CSF is the most likely candidate for "granulopoietin," a granulocytic analogue of the erythrocytic humoral regulator erythropoietin, and there has been an in vivo granulocytic response to partially purified GM–CSF injected into mice, there is not quite enough evidence to conclude that GM–CSF is the major humoral regulator for in vivo granulopoiesis.

There are probably both long-range and short-range control mechanisms for in vivo granulopoiesis. The monocyte-derived macrophage may act as a surveillance cell that is able to increase serum CSF levels in response to stimuli at any site, while bone marrow stromal cells probably mediate granulopoietic responses in the marrow microenvironment.

INHIBITION OF GRANULOCYTE–MACROPHAGE COLONY FORMATION

It has been postulated that the regulation of granulopoiesis in vivo is balanced between at least one set of inhibiting factors and stimulating factors. The search for the inhibiting factors in cell systems has centered around the concept of the presence of chalones—the tissue-specific inhibitors of DNA synthesis released from the most mature cells of each series. An active granulocyte chalone (M.W. 4,000 daltons) has been produced from extracts of mature granulocytes, which inhibits DNA synthesis in marrow granulocytic progenitor cells. Whether or not granulocyte chalone acts directly on hemopoietic precursor cells via a classical negative feedback system or through a suppression of GM–CSF production is not yet understood. It is, however, important to realize that many inhibitory responses demonstrated in vitro may be nonspecific effects caused by toxic metabolites. Certain lipoproteins in serum that inhibit in vitro GM–CFC growth and are decreased in sera from patients with acute leukemia have been studied; however, their in vivo significance is not known.

Recent reports that purified granulocyte chalone can be used therapeutically for remission-induction in acute myeloblastic leukemia add a possible new approach to cancer therapy. Further studies on the effects of granulocyte chalone are imperative, and the in vitro agar culture technique offers many possibilities in this regard.

The humoral and cellular interactions mentioned in this chapter are depicted in Figure 1.

GM–CFC IN HUMAN BONE MARROW

Although precise quantitation of GM–CFC (e.g., GM–CFC/femur) is possible in mice, GM–CFC numbers in human bone marrow are generally reported as a cloning efficiency (e.g., GM–CFC/2×10^5 nucleated marrow cells cultured). Consequently many reported increases in GM–CFC concentration, when there is also a generalized bone marrow hyperplasia (e.g., in megaloblastosis), have probably underestimated the increase in total GM–CFC's.

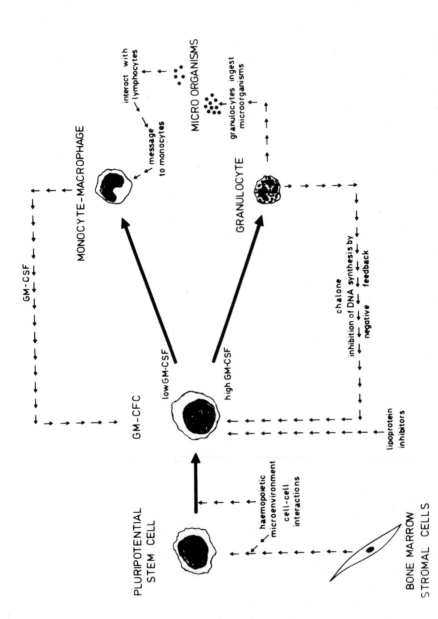

FIG. 1. Proposed model of the humoral and cellular interactions involved in granulocyte and monocyte-macrophage formation. Heavy unbroken lines indicate cellulare development while broken lines with arrows indicate possible regulatory mechanisms.

An adapted flash labeling technique, which determines the proportion of GM–CFC in the DNA synthesis phase of the cell cycle, can be used to demonstrate the proliferative status of GM–CFC and the GM–CFC proliferative response to various stimuli. Cell separation techniques, especially using velocity sedimentation, density gradient, and adherence procedures, have been useful to concentrate the GM–CFC population and to determine various biophysical characteristics of GM–CFC.

Although many different sources of GM–CSF have been utilized, few preparations have provided the necessary stimulus found in the plateau region of the GM–CSF dose-response curve. One-milliliter feeder layers containing 1×10^6 peripheral blood leukocytes and human placental conditioned medium concentrate have been the most reliable sources of the human GM–CSF.

GM–CFC IN ACUTE MYELOBLASTIC LEUKEMIA

The outstanding feature of bone marrow cultures from patients with untreated acute myeloblastic leukemia (AML) or AML in relapse has been the absence of normal colony growth in most cultures and only a few colonies in others. Large numbers of clusters (3–40 cells) and an increased cluster/colony ratio occur in most cultures. Several workers have noted a correlation between various in vitro culture patterns and prognosis (Moore, 1974; Goldman and Sultan, 1975).

GM–CFC numbers rise to normal levels during clinical remission, but fall with the onset of relapse. The number of clusters and the differentiation of the cells in the colonies also return to normal in remission.

The proportion of GM–CFC in DNA synthesis is reduced in untreated AML, increased during marrow regeneration of early remission, normal during consolidated remission, and decreased with the onset of relapse.

Density gradient analysis of marrow from patients with AML has shown that GM–CFC are usually less dense in relapse than GM–CFC from normal marrow. Similarly, velocity sedimentation analysis has shown that GM–CFC from the marrow of patients with AML are much larger than normal GM–CFC. By applying Stokes' Law to the experimental data obtained from these studies, it has been demonstrated that GM–CFC from leukemic marrow have a mean cell diameter of 11.5 μ compared with 9.1 μ for GM–CFC from normal marrow.

In vitro culture studies have demonstrated that leukemic cells respond to and depend on stimulation by GM–CSF. Although there has been speculation that such GM–CSF must be abnormal, analysis of human urine and sera and the use of specific antisera have failed to demonstrate abnormal forms of GM–CSF in AML. When these findings are considered together with the recent demonstration of remission induction with granulocyte chalone, there is considerable evidence to suggest that leukemic cells will respond to normal control mechanisms. It is most likely that leukemic cells have a serious genetic derangement that causes a complete or nearly complete failure of progenitor cells to differentiate into nondividing cells. Computer-assisted models have shown that such an intrinsic defect could alone be sufficient to account for the progressive proliferation and subsequent growth advantage of a leukemic population of cells.

GM–CFC IN CHRONIC MYELOID LEUKEMIA

In patients with chronic myeloid leukemia (CML) the number of GM–CFC in the peripheral blood is greatly increased (up to 10,000 times normal). A number of workers have noted a direct correlation between absolute leukocyte count and the GM–CFC concentration in peripheral blood. Bone marrow GM–CFC concentration is usually increased, but not to same degree.

Perhaps the most useful studies involving patients with CML have been those determining the proportion of GM–CFC in DNA synthesis. While the proportion of GM–CFC in DNA synthesis is decreased in the chronic stage, this parameter rises to quite high levels (40 to 70%) during blastic transformation. Furthermore, it has been reported that during blastic transformation there is a direct correlation between the proportion of GM–CFC in DNA synthesis and the percentage of myeloblasts in the bone marrow. Such observations suggest that leukemic cell behavior in blastic transformation of CML is indeed different from that of acute leukemia. In cultures from patients with Philadelphia (Ph^1) chromosome positive CML, the colonies contained cells with Ph^1 chromosomes. These studies demonstrate that most GM–CFC from CML patients belong to the leukemic clone, and such cells respond to and depend on GM–CSF stimulation.

GM–CFC IN NEUTROPENIA AND APLASIA

The absence of mature neutrophils in the peripheral circulation may result from any one of a number of causes. In vitro culture studies offer a new approach to such conditions by measuring granulopoiesis at a very early progenitor cell level. The wide variation in the results of such studies indicates the heterogeneity of these conditions. However, bone marrow cultures can indicate whether the stem cell pool is intact and if a maturation defect is present. A good assessment of granulopoiesis in a neutropenic individual can be achieved by combining GM–CFC marrow studies and measurements of GM–CSF in the peripheral blood with traditional leukocyte kinetic studies using $DF^{32}P$ labeling.

In vitro culture techniques can play an important role in bone marrow transplantation programs. Continual failure of marrow cultures to grow colonies over a period of several months confirms that a patient with aplastic anemia has a stem cell deficiency. Such has been recently referred to as chronic hypoplastic marrow failure. Serial marrow cultures post transplantation have provided an early indication of "take" and regeneration. Furthermore, the agar culture technique is the best available method of monitoring the viability of bone marrow cells after storage in liquid nitrogen and to assay stem cell content of cell populations after fractionation of a heterogeneous bone marrow aspirate.

The introduction of in vitro cell cloning techniques into experimental hematology in the last decade has provided some valuable new tools for the study of hemopoietic cellular proliferation and differentiation. This has led to a greater understanding of the factors involved in hemopoietic cellular proliferation and its control. Although many concepts have arisen, there are still questions to be answered and new avenues to be explored.

References

Goldman, John M., and Sultan, Claude. Clinical applications of bone marrow culture. *Lancet,* ii, 696–699, 1975.

Metcalf, Donald. *Hemopoietic Colonies.* Berlin: Springer-Verlag, 1977.

Metcalf, Donald, and Moore, Malcolm A. S. *Haemopoietic Cells.* Amsterdam: North Holland, 1971.

Moore, Malcolm A. S. In vitro studies in the myeloid leukaemias. In *Advances in Acute Leukaemia.* Amsterdam: North Holland, 1974.

Stohlman, F., Jr., Quesenberry, P., Niskanen, E., Morley, A., Rickard, K. A., Tyler, W. S., Symon, M., Monette, F., and Howard, D. *Control of granulopoiesis.* In *Hemopoietic Stem Cells.* Amsterdam: Elsevier, 1973.

Immunopathology

STEWART SELL, M. D.
Department of Pathology
University of California at San Diego
School of Medicine
La Jolla, California

Immunopathology is the study of how immune mechanisms cause disease. The term, "immunopathology" contains opposite concepts: Immune means protection or exemption from; in legal terms, immunity is applied to individuals such as diplomats who are exempt from particular laws. On the other hand, pathology is the study of disease. Thus immunopathology is the study of the destructive or undesirable effects of reactions that usually serve to protect us against infectious diseases.

Immune mechanisms are directed specifically by two major components of the immune system that are produced after stimulation by contact with an appropriate substance: immunoglobulin antibody and specifically sensitized cells (lymphocytes). They are produced by stimulation of an indivudal with structures that are recognized as foreign, termed "antigens." Complete antigens are soluble molecules or cell surface structures that are capable of inducing an immune response and of reacting with the products of the immune response. A normal nonimmune individual does not have detectable antibody or specifically sensitized cells to a given antigen. Upon exposure to antigen, an individual develops these products (immunization) and the specific capacity to recognize and react differently upon re-exposure to the same antigen. Thus the individual has learned to respond differently to specific molecular structures (antigens) by immune mechanisms.

An antigen may be a foreign material not normally present in an individual (exogenous antigen), or it may be a normal component of the individual's own tissue (autoantigen or endogenous antigen). Normally an individual does not make an immune response to his own tissues, a situation known as "immune self-tolerance." However, under some circumstances this tolerance is broken, and the immune effector mechanism turned against the individual, a condition known as auto-allergic or auto-immune disease. To reiterate, immune mechanisms may be activated by reactions to foreign (exogenous) antigens or to self (endogenous) antigens.

The effects of an immune response are usually protective and beneficial (immunity). The most compelling evidence that immune mechanisms are protective is as follows: (1) following recovery from an infectious disease such as measles, influenza, and so forth, the individual is not susceptible to a repeated infection by the same organism; (2) immunization with nonpathogenic forms of infectious organisms or nontoxic forms of bacterial toxins results in specific resistance to infection or toxin exposure; (3) individuals with inability to mount specific immune responses (immune deficiency diseases) invariably succumb to fatal infections, in many instances by organisms that are not usually pathogenic in normal individuals.

Immune effector mechanisms are initiated by reaction of preformed specific antibody or specifically sensitized cells with antigen. Antibodies belong to five major related protein species collectively termed immunoglobulines (Table 1), which have in common receptor sites that recognize and react with antigens. Two antigen receptors are present in each individual unit of immunoglobulin, and some immunoglobulins are made up of more than one Ig unit. Antigen binding sites are structures that provide a close molecular conformation of ionic charges opposite to those of the antigen; the binding site and antigen fit together like a lock and key and are held together by noncovalent bonds. Upon reaction with antigen, tertiary structural changes take place, which activate some of the

TABLE 1.   Some Properties of Immunoglobulins

Property	IgG	IgA	IgM	IgE	IgD
Serum concentration (mg/ml)	12	2.5	1	0.0005	0.03
Size (mol. wt.)	140,000	320,000 (Dimer)	900,000 (Pentamer)	180,000	200,000
Antigen binding sites/molecule	2	4	10	2	2
Complement fixation	+	0	+++	0	0
Lymphocyte cell surface	0	0	+	0	++
Disease association	Neutralization Toxic complex Cytotoxic	Toxic complex (rare)	Cytotoxic	Anaphylactic	?
Antibody activity	Major antibody class precipitation, ab	External secretions	First formed	Binds to mast cells	Lymphocyte surface
Structure				Master Cell	B Cell

Immunoglobulin antibodies belong to a group of proteins with related and unique properties. The basic immunoglobulin molecule is represented by IgG, composed of two pairs of polypeptide chains, i.e., two heavy chains and two light chains, joined by disulfide bonds. The molecule is shaped like a Y with two identical antigen binding sites, located at the top of the branches of the Y, composed of folded parts of both the heavy and light chains. The stem of the Y is composed of heavy chains which are shared by antibodies of a given IgG class. This part of the molecule bears the structures responsible for the biologic properties of a given immunoglobulin class. Other immunoglobulin classes are IgA, IgM, IgE, and IgD. IgA is a dimer composed of two Ig units, and is prominent in external secretions such as saliva, milk, and nasal and gastrointestinal secretions. IgM is composed of five Ig units, IgE and IgI) are composed of single Ig units, IgE has particular heavy chain structures, which allow it to become bound to mast cells. IgD is frequently found on the surface of lymphocytes.

biologic functions of antibodies and initiate the appropriate effector mechanisms. The type of immunoglobulin antibody mechanism that is active in a given individual is determined to a large extent by the immunoglobulin class of antibody produced.

Immune effector mechanisms are also initiated by specifically sensitized cells (immune lymphocytes). Lymphocytes are small round cells that are found in lymphoid organs of the body (spleen, lymph nodes, and so on) and in circulating blood; immune lymphocytes also have receptors for antigens. Lymphocytes may be divided into two major classes, B cells and T cells. B cells are precursors of cells that produce and secrete immunoglobulins, whereas different T cell subpopulations have different functions (see Table 2). Two classes of T cells, T_H (helper) and T_S (suppressor) cells, interact with B cells to help initiate antibody production (T_H) or suppress the extent of antibody production (T_S). The T cells that are responsible for immune effector reactions belong to the T_K and T_D subclasses. T_K (killer) cells react directly with tissue target cells and kill them, whereas T_D cells are activated by reactions with antigen to release mediators (lymphokines), which attract and activate another cell population, macro-

TABLE 2.   Some Properties of T Lymphocytes

T lymphocyte subclass	Function
T_H	Helpers for B cell stimulation—cooperate with B cells to stimulate antigen-induced differentiation of B cells to antibody-producing plasma cells.
T_S	Suppressors for B cell stimulation—act on proliferating B cells to limit the extent of plasma cell production.
T_D	Delayed hypersensitivity—produce lymphokines upon reaction with antigen that activate delayed hypersensitivity reactions.
T_K	Killer cells—react with antigens on the surface of cells and kill them.
T_P	Precursor T cell—develops in the thymus and differentiates into different functional T cell populations in other lymphoid organs.

Lymphocytes belong to two major classes, T cells and B cells. Both cell lines are believed to be derived from stem cells in the bone marrow. B cell differentiation takes place in the liver or gastrointestinal tract; B cells have surface immunoglobulin and are the precursors of plasma cells. T cells differentiate in the thymus to Tp or T precursor cells; these cells leave the thymus and further differentiate into different functional populations in other lymphoid organs (lymph node, spleen). Four functional populations of T cells have been identified (see table). T cells have surface Ig that is difficult to detect, but may be identified by other markers. In man, T cells bind sheep erythrocytes to form rosettes (i.e., sheep cells surround and adhere to the T cell on incubation in vitro).

phages. Infiltration of tissue inflammatory sites with macrophages is associated with destruction of antigen-bearing cells; however, the reaction must be initiated by specifically sensitized lymphocytes that react with antigens in or on tissues.

Immune reactions also cause disease (immunopathology). The terms "allergy" and/or "hypersensitivity" are often used for deleterious effects of immune reactions. The prevalence of disease-producing immune reactions is now so widely recognized that by common medical usage the term "immune" does not always connote protection, as it once did.

Accessory mechanisms are activated by some immune specific reactions: complement in cytotoxic and toxic complex reactions, pharmacologically active mediators in anaphylactic reactions, and macrophages in delayed and granulomatous reactions. Complement consists of at least 20 different serum proteins Upon reaction with antigen, the structure of antibody is changed so that the complement system is activated. If complement-activating antibody (complement fixing) reacts with antigens on the surface of a cell, the cell will be destroyed. By a series of enzymatic cleavages and aggregation reactions complement proteins alter cells so that they are susceptible to destruction by digestion in phagocytic cells of the body (reticulo-endothelial system), or transmembrane channels are formed that permit release of intracellular components (cell lysis). Activation of complement by reaction of antibody with soluble antigens (immune complex reactions) results in the formation of cleavage fragments of complement that attract and activate polymorphonuclear leukocytes. These blood-born cells carry lysosomal enzymes that are released and digest tissue structures. Reaction of antigen with IgE antibody affixed to certain tissue cells, called mast cells, results in release of pharmocologically active mediators from the mast cells. These agents in turn act upon smooth muscle cells to produce constriction (anaphylactic reactions). Reaction of T_D lymphocytes with antigen results in release of a variety of lymphocyte mediators, termed lymphokines. Lymphokines act to attract macrophages (chemotaxis) and stimulate them to ingest antigen or antigen-coated cells (phagocytosis). This activity of macrophages in tissues is responsible for some of the damage associated with delayed hypersensitivity reactions. If the macrophages are unable to digest phagocytized material, the cells may transform into epithelioid cells (resembling epithelial or skin cells) or giant cells. These cells organize into characteristic ball-like masses (granulomas) and may accumulate in tissue sites sufficiently to impair the normal function of the tissue (granulomatous reactions). In summary, accessory mechanisms that help immune specific antibodies or lymphocytes express immune reactions include complement, polymorphonuclear leukocytes, mast cells and their pharmocologic mediators, and macrophages. These accessory components play essential roles in immune effector mechanisms.

TABLE 3. Characteristics of Immune Mechanisms—Protective and Destructive

	Neutralization	Cytotoxic
Immune reactant	Antibody, usually IgG	Antibody, IgM or IgG complement fixing
Accessory components	–	Complement, reticulo-endothelial system
Skin test reaction	–	–
Protective function	Inactivate toxins	Kill bacteria
Examples of protective states	Diphtheria Tetanus	Bacterial infections
Pathology	Inactivation of biologi-cally active molecules or loss of cell receptor	Cell lysis or phagocy-tosis
Examples of disease states	Insulin-resistant diabetes Myasthenia gravis	Hemolytic anemias Vascular purpura Transfusion reactions Erythroblastosis fetalis

CLASSIFICATION OF IMMUNOPATHOLOGIC MECHANISMS

A major advance in the understanding of how immune reactions cause disease was made by the classification of effector mechanisms by Gell and Coombs in 1962. The present classification is an expanded form of their classification. Six immunopathologic mechanisms may be identified (Table 3), four of them caused by immunoglobulin antibody and two by specifically sensitized lymphocytes.

Antibody-mediated mechanisms are: (1) *neutralization* or inactivation reactions—loss of activity of biologically active molecules by reaction with antibody; (2) *cytotoxic* or *cytolytic* reactions—destruction of cells of the blood system by antibody and complement; (3) *immune complex* (*toxic complex*) reactions—tissue destruction induced by antibody and complement activation of

Toxic Complex	Anaphylactic	Delayed or Cellular	Granulomatous
Antibody, IgG precipitating complement fixing	Antibody, IgE skin fixing	Cells, $T_D + T_K$	Cells $(?T_D)$
Complement, polymorphonuclear leukocytes	Mast cells, pharmacologic mediators, end organs	Macrophages	Macrophages
Arthus: peak 6 hr, fade by 24 hr	Wheal and flare: peak 5-10 min, fade by 12 hr	Delayed: peak 24-48 hr, nothing at 6 hr	Delayed—weeks, granuloma
Mobilize polys to sites of infection	Open vessels—delivery of antibody and cells to tissue sites	Destroy virus-infected cell Kill organisms	Isolate infectious agents
Bacterial Infection	Parasitic infections	Virus infections, Fungi, ?Cancer	Leprosy, Tuberculosis
Polymorphonuclear leukocyte infiltration and digestions by lysosomal enzymes	Bronchoconstriction, edema, vascular shock	Mononuclear cell infiltrate—target cell destruction	Epithelioid and giant cell replacement of tissue
Glomerulonephritis Vasculitis Arthritis Rheumatoid diseases	Asthma, hay fever, anaphylactic shock, mosquito bites	Thyroiditis Demyelination Graft rejection Viral skin rashes	Sarcoidosis Berylliosis Leprosy

acute inflammation due to polymorphonuclear leukocytes; (4) *anaphylactic* or *atopic* reactions—acute reactions caused by release of mediators (e.g., histamine) from cells coated with antibody, causing smooth muscle constriction. Immune lymphocyte-mediated reactions are: (5) *delayed* or *cellular* reactions—infiltration of solid tissues by immune lymphocytes and destruction of tissue by macrophages; (6) *granulomatous* reactions—the accumulation of modified macrophages into masses of cells that occupy tissue and interfere with normal tissue function.

Neutralization Reactions

If antibody is formed that reacts with and inhibits the activity of a biologically active molecule required for normal body functions, disease will be produced because of a lack of that function. In addition, antibody to cell surface receptors may block the normal function of that cell. Inactivation of biologically active molecules is caused by alteration of the tertiary structure of the molecule so that it is no longer biologically active; antibodies to cell surface receptors may block the receptors or cause them to be metabolically removed from the cell surface (modulation). The former situation may occur in diabetes (antibody to insulin), blood clotting disorders (anti-body clotting factor), endocrine dysfunction (i.e., antibody to thyroid hormone, and so on), and other diseases; the latter occurs in myasthenia gravis when auto-acetyl-choline receptor antibodies inhibit neuromuscular transmission. On the other hand antibody to thyroid stimulating hormone receptors on thyroid cells may stimulate the thyroid cells by mimicking the action of thyroid stimulating hormone (a form of hyperthyroidism).

Cytotoxic or Cytolytic Reactions

Cytotoxic or cytolytic reactions are mediated through complement activation on the surface of the target cell by antibody that reacts with antigens on the cell surface. The antigens are either structural components of the cell surface, such as blood group antigens on red cells in transfusion reactions, or passively absorbed antigen, such as drugs (e.g., penicillin), which adhere to cell surfaces. Complement, by a series of enzymatic cleavages and aggregations of proteins in the complement system, produces alterations on the cell surface that render it susceptible to phagocytosis. In addition, the accumulation of complement components on the cell produces an intramembrane channel and lysis of the cell.

The cell types affected by cytotoxic reactions are those that occur naturally in suspension, such as red blood cells, white blood cells, and platelets. The disease states are characterized by a loss of the function of the cell type being destroyed: red blood cells—hemolytic anemia; white blood cells—increased susceptibility to infection; platelets—purpura, bleeding. Transfusion reactions occur when blood from an individual of one antigenic type is transfused into an individual who has antibody to that antigenic type. They are essentially massive hemolytic reactions. Auto-immune cytotoxic reactions may occur by reaction of auto-antibodies with self antigens on the affected cells. Although infrequent, these usually are temporary states following infection or drug therapy.

Toxic Complex Reactions

Antibody reactions with soluble antigens in the blood may result in the formation of circulating soluble antibody–antigen complexes which deposit in tissue sites, fix complement, and initiate acute or chronic inflammation. In addition, antibody may react directly with tissue antigens, in particular vascular basement membranes, activate complement, and initiate inflammation. The activation of complement by antibody-antigen complexes results in the formation of cleavage products of complement which cause endothelial cell separation (expose basement membrane) and attract polymorphonuclear leukocytes (polys). Polys are white blood cells that contain in their cytoplasm small membrane-circumscribed organelles filled with protolytic enzymes (lysosomes). When polys engulf antibody-antigen complexes or antibody on basement membrane, these organelles release their enzymes, which digest the adjacent tissue causing disruption of the basement membrane. This disruption permits leakage of blood elements. The kidney and lung have capillary basement membranes that are not completely covered by endothelial cells. These organs are particularly susceptible to toxic complex-mediated damage (glomerulonephritis, interstitial pneumonia). The damage may occur rapidly and extensively (acute) or be protracted and gradual with proliferation of tissue cells and fibrous scarring (chronic). A similar mechanism is operative in producing inflammation of the joints (rheumatoid arthritis). In toxic complex arthritis, activation of complement occurs within the joint space, polys invade the joint space, and the smooth surface of the joint (articular cartilage) is destroyed by the poly lysosomal enzymes. Toxic complex or antibody-induced acute inflammation is responsible for a wide variety of human disease including glomerulonephritis, serum sickness, systemic lupus erythematosis (DNA-anti-DNA complexes), other rheumatoid diseases, a variety of skin eruptions, and lung diseases (Goodpasture's syndrome, cellular interstitial pneumonias).

Anaphylactic or Atopic Reactions

These reactions are those commonly referred to as allergy by most people. The term "anaphylactic" was employed because the immune reaction seems to be the opposite of that usually found after immunization, i.e., anaphylactic as opposed to prophylactic. The term "atopic" means "strange" and was used because of the bizarre responses sometimes observed. Anaphylactic reactions are initiated by reaction of antigen (allergen) with the IgE class of antibody that has become passively absorbed to tissue (mast cells) or blood (basophils) cells. These cells contain membrane-lined vesicles (lysosomes) filled with pharmocologically active mediators (e.g., histamine, serotonin, slow reacting substance), which act on smooth muscle cells, causing them to constrict. This constriction produces narrowing of air passages in the lung (asthma), increased vascular permeability due to separation of the cells that line vessels (edema or systemic shock), and increased gastrointestinal activity (food allergy). The nature of the reaction depends largely on the route of exposure and dosage. If large doses are swallowed or inhaled, acute food allergy reactions or severe acute asthma occurs; if small amounts of antigen are injected, there is a localized skin reaction such as occurs commonly following a mosquito bite (wheal and flare, hive); if small doses are inhaled over a prolonged period of time, there are recurrent chronic reactions exemplified by hay fever or seasonal allergic rhinitis. Certain individuals tend to react with one organ system, i.e., demonstrate food allergy but not asthma. The severity of anaphylactic reactions may be greatly modified by pharmacologic agents (drugs) that determine the threshold required for mast cell degranulation or end organ responsiveness. These agents act by controlling metabolism of the mast cell or end organ cells through intracellular levels of cyclic AMP. Acute anaphylactic reactions may be treated by drugs such as epinephrine, which lowers the responsiveness of mast cells or end organ cells. Chronic allergic reactions may be controlled by drugs that interfere with the action of the mediators (e.g., antihistamines). Injection of the offending antigen under controlled conditions can sometimes produce a specific clinically significant decrease in anaphylactic reactivity (hyposensitization). The exact mechanism of this effect is not clearly understood for each case, but it is a method of immunotherapy commonly used by clinical allergists.

Delayed or Cellular Reactions

Delayed reactions are initiated by specifically sensitized lymphocytes which recognize antigens on cells or within tissues. Two lymphocyte populations are active: T_K (T killer) cells, which react with antigens on target cells and cause their destruction, and T_D (delayed hypersensitivity) cells, which, upon reaction with antigen, release lymphokines. These lymphocytic mediators attract and activate macrophages, which phagocytize (engulf) antigens. Delayed hypersensitivity reactions are generally effective in solid tissues, whereas antibody-mediated reactions involve soluble antigens or cells in suspension.

The lesions of delayed hypersensitivity are characterized by perivascular mononuclear cell (lymphocyte and macrophage) infiltration. It is possible that antibody-mediated reactions (immune complex or anaphylactic) may open up vascular endothelium to permit mononuclear cells to infiltrate tissues. This mechanism may be particularly important in the brain, where the vessels are less permeable to cells than other tissues are. Injection of antigen into the skin of an animal sensitized in the delayed manner results in a skin reaction that peaks at 24 to 48 hours (in contrast to immune complex reactions that peak at 6 hours and cutaneous anaphylactic reactions that peak at 5 to 10 minutes).

Delayed hypersensitivity reactions occur to a variety of infectious agents, to self antigens, and to grafted tissues. The tuberculin skin reaction is a classic delayed hypersensitivity reaction to antigens of mycobacterium tuberculosis. The skin rashes seen in measeles are due to delayed hypersensitivity to viral antigens on infected epithelial cells. Certain post-infectious conditions, such as the demyelinating diseases (post-infectious encephalomyelitis) following viral infection or immunization, are caused by delayed hypersensitivity to viral antigens or to self antigens (auto-allergic diseases). A number of organs may be attacked by lymphocytes that react against self antigens (e.g., thyroid, adrenal, salivary gland, testes, and so on). Rejection of grafts (in particular kidney or skin grafts) is mediated by delayed reactions. Successful graft transplantation between different individuals requires suppression of the rejection mechanism, usually by drugs that interfere with delayed hypersensitivity. Grafts containing lymphocytes (such as bone marrow grafts) may react to antigens of the treated recipient (graft versus host disease) if the recipient is unable to reject the grafted lymphocytes. (immune-deficient, newborn, radiation-exposed, and so forth).

Granulomatous Reactions

Granulomatous reactions are also initiated by specifically sensitized lymphocytes (T_D cells) and macrophages. However, in contrast to delayed reactions, the antigen is not catabolized or destroyed after phagocytosis by macrophages. This results in a metabolic and morphologic conversion of the macrophages into large rectangular cells that resemble skin cells (epithelial cells) or even larger multinucleated giant cells. Giant cells are formed by macrophages that undergo nuclear division but not cytoplasmic division. These cells accumulate in the tissues containing the antigen and form characteristic ball-like clusters of cells known as granulomas, the cell accumulations of a granuloma serving to surround the antigen and isolate it from the rest of the body. Loss of tissue function occurs if the masses become extensive and replace enough normal tissue to cause symptoms.

The organ most frequently involved is the lung, most likely because the antigens responsible are inhaled, but other organs may also be destroyed. Granulomatous reactions occur to many mycobacterial organisms or fungi, in particular tuberculosis and leprosy. Most of these granulomas remain small and localized and do not produce symptoms. Granulomatous reactions are the major lesion of sarcoidosis, in which disease masses of granulomas in the lung may seriously impair pulmonary function. The antigen responsible has not been identified. Similar reactions occur to beryllium, an inhaled heavy metal that interacts with host tissue to become antigenic. In leprosy, granulomatous reactions (tuberculoid leprosy) are associated with low numbers of organisms in the tissues, good prognosis, and favorable response to chemotherapy. The opposite is true for leprosy victims who do not exhibit granulomatous reactions (lepromatous leprosy).

PROTECTIVE FUNCTION OF IMMUNE MECHANISMS

In this chapter the destructive manifestations of immune effector mechanisms have been emphasized. However, each mechanism is believed to have evolved for its protective function. Neutralization or inactivation of toxic molecules by antibody permits the effects of bacterial toxins such as diphtheria or tetanus toxins. Cytotoxic effects of antibody and complement on bacteria will kill the infecting organisms. Antibody-initiated immune complex reactions deliver polymorphonuclear leukocytes to sites of infection where the poly enzymes can act on infecting agents. Anaphylactic reactions open up small blood vessels in tissues and permit exit of blood proteins or cells into sites of infection. Cellular or delayed reactions are effective in eliminating virus-infected cells, or fungal or mycobacterial infections. Granulomas form around infectious agents such as leprosy bacilli, isolating them from the rest of the body and preventing dissemination.

SUMMARY

Immune specific mechanisms exist for recognizing and protecting against the effects of infectious agents. In some instances, these reactions may cause disease (immunopathology). The immune system may be directed against self antigen (auto-allergic disease), or reactions with foreign antigens may result in tissue damage. Immune mechanisms are mediated by specifically modified proteins (antibodies) or cells (immune lymphocytes) which have the capacity to recognize and react with antigen. Six different mechanisms, four mediated by specific antibody and two by immune lymphocytes, are described, and examples of diseases given.

References

Bach, J.-F., ed. *Immunology*. New York: Wiley, 1976.
Gell, P. G. H., and Coombs, R. R. A. *Clinical Aspects of Immunology* (1st ed. 1962, 3rd ed. 1975). Oxford: Blackwell (Philadelphia: F. A. Davis), 1975.
Miescher, P. A., and Müller-Eberhard, H. J., eds. *Textbook of Immunopathology* (2nd ed.). New York: Grune and Stratton, 1976.
Sampter, M., ed. *Immunological Diseases* (2nd ed.). Boston: Little, Brown, 1971.
Sell, S. *Immunology, Immunopathology and Immunity* (2nd ed.). Hagerstown, Maryland: 1975.

Mediation of Cellular Immune Reactivity by Hormones and Neurotransmitters

TERRY B. STROM
MARY-ANN LANE
J. HAROLD HELDERMAN
Department of Medicine, Renal Division
Peter Bent Brigham Hospital, Harvard
Medical School, Boston, Massachusetts

Division of Immunogenetics
Sidney Farber Cancer Institute
Harvard Medical School
Boston, Massachusetts

Department of Internal Medicine
The University of Texas Health Science Center
Dallas, Texas

Lymphocytes express proliferative and cytotoxic responses following stimulation by cells bearing histoincompatible alloantigens. The transplantation antigens of the major histocompatibility gene complex (HLA, H-2, AgB) that stimulate the immunoproliferative responses mounted by allogeneic thymus-derived (T) lymphocytes in mixed lymphocyte cultures (MLC) and graft versus host (GVH) response are closely linked to, albeit separable from, the serologically identifiable specificities. At least two subpopulations of lymphocytes are able to lyse alloantigenic target cells. First, alloimmune cytotoxic T lymphocytes, bearing a receptor for cell-bound, serologically defined alloantigens, bind to and destroy target cells (lymphocyte-mediated cytotoxicity, Ab–LMC). In contrast, nonimmune lymphocytes designed K cells that express a receptor for the Fc portion of IgG, lyse target cells complexed with IgG anti-target-cell antibodies (antibody-dependent lymphocyte-mediated cytotoxicity, Ab-LMC). The ability of $3', 5'$-cyclic nucleotides to bidirectionally regulate the vigor of these proliferative and cytotoxic cellular responses against allogeneic cells and the dynamic changes in the lymphocytic membrane which perceive the messages of cyclic nucleotide active ligands are the subjects of this review.

The ability of sensitized cytotoxic lymphocytes to destroy target cells bearing donor alloantigens is regulated by cyclic AMP and cyclic GMP. The capacity of nonimmune T-independent lymphocytes bearing a receptor for the Fc portion of IgG to lyse target cells complexed with IgG anti-target-cell antibody is similarly modulated by cyclic $3'$, $5'$-mononucleotides (rev. in 1). The ability of cytotoxic T cells to lyse target cells is inhibited by a variety of agents that we and others have been demonstrated to elevate lymphocyte cAMP levels, including prostaglandins, isoproterenol, aminophylline, cholera toxin, and dibutyryl cAMP, whereas imidazole, cholinergic stimulation, insulin, or addition of 8-bromo cGMP enhances LMC[1]. Either adenylate cyclase activators (isoproterenol, prostaglandin, or cholera toxin) or methylxanthines, which increase intracellular cAMP by protecting cAMP from breakdown, inhibit LMC and Ab-LMC. The combination of adenylate cyclase activators and methylxanthines causes an additive attenuation of LMC or Ab-LMC associated with a syngergistic increase in cAMP. In order to establish conclusively that modulation of LMC may result from an effect exclusively upon the attacking cell, experiments were carried out with cholera toxin, a prolonged activator of adenylate cyclase that can be removed after its interaction with the cell without loss of adenylate cyclase stimulation. Cholera toxin (1 μg/ml) was preincubated with sensitized Lewis spleen cells for 10, 30, 60, 120, and 180 min; and the cells were washed three times before introduction of target cells. The cyclic AMP levels were determined at the time of introduction of the target cells. Cholera toxin had little effect on either LMC or cyclic AMP levels until 180 min of preincubation when both a marked inhibition of LMC and increase in cyclic AMP occurred. The consistent kinetic inverse relationship between cAMP and cytotoxicity (LMC or Ab-LMC) in systems in which the attacking cells alone are treated with cholera toxin in decisive evidence that elevations of attacking lymphocyte cAMP levels suppress their ability to kill target cells.

In contrast, 8-bromo cGMP, a lipid-soluble analogue of cGMP, enhances the ability of effector cells that mediate LMC and Ab-LMC to destroy target cells. Furthermore, cholinergic agonists, e.g., acelytcholine or carbamylcholine and insulin, agents that elevate cGMP, presumably, via activation of guanylate cyclase, also enhance LMC. The augmentation of LMC by insulin and cholinergic agonists is mediated by the activation of separate plasma membrane receptors, since atropine, a muscarinic antagonist, blocks the cholinergic, but not the insulin-induced, augmentation of lysis (rev. in 1).

Imidazole, an agent that decreases lymphocyte levels of cAMP, also enhances LMC. Recent investigations have demonstrated that imidazole and its derivative levamisole elevate human and murine lymphocyte levels of cGMP, in addition to decreasing cAMP. Thus, the ratio of cGMP to cAMP is altered in a manner that facilitates lymphocyte effector function. Both imidazole and levamisole enhance the proliferative responses of lymphocytes to phytohemagglutinin[2]. Levamisole and tetramisole have been demonstrated to potentiate a variety of in vivo immune responses in mice, rats, and humans. The therapeutic effect of levamisole on human tumor resistance is currently under study using a double-blind protocol. A total of 111 patients with primary pulmonary carcinomas were administered levamisole or placebo as an adjunctive therapy to surgery. The levamisole-treated group (51 patients) had 10 recurrences and 7 deaths after 1 year of follow-up, whereas the placebo group (60 patients) sustained 20 recurrences of tumor and 12 deaths. Since levamisole lacks tumoricidal effects in vitro, it is likely that this agent augments tumor immunity in man[3]. That in vivo immunopotentiation may be produced by a variety of agents that alter cyclic nucleotide metabolism is further supported by the provacative observation that transfer factor causes elevations of cGMP within monocytes (rev. in 1).

A brief preincubation of the attacking alloimmune cell population with carbamylcholine, insulin, imidazole, or 8-bromo cGMP prior to the introduction of target cells is a prerequisite for enhancement of LMC, an effect consistent with the transient increases in cGMP known to occur with carbamylcholine, insulin, or imidazole stimulation. Since these agents do not alter LMC when preincubated with the target cells, pharmacological augmentation of LMC is apparently the result of an effect on the attacking cells alone. Similarly, isoproterenol, prostaglandin, and cholera toxin attenuate LMC only when the attacking cells are preincubated with agents and at a time when cAMP levels are elevated. Taken together, these data indicate that the levels of cAMP and cGMP within the attacking cells at the moment of initial contact with target cells determine the extent of cytotoxicity.

Other investigators demonstrate that human polymorphonuclear (PMN) leukocytes that bear an Fc receptor are able to lyse antibody-coated tumor cells. The ability of these PMN effector cells is also governed bidirectionally by their intracellular cyclic nucleotides: cAMP inhibits lysis, whereas cGMP enhances target cell destruction. That cytotoxic T lymphocytes, K cells, and cytotoxic PMNs may utilize common mechanisms in target cell destruction is further suggested by the common requirement for divalent cations and energy.

It was recently shown that carbamycholine, acting via the muscarinic acetylcholine receptor, has the ability to activate murine effector lymphocyte populations from unsensitized spleen which were rendered cytolytic against syngeneic tumor target cells during in vitro interaction. These same activated cells exhibited only minimal reactivity against normal syngeneic target cells. The induced reactivity was inhibited by the muscarinic cholinergic antagonists atropine, scopolamine, and ioopropamide, but not by the nicotinic cholinergic antagonist d-tubocurare. Both T and non-T effector cells appeared to be activated, as treatment with anti-theta antisera plus complement only partially ameliorated this response.[4]

The precise mechanisms of cell-mediated cytotoxicity are unknown; however, attacking and target cell attachment is a prerequisite for lysis in all the systems outlined above. The mechanism by which cytotoxic T lymphocytes destroy target cells is the most rigorously studied cytolytic system. Three stages of this lytic mechanism have been isolated (Martz, 1975). First, cytotoxic T lymphocytes form firm adhesions with target cells; second, a lethal injury is delivered to the target cell; and finally, the target cell lyses in a process that does not require the continued presence of viable attacking cells. Henney[5] reported data indicating that the second stage of lysis is inhibited by elevations in cellular cAMP. Since our data (rev. in 1) indicate that cyclic nucleotides alter an early step in the lytic process, and the data of others provide evidence that the motility of T and B lymphocytes and PMNs are bidirectionally modulated by cyclic nucleotides (rev. in 1), we would speculate that increased attacking-cell levels of cGMP increase cell motility and enhance the opportunity for attacking and target cell adhesion. In contrast, cellular accumulations of cAMP inhibit attacking and target cell interaction. It is likely that multiple alterations in cell behavior regulated by the cyclic nucleotides account for changes in cell-mediated cytotoxicity.

We have also demonstrated that the ability of cGMP to enhance and of cAMP to inhibit the proliferative response made by lymphoid cells encountering allogeneic cells in vivo or in vitro demonstrates that both phases of cell-mediated alloimmunity, proliferative (recognition) and cytotoxic (effector), are regulated by cyclic nucleotides. These data are in concert with the mounting evidence that cGMP promotes proliferative events while cAMP opposes blastogenesis.

Fragmentary evidence gathered from several laboratories has indicated that the expression of lymphocyte cell receptors for ligands such as histamine, insulin and acetylcholine changes as a function of lymphocyte activation. As previously noted, insulin augments the effector function of cytotoxic T lymphocytes, whereas histamine, an activator of leukocyte adenylate cyclase, inhibits LMC produced by sensitized murine lymphocytes. Consequently, the functional appearance or disappearance of specific lymphocyte receptors for agonists that activate adenylate cyclase or guanylate cyclase constitutes a potential and intriguing mechanism for governing lymphocyte function. Obviously, a cell lacking specific receptors for acetylcholine, insulin, or histamine will not be directly influenced by alterations in concentration of these naturally occurring substances, since most polypeptide hormones and neurotransmitters convey their signals to target cells via interaction with membrane recognition units (i.e., specific receptors).

The distribution of insulin receptors among mononuclear leukocytes is incompleltely defined. Recent studies indicate that peripheral blood mononuclear leukocytes prepared by passage through glass-bead columns or by ficoll-hypaque gradient separation bear insulin receptors (rev. in 1). In contrast, rat splenic lymphoid cells or human peripheral blood lymphocytes prepared by filtration through nylon-wool columns do not specifically bind insulin. The primary consequence of passing mononuclear leukocytes through nylon wool is deletion of

B lymphocytes and macrophages. Subsequently, Schwartz et al. (rev. in 6) demonstrated that 85-90% of the insulin-binding cells found among human, ficoll-hypaque prepared peripheral mononuclear leukocytes are monocytes and not lymphocytes. Whereas normal peripheral T lymphocytes lack insulin receptors, stimulated T lymphocytes appear to express a receptor for insulin. Krug et al. (rev. in 6) demonstrated that insulin receptors are revealed on the membranes of lymphocytes prepared by nylon-wool filtration during, but not before, activation by concanavalin A. Since physiologic concentrations of insulin augment LMC produced by nylon-wool–filtered effector cells, alloimmune T lymphocytes also appear to develop an insulin receptor. This notion has been formally proved[6], since nylon-wool effluent, T-enriched spleen cells obtained from rats transplanted with histoincompatible skin grafts develop specific insulin-binding receptor sites, whereas normal T cells or T cells obtained following syngeneic transplantation lack insulin receptors. The T-cell insulin receptor site is of similar affinity ($K_d \simeq 1$ nM) to the insulin receptor expressed upon liver and fat cells. Subsequently, four additional protocols have demonstrated that activated lymphocytes rapidly develop an insulin receptor with nanomolar affinity. First, responder T cells in allogeneic, but not syngeneic or major histocompatibility complex matched, unidirectional mixed lymphocyte responses develop an insulin receptor. Second, T cells from rodents undergoing the graft versus host reaction also develop an insulin receptor. Third, purified cells, but not B cells, develop an insulin receptor subsequent to interaction with either of the T cell mitogens phytohemagglutinin or concanavalin A. Fourth, purified B cells, but not T cells, develop an insulin receptor subsequent to interaction with the B cell mitogen E. coli lipopolysaccharide. Thus, in all protocols the events of activation were linked to acquisition of insulin receptors upon the activated cell type, whereas the nonactivated population failed to develop these recognition structures. Furthermore, the emergence of the insulin receptor was an early event associated with activation, since the appearance of insulin receptors precedes discernable de novo DNA synthesis, and inhibitors of DNA synthesis or mitosis do not hinder the emergence of insulin receptors. Indeed, accurate and rapid assessment of rodent lymphocyte cultures has been accomplished by demonstrating the appearance of insulin receptors upon responder T cells within 16 hours of culture (Strom, Helderman, and Williams).

The potent muscarinic receptor antagonist 3-quinuclidinyl benzylate (QNB), previously used as a tritiated ligand to describe receptor binding in brain and heart, has recently been used to describe receptor binding in whole and purified rat spleen cell populations. Half maximal binding of ^{3}H-QNB (29.2 Ci/mM, New England Nuclear Corp.) to unfractionated spleen cells occurred at $2\text{-}5 \times 10^{-9}$ M, while half maximal binding to nylon-wool purified T lymphocytes occurred at 7×10^{-10} M. These levels are comparable to those found in brain[7] and heart[8] tissue by other investigators. Binding of ^{3}H-QNB is abolished by the muscarinic antagonists astropine and scopolamine but not by the nicotinic antagonist d-tubocurare. Preliminary studies with activated cell populations indicate that the level of receptor binding of ^{3}H-QNB obtained increases following allogeneic stimulation.[9]

Plaut et al.[10] reported that the cytolytic efficiency of murine splenic lymphocytes obtained 7 to 9 days after alloimmunization is unaffected by histamine in vitro, whereas out data show insulin to be effective at this time. From day 11 onward following allogeneic mastocytoma sensitization, histamine has an increasing ability to inhibit LMC. This study awaits rigorous confirmation by histamine binding studies. It would appear that early, alloimmune T lymphocytes (days 6-9 post sensitization) reveal an insulin receptor that allows the cGMP "go" signal to be transmitted, whereas the cells participating in the later immune response are more responsive to a cAMP-induced "turnoff" mechanism. Such dynamic changes on the lymphocyte membrane have obvious implications regarding acceleration of early immune events and exertion of negative control influences at a time when substantial tissue injury has been achieved. A further understanding of the regulatory influences of cyclic nucleotides on the immune response may allow rational and safe methods for pharmacological manipulation of the immune response. Indeed, immunomodulation has already been achieved in vivo utilizing agents demonstrated to alter lymphocytic concentrations of cyclic 3', '5-nucleotides.

References

Strom, T. B., Lundin, A. P. III, and Carpenter, C. B. The role of cyclic nucleotides in lymphocyte activation and function. In *Prog. Clin. Immunol;* Vol 3, R. S. Schwartz, ed. New York: Grune and Stratton, 1977, pp. 115-153.

Hadden, J. W. Coffey, R. G., Hadden, E. M., Lopez-Corrales, E., and Sunshine, G. H. Effects of levamisole and imidazole on lymphocyte proliferation and cyclic nucleotide levels. *Cell. Immunol. 20:* 98-103, 1975.

Study Goup for Bronchogenic Carcinoma. Levamisole in human breast cancer. *Br. Med. J. 53:* 461-464, 1975.

Lane, Mary-Anne. Muscarinic cholinergic activation of spleen cells cytotoxic to tumor cells in vitro *J. Nat. Cancer Inst. 61:* 923-926, 1978.

Henney, C. S. On the mechanism of lymphocyte mediated cytotoxicity. *Transplant. Rev. 17:* 37-70, 1973.

Helderman, J. H., and Strom, T. B. Emergence of insulin receptors upon alloimmune T cells in the rat. *J. Clin. Invest. 59:* 338-344, 1977.

Yamamura, H. I. and Snyder, S. H. Muscarinic cholinergic binding in rat brain. *Proc. Nat. Acad. Sci. 71:* 1725-1729, 1974.

Sastre, A., Gray, D. B., and Lane, M. A. Muscarinic cholinergic binding sites in the developing avian heart. *Dev. Biol. 55:* 201-205, 1977.

Lane, M. A., and Strom, T. B. Muscarinic cholinergic binding on lymphocytes. In preparation.

Plaut, M., Lichtenstein, I. M., and Henney, C. S. Properties of a subpopulation of T cells bearing histamine receptors. *J. Clin. Invest. 55:* 856-874, 1975.

Current Concepts of the Gastrointestinal Hormones

CHRISTOPHER S. HUMPHREY, M. B., Ch., B., F.R.C.S.

JOSEF E. FISCHER, M. D., F.A.C.S.

During recent years our knowledge of those peptides referred to collectively as the gastrointestinal hormones has increased considerably. Notable advances within this area include the recognition of an ever increasing list of peptides that may subserve a humoral role, and the realization that many of these compounds may not be hormones in the accepted sense of the word.

A common feature of the hormones and humoral candidates that have been found in gastrointestinal tissues (Table 1) is their peptide structure. The amino acid sequences of some of these peptides are sufficiently similar for them to be grouped into families. Thus gastrin and cholecystokinin (CCK) constitute one family, whereas another comprises secretin, glucagon, gastric inhibitory peptide (GIP), and vasoactive intestinal peptide (VIP). Such structural homologies provide one of the pieces of evidence suggesting that these peptides may have evolved from common ancestral molecules.

Some of the peptides, VIP and enteroglucagon, for example, have a fairly wide distribution throughout the alimentary tract, whereas others such as pancreatic polypeptide and CCK are more discretely localized. In many cases a combination of immunohistochemical techniques and electron microscopy has revealed the precise cellular origin of the gastrointestinal peptides. These endocrine cells are sufficiently characteristic and dissimilar from one another for them to have been individually named, as indicated in Table 1.

One of the most surprising discoveries of the last few years has been that some of the gastrointestinal peptides are not confined to the alimentary tract. Gastrin, VIP, and probably CCK have been found within the brain, whereas some other peptides such as somatostatin, substance P, neurotensin, and enkephalin, previously thought to be solely neuronal peptides, have since been found in the gastrointestinal tract. Outside of the central nervous system, VIP is located in peripheral neurones that appear to innervate muscular and vascular tissues of the alimentary and urogenital systems, and gastrin, too, may exist in some autonomic nerves.

This dual localization of peptides to endocrine cells and to neuronal tissue has been explained by the APUD concept, developed by Pearse. According to this theory the various peptides all possess a common origin in the primitive

TABLE 1.   The Gastrointestinal Peptides

Peptide	Tissue Source*	APUD cell†
Gastrin	Antrum, duodenum	G
Cholecystokinin (CCK)	Duodenum, jejunum	I
Secretin	Duodenum	S
Gastric inhibitory peptide (GIP)	Duodenum, jejunum	K
Vasoactive intestinal peptide (VIP)	Throughout gut	D_1
Enteroglucagon	Jejunum, ileum, colon	L
Pancreatic polypeptide	Pancreas	PP
Somatostatin	Stomach, duodenum, jejunum, pancreas	D
Motilin	Duodenum, jejunum	$?EC_2$
Substance P	Throughout gut	$?EC_1$
Neurotensin	Ileum	N
Enkephalin	Antrum, duodenum	?
Bombesin	Antrum, duodenum	P

*Tissues possessing highest concentrations and/or greatest numbers of endocrine cells. Species variations exist.

†Based on the Lausanne 1977 classification. In some cases the identification of cell type has been made in certain species only.

embryonic ectoblast. During development, clones of neuroendocrine programmed cells serve to populate such seemingly diverse tissues as the alimentary tract, thyroid gland (C cells), carotid body, adrenal medulla, hypothalamus, pituitary, and lung. The differentiated cells in these sites produce the various peptide and amine hormones. The cytochemical characteristics of these cells include the uptake of amine precursors and their subsequent decarboxylation, properties that have led to the acronym "APUD" cell.

Almost all of the gastrointestinal peptides under consideration exhibit widespread pharmacological actions when infused into either man or an experimental animal. These actions include both stimulation and inhibition of secretory and motor activity within the alimentary tract, as well as metabolic effects such as the production of hyperglycemia and the stimulation of insulin release. There is a considerable overlap between the actions of the various peptides, and in particular structurally related compounds often possess very similar properties. In addition, the effects of one peptide may be altered by the concurrent administration of another. Such interactions may be either potentiating or inhibitory, and similar neuroendocrine interactions are observed when parasympathetic stimulation or ablation is coupled with the administration of a peptide.

The actions and interactions of most of the peptides have been well documented. What is proving much more difficult is to decide which actions are truly physiological and which are merely pharmacological. If one considers the peptides as circulating hormones, then the question becomes relatively easy to answer. Grossman has proposed guidelines that help to define the physiological roles of gastrointestinal hormones. The first step is to determine the physiological range of stimulated secretion. In most instances this will involve giving a standard meal and measuring the resulting change in plasma concentration of the peptide in question by radioimmunoassay. The second step involves reproducing the measured response by means of an exogenous infusion. Any effects produced by an infusion that reproduces the physiological plasma concentrations of the peptide in amount, time course, and molecular species (thus recognizing the fact that many of the peptides exist in different molecular forms) may be considered as physiological. Using such criteria, four of the peptides are thought to possess physiological roles as circulating hormones: gastrin, cholecystokinin, secretin, and GIP. An additional three peptides—motilin, enteroglucagon, and pancreatic polypeptide—may subsequently become part of this list, since plasma concentrations of these peptides rise in a fairly consistent manner after the ingestion of appropriate meals. The probably hormonal functions of these peptides are given in Table 2. It must be emphasized that not only is this list provisional,

TABLE 2. The Circulating Gastrointestinal Hormones

Hormone	Releasing Stimulus	Function
A. *Probable hormones*		
Gastrin	Protein meal. Antral distension.	Acid and pepsin secretion. ?Trophic.
Secretin	Acid in duodenum.	Pancreatic HCO_3 secretion. Potentiates CCK.
Cholecysto-kinin	Protein and fat.	Pancreatic enzyme secretion. Gall bladder contraction. Potentiates secretin. ?Inhibits gastric motility. ?Trophic.
Gastric inhibitory polypeptide	Protein, fat, and carbohydrate.	Inhibition of gastric secretion. Glucose-dependent insulin stimulation.
B. *Possible hormones*		
Enteroglucagon	Carbohydrate and fat.	?Hepatic glucose production. ?Insulin stimulation.
Pancreatic polypeptide	Meal (especially protein). Probable vagal component.	??Inhibits pancreatic secretion. ??Stimulates GI motility.
Motilin	Meal response variable (?fat stimulates and carbohydrate inhibits). ?Duodenal pH.	?Stimulates GI motility.

but also the status of each of the peptides as a true hormone, and its ascribed functions, are still debated. Gastrin and CCK have been listed as possessing possible trophic effects. This potentially important property, which other peptides may also possess, implies that the presence of these substances is necessary for the continuous growth and replacement of alimentary tissues.

The remainder of the peptides may not function as true hormones. In some cases this is so because physiologically stimulated secretion of the peptide has not been found. VIP is a good example here, for the plasma concentration of this peptide does not rise after a meal, and indeed no truly physiological stimulus has yet been shown to cause VIP secretion, although acid perfusion of the canine duodenum does cause an increase in plasma VIP as well as gastric acid inhibition and intestinal secretion. In other instances the argument that a peptide is not a circulating hormone assumes more of a philosophical character. For example, somatostatin secretion occurs in response to a meal. However, the action of somatostatin is to produce widespread inhibition of the secretion and actions of almost all of the remaining peptides. Since it is difficult to conceive of a situation in which such widespread inhibition would be needed, somatostatin is currently thought to act locally on individual tissues on the basis of local release (paracrine action).

The presence of some of the peptides in nerve endings of peripheral nerves that run in the gut plexuses suggests that some of their biological potential may be realized through actions as neurotransmitter substances, or at least as substances that modulate neural activity. The third mode of action that peptides may utilize is that of a paracrine agent. Here, release from endocrine cells raises the tissue concentration of the peptide sufficiently to produce a local response. Peptidergic control of the alimentary tract may thus be considered to result from a combination of these three types of action: hormonal, neural, and paracrine (Figure 1). This concept is as yet in its infancy, and it must be admitted that much of the evidence for paracrine and neural peptidergic actions is circumstantial. Table 3 lists the possible functions of the remaining peptides that are believed to act in this way.

If this tripartite system of humoral control of alimentary function is as important as it seems to be, the potential for its involvement in diseases of the alimentary tract is enormous. The best-described examples of humorally mediated disease within the gastrointestinal tract are the syndromes resulting from excess secretion of one or more of the peptides by tumors. These tumors, for which the general term "apudoma" has been coined, may be single or multiple and vary from benign to malignant and metastasizing. The syndromes that result from tumorous peptide secretion include the Zollinger-Ellison syndrome caused by gastrinomas, the syndrome of profuse watery diarrhea which in some cases is associated with a VIP-secreting tumor, and spontaneous hypoglycemia resulting from an insulinoma. A glucagonoma syndrome comprising mild metabolic

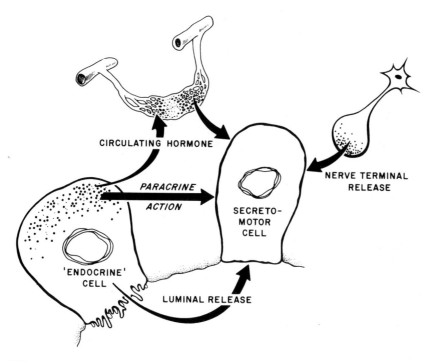

FIG. 1. Peptidergic control of the gut. Illustration of the potential for interactions between circulating hormones, locally released peptides (paracrine actions), and peptides released from nerve terminals (neurocrine actions). The significance of luminal release, which has been shown for some peptides, is unclear.

disturbances, weight loss, and a peculiar migratory skin rash has been described, and a few reports of somatostatin and pancreatic polypeptide–producing tumors have appeared in the literature. The term "apudoma" is perhaps an ugly one, but its usage is justified by the fact that it emphasizes certain common character-istics of the peptid-producing tumors. In large part these are due to the fact that the tumors arise not from the differentiated apud cells, but rather from the pre-cusor cells. The totipotential nature of these more primitive cells explains not only the varied pathological picture that may be produced, but also the fact that the presence of an apudoma often indicates a more generalized tendency to neoplasia in the individual. Occasionally more than one tumor may be present; if so, the pituitary or parathyroids are often implicated in addition to the gastro-intestinal tumor. Perhaps more commonly an alimentary apudoma will contain and secrete more than one peptide. A high proportion of pancreatic apudomas appear to contain somatostatin and pancreatic polypeptide in addition to the

TABLE 3. Gastrointestinal Peptides without Circulating Role

Peptide	Possible Function (paracrine or neurocrine effect)
Vasoactive intestinal peptide	?Stimulation of pancreatic and intestinal secretion. ?Control of smooth muscle tone and visceral blood flow.
Somatostatin	?Inhibition of secretion and actions of other peptides.
Bombesin	?Stimulation of gastrin release.
Substance P	??Stimulation of motor activity.
Enkephalin	??Inhibition of motor activity.
Neurotensin	?

symptom-producing peptide, a fact that is being increasingly utilized in screening and diagnosis.

The roles of the gastrointestinal hormones in producing other disease is less clear. In duodenal ulceration, for example, we know that the characteristic hypersecretion of acid is associated with increased meal-stimulated gastrin secretion as well as an increased sensitivity of the parietal cell mass to gastrin. The increase in stimulated gastrin release appears to have two components: increased G cell activity and decreased inhibition. Tentative suggestions have been made that these two properties may reflect abnormal local stimulation by bombesin and reduced control by somatostatin respectively, but these hypotheses are as yet unproved. Hypersecretion of acid also occurs in the face of extensive small bowel resection. Although this phenomenon is almost certainly humorally mediated and involves gastrin, the precise mechanism is unclear. Decreased removal of circulating hormones may be a factor to consider in some diseases. Perhaps the best example is the hypergastrinemia that may accompany chronic renal failure and reflect impaired renal removal of gastrin. Increased circulating concentrations of gastrin may be one of the reasons for the fairly high incidence of gastroduodenal disease in patients with renal failure. Hepatic failure may be accompanied by increased VIP concentrations, but the significance of this is unclear.

Our techniques for investigating abnormalities of hormone secretion are fairly well established. Unfortunately, we do not yet possess the same degree of expertise when it comes to evaluating possible disturbances of paracrine or neurocrine secretion, a fact that may explain the relative poverty of knowledge in the area of humorally mediated gastrointestinal disease. One of the most exciting prospects to be investigated as techniques are developed lies in the area of gastrointestinal motility disorders. These conditions, which include the aganglionic diseases such as achalasia of the gastric cardia and Hirschprung's disease as well as the "functional" disorders like spastic colon, diverticular disease, and biliary dyskinesia, may prove to be due to disturbances of paracrine and/or neurocrine control. Such slender evidence as there is for this statement comes from evidence that tissue concentrations of substance P and VIP are lower in the aganglionic segments of Hirschprung's disease, and that the diseased esophagus of achalasia shows increased sensitivity to gastrin.

In the area of patient management the gastrointestinal hormones have assumed a small but important role. At the present time this is largely confined to diagnosis, but in the future we may see an increasing use of these peptides in the area of therapeutics. The use of pure or purified hormones or synthetic derivatives as stimuli for diagnostic gastric or pancreatic function tests is far from new, and today pentagastrin, secretin, and cholecystokin are widely used. A word of caution should be interposed over the interpretation of results of, particularly, pancreatic function tests. A "normal" response to the infusion of secretin and/or cholecystokinin merely implies that the pancreatic exocrine tissue is capable of responding to the exogenous stimulus. There remains the possibility of pancreatic insufficiency due to a failure of food and acid to produce secretion of CCK and secretin from the intestinal mucosa. This may be the mechanism of the pancreatic insufficiency sometimes associated with mucosal damage, as in celiac disease, and also that found on occasion after truncal vagotomy.

Measurement of circulating hormone concentrations by immunoassay finds its greatest application in the diagnosis of the apudomas, and in particular the diagnosis of the Zollinger-Ellison syndrome. Here the mere documentation of elevated fasting gastrin concentration is not sufficient, for hypergastrinemia can result from hyperplasia of the antral G cells or from a retained antral remnant after gastric resection, as well as occuring after extensive intestinal resection or in renal failure. Current practice is to determine the pattern of hypergastrinemia in response to a standard meal, an infusion of calcium, and an injection of secretin. The autonomous secretion of gastrin from a gastrinoma is distinguished from that due to other causes by the insignificant response to a meal and the large response to calcium and secretin (Figure 2).

Similar provocative tests of hormone secretion have not been developed for the other gastrointestinal peptides, and reliance is usually placed upon the discovery of elevated plasma concentrations in the fasting state. Insistence on the patient's being fasted may not be important in some cases, but it is vital in the case of assessment of hypoglycemia. Here the demonstration of increased insulin secretion in a fasting patient (if necessary the period of fasting being continued for up to 72 hours) is necessary to distinguish an insulinoma from reactive hypoglycemia which is a postprandial entity. Any patient with unexplained diarrhea, particularly if it is of a secretory type, should have a VIP estimation performed. Elevated concentrations of VIP indicate the need for

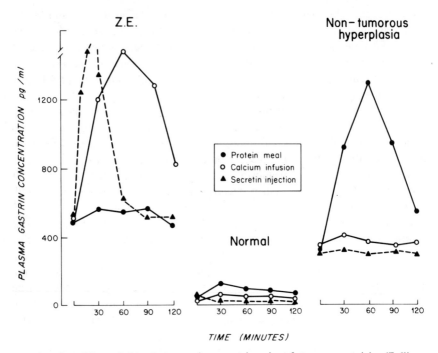

FIG. 2. The differentiation between hypergastrinemia of tumorous origin (Zollinger-Ellison syndrome) from that due to antral G-cell hyperplasia using provacative tests of gastrin release.

thorough investigation for a VIP-secreting tumor. It should be appreciated that VIP is not the only peptide that may be associated with the watery diarrhea syndrome, although when a humoral agent has been identified, VIP is the peptide most commonly involved. Ideally, any patient who is suspected of harboring a gastrointestinal endocrine tumor should have plasma samples analyzed for as many peptides as is feasible. Pancreatic polypeptide and somatostatin are found so frequently in other gastrointestinal apudomas that measurement of concentrations of these peptides provides a useful screening test, and also a possible means of monitoring subsequent treatment.

The field of therapeutics has yet to experience the impact of the gastrointestinal hormones. However, recent experience with somatostatin suggests that this may be remedied. Somatostatin exhibits profound inhibitory effects upon the release and actions of many of the other gastrointestinal peptides. This property has been successfully used in the short term to control symptoms due to tumor secretion in patients with unresectable apudomas. Synthetic analogues have been developed that possess not only longer actions but also a degree of specificity. Optimistically, this may herald the beginning of the use of a number of peptide analogues that, acting as agonists or antagonists, will enable the physician to manipulate a variety of gastrointestinal functions. The potential benefits in terms of both treatment and investigative physiology are enormous.

References

Barrington, E. J. W., and Dockray, G. J. Gastrointestinal hormones. *Endorinol. 69:* 299–325, 1976.

Daniel, E. E. Peptidergic nerves in the gut. *Gastroenterology 75*: 142-145, 1978.

Pearse, A. G. E. The diffuse neuroendocrine system and the APUD concept. *Med. Biol. 55*: 115-125, 1977.

Pearse, A. G. E., Polak, J. M., and Bloom, S. R. *Gastroenterology 72*: 746-761, 1977.

Straus, E. Radioimmunoassay of gastrointestinal hormones. *Gastroenterology 74*: 141-152, 1978.

The Feasibility of an Artificial Endocrine Pancreas

J. DUPRE
Departments of Medicine and Physiology
The University of Western Ontario

The role of the pancreas in regulation of the concentration of glucose in the blood was discovered accidentally by Von Mering and Minkowsky in 1889, in studies of the digestive functions of the gland. Removal of the gland resulted in a metabolic disorder closely resembling spontaneous diabetes mellitus in man. This finding generated ideas about the control of blood glucose and provided a model for experimental studies of diabetes. New concepts of hormonal regulation of physiologic functions originated soon afterward from further studies of digestive functions of the pancreas. In 1902 Bayliss and Starling identified an agent in the intestinal mucosa of animals that elicits secretion of digestive fluid from the gland. They named this activity "secretin," and suggested that it functions as a blood-borne factor in physiologic regulation of pancreatic secretion. The general term "hormone"was invented for agents of this type. The notion of interactions between the pancreas and other factors in regulation of the blood glucose led to the hypothesis that the pancreas produces a glucose-regulating hormone subject to control mechanisms originating in other tissues. The search for the glucoregulatory factor of the pancreas culminated in the preparation of insulin by Banting and Best in 1921. The dramatic effects of insulin in diabetes, and the later finding that the pancreas contains abnormally small quantities of extractable insulin in this disease in its juvenile-onset form, suggested that deficiency of insulin is probably the proximate cause of the condition.

Recently there has been growing interest in the possibility that an artificial device might be capable of regulating metabolism in diabetic subjects by delivering insulin continuously in response to signals based on measurement of the concentration of glucose in the blood. Two kinds of evidence have provided the rationale and the stimulus for these efforts. First, in spite of the recognition of increasing complexity in the mechanisms controlling the secretion of insulin under physiologic conditions, it appears that the blood level of glucose provides a dominant regulatory signal affecting insulin secretion under a variety of physiological conditions; and it also seems most unlikely that metabolism in diabetes can be restored to normal unless insulin is delivered according to a physiologic pattern of supply. Second, clinical evidence and recent studies in animals with experimental diabetes have suggested that imperfect control of metabolism may be related to the long-term deleterious effects of the disease. These two kinds of evidence will be briefly reviewed before consideration of the development of instruments capable of simulating the functions of the endocrine pancreas.

PHYSIOLOGIC CONTROL OF METABOLISM AND THE FEASIBILITY OF AN ARTIFICIAL ENDOCRINE PANCREAS

Physiologic Regulation of Insulin Secretion

Since the development of techniques capable of measuring insulin in body fluids there have been great advances in understanding of the role of insulin in metabolism and of the regulation of secretion of insulin itself. The endocrine pancreas also secretes a second important glucoregulatory hormone, glucagon, which mobilizes glucose from storage as glycogen in the liver, and stimulates production of new glucose from tissue proteins, thus maintaining the blood glucose levels during intervals between meals. In studies of the functions of the endocrine pancreas in intact animals and man, and of the isolated endocrine tissue, it has been established that the hormone-producing cells respond directly to local changes in the concentration of glucose. The release of insulin from the beta cells is stimulated by a rise and suppressed by a fall in blood glucose concentration, and the release of glucagon from the alpha cells responds in a reciprocal fashion.

It is also clear that other nutrients and metabolites affect insulin and glucagon secretion, apparently in physiologically appropriate ways. Thus amino acids derived from protein can stimulate insulin release, and they can also stimulate glucagon release. The stimulation of insulin secretion by amino acids is enhanced in the presence of elevated concentrations of glucose, while the stimulation of glucagon by amino acids is suppressed under these conditions. Teleologically these responses are appropriate because insulin is important in the disposal of amino acids, and its secretion in the absence of incoming glucose must be counterbalanced by the glucose-producing effects of glucagon. These direct responses to local concentrations of glucose and amino acids are subject to further interactions with other nutrients, with regulatory hormones, and with the nervous system. Therefore it may be concluded that while a dominant signal affecting insulin and glucagon secretion is provided by the plasma concentration of glucose, this signal is not the sole determinant of endocrine responses of the pancreas, which must vary with the pattern of nutrition and according to other physiologic conditions.

It has also emerged from studies of pancreatic endocrine secretion that the release of insulin may be extremely rapid. An abrupt rise in plasma glucose concentration results in an initial very rapid phase of insulin release, followed by a second slower phase. Other stimuli, such as those mediated by the nervous system or provided by hormones secreted by the intestine during absorption of meals, also appear to enhance the rapid response, and it has been inferred that the early release of insulin from the gland is important in determining normal metabolism of glucose.

The Endocrine Pancreas in Diabetes Mellitus

Studies of insulin secretion in patients with severe diabetes have confirmed the suspicion that insulin is virtually absent from the blood and the gland under these conditions. In the milder form of diabetes with slight or stable elevation of blood glucose in the fasting state, the picture is more complex. However, even in this situation there is evidence of a relative deficiency of insulin, and the secretion of the hormone in response to physiologic stimuli appears to be characterized by a diminished or absent early phase of release. In addition to the abnormalities of insulin secretion in diabetes, it has been recognized that the secretion of glucagon is abnormal. The blood levels of glucagon are generally inappropriately high in relation to the blood glucose concentration. It has yet to be determined whether this defect is secondary to the disorder of insulin secretion, or whether it represents an independent abnormality. Whatever the mechanism of the hypersecretion of glucagon, the available evidence suggests that the metabolic effects of disordered glucagon secretion are added to those resulting from deficiency of insulin as factors contributing to elevation of the blood glucose and other abnormalities of metabolism.

Further Physiologic Considerations Related to Regulation of the Blood Glucose

In normal animals and men the concentration of glucose in arterial plasma is maintained within quite narrow limits for a period of many hours after complete absorption of the preceding meal, by mobilization of stored glucose and by production of new glucose. Under physiologic conditions the other major challenges to regulation of the blood glucose concentration are the ingestion of meals and physical exertion. The responses of the pancreas to incoming nutrients restrict the rise of glucose in the blood, so that it rarely increases more than 50% above the basal (or fasting) level and is restored to this level within one or two hours of a meal. Studies with radioactive tracers for glucose show that this regulation results from accelerated removal of glucose from the plasma, and from efficient suppression of endogenous production of glucose. The resumption of endogenous production of glucose is closely adjusted to provide a normal rate of appearance of glucose by the time that absorption is completed, with no apparent need for temporary overproduction. However, it is notable that the magnitude and duration of the excursion of the blood glucose concentration after ingestion of a carbohydrate meal are not simply proportionate to the quantity of glucose in the meal. The integrated homeostatic mechanism appears to tolerate a certain perturbation, but meals with progressively larger glucose content are more efficiently "buffered," with increasing outputs of insulin apparently serving as the most important effector. These observations again suggest that the relationship between the concentration of glucose in the blood and the output of insulin from the pancreas is complex.

The challenge to glucose homeostasis presented by physical exertion is of a different nature. Under these conditions the plasma glucose concentration changes very little, but it can be shown with radioactive tracers for glucose that the rate of removal of glucose from the plasma is greatly increased, and that this is delicately matched by an increase in the endogenous production of glucose. Thus glucose "turnover" is raised, while the plasma glucose concentration is stabilized. In relation to the development of an artificial endocrine pancreas, this pattern of response might present difficulties, since it is associated with little change of the plasma concentrations of insulin and glucagon. It has been established in diabetic subjects receiving conventional treatment that insulin may be mobilized from depot sites during exercise, leading to suppression of endogenous production of glucose and resulting in troublesome depression of the blood glucose concentration. Thus it could not be predicted whether an artificial endocrine pancreas responding to a glucose sensor would permit a normal response to exercise.

The Delivery of Pancreatic Endocrine Secretions to Their Target Tissues

The pancreas derives its blood supply from a systemic arterial source, and its venous drainage passes directly to the liver by way of the hepatic portal vein, together with blood from the greater part of the stomach and the small intestine. Thus under physiologic conditions newly absorbed nutrients and the pancreatic hormones active in regulation of their disposal enter the systemic blood only after first passage through the liver. The liver is a major site of metabolism and effective storage of carbohydrate and of digestive derivatives of protein, though a major portion of the absorbed form of fat, packaged in particles of triglyceride, travels to the systemic pool by way of the lymphatic drainage of the gut and thus bypasses the liver. As a consequence of these anatomical arrangements, the liver is exposed to incoming plasma with relatively high concentrations of carbohydrate and protein nutrients, and of pancreatic and intestinal hormones. Variable fractions of the insulin and glucagon delivered to the liver in this way are cleared from the blood in this organ, and the balances that emerge are ultimately diluted in the systemic outflow from the heart. Thus the secretion of pancreatic hormones into the portal venous system may have important effects determining the distribution of their actions in different target tissues, and their net effects.

Feasibility of an Artificial Endocrine Pancreas

These physiologic considerations suggested that it might be possible to construct an artificial device responding to continuous monitoring of the concentration of glucose in the blood by appropriate delivery of insulin, and perhaps also of glucagon, in such a way as to maintain the blood glucose within an arbitrarily selected range approximating the observed normal, under various conditions. However, the same considerations suggest that it is unlikely that such a device would simulate the normal control of metabolism exactly, even if the physiologic route of delivery of the exogenous hormones by way of the portal venous system were used. Nevertheless the distortions that might result from subjection of the system to regulation solely by the glucose concentration, and from deviations from the normal timing and route of delivery of the hormones, could not be predicted. The benefits that might accrue in the form of better physiologic understanding and possible development of therapeutic approaches in diabetes justify the empirical approach to the problem that has been taken.

PATHOPHYSIOLOGY OF DIABETES MELLITUS IN RELATION TO THE NEED FOR AN ARTIFICIAL ENDOCRINE PANCREAS

The Long-Term Effects of Diabetes Mellitus in Man

Virtually all persons with insulin-dependent diabetes mellitus gradually develop evidence of disordered function and structural changes in the eyes, kidneys, and nervous system. The changes affect particularly the blood vessels, large and small, and show very widely variable rates of onset and progression. These so-called complications of the disease are associated with significant reduction in the mean expectation of life, attributable mainly to premature myocardial infarction or to kidney failure. Furthermore the effects of these processes on blood vessels are major causes of blindness and loss of limbs in long-term diabetes mellitus. The recognition of these complications in surviving insulin-treated diabetics led to speculation about their relationship to the metabolic disorder. It was argued that if they result from some aspect of the abnormality of metabolism, they should be influenced favorably by its correction. In spite of more than 50 years of clinical experience and experimental study this proposition remains unproved. Attempts to settle the question have necessarily been based almost exclusively on retrospective examination of the medical records. Many clinicians believe that the complications are less frequent or severe in diabetic persons with well-controlled blood glucose concentrations, but careful reviews of the available evidence lead to the conclusion that the matter cannot be settled definitively in this way. The difficulties of appropriately designed and executed prospective trials of optimal control of blood glucose with insulin in human volunteers are formidable and may indeed be insurmountable. Furthermore, the degree of correction of the metabolic defects attainable by means of intermittent injection of insulin according to current practice may be inadequate for the purpose. Thus the conclusion that the question may not be testable in the absence of advances in the mode of administration of insulin is a major reason for interest in the development of the so-called artificial pancreas. Meantime, further impetus has been given to these inquiries by the results of recent studies with animal models of diabetes mellitus.

Animal Models of Long-Term Diabetes Mellitus

After many years of debate about whether structural abnormalities in the blood vessels of animals with experimental diabetes correspond to those observed in the spontaneous disease in man, increasingly convincing evidence of small-blood-vessel disease in experimental diabetes similar to that in human diabetes has been obtained. Moreover, there is good evidence that these changes can be prevented or reversed as a result of good control of the metabolic disorder in experimental animals. This control has been achieved with intermittent injections of insulin, or by means of transplantation of pancreatic endocrine tissues. Such findings strongly suggest that the complications of diabetes mellitus are susceptible to prevention or amelioration as a result of optimum control of intermediary metabolism, and the studies in which animals were treated with injections of insulin suggest that "perfect" restoration of metabolism to normal may not be essential to these beneficial effects.

STUDIES WITH THE ARTIFICIAL ENDOCRINE PANCREAS

General Description of Current Devices

The artificial endocrine pancreas has been assembled as a bedside research device in a number of versions designed to maintain the blood glucose concentration within arbitrary limits approximating the normal range of responses to physiologic challenges. These devices have three elements: a sensor, a computer, and a delivery mechanism. The sensor is an analyzer into which blood is continuously drawn for measurement of the glucose concentration, and which delivers the signals thus generated to the computer. The computer is programmed to respond with instructions to the delivery mechanism, determining the rate of administration of insulin, and in some devices also determining the rate of administration of glucose or glucagon in order to prevent unwanted depression of the blood glucose. In the empirical approach that has been adopted, the internal control functions, or algorithms, of the computer are programmed with parameters related to the expected insulin requirement of the subject as well as to the blood glucose concentration and to its rate of change. The parameters may be manipulated by intervention of the programmer, or in more sophisticated usage the computer may be programmed to explore the effects of various approaches to optimization. In addition to the more or less arbitrary quality of this optimization, there are limits to the degree to which these devices as constructed and used at present can simulate the physiologic mechanisms described above, and some further limits are imposed by the current technology.

It has been pointed out that the endocrine pancreas functions as its own sensor, exhibiting extremely rapid responses to changes in the local concentration of glucose. With the artificial endocrine pancreas as described, the need for continuous aspiration of blood to the sensor results in delays in generation of signals to the computer. The reaction times of the chemical processes employed in the sensor are brief but must be added to the interval that occurs between ingestion of food and a use in blood glucose, for a total delay of several minutes. Furthermore it is more convenient and safe to draw the blood from a peripheral vein, rather than from an artery. Since there is normally a small arterial-venous concentration gradient of glucose, which varies with physiological conditions from tissue to tissue, the device used in this way regulates regional venous glucose concentration. Thus even perfect simulation of physiologic excursions of glucose concentration in that vein might be achieved by patterns of effect of insulin different from those that would be elicited by physiologic sensors. Nevertheless, it seems unlikely that distortions attributable to minor shortcomings would be important. A further problem depends on the difficulty of administering insulin by way of the physiologic portal venous route. However, these questions, and that of the degree to which administration of insulin alone, or insulin and glucagon, can reverse identified disorders of metabolism and its regulatory mechanisms in diabetes mellitus, can be approached in an experimental fashion by use of these bedside devices. In this way a considerable body of useful findings has accumulated in studies limited to one or two days' duration.

Short-Term Studies with the Artificial Endocrine Pancreas as an Experimental Tool

It has been shown that these devices, with access to peripheral veins, can maintain the blood glucose within the defined limits in animals and in human diabetic subjects eating normal meals and taking exercise. In order to achieve control of blood glucose after ingestion of glucose or of a carbohydrate-containing meal, it has proved necessary to program the system to deliver insulin at rates determined not only by the absolute concentration of glucose in the blood but also by its rate of change. This is achieved by addition to the control algorithms of a "difference factor" providing a response to the rate of change of glucose concentration, augmenting the delivery of insulin at a time when blood glucose begins to rise, and attenuating the delivery of insulin when the blood glucose concentration begins to fall. With such programming, a smaller quantity of insulin is required by comparison with that delivered at rates proportional to the glucose concentration, and it appears that administration of glucose or glucagon may be avoidable. It is notable that this empirically determined response of the device results in a pattern of insulin release in timing to that demonstrated by the endocrine pancreas itself, but that the concentrations of insulin in the blood that result from this treatment are in excess of the normal physiologic levels.

The question of whether it is necessary to deliver insulin by the physiologic portal route has also been addressed in experimental studies with the artificial pancreas in animals. In studies with dogs with experimental diabetes it has been shown that equivalent amount of glycemia can be obtained with intraportal and peripheral vein routes of administration of insulin. However, the physiologic considerations discussed earlier, and the observation that the concentrations of insulin in peripheral blood were higher when the peripheral route of administration was employed, raise the question of whether the nature of the effects of insulin under these two conditions may be different. It has also been shown with the artificial endocrine pancreas that severe physical exercise can be undertaken without a fall of blood glucose concentration, and that the normal physiologic increase of production and removal of glucose is permitted under these conditions.

These devices are currently being used to determine whether the control of the blood glucose achieved in this way is accompanied by correction of glucose disappearance and appearance rates, and of abnormalities of other aspects of metabolism, and whether disorders of regulatory mechanisms such as the secretion of glucagon are likewise reversed. There are already indications that normalization of all functions other than the concentration of glucose in the blood may not be attained. These findings and the deleterious effects of diabetes mellitus in the long term, discussed above, direct attention to the question of the longer-term use of the artificial endocrine pancreas in experimental or therapeutic programs.

Long-Term Applications of the Artificial Endocrine Pancreas

Formidable technical problems have yet to be dealt with before long-term use of an artificial endocrine pancreas can be undertaken. The major difficulties relate to the glucose sensor and to the route of delivery of insulin. In order to permit long-term studies under physiologic conditions, and in any therapeutic program, the system would have to be miniaturized. The sensor might be placed in an interstitial location, where the fluids are in rapid equilibrium with blood plasma, but no suitable device is at present available. There have been advances in the use of specific enzymes on solid phase, or isolated by membranes. With suitable transducers these enzymes can generate electrical signals proportionate to glucose concentration, but such devices are not yet sufficiently reliable for long-term use. Similar problems beset systems in which regeneratable noble-metal catalysts are employed, though such applications of glucose electrochemistry have yielded promising results. At present the application of such techniques to the problem of long-term management of diabetes mellitus in man is not practicable.

Possible Therapeutic Implications of Studies with Continuous Administration of Insulin

It has been pointed out that the most sophisticated artifical endocrine pancreas so far devised may not be capable of correcting all disorders of metabolism in diabetes, though such an instrument may successfully regulate the blood glucose concentration. Proponents of the use of the instrument to study the effects of long-term control of blood glucose in diabetes would accept this compromise. It may be worthwhile considering further compromises, and examining the effects of attainable improvement in control of the blood glucose that can be objectively demonstrated by comparison with the results of conventional therapy. It appears that such improvement can only be obtained with continuous administration of insulin, and with increased rates of administration early in the course of absorption of meals.

In view of the practical difficulties in development of a reliable glucose sensor, a number of workers have investigated the use of predetermined programs of insulin infusion. The effects of some of them have been encouraging, and in preliminary studies with intravenous infusion of insulin there is evidence that the control of blood glucose can be improved in comparison with that obtained with intermittent subcutaneous injections. This has been achieved in subjects wearing portable infusion pumps programmed to deliver background rates of infusion of insulin, with increased rates on ingestion of meals. These supplements are empirically determined and initiated manually by the subject without immediate reference to the blood glucose concentration. Similar studies have also been undertaken with continuous subcutaneous infusion of insulin, which is quite rapidly cleared from the tissue when the volume-rate of delivery is low. The subject can voluntarily initiate the delivery of supplementary insulin before each meal, this substituting for those physiologic mechanisms that provide for the rapid insulin response and in practice reducing the doses of insulin employed. With the recent advent of simple instruments for the rapid estimation of glucose in small volumes of capillary blood obtained by skin puncture, it becomes possible for the subject to monitor his own blood glucose concentration. He can then respond by delivering signals to the infusion system, and the technique thus matched the working definition of an artificial endocrine pancreas.

If these therapeutic approaches prove to be applicable to longer-term studies in diabetes mellitus in man, the task of settling the question about the interaction between disorders of metabolism and the so-called complications of the disease will remain a formidable one. The application of the technique on the necessary scale will be an enormous and expensive undertaking. It is almost certain that a major factor determing the clinical course of the disease in an individual is his susceptibility to the complications, as a factor separable from the severity of disorder of metabolism. Thus progress with the development and application of these new means of administration of insulin, and also with the alternative potential solution provided by transplantation of pancreatic endocrine tissues, will probably depend on the recognition of the heterogeneity of the disease and selection of appropriate management for different groups of subjects. The therapeutic techniques may also involve additive or preparative modifications of food. It is also possible that new preparations of insulin for parenteral or even oral administration will prove useful. Progress will be expensive and the outcome uncertain, but the scale of the problem, the potential benefits, and a judgment that the technological difficulties can be overcome, suggest that these are worthwhile areas of investment in goal-oriented medical research.

Bibliography

Albisser, A. M., Leibel, B. S., Zinman, B., Murray, F. T., Zingg, W., Botz, C. K., Denoga, A., and Marliss, E. B. Studies with an artificial endocrine pancreas. *Arch. Intern. Med. 137*: 639–649, 1977.

Champion, M., Shepherd G. A. A., Rodger, N. W., and Dupre, J. Continuous Subcutaneous infusion of insulin in the Management of Diabetes Mellitus. *Diabetes 28* February 1980.

Knowles, H. C. The problem of the relation of the control of diabetes to the development of vascular disease. *Trans. Am. Clin. Climatol. Assoc. 76*: 142–147, 1964.

Lacy, P. E. Beta cell secretion. *Diabetes 19*: 895–905, 1970.

Rotter, J. I., and Rimoin, D. L. Heterogeneity in diabetes mellitus–Update 1978. *Diabetes 27*: 599–605, 1978.

Soeldner, J. S., Chang, K. W., Aisenberg, S., Hiebert, J. M., and Egdahl, R. H. Diabetes mellitus: A bioengineering approach: An implantable glucose sensor. *Fogarty International Series on Preventive Medicine,* Vol. 4. Washington, D.C.: DHEW, PHS, NIH, 1975, pp. 267–277.

Unger, R. H. Diabetes and the alpha cell. *Diabetes 25*: 136–149, 1975.

Learning and Memory –
Some Recent Approaches
and Some Old Themes

SHIVAJI LAL, L.R.C.P.I. and S.I., B.Sc., Ph.D.
Department of Physiology
Chelsea College
University of London

Neurobiological research into the problems of learning and memory has accelerated greatly in the last few years. An enormous amount of data—psychological, physiological, biochemical, histological—has been accumulated. But satisfactory interpretations of these findings (and, more important, their welding into a firm and widely accepted understanding) are nonexistent. A variety of reasons can be advanced for this unsatisfactory state of affairs. There is, for example, the problem of designing clear-cut learning experiments in which the parameters of the learning experience can be clearly and unambiguously specified. There are the related difficulties of individuating and characterizing learned forms of adaptive behavior and of distinguishing them from nonlearned forms; for clear behavioral indices of learning are difficult to specify. Nor does there exist any definite method for separating the morphological and biochemical changes that are essential to the learning process from those that are incidental concomitants. Another enormous handicap is the lack of knowledge, both descriptive and explanatory, of the functional and structural organization of the fully developed, normally operating nervous system; consequently the identification and definition of neural changes that mediate learning in the adult organism are bound to be incomplete and fragmentary.

A final very important reason for the slow rate of real progress is the lack of a widely subscribed-to functional conceptual framework in terms of which problems of learning and memory can be properly discussed. It is sadly true, for example, that the phrase "short term memory" is often used to denote very different phenomena—at least in temporal terms—by biochemists, psychologists, and physiologists. Thus to the biochemist the span of short term memory processes is to be measured in hours; to the psychologist such processes extend over periods of many minutes; while to the physiologist a short term memory process is a matter of milliseconds. Another indication of the lack of conceptual clarity and disagreement is manifested in the differing classifications offered of distinctive types of learning. Even the terms "learning" and "memory" are used in multiply ambiguous ways.

As this is a rapidly changing area of research, vast in scope and confused in character, this essay will (after a short prelude in which an attempt will be made to clear up some terminological and conceptual ambiguities) only try to review some of the newer experimental approaches to some old and long-standing problems.

LEARNING AND MEMORY: PROBLEMS OF DEFINITION AND LEARNING

The terms learning and memory are general terms of a multiply ambiguous character; they are used to denote a variety of different neural and behavioral phenomena. The notion of learning initially derives from observation of human behavior. It is a common, well established experiential and observational fact that human beings can learn (for example) facts and skills, and that these things can be retained and recalled. It is also well known that such learning depends upon the nervous system. Put in other words, human beings can modify their behavior as a result of individual experiences, and these changes depend on certain plastic properties of the nervous system. The process whereby behavior is modified as a result of experience is commonly referred to as learning. The ability to learn is not confined to *Homo sapiens*—in a loose sense all species can learn; but the ability is most clearly exhibited by certain warm-blooded mammalian species.

Since it is the nervous system that confers the most important learning abilities to an organism, we have to consider the responses of the nervous system to experience. Put in more physical language, learning means that as a result of past activations (past inputs) the system's responsiveness (its outputs) has changed. Thus if a specific input recurs, the response it elicits is different from the one that it originally elicited. This change may be due to the storage of information about the past input and its consequences, so that when the same input recurs the response is modified. This entails the ability to make a comparison between successive stimuli and the ability to make the response contingent on that comparison. Hence the original input must leave some "trace" or "record" that permits the successive inputs to be related to it. Thus we must have some memory—a more or less maintained store of information that can be retrieved and used to direct the response. Learning, in this case, depends on memories, i.e., on records of the past events and stimulations. But learning can be defined in a broader way. It can be said that any time the nervous system behaves differently as a result of previous activity, a kind of learning has occurred. Defined in this broad way, learning becomes almost synonymous with the notion of plasticity of the nervous system. For a past input can lead to a modified response to succeeding inputs if it produces a structural change in the system, i.e., alters the system's characteristics to a significant extent. This could be due to a hysteresis-like effect; or it could be due to a differentiation of a totipotent system into a specific form and state as in development; or it could be due to a more massive structured change imposed by the energy content of the stimulus.

Whether or not the functional recovery of the nervous system (especially in mammals) from irreversible structural damage should be considered a form of learning is a moot point. Obviously this is an example of a certain kind of plasticity; but it cannot easily be construed as a change resulting from some "memory" of a past input.

It might be thought that all changes on adaptive behavior result from "learning" and from "memories" in a broad sense. This is not so. Fatigue, sensory adaptation, aging, and hormonal changes, for example, can lead to changes in adaptive behavior. As has been pointed out, there is no need to suggest that the disappearance of copulatory behavior in a pregnant rat is due to memories of events during the previous estrous cycle. There may be memories, but they do not control behavior.

The notion of learning in a broad sense has not only been applied to the adaptive behavior of whole organisms but also to the "adaptive behavior" of neural networks and individual neurones. When employed in this way the term merely refers to any relatively sustained change in output resulting from a single or multiple past activation. Thus post-tetanic potentiation can be considered to be a model for learning, and the neuronmuscular junction a model learning system.

NEURAL LOCI AND NEURAL CIRCUITS
INVOLVED IN LEARNING

On a behavioral level a number of different kinds of learning have been distinguished by experimental psychologists. The most important varieties that have been studied are: Habituation, Pavlovian or classical conditioning, operant or instrumental conditioning, and latent learning.

As some of these types of learning may not be familiar to all readers, very brief descriptions and definitions will be presented before an account is given of some of the techniques that have recently been employed to investigate their neurophysiological basis. Briefly then, it may be said that habituation refers to the relatively sustained waning of a response that occurs as a result of continuous or repeated stimulation that is not followed by any kind of reinforcement. The organism has "learned" that the response is unnecessary. Such a reduction in response may be difficult to distinguish from that resulting from fatigue, a reduction in attention level, or sensory adaptation. In Pavlovian conditioning the repeated pairing of the sensory stimuli (the conditioned stimulus, or CS, followed by the unconditioned stimulus, UCS) leads to a change in response to the first of the pair. The temporal separation between CS and UCS and the ordering are critical to the establishment of the conditioned response. In most animals an interval of about half a second is the most effective one; longer intervals are less effective. If the sequence is reversed so that the CS is applied after the UCS, then learning may become impossible. In operant conditioning an active response by the animal is essential to learning, for it is the occurrence of this response that determines whether it is rewarded or not. In other words the response has to be rewarded in order for it to be established. Note that in Pavlovian conditioning the response is incidental and not essential to learning. In latent learning, which occurs as for example in place learning (learning about the geographic features of an environment), a response is learned without apparent reward. The mere contiguity of a novel sequence of stimuli is sufficient to give rise to a new pattern of behavior, i.e., for learning to take place.

Ever since these types of learning were distinguished, attempts have been made to identify the neural circuits involved in setting up the new behavior and the neural loci at which information might be stored. Two main strategies of research have been employed. In the first kind an animal is trained to perform a response and the effects on that response of selective brain lesions are studied. In the second kind, direct electrical stimulation of neural masses and pathways is attempted. Work along these lines has continued and been extended. It has also been augmented by biochemical and electrical recording methods which have attempted to assay the biochemical and electrical correlates of learning. Some of this recent work will now be briefly described.

Early work, on the critical path taken by neural activity to link sensory input to motor output in conditioning, had seemed to establish that the connection between CS and UCS occurred somewhere between the sensory and motor cortex; it had also seemed to establish that the cerebral cortex was necessary for conditioning. For the early investigators had shown that electrical stimulation of the cerebral sensory cortex and of the spinal afferent pathways could serve as a conditioned stimulus for salivation or leg flexion; and that stimulation of the motor cortex was ineffective in establishing a conditioned response. Recent work has shown that the cerebral cortex is not necessary for the establishment of a learned response. For example, in a decorticate animal a conditioned response can be established, albeit rather slowly; and although the experimental evidence is contradictory and confused, it seems that the spinal cord can be conditioned, i.e., it can "learn" in a very limited way.

The modern technique of electrical recording of neural activity in chronic experimental animals has not proved as fruitful as it once seemed in the investigation of the neural circuits involved in learning. The idea underlying the approach is to use a low frequency stimulus, such as a 10/sec flickering light, as a tracer to identify neural systems and cricuits involved in processing the conditioned stimulus. If electrical activity at the frequency of the tracer stimulus is detected in a given nucleus or tract, then that constitutes prima facie evidence of its involvement in the learning process.

It must be said that the variety of electrophysiological and anatomical techniques so far employed have not provided any conclusive evidence as to the route taken by a CS to link up with a UCS or of the locus or loci at which they interact.

A very promising new technique which may shed light on these issues is the biochemical one of injecting a radioactive analogue of glucose into the bloodstream of animals undergoing specified stimulation procedures. This glucose analogue is taken up by nerve cells but is not metabolized by them; so it remains there. Since the uptake of glucose is an index of energy metabolism, it is the active stimulated nerve cells that take up most of the analogue. Autoradiography then makes possible a quantitative estimate of the amount of the analogue in a specific region and therefore of the group of nerve cells specifically excited by the stimulation used.

THE EFFECTS OF ENRICHED AND IMPOVERISHED ENVIRONMENTS

The classical methods of observing learning and memory processes in the whole animal and interfering with them do not give a great deal of insight into the physiological processes involved. The more modern approaches which have flourished recently have attempted an analysis of the physiological and biochemical processes involved in learning by trying to correlate neuronal changes (electrophysiological and biochemical) with whole animal stimulation and learning procedures. Typically, animals are exposed to enriched or impoverished environments of various kinds or subjected to specific training procedures, and the physiological, biochemical, and morphological changes induced are examined. For example, kittens have been reared from birth in restricted visual environments where the only form of visual stimulation they have is that of horizontal or vertical strips. When the firing characteristics of the neurones of the visual cortex of such animals are examined, they are found to differ from those of normal kittens. The changes observed are long-lasting, and, depending on the period of rearing, and so on, can be irreversible. In other experiments, the effects of the onset of visual experience on specific parts of the nervous system of rats reared in the dark have been examined. Both transient and long-lasting changes in certain neurotransmitter enzymes and in the rates of synthesis of certain neural proteins have been observed.

Certain variants of the above types of experiments have involved the training of rats, guinea pigs, or fish to perform some task and then examining the animals for changes in RNA and protein synthesis. The finding of such changes has led to the development of theories to the effect that specific memories were encoded by unique sets of RNA or protein molecules. Such theories have been not only controversial but also difficult to assess. Partly this difficulty has been due to the complexity and the stimulus ambiguity of the training procedures used; partly to the crudity of the biochemical methods of detection, extraction, and assay; and partly to the nonspecificity of the correlations observed. Certainly failure to replicate such findings is commonplace. Moreover, it seems a bit premature and megalomaniacal to try to develop a full-grown theory of learning and memory on the basis of changes in the levels of a few enzymes or proteins.

DEVELOPMENT AND PLASTICITY IN THE NERVOUS SYSTEM

Perhaps the most widely held view—it can hardly be called a theory—about the neurophysiological basis of learning is that it is mediated by changes in synaptic effectiveness. Such changes could be due to the formation of new synaptic connections, potentiation of existing ones, or the selective repression or dissolution of connections. Such thinking has led to increased interest in and increased research effort on the problems of developmental determination of neural connections and repair of neural connections following trauma.

Early work involving the wiring-up of motor nerves and muscles and of optic nerves and optic lobes in amphibia has been extended and refined. Earlier theories concerning the mechanisms of labeling and signaling between sets of nerve cells or nerve cells and muscle fibers have been either rejected or extensively modified. But the general principle that connection formation depends upon a set of functionally (embryologically) marked neurones making connections with another (embryologically) marked set of neurones or muscle cells seems firmly established. Whether the connection-specifying markers are positional (co-ordinate or rank–ordered), temporal, or chemical is not clear. Nor is it clear whether the signaling mechanisms are primarily chemically or physically mediated. It is clear, though, that some, perhaps most, of the formation of specific synaptic connections does not require use or practice but rather hinges on developmental signals that serve to match up neuronal populations. In fact there seem to be, from a developmental point of view, three kinds of neurones. First, there are those that are epigenetically rigid in the sense that they are unlikely to show changes in connectivity during development and in later life. Second are those that are epigenetically plastic; that is, during development they can change into any one of a number of possible, differing configurations and wiring patterns, and which actual state they crystallize into depends upon the environmental situation obtaining during the critical choice period. Subsequently these neurones remain, so to speak, relatively hard-wired. Third are those neurones that show plasticity in later life, that is, are capable of "rewiring" and changing their responsiveness on the basis of the information they receive.

In concluding this section it should be pointed out that there is no direct, firm evidence to the effect that new synaptic connections form in the adult CNS as a result of learning, memory, or experience. However, it now seems clear that the CNS of warm-blooded animals (like that of cold-blooded animals) is capable of some degree of regeneration and synaptic rearrangement following lesions.

PHYSIOLOGICAL STUDIES OF SYNAPTIC EFFECTIVENESS

The various difficulties associated with the experimental approaches outlined previously have led some investigators to search for a simple experimental situation in which "learning" in a "simple" neural system can be studied. Such neural systems as isolated slabs of cortical tissue, invertebrate ganglia, and invertebrate and mammalian neuromuscular junctions have been examined for plastic behavior resulting from (usually) electrical stimulation. The view has developed that anything discovered about long-lasting changes in synaptic transmission is applicable to the phenomenon of learning. Such an approach at least has the merit of focusing attention on changes and events that (a) outlast the period of stimulation and (b) extend over time scales greater than milliseconds.

One of the more interesting recent findings is that it is possible to produce long-lasting changes in the firing patterns of neurones in the rat cerebral cortex by passing (for a few minutes) a weak current through it in the right direction. These charges last for hours and are sensitive to metabolic poisons acting on the mechanisms of protein synthesis.

Such studies, though they do not shed direct light on learning mechanisms, at least direct attention and thought toward the study of *modifiable* neural functions. The investigation of plasticity of the nervous system becomes as important as that of its reactivity.

CONCLUSION

Information, then, on the chemical, electrical, and morphological correlates of learning and memory accumulates apace. But the integration of this information into reasonably precise theories about the physiological substrates of learning and memory is still a slow and uncertain affair. And the greatest lack of progress still lies in the lack of plausible and rigorous theorizing and investigation into the organizational and functional aspects of learning and memory. How does the nervous system store and retrieve information? Is the information indexed in any particular way? Are there universal learning mechanisms and procedures? Is remembering a matter of constructive rendering or of recalling a duplicate?

No doubt these questions and many others will find some sort of plausible answers in the foreseeable future.

References

Ansell, G. B., and Bradley, P. B., eds. *Macromolecules and Behaviour.* London: McMillan Press, 1973.

Bindman, L. J., Lippold, O. C. J., and Redfearn, J. W. T. Long lasting changes in the level of electrical activity of the cerebral cortex produced by polarising currents. *Nature 196*: 584–585, 1962.

Mark, R. *Memory and Nerve Cell Connections.* Oxford University Press, 1974.

The Control Theoretic Approach to Neurophysiology – Problems and Opportunities

SHIVAJI LAL, L.R.C.P. and S.I., B.Sc., Ph.D.
Chelsea College
University of London

Any reasonably well-developed field of scientific inquiry is based upon a coherent conceptual framework in terms of which focal problems are specified, facts relating to these problems characterized, explanatory goals and expectations delineated, methods and techniques of investigation defined, and laws and theories articulated. Such conceptual schema are not static. As a result of the action of a complex, heterogeneous mix of "pressures" and "needs"—factual, theoretical, technological, philosophical, social, and ideological—there is conceptual evolution and, in some cases, conceptual revolution. It is the revolutionary, conceptual changes—revolutionary coups d'etat—that really motor the sudden rapid development of a science.

Since World War II a radical transformation has been occurring in the way in which neurophysiologists perceive and define the problem fields relating to the structure, function, and organization of the central nervous system. A paradigm shift has been taking place, and it is the aim of this article to try to explain and to some extent evaluate some facets of this important change. More precisely this paper will: (1) describe in qualitative terms some of the key ideas of the new framework and of the problem-identifying and problem-solving strategies associated with it; (2) review some of the difficulties, theoretical and practical, that currently beset attempts to employ the new approach; (3) identify some of the "dangers"—forms of conceptual imprisonment and conceptual bedazzlement— that need to be recognized if the maximum benefits of the new strategy are to be realized.

In simplicistic, unqualified, sloganlike terms, which is all that is really possible in a compressed account, it might be said that the old ways of thinking about the central nervous system were dominated by quasimechanical metaphors and models. The behavior of neurones and of neural arrays was visualized in terms of passive reactions of complex, machinelike, physical objects to external stimuli. The dominating implicit metaphor was that of a telephone network—of telephone exchanges linked by fixed lines. Electrical events traveled along cables to discrete centers where they were relayed and distributed to other centers. The central nervous system was a complex switching network; behavior was a matter of compounding reflexes, of compounding triggered, automatic, stereotyped actions. In other words, neural entities, simple or complex, were considered primarily as physical event-handling devices rather than as information-processing systems, and neural processes were considered primarily as processes in which physical quantities were transformed, that is, as involving energy exchange, rather than as processes in which patterns were transformed, in which information exchange took place.

The postwar outlook has become increasingly dominated by metaphors and models based on information handling, of devices and systems that acquire, transmit, store, and use information—the computer, the communication network, the control system. To some extent, of course, such ideas as information, control, and computation have been around for a long time and have been foci for debate and argument. But only relatively recently have these notions been developed into the intelligibly related parts of systematic, mathematically articulated theories that can be used to (a) describe and model entities and processes of various kinds and (b) make exact, often quantifiable, predictions and inferences about structure and behavior of such items.

SYSTEMS SCIENCE AND CONTROL THEORY

The new rapidly growing and, what is more important, rapidly evolving outlook, is sometimes referred to as the systems approach and sometimes as the control theoretic approach, for the terms control theory and systems theory are often used loosely to denote the same subject matter and the same body of mathematical techniques. It is probably more useful to consider control theory to be a specialized part of systems theory; it is that part concerned with the dynamic responses of systems to commands and disturbances. The reason for making this separation will become apparent later.

SYSTEM, INPUT, AND OUTPUT

In order to understand the control theoretic approach we need some sort of intuitive purchase on the notions of system, input, output, control, and information. The next few paragraphs will be devoted to an intuitive, verbal explanation of these key ideas, as they are rather more subtle than one might, on first acquaintance, take them to be.

As an initial rough definition we can take a *physical* system to be a collection of elements linked and interrelated in such a way as to form and act as a whole. A system then is an organized structure that can be isolated, or rather differentiated, from its environment by a boundary or an interface. It can be pictured as a block, that is, as an enclosure containing a structure; the system and the block are then imagined to be physically equivalent. There may be sufficient information available about the system so that a complete description can be given of it; that is, we can portray in the form of a schematic diagram the relationships and interconnections of the components of the system, and we can write equations describing the behavior of each component and how it affects other components. The box, in other words, is transparent. Now each component can itself be considered to be a system—a subsystem. In the same way the original system can be considered to be a subsystem of a larger enclosing system. There is, however, no unique way of partitioning a system into subsystems or of combining subsystems into systems. A given system such as a neurone can be partitioned into subsystems in many different ways; several possible systems can thus be derived. In many cases we may have very little knowledge about the system, and it presents itself as a black box with an unknown internal structure. Whether the box is transparent or black, the investigator is usually interested in describing the behavior of the box and explaining how this behavior is brought about. An understanding is sought of the way in which the collection of variables and parameters defining the system changes with time. This understanding is achieved when cause-and-effect relationships between system components can be precisely specified.

The notion of a system needs to be loosened from its connotation of a structured material object with a continuous sharply defined boundary; for this restricts the flexibility and usefulness of the concept. It is more useful to consider a system as a functional entity, as a collection of systematically related variables that constitute the external characteristics of a "box." The behavior of the system can then be described by stating how each of these variables changes with time. Now such changes can only be due to the influence of other variables which are independent of the system and which may be internal or external to it. The variables influencing the system from "outside" are normally called inputs; whereas the variables defining the system, or rather the subset of these whose behavior is being investigated, are called outputs.

Thus in the most general sense, the concept of a system can be identified with the notion of a stable, reproducible, input–output relation between two physically linked variables. Mathematically a system is an *operator* that maps functions onto functions. Physically it is a process by which a variation in a physical characteristic causes a systematic variation in some other physical characteristic.

From this it follows that the concept of a system is inextricably and ineluctably linked to the notions of input and output. Hence a single input, single output system is normally pictured as a box with an incoming arrow (representing an input signal) and an outgoing arrow (representing an output signal). Such a representation (see Figure 1) can confuse the picture-loving imagination; it may lead the unwary to think of inputs and outputs in terms of specific channels or terminals through which signals are taken into and out of the system. But the arrows are merely symbolic devices that indicate the simultaneous and instantaneous application of a stimulus to the whole system and the simultaneous and instanteneous response of the whole system. If one likes, this may be envisaged as if the system possessed a fictitious input and output terminal. Stimuli can only act at the input terminal, while responses can only be recorded from the output terminal.

INFORMATION AND CONTROL

The two other key ideas that need some explication are those of information and control. The concept of control is perhaps easier to grasp; in a way it can ease the path toward understanding the notion of information. Intuitively, the idea of control suggests the ability to change something in a prescribed manner. More precisely, control can be said to be exerted whenever the magnitude of one physical variable (usually dynamical) determines uniquely the magnitude of another physical variable (again, usually dynamical). Hence, if the output of

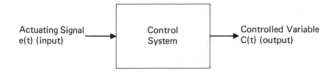

FIG. 1. Schematic diagram of a basic control system.

a system can be changed in a determinate way by changing the input in a determinate way, then the input can be said to control the output. Such an abstract, functional definition allows virtually any structured, material object to be regarded as a control system; for every such object interacts with its environment (i.e., possesses inputs and outputs). Under this definition a mirror deflecting a beam of light becomes a control system. The definition needs refining; and we will now do this in two linked ways. For a system to be a control system it must *actively* command, direct, or regulate itself or some other system. Thus a passive system, strictly speaking, cannot be a control system, since the output of such a system is a reflection of the power applied to the system, that is, the energy content of the input. Ideally, then, control is exercised when a variable representing a smaller energy regulates a variable representing a larger (in the limiting case a similar) energy. A classical example of a control system is a valve that regulates the flow of water in a pipe. The rate of flow of the water can be adjusted by altering the valve position. The amount of water delivered per unit time is a function of, and controlled by, the valve position. A neurophysiological example is the way in which the rate of firing of a motor neurone determines the tension developed by the muscle fibers to which it is connected.

The notion of control, then, is related to the directionality, determinativeness, and energetic aspects of the input–output relation. Another way of indicating the control character of a system's actions is to say that the system acts on or processes signals rather than is acted upon and responds to forces.

What is meant by the term information is a subtle and difficult question admitting of no easy answer. The technical definition given it in information theory relates information to statistical rarity; to a measure of freedom of choice when a message is selected from an available set of messages. For our purposes, information is best thought of as data or measurements that indicate for a receiver (sink) something about the state of a sender (source). This intuitive notion presupposes the idea of a communication link and an exchange of "intelligence." The important thought to grasp is that the signals (the information-carrying events) are not to be identified with the symbols, i.e., with what is being transmitted and processed; and that symbol processing rules cannot be put into one-to-one correspondence with physical processing laws.

LINEAR, LUMPED, CONTINUOUS DATA DETERMINISTIC SYSTEMS

Control systems can be classified in a number of different ways; these classifications depend on either the characteristics of the signals handled or on the system characteristics.

Since the mathematical techniques and methods for analyzing and designing control systems have been most fully developed for univariable, linear, lumped, time-invariant, continuous data deterministic systems of the open loop or closed loop variety, the meaning of these terms and the properties that these meanings embody need some degree of explication.

The term univariable is reasonably self-explanatory; it refers to single input, single output systems. Obviously a multivariable system is a multiple input, multiple output system. Open loop and closed loop are also relatively trans- parent terms. In an open loop system the control action—the input quantity that brings about the system response—does not depend on the output. For a closed loop system the control action is a function of the output, i.e., there is some feedback so that the control action depends on both a reference input signal and a feedback signal. Schematic diagrams of the two types of systems are displayed in Figure 2. Note that in the open loop system diagram the actuating or control input to the controlled process (sometimes called the plant) is en- visaged as being derived from a controller that is itself driven by an externally applied or an internally generated reference input. The controller is sometimes modeled as a separate element in the open loop system, as in the diagram; at other times it is considered to be an integral part of the system being studied, and the reference input becomes the input to the undifferentiated single block.

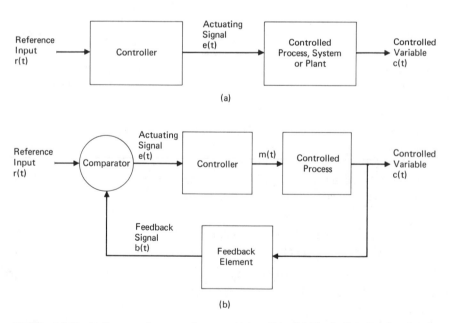

FIG. 2. (a) Block diagram of an open loop control system. (b) Block diagram of a closed loop control system.

Whichever representation is chosen, the performance of the system is specified in terms of the relationship between the reference input and the controlled output. For the closed loop system note that control is exercised by means of a comparator and a controller; both actually constitute the controlling system, and a separate controller is not necessary—a comparator alone will do. Note also that it is possible to put the whole closed loop into a box and treat it as an open loop system. Again, performance of a closed loop system is specified in terms of a relationship between the reference input and the controlled output.

Questions about feedback and its advantages and disadvantages cannot be gone into here. But the existence of two types of feedback, negative and positive, must be noted. A negative feedback control system is concerned with making the controlled output follow as closely as possible reference input commands. In positive feedback systems the aim is to change the controlled output as rapidly as possible—"explosively"—toward some constrained value. Note that positive feedback control systems are not pathological; they serve useful functions. However, the occurrence of positive feedback in a negative feedback control system is a pathological event.

A linear system must possess two main characteristics: additivity and constant scaling. The additivity condition implies that if an input $S1(t)$ elicits a response $R1(t)$ and another input $S2(t)$ the response $R2(t)$, then the response to the sum of $S1(t)$ and $S2(t)$ will be the summed response $R1(t) + R2(t)$. The constant scaling condition entails that if an input signal $S1(t)$ is multiplied by a factor K, then the response $R1(t)$ is scaled by a factor K.

A lumped system is one in which the physical characteristics can be considered to be concentrated into a lump. This means that if any input is applied, then the whole system is simultaneously and instantaneously activated; the response is also a simultaneous and instantaneous one of the whole system. Thus, as far as the system's behavior is concerned, positional effects and time delays due to propagation effects can be neglected.

Time invariance refers to the fact that the properties of the system do not change with time; and time-shifting an input either by advancing or delaying it merely results in an equivalently time-shifted response.

In a continuous data system, signals are always continuous functions of the continuous variable time. Intuitively they are continuous graphs. Discrete data systems then are a system in which signals are not continuous signals but are intermittently occurring either at specific instants or during short intervals separated by instants or gaps.

The final term mentioned was deterministic. It can best be thought of in terms of predictability. For a deterministic system a knowledge of the input, the initial conditions, and the dynamic equation defining the system operation enables the value of the output to be predicted (determined) uniquely. This is not the cast for stochastic or probabilistic systems.

IMPULSE RESPONSES AND FREQUENCY
RESPONSE FUNCTIONS OF LINEAR
SYSTEMS

Since three basic quantities are involved in describing a system's behavior fully, a knowledge of two of them enables the third to be specified. From a knowledge of the system as operator and the input, it should be possible to predict the output; from a knowledge of the output and the system operator, it should be possible to retrodict the input; and from a knowledge of the input and output, the system can be identified.

But what is the best way of describing the system's action on inputs? Only two methods will be described here: the impulse response and the frequency response.

An impulse response may be defined as the response of the system when the input is an impulse function. This can be thought of as a sudden instantaneous excitation, or one that lasts for a negligible amount of time. Although a true impulse function cannot be physically generated, a pulse with a very narrow pulse width provides a suitable approximation. In fact, if the duration of the excitation is an order of magnitude less than the time scale of the response, then the stimulus can be considered to be an approximate impulse function. The total response of a linear system to an impulse will consist of two factors. The first portion of the response will occur while the impulse is being applied; the second when the impulse has terminated. For this reason, the latter response, which occurs during the period when the system is not driven by a stimulus, is known as the "free" or "transient" response. As this response takes place while the system is unstimulated, the response will depend on the system properties and not on the form of the excitation; it is thus a measure of the stimulus properties and defines the system operator. Now any continuous or discrete input signal can be dissected into a sequence of impulse excitations, the strength of each impulse being equal to the magnitude of the input at the corresponding instant of time. For a linear system the response is merely a superposition of the individual impulse responses. The impulse response, therefore, completely describes the way in which the system responds to excitation.

An equivalent way of describing the response of a linear system to any input is by means of the frequency response function. Empirically, the frequency response function can be obtained by applying sinusoids of different frequencies to the system in question. A linear system responds to a sinusoid at a given frequency by producing a sinusoid of the same frequency but with a changed amplitude and with a phase shift. Since it is possible to describe virtually any physically realizable signal as a discrete or continuous sum of sinusoids, we can characterize the system by the amplitude and phase shift it imposes on all possible sinusoids.

NEURONES AND NEURAL SYSTEMS AS CONTROL SYSTEMS

Obviously if neurones and other neural systems (e.g., networks and pathways) can be modeled as linear, lumped, time-invariant, continuous data, deterministic systems, then several problems facing neurophysiologists have in principle, been solved. The only difficulties are the purely technical ones of obtaining the impulse response or the frequency response function of the systems in question. But can control theory be applied to neural systems? What are the problems and difficulties encountered in applying control theory techniques to the understanding of neural system behavior? The next few paragraphs will address themselves to these two questions.

It does not require any great perspicacity to see that may aspects of neural behavior at a number of different structural and descriptive levels can be conceptualized in control theory terms. For example, any single neurone constitutes a definite structured unit possessing a number of input channels and usually one single output channel. A typical cat motor neurone has about 15,000 presynaptic axons contacting it; it emits a single axon which, after giving off a number of collaterals, synapses with a number of muscle fibers—about 200 in the case of the cat soleus muscle. The cat motor neurone, therefore, can be visualized as a black box with 15,000 input channels and a single output channel. The incoming signals will be patterns of action potentials, while the output will be a patterned train of action potentials.

In a similar way a motor neurone pool such as that of the cat soleus muscle, for example, can be represented as a box containing some 250 motor neurones. Impinging on the box would be tens of thousands of presynaptic fibers derived from sensory neurones, interneurones of the spinal cord, and neurones whose cell bodies are located at higher levels of the CNS. Emerging from the box would be 250 axons, collaterals of which would feed back via interneurones to influence motor neurone behavior.

This example should make it obvious that any neurone pool or neural network or a whole nucleus can be conceptualized as a system with multiple inputs and outputs. By extension, so can neural pathways, such as those that mediate reflexes, and whole nervous systems. Consider one possible conceptualization of the stretch reflex system, as in Figure 3. It must be borne in mind that each box in the diagram represents a complex network of elements with multiple inputs and outputs. In fact the diagram represents a gross idealization and oversimplification. A few of these simplifications must be mentioned. Nothing in the diagram indicates that time delays are involved. Distributed networks have been lumped; multiple inputs and multiple outputs have been reduced to single inputs and outputs; the presence and effects of other feedback loops such as those from the tension control system are not indicated.

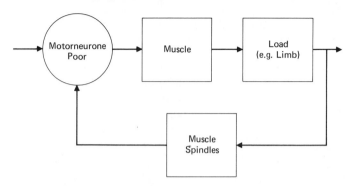

FIG. 3. Schematic, highly simplified model of the stretch reflex.

These simplifications are not merely due to the technical difficulty of embodying this information in a simple, visually intelligible diagram; they have to do with the necessity of certain kinds of idealization if the full mathematical apparatus of *classical* control is to be successfully employed.

But to what extent do such idealizations produce mathematically tractable but physiologically irrelevant models? And can *modern* control theory provide techniques for handling more physiologically relaistic models?

To be physiologically realistic, many neural systems in many situations must be treated as *multivariable nonlinear stochastic distributed adaptive* systems. Mathematical techniques for handling systems possessing all these characteristics are, for all practical purposes, nonexistent. Modern control theory has been mainly concerned with the development of methods for dealing with multivariable nonlinear systems and with linear stochastic systems. And the procedures developed have nothing like the power or generality of those that have been elaborated for classical linear deterministic control theory. But although there will almost certainly be difficulties, hazards, and setbacks, and although progress will be slow and is by no means inevitable, there still seems to be no good reason why the requisite control theory methods for handling neural systems should not emerge in the foreseeable future. As it is, linear control theory, both stochastic and deterministic, has made and is increasingly making contributions to the solution of some neural problems.

Nor do the experimental difficulties seem insuperable; for they are the mainly traditional, biological ones of getting effective isolation of the system, of obtaining effective isolation of the forcing applied to the system, and of acquiring "noise-free" recordings.

OPPORTUNITIES AND DANGERS

To close this discussion a few comments will be made on some of the possible general costs and "benefits" of the control theoretic approach to neurophysiology.

Two major advantages at once suggest themselves. The first relates to the clarification and redefinition of existing problems and of the strategies that can be employed to tackle them. The second relates to the precipitation of vaguely sensed perplexities into reasonably well-specified, discussable problems capable of, in principle, some kind of experimental investigation.

The first advantage can be manifested in two main ways. Thinking about neural systems in control theory terms brings a whole class of previously vaguely defined questions about the causal behavior of neural entities into precise focus: What are the inputs to a system? Are there feedback loops? How does feedback affect the stability of the system? What are the magnitudes of steady state error and parameter sensitivity? Is the system controllable and observable? What sorts of impulse response does the system have? But not only does control theory lead to the asking of precise questions, it also supplies quantitative methods of answering these questions. The second way it facilitates the solving of existing problems is through its qualitative effect on theorizing about neurophysiology. Thus, previously acceptable theories and techniques become viewed in a new light and become, to some extent, elaborated, specified, and redefined to take account of the new qualitative insights provided by specific control theory strategies. There is clarification without replacement, and new problems become identified.

The second advantage is, perhaps, best illustrated by looking at the effect control theory is having on the way in which we think about the nature and structure of mental functions and the relationship they bear to the functional and structural organization of the nervous system. For an illuminating, though not necessarily true, analogy can be drawn between the CNS and a computer (i.e., a control system of a particular kind). Psychological processes can be construed as software, the programs that specify what the computer is doing. The programs are, of course, arrangements of physical events (electrical events) that are taking place in the hardware of the neural computer. Thus, in understanding the functioning of the neural computer we are interested in information processing, in the logical structure and rules of operation as much as in physical structure and functioning. We are interested in physical events as carriers of information and physical processes as symbolic processing rules. We can begin to have, to some degree, explicit, investigatable, and empirically testable theories about various age-old philosophical and scientific problems. The analogy between computers and the nervous system can also illuminate and direct investigations into the problems of memory. For we can begin to think of testable theories about the storage of information and about the character of information retrieval.

But, of course, such analogies can be dangerous. For some people may begin to think that analogies, instead of being heuristic tools for stimulating thinking and theorizing, are explanatory theories that have in some sense solved a range of problems. In other words, premature, facile, physiologically or psychologically or philosophically naive formulations become accepted—because they are formal and exact—as substitutes for genuine theories based upon experimental insights and information gained from traditional approaches.

This points to a related danger, that of neglecting traditional approaches and modes of theorizing and conceptualization. Attention becomes directed toward forms of input-output explanations that can be expressed mathematically. But, of course, many problems cannot be naturally cast into an input-output control vocabulary—questions, for example, about the changing potentialities and adaptive significance of structural and functional features of the nervous system. The question of how, in a biological sense, a particular neural tract has developed and the contribution this makes toward the success of a species in a particular environment does not arise naturally in the current control theoretic framework. Too much emphasis on functional input-output linkages may lead the investigator to neglect the "obvious experiment" of looking into the box and directly observing the physical structures and processes that bring about the linkage; that is, it may lead to a neglect of physical investigations and theorizing of a valuable kind such as those based upon the use of a microscope.

The burden of these reflections, I hope, shows the value of methodological, conceptual, and theoretical pluralism in any scientific field. It is probably neither possible nor desirable to reduce the variegated jungle of "brute facts" and natural scientific problems into a featureless grassland grazed by placid ruminants.

Further Reading

Barrett, J. N., and Crill, W. E. Specific membrane properties of cat motorneurones. *J. Physiol. 239*: 301-324, 1974.

Barrett, J. N., and Crill, W. E. Influence of dendritic location and membrane properties on the effectiveness of synapses on cat motorneurones. *J. Physiol. 239*: 325-345, 1974.

Keller, D. J., and Lal, S. Membrane voltage changes in a compartment chain model of a neurone. *Biol. Cybernetics 24*: 211-217, 1976.

Marmarelis, P. Z., and Naka, K. I. Identification of multi-input biological systems. *IEEE Trans. Bio. Med. Eng. B.M.E.-21*: 88, 101, 1974.

Stark, L. Neurological Control Systems. *Studies in Bioengineering.* New York: Plenum, 1968.

II
ECOLOGICAL PSYCHOLOGY, MEDICINE, AND DISEASES RELATED TO THE BIOSPHERE AND TO THE ENVIRONMENT

Racial Equity in the Health Care Fields During the Coming Age of Limited Technical Growth

ROBERT SCHLEGEL, M.D.
Professor and Chairman
Department of Pediatrics
Charles R. Drew Postgraduate
Medical School and Martin Luther
King, Jr. Community General Hospital
of Los Angeles County

The major world question of today is how to regulate high technology in advanced industrial nations.[1] While many of the earlier advocates of controlled technical growth viewed the health sciences as a benign alternative to hazardous industrial technologies, recently there has been a rising tide of criticism directed against inflationary costs, inhumane practices, and wasteful use of resources in the medical-industrial complex, just as there has been in other sectors of the American economy.[2] Consequently, some new public controls have already been imposed on the health care fields,[3] and many others are under consideration.[4]

Similarly, early advocates of limited technical growth specifically exempted from proposed controls third-world peoples who are struggling to establish decent standards of living through the use of high technologies.[5] They recognized that across-the-board application of rules limiting technical development would create intolerable world tensions between haves and have-nots. In the United States, identical considerations apply with regard to historically oppressed racial minorities who are attempting to establish parity in employment, careers, and public services.

Hence, the question of equity in the health care fields for America's racial minorities is part of this larger public policy issue, and answers derive from general principles established in that larger arena.

What then does equity mean in the health care sector of our American economy? It means the attainment of equal access to employment (including professional careers) and products (in this case, service benefits), just as in any other part of the economy. Looked at in this way, the importance of the question takes on staggering dimensions. Today, the health care fields form one of

115

the nation's largest and most rapidly growing economic aggregates. This aggregate is the nation's third largest employer, providing jobs and professional opportunities in thousands of fields and dozens of industries; pharmaceuticals, medical instruments, health insurance, and hospitals, to name a few.[6] All are proliferating and growing with exponential speed. This year we will spend over $150 billion on personal health care, up more than $30 billion from 1976.[7] The exponential doubling time of personal health care expenditures is, at present, less than seven years, whether taken in the aggregate or calculated on the basis of what we spend on each man, woman, and child[8]. Further, these fields have increased their share of the total goods and services produced by our nation from 4.6 to 8.5%.[7]

How can we achieve racial equity in the health care system? One way is to examine the impact of existing public programs on racial minorities at the local community level. Unlike Henry Adams, we do not grieve over having to seek unity from multiplicity,[9] but accept the burden of realism. In this pragmatic approach we examine the real-life situation of the people involved, sifting the program wheat (what works) from the program chaff (what does not work).

The greater Watts community of Los Angeles has much to teach the public policy-maker. Like all minority populations in major metropolitan areas of America[10] the people of this community have many preventible sicknesses, and are more likely to die unnecessarily at early ages than other Americans.[11] Many sicken and die for reasons different from those causing disease and death in the nation as a whole. For example, babies are more likely to die in later infancy from malnutrition, trauma, or infection.[12]

There is a considerable body of evidence indicating that these excess rates of disease, disability, and death would yield to the social and economic betterment of people[13] that could be provided by the enormous resources of the health care field. There is even evidence that currently available medical technology would reduce the burdens of illness, were it made accessible to the people.[14] Were the medical care system flexible enough to address the special causes of poor health alluded to above, it might make even more of a difference.[15]

Yet, prior to 1972, the 360,000 black people of Watts had available only a few substandard private hospitals in their community.[16] There were only 164 physicians in full or part-time practice in the area—one for every 2200 citizens, compared with one for every 500 in the state of California as a whole.[16] Some of the most fundamental types of care were unavailable. For example, there was only one primary care pediatrician in full-time private practice—this despite the fact that the mean age of the black population in Watts was less than 16 years.

Public programs to lessen the disadvantages of people living in Watts and similar American communities have not been an unmixed blessing. Programs aimed at improving one aspect of the health care system (e.g., financing services) have canceled out the benefits of others (e.g., developing resources). Coercive approaches have contributed to the present public backlash and charges of reverse discrimination.

Medicaid, mandated in 1966, is the nation's most expensive public program in the health care field for the poor, with estimated dollar outlays of more than 14 billion in the fiscal year 1978.[17] It pays on a fee-for-service basis for physician visits, hospital care, and nursing home services.[18] While these services have benefited many of those in most desperate need, the program does not cover the many "near poor" (e.g., small businessmen, ministers) in our community who are part of a large national population not covered by private health insurance,[19] and who pay a disproportionate amount of out-of-pocket expense for health care.[20] With health care expenses rising at an annual rate of more than 15% on the consumer price index,[21] there are predictable effects on the use of health services by the near poor.[22]

There has been another more important negative effect of Medicaid on communities like Watts. The program has, by virtue of its exclusive concern with financing, favored services by private vendors located in affluent communities.[23] This situation has promoted the destruction of public hospitals and clinics in poor communities.[15] California lost more than a third of its public hospitals between 1969 and 1973, following the full implementation of its Medicaid program.[24]

Although some, doubting the quality of services in public institutions, might see this as beneficial, the loss of these resources has both immediate and distant negative results. First, and least important, the loss of health care providers in local communities makes the benefits of other programs like Medicare less accessible.[25] Second, and more important, minority communities lose their share of jobs, leadership training, and professional career opportunities in institutions of health care. Journey to any medical school in America, and you will see a social and economic powerhouse. There are, of course, classrooms, research laboratories, clinics, and hospitals (including affiliated Veterans Administration hospitals mandated to serve the poor). In addition, the school is ringed by pharmaceutical houses, electronic industries, and other health-related private enterprises which provide social and economic strength to surrounding communities.

A number of smaller federal programs provide health care resources (e.g., multipurpose community health centers of the former Office of Economic Opportunity). At their best, these are a source of local employment on a small scale, as well as services of the kind that are needed in disadvantaged communities. Since they are not empowered to conduct medical and health professional educational programs, increasing difficulties have been encountered in recruiting health professionals. Increasingly too, the special services required for health education (e.g., teaching local mothers how to shop for a nutritious diet to feed their families) are being lost as the clinics fight to survive in a system of medical fee-for-service cost reimbursement.

The Health Planning and Resources Development Act of 1974 mandated a redistribution of resources favoring poor and minority people. The means for achieving this and other purposes of the act (e.g., cost control) was to divide the United States into more than 200 Health Service Regions, establishing in each a Health Systems Agency empowered to review and recommend approval or disapproval of all federal grants and contracts, excluding those of the uniformed military services and Veterans Administration. Unfortunately, the intent of Congress was not followed in administrative rule-making. As a result, the Health Systems Agency in Los Angeles is dominated by local, political, special interests. Under this arrangement, the people of Watts will lose an ever larger share of the federal health dollar, on which they are more dependent than other citizens of Los Angeles.

The Health Professions Assistance Act of 1976 mandated, among other things, increases in the number of minority students admitted to American medical schools. The mandate seeks to remedy a situation in which 11% of the American population (black) is served by less than 2% of its physicians.[26] There is currently one white physician for every 538 white Americans, while there is only one black physician for every 4100 black Americans.[27] Yet, only 6.8% of American medical students are black, despite the fact that American medical schools, private and public alike, are almost entirely supported by the tax dollar.[27] In 1976 there was, instead of a further increase toward at least the necessary parity number of 11%, an absolute drop in the proportion of black medical students from 7.1% in 1975 to 6.8%.[27]

Like other coercive federal legislation, the equity provisions in this Act will be, and have been, challenged. In the state of California, a white student, Alan Bakke, charged the University of California at Davis with reverse discrimination, in a case that was reviewed by the Supreme Court of the United States. Despite the fact that the school he challenged is one of the more than 40 new medical schools to be developed, based in part on the evidence of excess sickness and death in American minorities, and despite the 27% increase in white students enrolled in American medical schools since 1971, compared with less than a 5% increase in black student enrollment,[27] the Court ruled in his favor.

The Emergency Health Personnel Act of 1970 established a National Health Service Corps (NHSC) of physicians who would settle in areas like Watts to practice medicine for at least three years. Every evidence is that this is a well-run program, although small in scale. However we currently have no NHSC physicians in Watts. Further, the physicians employed by the NHSC are not educationally prepared for the special conditions of practice they will encounter in a community like ours.

The only unqualified success from the vantage of Watts is the American community-based minority medical school—Howard University School of Medicine, Meharry Medical College, and the recently founded Morehouse College

School of Medicine. These schools bring to the impoverished communities in which they are located the economic and social strengths of a major medical complex. They train students who will be comfortable leading professional careers in underserved minority communities, and they educate them appropriately for this purpose. As a result, more than 80% of the graduates of Meharry Medical College are known to be established in rural or minority communities.[26] Almost all of our physicians in private practice in Watts are graduates of the medical schools at Howard and Meharry.

These schools also carry out special programs preparing local high school and college students for the scholastic demands of medical school, or of graduate school programs providing doctoral degrees in the biological sciences. In this way they help to ameliorate the manpower shortage of qualified applicants to professional schools from rural or inner city minority communities. They are aided in these activities by two small federal programs—the Minority Biomedical Science program and the Minority Access to Research Careers program, both of the National Institutes of Health.

Although they suffer the consequences of the great and growing gap in racial equity affecting the health care fields on a national level, the people of Watts are more fortunate than most minority people in possessing at least part of a modern medical education complex. Together, the Charles R. Drew Postgraduate Medical School and the Martin Luther King, Jr. Community General Hospital of Los Angeles County provide more than 3000 jobs in an area characterized by one of the highest unemployment rates in the country.[28] More than 90% of the employees are from minority populations, and the school and hospital bring a $60 million annual budget to one of the nation's poverty areas.[28] In addition, they offer responsible grants and contracts management, allowing the award of federal and state funding for service and manpower development. Thus, a department like Pediatrics, which operates on an annual county budget of about $1.5 million, carries thrice that amount in addition grants and contracts.

This new medical center is strengthening the private sector of medical practice and allied health care in Watts. More than 75% of the 205 postgraduate physicians and 123 allied health personnel in training remain to practice in the area following graduation—an area defined as underserved by the Federal Health Resources Administration. Many programs of continuing education improve the quality of care by physicians, nurses, and other health professionals in hospitals, clinics, and physicians' offices throughout the region.

Educational programs have as their objective the learning of urban health care. They are based on an extensive array of clinical services in community settings as well as clinics and hospitals. Hence, a primary care department like Pediatrics operates 28 community-based programs to give students experience in citizen health education and child development services. That department also teaches sick-child care in a busy municipal hospital setting.

Unfortunately, this review shows that the opening round of "era of limits" legislation (circa 1970-) has especially disadvantaged racial minorities in Watts and throughout the nation in the health care fields. The proportion of the federal health dollar going to the poor dropped from 40¢ to 32¢ between 1969 and 1974.[29] Efforts have concentrated on reducing federal and state spending, while failing to control the steep inflation of private health care and health care commodity prices. Consequently, the health care interests of the poor and racial minorities are being squeezed in a vise between rising prices and a lesser rate of increase in fiscal outlays.

Liberal legislators have been misled into thinking they attack vested interest technologies, when in reality public controls have merely worsened the conditions of life for the poor. Coercive social legislation affecting private individuals or institutions is seldom practical in a nation devoted to civil liberties for all. For example, medical schools will respond to public interference in academic processes by political or legal action, as they are currently demonstrating in the controversy over enrolling third-year American medical students who have received their preclinical education in foreign medical schools.

Several principles emerge from this brief overview for developing a prudent and fiscally sound public policy on racial equity in the health care fields during the coming era of limited technical growth. These principles are based on empiric observation of success and failure in public policy measures affecting a community of racial minorities.

Public programs should coordinate equity provisions affecting community development, educational opportunities in the professions, resource availability, employment, and financing for personal health services. Mandates limited to assuring equity in one feature (e.g., a health care financing program such as National Health Insurance) can create serious dysequilibria in another arena (e.g., the equitable distribution of employment opportunities in health care institutions).

Second, equity provisions must be detailed and specific. For example, regional shortages of physicians in poor and minority communities will not be met by merely increasing the number of medical students enrolled in American medical schools in general. An educational system must be created that is charged with the specific responsibility of enrolling those types of students known to settle in minority communities for their professional careers. In addition, it must educate them to solve the types of practical health problems they will encounter in those areas, as opposed to affluent communities.

Third, public mandates should be compatible with both the spirit and the substance of American civil liberties for all. For example, it is unnecessary to conscript students or physicians into unwilling servitude in Watts or similar communities. The expansion of our existing system of community-based minority medical schools would solve the physician shortage and many other problems of social and economic equity.

The community-based minority medical school is the foundation on which to build a workable and just public policy for the nation's racial minorities. It is the only social institution having a mission broad enough to include all of the factors involved in the provision of equity throughout the highly diversified but interlocked elements of health care. Expansion of this strong foundation through the creation of new institutions and supportive legislation (such as the Minority Biomedical Science and Minority Access to Research Careers programs) is a fiscally sound and effective public policy for American racial minorities.

Should legislation during the coming age of limited technical growth continue to feature the indiscriminate application of public controls, regardless of the health status of our social minorities or their health care institutions, disastrous long-lasting effects can be anticipated on the social stability of our nation. The magnitude of the health care field as a social and economic entity in America makes it one of the nation's most important arenas of civil rights. It has been pointed out here that both current and future policy problems can be solved through tested programs which assure equity in employment, professional opportunities, and service benefits.

References

Kahn, H., Brown, W., and Martel, L. *The Next 200 Years.* New York: Morrow, 1976.

Illich, I. *Medical Nemesis.* New York: Morrow, 1974

Mott, B. J. F. The new health planning system. *Proc. Acad. Pol. Sci. 32*: 238, 1977.

Kissick, W. L., and Martin, S. P. Issues of the Future in health. *Ann. Am. Acad. Pol. Soc. Sci. 399*: 151, 1972.

Brown, H. *The Challenge of Man's Future.* New York: Viking, 1954.

Committee on Ways and Means, U.S. Congress. *National Health Insurance Resource Book.* Washington, D.C.: U.S. Government Printing Office, 1974.

Nelson, H. The rising cost of health care. *Los Angeles Times,* July 18, 1977.

Keintz, R. *National Health Insurance and Income Distribution.* Lexington, Massachusetts: Heath, 1976.

Adams, H. *The Education of Henry Adams.* Cambridge, Massachusetts: Houghton Mifflin, 1918.

American Medical Association. *Socioeconomic Issues of Health.* Chicago, 1973.

Haynes, M. A., Gottlieb, S., and Lewis, S. Health problems in the Martin Luther King, Jr. Hospital service area. *Cal. Med. 118*: 105, 1973.

Schlegel, R. J. The formulation of health policy. In *Public Policy and Biomedical Science, Science,* Vijaya Melnick and Franklin Hamilton, eds. New York: Plenum, 1977.

Kessner, D. M., and Kalk, C. E. *A Strategy for Evaluating Health Services.* Washington, D.C.: *Institute of Medicine, National Academy of Science, 1973.*

Kessner, D. M., Singer, J., Kalk, C. E., and Schlesinger, E. R. *Infant Death: An Analysis by Maternal Risk and Health Care.* Washington, D.C.: Institute of Medicine, National Academy of Science, 1973.

Schlegel, R. J. How to think about health policy. In *Public Policy and Biomedical Science,* H. Hugh Fudenberg and Vijaya Melnick, eds. New York: Plenum, 1977.

Lewis, S. Background information: Service area of the Los Angeles County Martin Luther King, Jr. General Hospital. Series 2, No. 1, 1971.

Executive Office of the President. *Special Analysis Budget of the United States Government, Fiscal Year 1978.* Washington, D.C.: U.S. Government Printing Office, 1977.

Weikel, M. K., and Leamond, N. A. A decade of Medicaid. *Public Health Rep. 91*: 303, 1976.

Davis, K. *National Health Insurance in Setting National Priorities, the 1975 Budget,* B. M. Blackman, E. M. Gramlich, and R. W. Hartman, eds. Washington, D.C.: Brookings, 1974.

U.S. Department of Health, Education and Welfare. *Health in the United States.* DHEW Pub. No. (HRA) 76-1233, 1975.

Greenberg, D. Health care review: Prices go out of sight. *Los Angeles Times,* July 8, 1977.

Davis, K. *National Health Insurance.* Washington, D.C.: Brookings, 1975.

Stuart, B. Who gains from public health programs? *Ann. Am. Acad. Pol. Soc. Sci. 399*: 145, 1972.

Blake, E., and Bodenheimer, T. Hospitals for sale. *Ramparts 12*: 28, 1974.

Davis, K. *Lessons of Medicare and Medicaid for National Health Insurance.* Washington, D.C.: Brookings. 1975.

Sullivan, L. Testimony before the Subcommittee on Health of the Committee on Labor and Public Welfare, U.S. Senate, 1975.

Locke, G. E. Testimony before the Select Committee on Health Services Education of the Assembly of the State of California, 1977.

Spellman, M. W. Testimony and information report before the Select Committee on Health Sciences Education of the Assembly of the State of California, 1977.

Center for Health Policy Studies. *Chartbook of Federal Health Spending 1969-74.* Washington D.C. 1974.

Cultural Transformation and Cultural Diversity in Technological Societies

STACEY B. DAY, M.D., Ph.D., D.Sc.
Professor and Member, Sloan Kettering Institute for Cancer Research
Head, Biosciences Communications and Medical Education,
Sloan Kettering Institute
New York, New York

If not speculatively simple, the question posed by this paper may be simply stated: *What are the operational changes in social history of men today, and how do they determine the quality of life?* As with many simple questions the nature of the language used opens up a veritable *lebensform* of interdisciplinary constructs that virtually, like the tentacles of an octopus, grasp an extraordinary range of dominants that relate to the quality of life and the outlook of generations of men. Recognizing this situation, and the truth that each man lives with and among other men, and that each individual interprets events that surround him, and conducts himself according to sets of values, *transformations* such as this writing explores may be represented by hierarchical tiers that one might effectively consider *vocabularies of communication,* languages distinct and operative on several diverse planes, some regional, some national, some international, and others intercultural, by which variable sets of expression are analyzed and evaluated.

The content of the present discussion crosses several boundaries and includes or integrates parts of several disciplines, including population (numbers), cultural and genetic diversity, integrative strategies of learning and education, and communication faculties such as use of symbols, rhetoric, and the capacity for thought and speech. Transformation via such interdisciplinary or integrative growth requires painstaking work among the interstices in the matrix of society, rather than the agitated frenzy of constant perambulating up and down interdigitating matrix fibers. It should be recognized that the interdisciplinary strength is manifest as the cement, the filling of lacunae between cell structures that gives solidity to the matrix at the "grass roots" level. Such filling of the lacunae makes possible the building of a solid edifice on a reliable foundation. The secret of interdisciplinary strength lies in the ability of perceptive scholars and communications scientists to build in the "holes," to create a *wholeness* from "spaces" between anchoring fibers, and so to give form to a powerful base for future development. It is therefore the *effort* in these "intercellular spaces"

123

that one sees as the essential payoff of the interdisciplinary method. By binding the "holes" with an intellectual cement, a construct is established anchoring a future integrated holistic one, which functions as a whole of many parts. Parenthetically it might be said that those, who like ants, busy themselves scurrying from tendril to tendril on the system to be conjoined, while eminently visible, contribute little to the real organization or to the building of the base foundation, the root strength on which future stability of the whole will rest.

This integrative philosophy is a keystone of *biosocial development*. It is able to achieve a synthesis that accommodates both the classical notion of Darwinian evolutionary biology—while transcribing in terms of social evolution constructs that include ecological psychology, comprehension, and appreciation of state-power politic (democracy, technocracy, etc.)—and such perspectives as control, order, and regulation within the state, numbers (population) factorials, the *convivial tools* of Ivan Illich, and the biological and social imperatives that can be encompassed by such modern-day life strategies as, variously (and not necessarily correctly named), *techno-fascism, military intellectualism,* and *culture constructs* aimed to absolve contemporary stresses of life, to facilitate power sharing and power transfer to the benefit of *survival* of the group, and to permit a reshaping of balance of power between biologic evolutionary and sociologic evolutionary forces, as well as a wise reorganization of human life under the dominating power of the machine.

HISTORICAL EVENTS LEADING TO THE ESTABLISHMENT OF CONTEMPORARY TECHNOCRACIES

Harold Laski, as convincingly as anyone else, argued that in Europe the overthrow of the feudal state was accomplished by an alliance, principally in France and England, between the middle and working classes. If democracy was a desirable form of government, then expansionism, trade, and economic interests made this as elusive as any goal that could be expressed by any society relying on class structure to serve its will.

Western civilization with its theocratically based culture has essentially witnessed three remarkable unfoldings (two of which were noted by Laski) since the Middle Ages: first, the spread of the reformation and the disestablishment of power including the military power of the Holy Roman Empire (replacement of a single sovereign faith by a multiplicity of secular faiths); second, toward the end of the eighteenth century the extraordinary social impacts of the Industrial Revolution in Great Britain, and the French Revolution on the continent of Europe; and finally and latterly, in our day, the advent of technocracies.

These major social transformations achieved first what was in fact an emancipation of a new middle class, a transition of social values in an order that was essentially, in its naissance, an industrial creation, and a reorganization of economic power based on trade and production. The state, as much as institutions of state, and society, had inevitably to find new compatibility with changed economic order. Acquisition of property, manufactured goods, political reconstruction of states, was the hallmark of "democracies." But with time, newer perspectives evolved. In the Soviet Union ownership of production by the state itself became the manifestation of the social spirit. The advent of World War II and the remarkable advances in science and technology (development of atomic power, fission, energy, space exploration, and satellite potential) have possibly laid to rest permanently notions of democracy, if ever such systems *did* pragmatically function. All roots of all society have been affected by technology. For the main, in the contemporary adversary confrontation between power nations, we find ourselves living in technocracies. National, sovereign, and transcultural habits have been affected, personal and collective security has been ransomed, and machine and man relate in such a prescriptive way that the dimension of the intellectual world has been forever altered—though whether favorably or to a more critically debilitating degree few would care to say. World War II and science/technology have changed the basis of all institutions. The postindustrial world has been shaped by the most imperial force that the social history of people has witnessed since the onset of the Middle Ages—this must certainly be the contemporary evolution of life shaped by technocracies. The ethic and conduct of life as a social dimension of people has changed with the concentration of power into a machine-reality in a new age, the *Age of Information*. It is within this power that the lives and claims of persons must now be shaped.

EVOLUTION OF EDUCATION WITH
TRANSVALUATION OF POWER

It is useful to try to understand relationships in society as it undergoes transformations or movements in its governance. This is especially so for matters of educational and cultural value. Thus the word revolution, while implying fundamental change, may in fact represent a broad spectrum of possible strategies for change. In Great Britain within the 20-year period 1765–1785, important textile inventions appeared, and experimental changes contributing to industrialization were being made. Change was peaceful and orderly so that the Industrial Revolution was in fact a change that took place without bloodshed. The comprehension of these relationships is more than a matter of semantics; for as a social revolution is a change in the relative importance of social classes, so does it mark a change in ways of life, architecture of towns and cities, symbolism as a psychological backdrop in the life style, religion, mythology, and everyday culture of the people and their national "inheritance," as well as the manifest of change from sowing, reaping, and ploughing, to new orders of life. Urban living, the mobile society, factories, inventions, innovation, new demands from abroad, migration, emigration, intermarriage, the changing common gene pool selected for survival—all encourage new social and spiritual emotions in the workpeople. In the case of the Industrial Revolution, transformation of industry resulted in innumerable paradoxes; on the one hand political and financial stability was forthcoming, freedom from invasion was more assured, accumulation of capital brought "cultural" acquisitions as well as material benefits, yet "wage-slavery" was an increasing misery in factory life, massing of people in towns brought appalling problems of hygiene, and unsanitary conditions fostered dirt and disease. New "personal awareness," often militant, arose, as with the Chartist Movement of 1848; and if coal, iron, and engineering brought profit, they also brought need for new social conscience. Such movements as these led slowly to social legislation, codification of work laws, regulatory acts of Parliament, and the growth of trades unions. Underlying all was a deeply felt need for education with reconciliation of interests among society on a broad base. As industry developed, so also did the need for general price movements and the growth of banking systems emerge as national institutions—inevitably bringing what might be termed a counterculture paradox, no less real because it was controversial and adversary. Wealth was destroyed, and to be destroyed, in wars; soil conservation increased in importance as harvests became deficient, and improved arts of agriculture were needed; the opening up of America and Australia under the psychological imprint of land for homesteading, freedom from class bondage, religious emancipation, and wealth to be gained from the gold rushes of the 1850s, encouraged European emigration to North America, and the westward opening of a new continent under the turbulent thrust of a new and constantly changing population mix that became a new common gene pool.

Under these influences, in England and on the continent of Europe, trade depressions, unemployment, and heavy national taxation served only to repress education and social reform. If anything a circular paradox saw that as things got better, for some they got considerably worse! The English situation was reasonably typical. Unrest was general throughout the mining and manufacturing towns of the Midlands and the North. Emotion, anger, and pain, and the "curs'd Corn Laws," led to rude blasts for *people's strength*. Unrest was familiar on a daily basis, and such newfound newspapers as the *Northern Star* became the watchdog for the underprivileged, devoting issues to both reason and unreason, as often as not in rhyme:

> Who are that blustering, cantering crew,
> Who keep the cheap loaf in our view,
> And would from us more profit screw?

In France conflagrations in 1848 were a signal for the whole of Europe to arise in unrest. In Vienna the barricades were raised, and the Hapsburgs, with their empire of a thousand years, were rocked under the strain of movements such as the Croatian demands for a new constitution; in Hungary Louis Kossuth led an uprising demanding an independent Magyar state, and all through the civilized world of central Europe a theretofore unseen rise of serfdom began to swell. The abolition of privilege of the nobles was in the offing, never again to be restored. Essentially all these transformations followed in the wake of the new economic balance of power. Society generally had to resolve new conflicts, which one may suggest were not without certain parallels to the circumstances of a modern machine-ordered society under conflict and testing from new life evolutionary situations.

Curiously enough, while education was at a rare premium in the European upheavals, in the United States, a rough uncharted continent, progressive visionaries of the character of Horace Mann could and did undertake innovative pioneering educational work. Mann, an educator of classic bent, was—at the time when the "rabble" of Vienna were causing Metternich to flee the Chancellory in Austria—on a far different frontier, the far west of America (Dayton/Yellow Springs, Ohio), engineering the philosophy of an educational system to be built on *moral tone of the highest order, advocating an instinct for knowledge based on social rather than on pragmatic goals!*

If a lesson is to be derived from these events, it is surely that educational action and cultural comprehension, including the social significance of revolutionary changes, come slowly, as an after the fact emergent human need. Change begets change. Addressing one new balance in society perforce obliges attention to other changes in and for national, as well as international, societies. To the degree that wise leadership can foresee these changes and anticipate and direct concurrent imbalances—recognizing that if historical precedent has any truth, then wise anticipatory action is as likely as not to assure *less* social turmoil and hazard than decadent or metered vision—then the problem of haplessly waiting for a future may be resolved!

DEMOCRACY, TECHNOCRACY, AND HUMANISM

The general thrust of this paper has been to advance the argument that cultural transformation is an imperative for the survival of technological societies. Yet having created the thesis, one is almost immediately constrained by the dimensions of the problem and the need for cogent and useful understanding of the case one is arguing. Contemporary societies are in a dynamic of constant change. Ideas change as frequently as do clothing fashions! The grass roots of societies generally, in the West, are so mobile, and in the United States there is so clearly a two-generational society, that few assumptions even on basic beliefs can be allowed. What is democracy? What is meant by humanism? Who defines technocracy, and what are the definer's qualifications for so onerous a task? Are there limits to evolutionary biology? Can these thresholds, or limits, be extended by biotechnology? Can biotechnology serve as a control device? What are the relationships between biotechnology and bioengineering? Few would disagree with Gabor that medical and biological innovations in future decades are likely to interfere powerfully with social life; but is that circumstance alone sufficient for an understanding of biotechnology? Almost any biological truth has consequences of social and ethical concern. How then do we organize, rate, calibrate, these events? How do we react to them? *Can* we indeed intelligently provide for or interact with such events?

It has been argued that the question best raised in this writing relates to change—operational change in social history. Such changes as do occur, or as may occur, are seen through individual cultural blinkers, each of which should be considered as variable. The most important cultural perspectives perhaps relate to (1) democracy and (2) quality of life.

Democracy

If the democratic view of man is a concept of equality, to this observer, while it is conceivably morally just, the concept in its application has seldom been truthfully applied. No less a saint of democracy than Jefferson recognized the obvious inequalities common in the lives of most people. Indeed, totalitarian as well as parliamentary states could probably with equal self-justification argue their case for being "democratic states," and each would, in all probability, make much of the premise that prestige and position determined *before* birth bring relatively less recognition than do personal ability and the advantage earned by meritricious capacities. Even if this *should* be so, one finds it unconvincing that "democracy" can exist, or indeed has existed in the "technocracies" of the last 25 years! Both democracy and humanitarianism have undergone extraordinary changes in the face of concepts of *order, regulation,* and *control,* which are the marks of technological societies of our times. For us, utilization of power is based on machines and on machine intelligence in a hierarchy of systems that today, in different nations, while similar in logical content, are as frequently as not in adversary roles, as varying societies are obliged to face down each other as "competing technocracies"!

The technological society, in the sense that we know it, is a spin-off from World War II scientific development. We are now presented with the critical choices of understanding and accounting for basic human needs in harmony with a machine society, or with challenging the construct of the society we have founded on the very basis of its philosophy *as* a machine society. Technocracies have now gone byond endeavors to design, operate, and control machines and machine resources. What is critically at stake is the dimension of human lives, and the nature of the society in which those lives are pursued.

In my view, democracy and technocracy are incompatible in the sense of human equality. Technocracy encourages certain inequalities, which in turn secure inequities not comprehensible or inherent in the concept of democracy. While to the popular mind democracy is morally and ethically just, and while it appears to serve equality, no pattern of social organization in today's developing technocracies can reasonably incorporate infallible and rigid egalitarian concepts— one equality for all. Equality is, in itself, a danger, and in a technocracy it is nonexistent. And this I believe must hold up irrespective of ideology—whether the dialectical-materialist position, or the so-called bourgeois sociologist proposal that there is a gradual rapprochement between the communist and Western systems, that the present capitalism has changed and become more human, that modern technology and management either could, or have, transformed certain social problems, thus integrating all within the capitalist system! Irrespective of the action of society to itself, irrespective of existential influences, objective historical necessity, ideology or anti-ideology, and remarking that spatial solutions for life on earth are becoming more and more restricted, with men living as they do in an increasingly smaller and smaller dimension in terms of communication—irrespective of all this, it appears to me that no one argument qualifies as an exception in terms of this understanding of technocracy and control via order and regulation.

Science can approach goals, but it cannot determine ends. Science and technology may predicate possibilities, but predictability is no certainty. Ends are determined by human agency; adaptation and diversity bespeak variabilities in ends. Regardless of our choice, hierarchies of value must exist, and variations of station or inequalities must characterize the technocratic state. This is acceptable within the limitations that we place upon human life. It is useless to dwell on technocracy solely by its perceived justifications. Computers in medicine, artificial kidneys, and renal dialysis membranes are good; cardiovascular bypass instrumentation is life-saving and a technological wonder! These things are true— but in themselves they do not justify or explain the evolution of society toward technocracy, with its potential choices of self-advancement or self-annihilation. To appreciate human and national affairs over these last few years, one must consider scientific methodology crucial to the technocratic state as a *regulatory* method, which, in both science and technology finds inevitable expression in various forms of social policy (Day, in press). Democratic egalitarianism seldom can exist in regulatory situations. Society applauds the *control* that on command launches a rocket and lands it upon the surface of the moon. But that same society does not see fit to recognize that the idea of the control of power, of scientific method, even of scientific purpose in regulatory methodology cannot be conceded to be within the domain of every person (Day, 1979). That which is of equal benefit to all in a technocracy may be unequal in its demands upon some in the same society. Hence the same regulatory power may be at one and the same time equal in some circumstances, and from another point of view deliberately infringe on so-called human rights. Therefore technology and science can resolve urgent problems and primary needs of society, while at the same time represent potential destruction to the society. These questions are basic and important.

Quality of Life

The problems suggested recognize power and political sense in addition to resources of technology, science, and learning. As previously discussed, these factors together with a broad range of *people* actions and shared social constructs comprehend biosocial development—a sociocultural and biocultural augmentation of biologic and sociologic evolution.

Various factors beyond those discussed also interface with quality of life: the nature of health; the scope and content of professions and their dominion and interaction with government and governance; the conditions of work, labor, and leisure; the essence of freedoms and human choice *within the constraints of an ordered society;* decisions, strategies, and milieus for action; and development of standards to ensure quality of life.

The actual relationship of technology of life may be understood in many ways—in the relationship of air, water, and sunlight to arable land as essential resources for agricultural production; or in the rather pessimistic view of Ivan Illich (1976), who has proposed that we name the mid-twentieth century the *Age of Disabling Professions* that would have "physicians transmogrified into biocrats, teachers into gnososcrats, morticians into thanocrats . . ." so that for all practical purposes we are living within a system of inquisitorial and recalcitrant clergy! If not exactly true, this proposal is neither false nor invalid as a call against social folly. The point is, of course, that change is the one true dynamic that is a constant. We find ourselves in an age of technocracy, springing as it has from the womb of war and destruction, uncertain in the nature of its growth in an unstable world of extraordinary diversity and inequality. Even capitalism, vaunted as a citadel, is under fire, and developing and third world nations have rapidly learned that *reverse capitalism,* ownership and control of raw materials (say petroleum), can effectively spike the best laid plans of automobile producers a technology and a world away from desert sands. Or African copper could, certain variables being operative, effectively destroy present general copper prices and world market! Whatever the presumptive power, Illich's "techno-fascism" of the industrial world, the ownership of the means of production by the state, or the control of raw resources by developing nations, technocratic power and any dicta, authoritative or not, sit poorly upon the head of troubled and uneducated populations, massed as numbers, not comprehending technocracy or democracy, but concerned more with *survival*. It is difficult in these paradoxes for man to detach himself from life, and in detachment, observe it. Yet this is absolutely necessary if man *is* to survive!

ECOLOGICAL PSYCHOLOGY, INTERCULTURAL COMMUNICATIONS, AND THE MILITARY INTELLECTUAL

In the planning of contemporary societies (communities, towns, rural settlements) in harmony with present-day concepts of living, the keywords of strategy are *ecological psychology,* awareness and understanding of all of the variables for man's survival in the present world—including numbers, location on global bases, Illich's *convivial* (and not so convivial) tools, fiscal and organizational strategies, and anthropologic and sociologic insights into evolution, natural selection, and survival.

Consider, for example, the food chain. Overall energy consumption in support of technological agricultural systems is estimated to be 12.8% of the total energy consumption in the United States—much of which is primarily to replace labor *and does not increase yields per unit acreage of the land.* In a future time, for survival, one could reasonably expect to *synthesize* foods from raw materials, carbon dioxide, water, and nitrogen. Technological considerations notwithstanding, one must still take note of closely related social problems. Even given that chemical processes for conversion of fossil fuel raw materials to food are technically feasible, and they are (fats, amino acids, vitamins may yet be manufactured onboard space stations!), such systems, even if they do have advantages over land agriculture, require time for social and cultural acceptance. First studies in Japan show little true public tolerance of such chemically produced foods! Algal culture and biologic conversion to synthetic foods must also be considered from the point of view of their biologic effect on the person. Would a biologically different individual be in the potential offing? Such strategies are clearly vital as methodologies for leap-frogging third world nations into the technological twenty-first century, but, it might be added, are not without considerable risk from variables beyond guesswork.

Little is known and nothing is published of the economics of these bioconversion processes for survival, especially on the order of magnitude of survival of nations, or of their psychological effect on survival following war. Whether this suggests that leadership is little concerned with the real possibility of survivals following global conflict in terms of *real money spent* is unclear! What is the monetary value of the lands to be destroyed? What is the monetary value of those who survive, and what is the monetary cost of the technology to support that life? Will life be independent of other national communities and nations, of other regional food areas, of other animal systems of life? How can one define an environment not yet seen, not yet experienced or known? Who will plan architecture, and construct cities for survivors? These are all issues of ecological psychology and include issues of survivorship, organization, control, and rule. If we spend now on construction of food energy plants, dwellings, and so on, are we developing with a view of problems to be encountered in the survival-of-the-future, or are we constructing on the basis of education relevant to survival in the past? Do we take into account conversion *efficiencies* both for man and for production? How are these efficiences appraised, and how can they be implemented under conditions of *who will die* and *who will survive?*

With no oracle to advise us, no profound answer can be immediately given. But the handling of knowledge, wise foresight, and discipline in terms of order and regulation may provide a frame of reference in which man may work *with,* rather than against, Nature.

In approaching this understanding I argue that science must be seen as a culture, and understood through relationships that are in effect *intercultural.* He who would bully Nature loses mastership of his own destiny, for he has failed to understand his own limitations. Insensitive or irrational demands of Nature jeopardize man himself. There is a threshold beyond which man cannot go, save at his own peril: the extermination of a life species, the depletion of nonrenewable resources, or the disruption of the ecosystem to the glorification of economic expansion as the *sine qua non* of progress and perfect living becomes dangerous not so much because of the technology involved, as the realization of man's failure to understand the limitations of his actions. There is need too for spiritual and human value structures to equalize quality of life, now no longer within a vision of uniform equality, but within a concept of ordered conduct in human affairs and a democracy of inequalities. It must also be understood that technologic and scientific concepts can and do enter the world of cultural and social experience. It is quite impossible to read these lines from Louis McNeice's *Passage Steamer* without an awareness of a felicity of synthesis between art and science:

> The great cranks rise and fall
> The great cranks rise and fall
> like Assyrian feet.

To one unfamiliar with the historical background, the term "Assyrian feet" is likely to mean little. But to a generation familiar with technology of steam ships and passenger steamers, who could not visualize the great cranks rising and falling like "Assyrian feet" when viewing the engine room from the ship's deck?

Survival itself in its biologic and sociologic expression can be supported and guided by *cultural diversity,* a strategy that not only favors the genetic pool but also assures best options for survival by selection. Irrespective of the inevitable uniformities provoked by technological routines, society and its cultures should preserve forms that are diverse and free from uniformity. Such diversity will offset restraints imposed by technology and work toward the ultimate good of the society. Change is a part of survival. Change is desirable through migration, intermarriage, and selection based on the best qualities and merits of the common gene pool. It is not unreasonable to anticipate that the species will improve socially and psychologically on an ecologic front as well as on purely selective anatomical traits. Irrespective of state politic and philosophy of power, cultural diversity can serve as a potent fundamental strategy in evolutionary survival, and offers the possibilities, in the face of technological discipline requiring order and regulation, that certain freedoms can be maintained and expressed as suitable safeguards for mankind.

A final word may not be inappropriate on the subject of control and the concept of *military intellectualism.* The rise of technology itself was never of course a sudden event. Nor was it simply a matter of the design and implementation of machines that can simulate the human brain. Among the most serious of the dilemmas fueled by changing events, as Western societies have gradually changed from democracies to technocracies, has been the nature of leadership, and the quality of those in power, and their credentials for leadership rights. It is probably reasonably true to say that of all groups exposed to the new power quotients, implications of new technologic knowledge for economic and societal growth was grasped early by the military, who recognized the impact that the techno-sciences would have when applied to complex military systems and strategies of diversified military potential. Unhappily the academic professions seem never to have grasped the same insight. Established leadership in the universities (presently at least three computer generations away from leadership as exemplified by the military—conceivably because of age, lack of education and technological training, general unpreparedness to accept new constructs, and an ossified pedagogy, as often as not—has not, by and large, recognized the creature of power and politics that has been spawned from its fastness. Hence, unalert, academicians could not advise, and have not advised—nor have they been in a position to advise—the military-industrial complex. So inept, they have been unable to *intellectualize* these forces. This is regrettable because in a machine society, in an age of expanding technocracies based on a multiplicity of philosophic ideologies, with urgent need to comprehend and to respond and interact with sophisticated information-communication systems in relation to knowledge, and in respect of people, an intellectual military complex may be best placed to articulate the way through many of the seeds of distress—social, political, human, and global—that all nations have, willingly or unwillingly, inherited.

Technocracy is here to stay for the foreseeable future—and with it, *order, regulation, and control.* Economic and political organization might do well to appreciate that such freedoms as men will and wish to preserve can and should move from individualistic rights to more *collective* value orientations, within a sustained cultural diversity of options. Historically, I see no conflict in the personality of the military intellectuals. These are men, in my judgment, eminently qualified to lead. I would argue that both Julius Caesar and Alexander Hamilton could be described as military intellectuals. The former was, in addition to being a soldier, an orator, poet, legislator, and statesman who ordered and commanded an empire—successfully. The latter was a man of letters, a scholar of note, an eminent statesman and founder of the American republic. No small part of the success of the American Revolution was due to his efforts. It is of men of this quality, incomparably fit to lead, that I write.

Further Reading

Day, Stacey B. *Applied Health and Communications.* In *Health Communications.* Published by International Foundation for Biosocial Development and Human Health. NY. 1979. (ISBN: 0-934314-00-4).

Gabor, Dennis. *Innovations. Scientific, Technologic and Social.* London: Oxford University Press, 1970.

Illich, Ivan. Disabling professions: Notes for a lecture. *Biosci. Commun. 3*: 269-280, 1977.

Laski, Harold J. *The State in Theory and Practice,* 6th printing. The Vail-Ballou Press, 1968.

McHale, John, and McHale, Magda Cordell. *Basic Human Needs: A Framework For Action.* New Brunswick, New Jersey: Transaction Books, 1978.

Sitaram, K. S. Intercultural communication: An overview. *Biosci. Commun. 4* (6): 334-347, 1978.

Straker, Robert Lincoln. *Horace Mann And Others.* Chapters from the *History of Antioch College.* Yellow Springs, Ohio: The Antioch Press, 1963.

Project For a "Guide to Use-Value Oriented Convivial Tools—and Their Enemies"*

VALENTINA BORREMANS
Cuernavaca, Mexico

With an Introduction by Ivan Illich

INTRODUCTION, BY IVAN ILLICH

Alternative administrative styles of medicalized health must be clearly distinguished from a reversal in the existing trend of medicalized sick and health care. The former represents a move toward an even more commodity-intensive utopia than that which guided public policy-making in the post World War II period. The second is part and parcel of a new social vision in which technical progress is valued primarily, insofar as it increases the power of individuals and of primary groups to satisfy their own needs by autonomous activities. I call "autonomous activities" those by which people define their own needs in the process of creating the values that satisfy them. The choice within medicine— in Greek, medicine's "crisis"—cannot be understood without making this philosophical distinction.

The appearance of multiple, very new, and often compatible styles of health-oriented *professional* activities has been the prevalent reaction to the breakdown of the military paradigm of a war for health that had prevailed among practitioners and administrators in the fifties and sixties. Public health management, centrally planned health protection, professional training for decentralized feeders into the medical system, and compulsory health education were increasingly compounded with a medical mania for "wellness," for "holistic health" and the incorporation into the medical armamentarium of folk, as well as occult, practice. The crisis in medicine has thus served—at least to a large extent—to expand the reach of university-trained professional health-officers over new groups of patients, new conditions that require regulation and supervision, and new forms of social control. Though in this process the first-line practitioner might have seen some of his functions pruned, the trend toward new compatible styles of "health provision" has in fact increased professional dominance over health care during the seventies. At the cost of the physicians who continued to practice as they had learned that they should, at the time

*To be published as a special issue of Library Journal in Nov. 79, ed. Karl Nyreu, 1180 Ave of the Americas, New York, N.Y.

when they graduated in the forties and fifties, new kinds of innovative health-professionals and their welfare-oriented political allies have discovered new types of pastures.

On the other hand, the last three or four years have brought us a new crop of social proposals that oppose the idea that a postindustrial age would have to be one in which services abound and in which professionally managed welfare predominates. How competent, rational, and innovative—but also how dispersed, varied, and unprecedented—social experimentation on new kinds of decentralization is, I for one understood only when I recently had the opportunity to study the manuscript of Valentina Borreman's new *Guide to Reference Books on Use-Value Oriented Modern Tools*. Consistent with this alternative view about the relationship between human beings and their modern tools, health consists precisely in the independence from, and not in access to, service. The ideas of Dr. D. Banerji and his colleagues, embodied in the introduction to the *Shrivastava Report* (Ministry of Health, New Delhi), summarize on a high governmental level and in elegant sentences insights that are brought forth, in very different terms, by women's self-care movements, cripples' cooperatives, and literally thousands of groupings all over the world.

Both trends, that toward diversified and radical professionalism which paternalistically concedes responsibilities to its wards and the other one, directed toward prudent, yet radical deprofessionalization, are fueled by the anguishing loss of credibility that has quite suddenly affected the post–World War II framework of worldwide medical policies. In no other major sector of the industrial system has the institutional rationality of a functional ideology been eclipsed so suddenly as in the field of world health. No doubt the times were ripe, and it was suddenly easy to recognize the pseudoreligious character of the health concept that had been enshrined in the WHO constitution. But we owe it to a new breed of philosopher-bureaucrats, of whom—in my opinion—Dr. Halfdan Mahler is the most noticeable example, that this crisis of an ideology could evolve into a crisis of much deeper nature, the public opposition between two incompatible perceptions of health itself: on the one side primarily operationally verified well-being that is overwhelmingly professionally fostered, protected, and managed, and on the other side primarily personally defined and pursued health, which is health that flowers where not only the right to commodities but equally the freedom to use-value generation is politically protected.

The following article, to which I was asked to write an introduction, was prepared by Valentina Borremans for a consultation among a dozen persons convened in June 1977 by the Hammarskjöld Foundation to discuss "Another Development in Health." Some of the misunderstandings to which my book *Medical Nemesis* has given rise, could have been avoided had I in that book used the language and terse distinctions of Valentina Borremans.

PROJECT FOR A "GUIDE TO USE-VALUE
ORIENTED CONVIVIAL TOOLS–AND
THEIR ENEMIES"

This is a draft for an International Library Guide to a field of study which is now emerging as a distinct subject or discipline and which is based on contributions from a wide variety of traditional fields.

The new area of investigation focuses on the evidence that "tools," in their technical development, occasionally reach thresholds that are societally critical. When a tool acquires such a critical character, it inevitably affects the culture, social structure, and distribution of political power of the community that uses it.

> The new discipline first identifies those tools that make an industrial market-intensive society inevitable—that is, a society in which the needs of people are increasingly correlates of goods and services designed and prescribed for them by dominant professions.

> Second, the discipline explores old, new, and possible tools that enable people and primary groups to shape their needs in the activity by which these needs are also satisifed. Such tools are overwhelmingly those that enhance the generation of use-values rather than the production of commodities.

> Third, this new discipline deals with the cultural, social, and political conditions under which use-value oriented modern tools can and will be widely used, and with the renewal of ethics, politics, and aesthetics that is made possible by the democratically decided limitation of the industrial mode of production.

This area of investigation is not confined to one new society in particular, but encompasses the prevalence of convivial over industrial tools in any modern society, and deals with the wide range of options in life style, governance, and economics that would be fostered by this prevalence.

The vision of these new possibilities requires the recognition that scientific discoveries can be used in at least two forms. The first leads to specialization of functions, institutionalization of values, centralization of power, and turns people into accessories of bureaucracies or machines. The second enlarges the range of each person's competence, control, and initiative, limited only by other individuals' claims to an equal range of power and freedom.

The term "tool" is used here with the meaning given it by Ivan Illich in *Tools for Conviviality*.

> I use the term "tool" broadly enough to include not only simple hardware such as drills, pots, syringes, brooms, building elements, or motors, and

not just large machines like cars or power stations; I also include among tools productive institutions such as factories that produce tangible commodities like corn flakes or electric current, and productive systems for intangible commodities such as those which produce "education", "health", "knowledge", or "decisions". I use this term because it allows me to subsume into one category all rationally designed devices, be they artifacts or rules, codes or operators, and to distinguish all these planned and engineered instrumentalities from other things such as basic food or implements, which in a given culture are not deemed to be subject to rationalization. School curricula or marriage laws are no less purposely shaped social devices than road networks.

Tools are intrinsic to social relationships. An individual relates himself in action to his society through the use of tools that he actively masters, or by which he is passively acted upon. To the degree that he masters his tools, he can invest the world with his meaning; to the degree that he is mastered by his tools, the shape of the tool determines his own self-image. Convivial tools are those which give each person who uses them the greatest opportunity to enrich the environment with the fruits of his vision. Industrial tools deny this possibility to those who use them and they allow their designers to determine the meaning and expectations of others. Most tools today cannot be used in a convivial fashion.

A convivial society should be designed to allow all its members the most autonomous action by means of tools least controlled by others and use-value oriented. The growth of tools beyond a certain point increases regimentation, dependence, exploitation and impotence and cannot but produce exchange-values.

By publishing this guide, I intend to "establish" the field of study that deals with convivial tools by providing it with a niche in every respectable library. As a librarian, I believe that the library—today more than ever—is the place where a dissident worldview can first take shape and consistency. By properly labeling a new kind of perspective and by putting a new kind of material on the shelves, a new social reality can be fostered that will be confirmed even by those who impugn its legitimacy.

But a field needs a name if it has to mature. It would be a mistake to call this new and systematic pursuit of practical wisdom about tools "futurism." The term futurism has only recently found acceptance, but already designates one more academic discipline in which hierarchically organized professionals use prestigious procedures to forecast, plan, and make policy about people's needs and the services by which these needs shall both be shaped and satisfied. Convivial research does precisely the inverse: those who pursue it explore new ways and means by which they themselves and the members of their primary communities can satisfy those needs which are shaped and limited in the very same process by which they are satisfied. This approach to renewal and progress is conspicuously absent from the many excellent guides to the literature on futurism. I would rather follow Peter Harper in calling the study of convivial tools "radical technology."

> We wanted to express an ideal of technological organization that was part of a totoal movement towards a new form of society; but at the same time to assert the belief that technology itself matters, not *just* who controls it—that, in other words, not only the relations of production, but the *means themselves* must be changed to permit the achievement of a just, stable and fulfilling society.
>
> Since this last is a notion that most radicals would not accept, we adopted the word "radical" with some diffidence, reinforced by the fact that most of the material in the book is purely technical and has no overt political content at all. But other explicitly political labels were even more misleading or susceptible to misinterpretation. "Socialist Technology", "Anarchist Technology" or "Utopian Technology" could all have done at a pinch (let no one call us sectarian!) but the terms are so muddied that the relatively anodyne "Radical Technology" was wheeled in *faute de mieux*. (*Radical Technology,* ed. by Godfrey Boyle and Peter Harper, New York: Pantheon Books, 1976)

This is definitely not a guide for the study of "Alternative Technology" in the broad sense. Feeding high voltage networks from renewable geothermal sources, ocean waves, or the burning of alcohol—defensible under some possible set of assumptions—is clearly an alternative to coal, fission, or fusion. But the fact that such production may be less destructive of the physical milieu does not necessarily mean that it is also a convivial tool. Therefore, references to oil, coal, or "alternative" feeders of high voltage networks are listed as aids to clarify the differences between these and specifically *radical* technologies.

This guide must also be distinguished from an access tool to "Soft Technologies." The ecological movement has enormously contributed to the critical atmosphere that has made radical technology possible and acceptable. Most of the research, both critical and creative, that has resulted from the new emphasis on environmental studies, constitutes a precious source for the radical technologist. In many cases, the best test for the long-range ecological feasibility of a technique is its acceptability according to the criteria of soft technology. The emphasis of this guide, however, is not ecological. The radical technologist, in the design and selection of tools, primarily utilizes criteria that ensure the ability of individuals and small groups to generate use-values. Secondarily, environmental requirements are considered. In many ecological projects, priorities are reversed: the preservation of "nature" comes first, and specifically human needs are either ignored or slighted.

In a similar manner, reference material on "Soft Bureaucracies" and their organizational tools will help the radical technologist to define and clarify his research in a new dimension. But this is not a guide to radical professionalism. No doubt, adult education is an "alternative" to schooling; no doubt, the participation of the pupil on the board of his "college without walls" renders his educational management sweeter and more persuasive; no doubt, public television has pioneered some techniques that can be used in convivial frameworks. But the radical inverse of schools is not some new form of education; rather, a structure of tools that fosters more widespread, satisfying, and stimulating learning. References to policy alternatives and new techniques in the areas dominated by the great professions of medicine, education, and the administration of law have the same purpose as references to alternative urban sewer systems, insecticides, or computers.

This is a guide to "Use-Value Oriented Convivial Tools—and Their Enemies." It is meant primarily as an *instrument for the selection of reference materials* for a library and, secondarily, as a *research guide*. The persons whom I want to assist are of three kinds:

1. From Fiesole in Italy and Arequipa in Peru, Puna in Maharashtra, and Corte in Corsica, I have been asked to help in the creation of reference collections for the study of radical technology. This guide, then, has been prepared for the librarian who must build up a specialized research tool far from any large and well-rounded general library. My emphasis is on those materials that allow the researcher to identify his needs, so that the librarian can then order these items, thereby enlarging the library's collection in the special fields actually used by researchers.

   In two decades of experience as a librarian in Latin America and, with some experience in Africa, I have had to work with people who wanted to do research outside of the capital cities which monopolize documentation. I have come to the conviction that the one way to build up a good library in such conditions is this: let the librarian splurge on access or reference materials, and only later stock his shelves with what the few researchers who regularly use the library request. I am convinced that a thousand dollars for the acquisition of reference materials will enable a part-time librarian in most countries of the world to provide a first rate access and research tool for the study of radical technology.

2. The lack of research facilities in the libraries of poor countries is notorious. But even more scandalous is the absence of materials covered by this

guide in the university libraries of the rich. Therefore, the guide is designed to remedy this lacuna. The well-equipped librarian can use the guide to expand his reference section both on radical technology and in the fields that relate to it.

This professional librarian might be surprised to find some of the most basic tools of his trade in the guide. But it must be remembered that the nonprofessionally trained librarian in a Colombian town, asked by three schoolmasters to use one fourth of each man's salary to create their research tool, will be delighted to discover a general guide to reference books in both English and Spanish.

3. There is a third kind of user whom I have in mind: the individual researcher who has no access to any significant library at all. He might be a journalist in the Northeast of Brazil who wants to argue his case against a new power station, or the union member in Italy seeking a list of others who have organized worker control over jobs in a plastics plant. For the sake of these readers, I have made many exceptions to my general rule to include second-level reference tools, guides to literature, to organized activities, and to sources of documentation, and some other materials significant enough to retain their value as historical documents even though they have been replaced by more comprehensive new books.

For the sake of the individual and isolated researcher, I have listed also a few more ephemeral items.

The dominance of English in this bibliography highlights the urgency of its international use. Today the need for "radical technology" is recognized in the English-speaking world, from India to Canada, more than elsewhere—with the possible exception of China. This is partly due to a political and historical tradition, and partly to the resources for systematic analysis and publication of experiments in the Anglo-Saxon countries. Thus English has become both the "uniquak" of corporate and professional multinationals extending their global reach and the "koiné" by which the housewife in Lima can establish contact with a women's health collective of London or Boston.

Today, it is abundantly clear that the Peruvian or Dahomelian who does not acquire a reading knowledge of English is condemned to be the victim of translators. He will have to depend on what his tutors, large corporations, or governments decide to translate into Spanish, French, or Quechua. The multinational industrial system defends its global power by this monopoly on access to the written word. This guide to reference tools can help people all over the world raid the centers where research on radical technology takes place, research published overwhelmingly in English. For this reason, I include a rather detailed section on language learning. In addition, vernacular language is the prototype of a radically convivial tool.

Most of the key items to which I would like to lead the user of this guide are of very recent vintage: they are being constantly criticized, improved, or superseded—and the information on this lively process cannot be obtained from materials now commonly found in libraries. My guide is of limited usefulness unless it is complemented with a few other tools, among which I would give priority to the following:

1. The *Rainbook* complemented with *Rain* magazine
2. Peter Harper's bibliography in *Radical Technology,* edited by Boyle and Harper
3. The *Appropriate Technology Sourcebook,* edited by Darrow and Pam
4. *From Radical Left to Extreme Right,* Vols. 2 and 3, by Theodore Jurgens Spahn and Janet Peterson Spahn
5. *Workbook* magazine
6. *Alternative Sources of Energy* magazine

The arrangement of my guide to reference tools reflects the specific purpose for which I have destined it.

In *Section A* I list under 18 conventional headings a selection of 80 easy to use and comprehensive—mostly annotated—guides to research. This 7% of the total alphabetical list given in Section B will very frequently be sufficient to answer reference questions. Section B is an alphabetical list of 698 entries. I list entries under the personal name of the first given author or editor, rather than under the name of the impersonal agency, publisher, or collective. All coauthors as well as institutes, sponsors, and publishers (unless these are major commercial firms) are listed in the index. *Section C* lists periodicals. *Section D* provides addresses of small, special, or unusual sources of the literature mentioned. *Section E* is a name and subject index which includes some titles. The subjects are listed as the authors would define them. Thus Section E can be used not only as index but also as glossary to the new field and as "Who's Who."

Biotechnology and Cultural Transformation as Imperatives in the Health of Contemporary Societies

STACEY B. DAY, M.D., Ph.D., D.Sc.
Professor and Member, Sloan Kettering Institute for Cancer Research
Head, Biosciences Communications and Medical Education,
Sloan Kettering Institute
New York, New York

The construct of this paper is to view the nature of health as being based on contributions from a wide variety of traditional and nontraditional disciplines, which under thrusts, sometimes volatile, sometimes latent, from a multiplicity of changing socioeconomic pressures have become increasingly unstable and unpredictable, not only in terms expressing their orientation and development, but also inevitably in their efficiency.

It is the view of the writer that the heretofore preeminent concentration of clinical autonomy and power in the hands of the physician, who is presumed to have superior knowledge and skill in the concepts and management of health, has become in modern society a less and less valid proposition. There are also reasonable arguments that the psychological and philosophical premises for such direction little serve a society in the wake of marked technological change accompanied by the emergence of new institutions of social power. Irrespective of ideologies, societies in general are now moving toward living systems in which person and patient are becoming increasingly responsible for the production, maintenance, and restoration of their own health. In this view, people as communities are responsible as *producers of health* within the social and political conditions of their own environment.

Considered from this point of view then, health becomes but one of the several priorities of nations, and as such is one of the optional alternatives for survival. In dealing with problems of health it is essential to identify the basic organizing *needs* of the community and/or society, and these may be supposed to vary in respect of efficiency, equity, and distribution, as do the distribution of wealth, the distribution of power, the infrastructure and matrix of the culture, and the level of technology within the understanding of extant scientific and applied industrial potentials.

Considering the biosphere as a whole and given the various options for quality of life, it must be recognized that the world population is increasing by 60 to 70 million people per year. Realistically this increase in population cannot be restrained within at least the next 20 to 30 years. The major task of nations therefore, irrespective of any particular disease, must be one of *nutrition*—the feeding of this magnitude of people, who presently are consuming over 900 million tons of food per year. Thus disease and the conditions of health should be recognized within an order of priority that views food (agriculture), overall energy resources, and energy conversion processes, as well as matters of modernization in terms of cost-efficiency and cost-benefit, as demanding even more prior resolution. Together these several variables reflect ecological changes in the environment, which in turn effect the well-being of the individual, no matter from what region, class, or society he/she may come.

Since power and politics have historically described the wealth of nations, and in this context the wealth of the biosphere as a whole, both fiscal and physiological, must be considered fixed, a given group or society is wealthy only within its bioresources, the developmental capacity of that society, and the way that it manages the use of its wealth (money). The ordering of its priorities may include health, in terms of ultimate survival for the group as a whole. Decisions brought to bear on this priority rating are effectively related to the nature of the culture and the goals of its individuals. For the society, as for each individual in the society, as I have argued elsewhere, health including freedom from disease may require such a methodological or philosophical approach as is resolvable through the intellectual device of the *General Principle of Parsimony*. In fact in underdeveloped societies, and for developing nations facing extraordinary problems, including the need to leap-frog into an age of technology while simply not possessing immediate technological means, this principle may be critical in application. The general principle states that, in a given problem-solving situation *if one chooses the smallest number of criteria to effect the solution, then efficiency and equity will approximate as a function of a situation dealing with variables.*

The ecological viewpoint and bioresources are really expressions of the organization of the *ecology of people*, who one might suppose are more commonly portrayed as all the bland nonentities of the census report—the *numbers* on parade each decade: population, its age and sex, content by ethnicity, its distribution, its appetites, rates of growth—in fact so many faceless numbers aging and dying, transforming and being transformed within and by the multitude of variable factors influencing the biosphere. Within this faceless multitude all the variable links of culture are at play, work habits and preferences, ethnicity, prejudice, educational background, class structure, generation and deontological peer groups as may be the case, and all these are weighted to varying degrees by the economic and sociocultural milieu summarized as growth curves, per capita incomes, balance of trade revenues, and religious beliefs, as well as economic and noneconomic descriptives consequent upon transformation in society.

Most relevant for us clearly are those changes that have been wrought in global spheres over the last century and a half. In a critical sense, based on fire, coal, and oil, modern scientific and technologic society is barely a kindergarten expression beyond a century in a time frame reference of 100 billion years. The expression of this circumstance has been splendidly stated with analytical insight and understanding by Stanford:[6]

> We believe that this galaxy is about 100 billion years old, and that our earth formed up in less than half that time—about 50 billion years ago. Life began about 30 million years ago, and man first appeared after 9/10ths of that time had elapsed—he is a newcomer, only 3 million years old. Only in the last tenth of his period, about 40,000 years ago did man learn to use fire for cooking; and he began purposive agriculture much later than that—about 12,000 years ago.

It takes little imagination to understand that culture, expressed in knowledge forms, is a relatively recent human acquisition, and health and disease existed long *before* man had devised strategies for his benefit and welfare.

Granted that political philosophies will invite differing interpretations of the consequence of expansion of industrial change for society, technology, and professional dominance, the concept of *convivial tools* as advanced by Ivan Illich (and described by his associate Valentina Borremans[2]) provides critical insight into strategies evaluating effects of culture, social structure, and the distribution of power, both political and fiscal, as these function in societies in our times. Illich broadly defines a tool as:

> to include not only simple hardware such as drills, pots, syringes, brooms, building elements, or motors, and not just large machines like cars or power stations; I also include among tools productive institutions such as factories that produce tangible commodities like corn flakes or electric current, and productive systems for intangible commodities such as that produce "education", "health", "knowledge", or "decisions".

In this sense *tools* are intrinsic to all human situations and to all human conditions including the maintenance of health, as well as for measures appropriate in society toward solutions of its problems. Illich and Borremans can hardly be said to share the conventional North American science fiction view of engineering the "six million dollar man" and his "bionic woman." That is not the issue. For them their convivial tools may well be unconvivial, but the impact at the cultural level is far-reaching, especially in underdeveloped nations. Technology is vitally and forcefully brought home. The political implications of science, technology, and culture, inclusive or not of health considerations, can be disregarded at the peril of interrelated human values and reciprocal existence.

The truth is of course that technology and culture have always been related. Man is *Homo faber,* the tool-making animal. At the core of the life systems upon which man functions, these imperatives have always been of cardinal importance.

In the same sense that spontaneous mutations, hybridization, and selection fortify and improve genetic variability, so in human societies, migration, inter-marriage, and preselection from a common gene pool, based on cultural diversity, support and improve prospects for enhanced quality of life and survival of the human species. "Spaceship earth" may be a catch-all phrase describing the reduction in perspective of our biosphere. Whatever advantages may accrue, there is also presaged, among many other problems, the serious jeopardy of rapidly decreasing genetic diversity in our biosphere. In this respect the cost of breeding is raised in both a philosophical and a fiscal respect. Unless greater diversity can be preserved, the ultimate fate of the common gene pool may be limitations that seem at this time undesirable. Good health, and prospects for enhanced better health, must be considered problems not solely of technology or of economics, but rest seriously in part on culturally related aspects of this whole growth-related problem. In the absence of diversity, with or without disease, predictable limitations to human advance must inevitably occur.

How then might we reasonably view biotechnology and cultural transformation, in respect of disease and maintenance of health in our contemporary societies? If the thrust of the present argument be admitted, it will reinforce similar thinking of such observers as W. H. C. Simmonds of Ottawa, Sir Geoffrey Vickers of Great Britain, and others of like mind, that a new ecological viewpoint must be introduced that permits societies a certain resilience and collaborative independence in directing *change* so as to optimally utilize cultural diversity and naturally occurring bioresources. Economic, demographic, sociologic, and cultural perspectives will suggest that technological advances of the same magnitude are not possible, nor are they desirable, in all regions of the biosphere at a simultaneous fixed point in time. Rates of time frame to introduce technologic change become critically important. Appreciation of this is emphatically brought home by a precise understanding of Stanford's *time-scale of events in evolution.* Consider the introduction of technology in terms of Stanford's work—imagine that all life began just 10 years ago. "If that were so, using log scale factors, then men first appeared on earth about one year ago. Fire for cooking was introduced 5 days ago. Agriculture commenced 1½ days ago. City life as urban existence began 20 hours ago, and what we think of as *science* began in all our wisdom 6 minutes ago." On this scale we can begin to understand the magnitude of the variables we are handling and the insolence that we offer Nature. "Atomic energy as we know it (the atomic bomb) in the 10 year simile began 2 minutes ago." In terms of high technology, therefore, would it not be prudent to speak less of progress and consider better the nature of change? We would submit that *the understanding of change itself* becomes one of the cardinal features of technology. It is essential to minimally disturb the cultural harmony of the ecosphere that has over centuries itself been a child of Nature.

Possibilities for technologic change in two examples will be discussed here. One might refer to modernization and the bullock cart in post-British India. The other will consider a role for computer-assisted remote sensing devices to define temperature, altitude, and vegetative cover by satellite to assist in mosquito and insect control. Unquestionably technological research has refined remote sensing technics so that it becomes feasible utilizing satellite imagery to classify broad ecotypes of vegetation associated with insect development. Programs have in fact been designed to eradicate the screwworm fly, *Cochliomyia hominovorax,* from vast tracts of Mexico. No one would question that such technology could work to the benefit of mankind. But unless implementation is undertaken within the framework of priorities for the region, it may be more disadvantageous than advantageous. Thus is screwworm fly, of all diseases associated with insects, the most urgent one to remove? By removing these flies will there be adverse effects in the ecological harmony of the region? Have these effects been studied? What are the social and economic advantages of removing the fly? If there are no people in the region, or if the land so freed of insects is infertile and cannot be used in agriculture, could funds so spent have been better applied elsewhere? And with satellites, as sophisticated as they may appear to be, their use in developing countries is still subject to all the many hazards and difficulties that I outlined five years ago:

> But the satellite itself is only *one* component in a system which must include earth stations, . . . and staff and facilities on earth to establish connections . . . with those responsible for program preparation, production, . . . as well as organization, management, and socio-cultural feedback. . . . Unless feasibility studies are performed, the expenditure on *software* is likely to be far higher than on *hardware.* . . . No satellite ought to be launched until these potential circumstances are effectively gauged. . . .
>
> The potential for financial waste is high with satellite cable development. . . .

Problem solving is one thing—decision making is another. This discussion can be presented from an alternative viewpoint. Consider the bullock cart in India, a subcontinent in which there are estimated to be over 13 million such carts in operation. These vehicles are admirably adapted for poor road systems and transportation conditions subject to such hazards as heavy rains in the monsoon and intense dry heat as in the warm seasons. They do not pollute the atmosphere as would gasoline engines; they do not require the import of expensive oil reserves, or damage or add further crisis to an unfavorable balance of payments; and they annually provide 20 million people with employment in repair of such carts! In an age of high technology, such a system of transportation is inconceivable for the United States, but that in itself does not alone constitute an argument for developing precisely the same oil-dependent transportation systems in India as are used in America. Nor can American time-frame values be transferred without prior thought to a culture in which other standards exist as norms. Technological change should be brought about within rates of time changes based on national, ecological, and cultural, as well as fiscal and philosophical values in a society. Prudence recognizes that each cultural system has its own harmonies which might well be worth preserving. To locate mosquitoes by LANDSAT satellite and multiband aerial photography is a superior achievement. But such a technological potential carries with it per se no certainty that it may be the best or even a necessary strategy, merely because it is a new technology. Indeed, in a culture in which technology itself may be alien, far more problems may result than can be resolved.

Planning principles and resource-conserving in relation to cultural dimensions are well illustrated in present Chinese efforts to conserve energy. An example would be the conversion of sewage wastes and night soilage by microorganisms to provide energy in the form of fuel (methane gas) for domestic needs. In the same process hygienic control of parasitic ova that may transmit disease is effected. Use of biomass resource bases of household wastes for generating cooking gas, while hardly an immediate context for dominant planning in technological America, is a practical everyday solution for obtaining cooking gas in over 5 million homes in China. This system is becoming an increasing potential source of fuel energy in other developing countries where cost restraints prohibit import of expensive oil. This system of sewage-generated heat is being widely applied in India, and becoming increasingly so used in other countries, Egypt for example.

These cases demonstrate, perhaps as well as any, biotechnological resource applications for the well-being and survival of peoples, based on methodologies related to *cultural organization*. Such prospects defend the ecological balance of the biosphere, and in an age of often thoughtless technology preserve cultural diversity. It is this cultural diversity that fortifies the collective gene pool upon which ultimate human survival depends.

References

Barnes, C. M. Satellite and computer systems to aid in insect control. Presented at the International Conference on Bio-Resources for Development, Houston, Texas, November 5–10, 1978.

Borremans, Valentina. Project for a "Guide to Use-Value Oriented Convivial Tools—and their Enemies." *Techno-Politica,* Doc 78/12. Apdo. 479 Cuernavaca, Mexico.

Day, Stacey B. Space and communications. *Biosci. Commun. 2:* 65–72, 1976.

Day, Stacey B., Cuddihy, R. V., and Fudenberg, H. H. The American biomedical network:

Health care systems in America present and future. *Scripta Medica and Technica.* New Jersey, 1977. (see: Management in medicine: Parsimony and options, pp. 57–63).

Simmonds, W. H. C. New directions for economic and social growth: The ecology of change. Presented at the International Conference on Bio-Resources for Development, Houston, Texas, November 5–10, 1978.

Stanford, Geoffrey. The long term productivity of agricultural soils. Presented at the International Conference on Bio-Resources For Development, Houston, Texas, November 5–10, 1978.

The Economic Times, Calcutta, December 29, 1976, No matter for sneer (editorial referring to the oil crisis and the bullock cart. Problems of modernization).

Vickers, Sir Geoffrey. The future of culture. In *Futures Research, New Directions,* H. Linstone and W. H. C. Simmons, eds. Reading, Massachusetts: Addison Wesley, 1977.

Value Systems and Social Process. London: Pelican, 1968 (ecology of ideas, science of human ecology).

A Simple Man's Approach to Health Economics

ROBERT J. MAXWELL, MA., ACMA., J.P.
*Administrator, Special Trustees for Saint Thomas Hospital
London, England*

It seems self-evident that complex problems call for sharp wits. And few problems are more complex today than financing health care and using to the best effect the resources available for health. Thus the growing interest in health care from economists—many of them clever and some of them brilliant—is in principle to be welcomed. Unfortunately, much of the activity in health economics has gone into spinning elegant webs of theory comprehensible only to other economists. Few of the doctors and nurses looking after patients, or the administrators and politicians trying to enable them to do so, know what economists are writing or, if they did, would understand it. Consequently the sharp wits are not contributing.

Rather than starting from the theoretical end and trying to communicate economic theory to noneconomists, it is perhaps better to start with some of the facts about health spending and about the economic problems facing those who hold positions of responsibility in the health field. We can then see in what ways economic theory may illuminate these problems.

THE FACTS ABOUT EXPENDITURES

For at least the last 30 years, health expenditures have been rising throughout the developed world, not merely in money terms but as a proportion of national income (as measured by GNP or GDP). Thus in France, to quote Madame-Simone Sandier's paper presented in Milan,[1] health expenditures from all sources rose 33-fold in money terms between 1950 and 1975; and as a proportion of GNP, health expenditures were 2.9% in 1950 and 6.8% in 1975. In the United States in the same period, health expenditures rose from 4.6% of GNP to 8.3%. Although the levels of expenditure vary from nation to nation, this upward trend is echoed in every industrial country for which reasonably reliable figures are available, as Table 1 illustrates.

Why have these formidable increases in expenditure occurred? There are, I believe, five main causes:[2]

1. A changing pattern of disease toward chronic illness and handicap associated with aging, speeded or slowed by personal behavior, and toward psychiatric illness.
2. Advances in medical technology and the introduction of far more sophisticated patterns of care, particularly in the acute hospital sector.
3. Rising public and professional expectations as regards technology and as regards the less scientific aspects of care, such as what constitute appropriate and acceptable living standards not merely in general hospitals but for groups like the mentally ill, the handicapped, and the elderly, who have often been neglected in the past.
4. Higher wage and salary costs, caused in part by a "catching up" process of health sector wages but also the inevitable result of failures to achieve

TABLE 1. Health Care Expenditures (Public and Private) as a Percentage of GNP

	West Germany	Sweden	USA	France	Canada	UK	Australia
1950		3.4	4.5	3.4*	4.0		
1960		4.7	5.2	4.7*	5.6	3.9	5.0*
1965		5.6	5.9	5.8*	6.1	4.0	5.2*
1970	6.4	7.4	7.2	6.4	7.1	4.5	5.5
1975	9.4	8.5	8.6	7.9	7.1	5.5	7.0

* = Estimates

manpower savings in the health sector in a world in which manpower is becoming ever more expensive; in health care, technological advances have seldom resulted in manpower reductions.

5. A transfer of financing from direct payment by individuals to insurance schemes and to government.

Most of these causes will continue to operate in the future. It is true that in some countries, though not in all, the movement to public funding has gone as far as it can go, and that wages in the health sector have caught up with pay rates elsewhere. But the swing to an older population, afflicted with more chronic disease and handicap, is by no means finished. Still less have the pressures of medical technology and of rising expectations spent their strength. And the health sector remains, and is always likely to remain, personnel-intensive. Anybody who believes that health expenditures have increased simply because nobody was watching them and that, as in the children's game of grandmother's footsteps, the stealthy advances will stop once they are spotted, is fooling himself. The inflationary forces in health spending remain extremely strong and will mean that constant value health care dollars—at least as traditionally spent— will buy decreasing amounts and standards of care.

However, there certainly is more resistance to further rises in health expenditures than there was a few years ago, as I predicted there would be.[3] The inevitable clash with other priorities has come sooner and more sharply than I expected partly because of the sluggishness in the world economy. Thus governments are without doubt applying the brakes as firmly as they can to their health budgets. Canada, Sweden, France, and (for a short period) the United States all provide clear examples, let alone England, which has developed unparalleled skill at controlling health expenditures, to the point where the viability of its health service is in danger. For learning to control public expenditures on health is not by itself enough. Control can be achieved at the cost of equity or quality of care or both. The real task is much more complex and involves weighing health against other priorities in a rational way, and using all the resources available for health wisely and well.

INSIGHTS FROM ECONOMICS

Health economics is a relatively young field and one that is little illuminated by conventional free market economics. It is not that the market system *cannot* apply in the health field, but that there are two major snags about its application. The first is that the principal decisions about utilization are not made by consumers but by suppliers. Once we have asked a doctor for help, it is chiefly doctors who decide what services we require and who therefore are the prime determinants of how resources are used in the whole health sector. The United

States provides evidence that, for example, the incidence of surgery is strongly influenced by the availability, distribution, and motivation of surgeons. In the health field demand and supply are not independent forces reaching a point of equilibrium where marginal benefits equal marginal costs, as in the classic market system. Instead, when a market reimbursement system applies, the quantity and quality of medical services tend to rise to the point where, in the judgment of suppliers, the marginal benefit of further services is zero.[4]

The second snag is that governments, reflecting your and my instincts as electors, are not prepared to see the interplay of market forces carried to a ruthless conclusion in health care. For what happens through the free interplay of market forces, in this as in other fields, is that the resources go where people can afford to pay for them and where suppliers find operation attractive. This can be seen clearly in, for example, the share of medical resources taken by Northern Italy compared with the South, or by the Paris area compared with other parts of France. Those who cannot afford to pay, directly or through insurance, get less care. None of us, I suspect, is happy about this. We feel instinctively that in the health field the care given should be related to need rather than to the capacity to pay for it or to its prestige or profitability to suppliers. And as soon as governments intervene to secure equity in health care for the less fortunate, they disturb the interaction of supply and demand. You cannot at one and the same time remove the sting of deprivation and expect the market system to exercise constraint on the supply of medical care.

For analytic, not political, reasons I therefore believe that we cannot let the interplay of markets forces determine the total amount spent on health and the way in which health resources are distributed and used. We have to find some other approach. This does not necessarily mean adopting a national system such as the British NHS. But it does mean accepting that there is a shared communal responsibility—involving patients, their families, those working in the health field, and representatives of the public, including government—for health care and health expenditures. Whatever part may be played by private practitioners and by nongovernment institutions, health becomes indisputably a matter of public policy. Communities and governments have got to be concerned about the effectiveness and cost of the *total* pattern of health provision, not just about whatever part is directly provided by the government.

We thus have a different and little-studied field of economics, involving the allocation of scarce resources on a basis other than that of the free interplay of market forces. Conceptually the problem is how best to relate limited resources of different degrees of sophistication and cost to "needs" that are also heterogeneous, not homogeneous. I will come in a moment to the conundrum of what "needs" are, and turn first to the resource side. Simplifying, one can envisage a pyramid of resources like this:

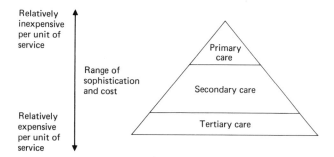

In reality, the boundaries between levels of care are not as tidy as this, nor is primary care always less expensive than secondary care, or secondary care cheaper than tertiary. Nevertheless the pyramid image is, I think, a helpful one to illustrate the fact that in terms of the sophistication of skills and hence of costs there is a hierarchy of resources to deploy.

Turning now to needs, the term is imprecise, and yet most people working the health field use it with fair concensus as to its meaning. I agree with M. H. Cooper[5] and A. J. Culyer[6] that the term implies a professional judgment that an individual or group of individuals has an actual or potential problem of handicap or suffering. I do not go so far as to assert, as some economists do, that the problem is not a need unless some form of treatment is available to avoid or alleviate it. A dying cancer patient has needs beyond our capacity to treat them. And yet this difference of definition is in practice not great, since as soon as one begins to try to relate the resource pyramid to needs one is asking "How can these resources be best used to bring benefit to these people with these handicaps?" The handicaps or health problems are not of course of one kind only, nor are they of one degree of severity, but they are heterogeneous. Thus there is a range of illnesses and handicaps that can again be represented in pyramid form:

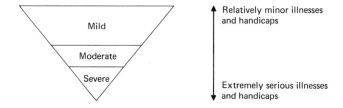

As with the resource pyramid, the boundaries within the pyramid are not nearly as precise as in the diagram, but there is a gradation from stark unambiguous needs (people involved in a serious road accident) to relatively mild conditions for which some people feel they need help, while others do not.

Putting the two pyramids side by side—which is what all managers of health service resources have to try to do, from the doctor managing his time to the minister of health—one is likely to find mismatches. For example, some health problems not calling for such a degree of sophistication, or that could be avoided or prevented, may be dealt with by the secondary or tertiary parts of the system:

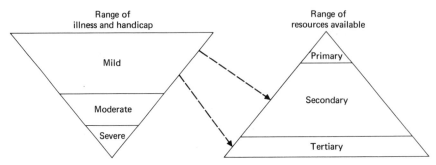

Other relatively serious conditions may be neglected. Still others are absorbing time, energy, skill, and money to little effect.

Looking at the resource allocation task for a nation in this way, one can at once see that the amount the nation is prepared to spend should radically affect the whole pattern of its services. It is lunacy for a poor country to try to duplicate the tertiary services of a rich one, for if it does (as many have done), the lion's share of its health budget will be eaten up in services for relatively few people. Meanwhile many people will go without simple, basic services with a high ratio of benefits to costs. Even among the developed countries the amounts available for health spending per head are so different that Britain, for example, has got to be more selective about what it tries to achieve than, say, Sweden or the United States.

It is also clear that the allocation of health resources is an extraordinarily complex task, requiring not only calculation but also insight and compassion. There is never likely to be any perfect, let alone permanent, "right" way to allocate these resources, but there is scope for most nations and local communities to do better than they yet do.

THE FUTURE

Economists will very properly continue to refine the theories of health economics; there is a long way to go before there is anything like the same grasp of the problems of need-related resource allocation as there is of the free market system. The problems themselves are much tougher, and the study of them is in its infancy. Interesting work is being done on relative indexes of need,[7] based on professional and consumer judgments: for example, "How important is it to ameliorate this problem compared with that one?" or "How much pain and inconvenience am I prepared to undergo to achieve a specified improvement in my condition?" My own belief is that the search for a single index of need, which can then be used to determine how much to spend on hernias as compared to coronary bypass surgery, is rather like the search for the Holy Grail. It will never, I suspect, reach its goal, yet it should produce benefits in terms of insights and usable applications, and no doubt in the wisdom and holiness of the searchers.

I also have high hopes for the epidemiologists. Unfortunately much bad work will no doubt be done in the name of health service studies, but Professor A. L. Cochrane[8] is unquestionably right to emphasize how much more attention should be given to scientific assessment of the effectiveness and efficiency of most health care activities.

Meanwhile, at the same time that the economists and the epidemiologists pursue their inquiries, it seems to me that there are three developments that would put people who have to make health care resource allocation decisions in a better position than they now are for the immensely difficult task they face. These developments are:

1. To decentralize resource allocation so far as possible to the service of a defined local population.
2. To encourage flexibility within a defined budget.
3. To help people question current resource uses and consider the implications of major decisions affecting them.

The economic climate for health care today is a chilly one, and the responsibility for applying restraint is coming from the center, particularly from ministries of finance. There is a grave danger that nations will try to undertake the whole resource allocation task centrally, and that will lead to immense frustration locally and among the members of the medical and allied professions. The alternative is to develop a structure and an environment in which people do the best they can with the resources available to them locally, for a community that is large enough to pose resource choices and small enough to have personal identity. It is astounding and deeply encouraging how constructively people respond when they know what community they are trying to serve and what the resource constraints are, and are confident that they are responsible for giving the best service they can within those constraints. Allowed maximum flexibility they will of course make some mistakes. But even if mistakes are avoidable, which I doubt, the price paid for doing so is too high. Good health care at reasonable cost depends on the combined skills of many people and their determination to use those skills for the benefit of others. That does not require a free market system—indeed a free market system will never achieve it for a nation, as opposed to certain individuals within a nation—but it certainly requires a decentralized one.

References

1. Sandier S. (the reference is to figures presented by Madame Sandier at the Milan Seminar).
2. For this list I am indebted to Professor Abel-Smith in *Health Care Planning* edited Burkens, J. C. J., van Nieuwenhuizen, C. L. C. and Wiebenga, A. H., Excerpta Medica, Amsterdam, Oxford, 1976.
3. See Maxwell, R. *Health Care: The Growing Dilemma,* 2nd Edition, McKinsey and Company, New York, 1974.
4. See Jeffers, J. R. (the reference is to his paper at the Milan Seminar entitled, I think, *Financial Mechanisms and Their Implications for Health Price and Cost Inflation: The U.S. Experience.*)
5. Cooper, M. H. *Rationing Health Care,* Croom Helen, London, 1975, especially pages 20 to 24.
6. Culyer, A. J. *Need and the National Health Service,* Martin Robertson, London, 1976.
7. See, for example, the references in Culyer, A. J. op cit, pages 37 and 38.

Depression in Children

MICHAEL KOCH, MD
Director of Child and Adolescent Psychiatry
Saint Paul-Ramsey Hospital and Medical Center
Saint Paul, Minnesota

Although descriptions of depression began with Hippocrates (Lewis, 1967), there is still considerable controversy about its nature. Symptoms of sadness in children are not difficult to recognize, yet depression continues to be a poorly understood disorder of childhood. There is no general agreement about its classification, phenomenology, and biological characteristics.

It is necessary to distinguish sadness from a depressive syndrome. A lowered mood is the central feature of both, and in a depressive syndrome is characteristically accompanied by insomnia, loss of energy, and either agitation, or its opposite, psychomotor retardation.

Depression in children can have several different manifestations: (1) as a normal lowering of mood that is an expected response to situational stress;

(2) as a persistent abnormality of mood that is severe enough to be a handicapping condition and can be regarded as a distinctive clinical syndrome or disorder; (3) as a disease with a specific etiology or pathophysiology, symptom pattern, prognosis, and response to treatment.

FREQUENCY

The classic description of manic-depressive illness states that it is a disease of adulthood. Kraepelin (1921) reported that in a sample of 900 patients, 0.4% had their first manic-depressive episode before the age of 10 years. Many authors have subsequently contended that manic-depressive illness is rare in childhood. Kanner (1948), in his textbook of child psychiatry, states that the full-fledged depressive illness seen in adults is very rare in children. Anthony and Scott (1960) used ten rigid criteria for the diagnosis of manic-depressive illness in childhood. Using these criteria they analyzed cases described over an 80-year period as prepubertal manic-depressives and found only 3 verifiable cases (out of 28), which fulfilled only five of the criteria and had age of onset under 12 years. A more recent review of adolescent patients who, since 1971, were initially admitted to the UCLA Neuropsychiatric Institute with the diagnosis of schizophrenia and subsequently diagnosed as having bipolar manic-depressive illness, found 6 such patients, with age of onset of first episode of illness from 12 to 16 years (Carlson, 1976). In this study the diagnostic manifestations of affective disorder were identifiable even at the onset of illness. There is, therefore, a consensus that bipolar manic-depressive illness is exceedingly rare in children but may begin in adolescence.

Instead of looking for manic-depressive illness, more recent studies have looked for a modified clinical picture of childhood. Rutter et al. (1976b) studied the total population of 10- and 11-year-old children on the Isle of Wight. In the first stage they administered questionnaires of known reliability and validity to parents and teachers. Children scoring above a defined cut-off point were then studied intensely along with a randomly selected control group drawn from the same population. Among some 2000 children they calculated a one-year prevalence for affective disorder of 1.4 per thousand. Overt depressive disorder was found in only three girls and no boys although a larger number of children were quite unhappy. In another study, 14- and 15-year-old children showed a threefold increase in the prevalence of depressive disorder; out of 2303 adolescents in the general population there were 9 with a depressive disorder and another 26 who had a disorder involving both anxiety and depression. Feelings of unhappiness were still more common, occurring in a fifth of the adolescents (Rutter et al., 1976a).

Completed suicide is a rare event in children before the age of 12 years. Shaffer (1974) found no cases younger than this in his study. Most of the suicidal children had psychiatric problems before their death, but they took the form of both antisocial and emotional disorders. There was also a high incidence of depression and suicidal behavior in the children's parents and older siblings. Shaffer questions whether depression in adolescence might initially present as antisocial behavior.

CHARACTERISTICS OF DEPRESSIVE DISORDER

Almost every symptom has been claimed to be associated with depression in children (Malmquist, 1971). Part of the problem is that children can have difficulty describing their emotional states and adults may be unaware that children are feeling miserable. Careful questioning often elicits depressive symptoms, but Rutter and Graham (1968) found the lowest inter-rater reliability for two items of their structured psychiatric examination of children that dealt with affect. They also found low reliability in evaluating depressive affect and thought content in different interviews with a mean interval of 12 days. They concluded that children's behaviors used to infer depression are unstable and inconstant.

Depressive mood change with low self-esteem and guilt is the main characteristic of depressive disorder. Although uncomplaining, the child may look sad and be hard to cheer up. Depression in children is also often expressed by somatic symptoms. Abdominal pain, headache, transitory migratory aches and pains may reflect feelings of depression. When such symptoms recur frequently and when a physical cause cannot be found, emotional conflicts in the child and family should be investigated. Glaser (1967) called attention to the occurrence of "masked" depression in children and adolescents. He argues that depression can present as behavior problems or delinquency and may not be recognized. Cytryn and McKnew (1974) also describe "masked" depression as a common but unrecognized variety of depressive disorder in children. Using a psychodynamic orientation, they studied fantasy, self-description, and drawings of children and found the manifestations of depression to vary with the age of the child. If the concept of masked depression is correct, one should find a higher percentage of adult depressives in a cohort previously diagnosed as masked depression in children. This has not yet been demonstrated in follow-up studies.

Poznanski et al. (1976), however, did follow a small sample of ten children who had been diagnosed as overtly depressed between the ages of 3 and 12 years. On an average of more than six years later, 50% of them were clinically depressed and resembled adult depressives. This study lacked blind raters and a control group to indicate psychopathology in nondepressed children who were similarly studied at follow-up. Nevertheless, in this sample, depression was not merely a transient phase of development.

McConville et al. (1973) also found that the manifestation of depression depends on the developmental level the child has reached. Using an inpatient sample of 75 children with the primary symptoms of depression, they were able to differentiate developmentally overlapping subtypes of depression. Six- to eight-year-old children displayed an affective subtype of depression. They could not verbalize their thoughts but showed sadness and hopelessness. Eight- to twelve-year-olds had a more common self-esteem depression with rather fixed ideas of low self-esteem, worthlessness, and being unloved and used by others. A third or guilt depression was found to be uncommon and generally followed a loss that began after the age of 10 years. These children felt wicked and that they should be dead either because they were bad or to rejoin a dead person. Frequently they expressed suicidal thoughts. The authors concluded that an affectual depression occurs in younger children and gives way in midchildhood to a negative self-esteem type. This was most commonly seen in children with multiple placements and chronic losses. A less common guilt depression occurs later and probably represents a newly emerged depressive picture in those old enough to experience an adult-type mourning response. They found it to be most common in older children who had recent bereavements.

DEPRESSIVE DISORDER

Pearce (1978) made a systematic study of 547 children between 3 and 17 years attending a child psychiatric clinic. Twenty-three percent were rated as having the symptoms of depression defined as "morbid depression, sadness, unhappiness, and tearfulness." This group was compared with a control group from the same clinic without depression. The depressed children had a number of symptoms that were significantly associated with depression and formed a characteristic pattern of symptoms that could be defined as a specific depressive disorder. They were significantly older than the other children, more emotionally disturbed, and had more disturbed relationships within the family but not with peers. They were more likely to be anxious and to have disturbances of sleep and eating, suicidal thoughts, obsessions, and school refusal. These symptoms show a notable resemblance to those associated with depression in adults. More than 50% of the depressed children had the disorder present for more than one year. Pearce also found that the pattern of symptoms changes with age and sex. Depressed prepubertal children were more likely to have abdominal pain and alimentary disorder, school refusal, and irritability. Older children were more likely to have sleep disturbance and phobias. Depressed girls were more likely to have abdominal pain and gastrointestinal disorder. Depressed boys were more likely to have sleep and eating disorders, phobias, school refusal, and hypochondriasis. In very young children depression was less clearly defined, but with maturity the emotional symptoms were more differentiated and specific. Pearce also contends that the physical and psychological stresses of puberty are probably important in lowering the threshold for developing a depressive disorder.

Certain symptoms commonly regarded as depressive "equivalents" or masked depression were found by Pearce to be negatively associated with depression. For example, this was true for aggression, truancy, and enuresis which had no diagnostic significance for depressive disorder in his sample.

This study shows that it is possible to study and demarcate the symptoms that serve to make up depressive disorders in children. In this condition there is a characteristic association of depressed mood with various symptoms. The symptoms must represent a change in the child's usual functioning and be persistent and severe enough to be handicapping. However, there are still many questions. What is the outcome of children so diagnosed? Does childhood depression predispose to an adult depressive disorder? Is it related to cyclical forms of manic-depressive illness, and what is the value of antidepressant medication?

TREATMENT

Depression in children is often associated with a variety of acute and chronic stresses both within the family and outside the home. Treatment usually focuses on improving relationship at home, in school, and with peers. Individual, family, and group therapy have been used both to help the child find successful ways of coping with stress and to improve family functioning. In addition, when there is a depressive disorder with imparied functioning, a trial of antidepressants may be indicated.

Frommer (1967) treated a large series of depressed children in London. She divided them into three categories; 54 enuretic depressives, 74 mood depressives, and 62 phobic depressives. She found they differed in response to monomine oxidase inhibitors, tricyclic antidepressants, and minor tranquilizers. The enuretic group had the least favorable response, 41% compared with 70% in the other two groups. However, it is difficult from her report to tell how the groups differ and were selected for treatment, and there was some overlapping use of medications.

A more recent study by Weinberg et al. (1973) diagnosed depression in 42 children selected from a population of 72 referred to a psychoeducational clinic. To be considered depressed, a child had to either have dysphoric mood or self-deprecatory thinking as well as two or more symptoms from the following eight categories: aggressive difficult behavior; sleep disturbance; social withdrawal; change in attitude toward school; somatic complaints; change in school performance; loss of usual energy; unusual change in appetite or weight. These criteria are also inclusive of other diagnostic categories such as conduct disorders, but using them 58% of the children referred to their center were diagnosed as depressed. This is a very high estimate of the incidence of depression in children and has not been confirmed by other investigators. Similarly, their finding of a very strong relationship between affective disorder in children and first degree relatives (40 out of 45 cases) has not been replicated (Welner et al., 1977).

Drug treatment (amitriptyline) was recommended for 35 children. Eighteen of the nineteen treated showed notable improvement in contrast to only 6 of the 15 non-drug-treated depressive controls. The study was not double blind, and it is not clear what the data sources were, that is, child self-report, parent, school, or direct observation of the child. At any rate, the improvement was marked and would certainly need to be replicated by others.

Lithium has a definite place in the treatment of adult depressive disorders and the prophylaxis of mania. It was used extensively by Annell (1969) in children and adolescents with a variety of symptoms including flagrant psychosis but all with periodic course. Eleven of twelve children showed marked clinical change with lithium. This was not a controlled study, but the changes were dramatic.

In summary, depression in children is more complex than in adults because it occurs in a developing organism. In most children the sadness and unhappiness occurring with common emotional or conduct disorders probably has no genetic or special psychopathologic link to adult depression and is best viewed as a reaction to stress. In the preschool period, diagnostic classification is less satisfactory than in later life, and no clear-cut depressive state analagous to that in adulthood has been identified. In later childhood a child's moods become less transient and with sufficient stress and vulnerability, a persistent depressive disorder can occur. These symptoms vary with age, sex, personality, and previous experience, and according to Pearce, can be expected in 10 to 20% of children attending a psychiatric clinic. In adolescence "pure" depressive illness and bipolar psychosis occur but are rare. The prevalence of childhood depression cannot be determined unless there is better agreement about the definition of the condition. To date there have been few adequately controlled drug trials, and there is little evidence upon which to make strong statements regarding drug treatment.

References

Annell, A. -L. Manic-depressive illness in children and effect of treatment with lithium carbonate. *Acta Paedopsychiat. 36*: 292–301, 1969.

Anthony, E. J., and Scott, P. Manic-depressive psychosis in childhood. *J. Child Psychol. Psychiat. 1*: 53–72, 1960.

Carlson, G., and Strober, M. Manic-depressive illness in early adolescence: A study of clinical and diagnostic characteristics in six cases. *J. Am. Acad. Child Psychiat. 17*: 138–153, 1976.

Cytryn, L., and McKnew, D. H. Factors influencing the changing clinical expression of the depressive process in children. *Am. J. Psychiat. 131*: 879–881, 1974.

Frommer, E. A. Treatment of childhood depression with antidepressant drugs. *Br. Med. J. 1*: 729–732, 1967.

Glaser, K. Masked depression in children and adolescents. *Am. J. Psychother. 21*: 565–574, 1968.

Kanner, L. *Child Psychiatry* (2nd ed.). Springfield, Illinois: Charles C. Thomas, 1948, pp. 731–732.

Kraepelin, E. *Manic-Depressive Insanity and Paranoia*. Edinburgh: Livingston, 1921, p. 167.

Lewis, A. Melancholia: A historical review. In *The State of Psychiatry: Essays and Addresses*. New York: Science House, 1967.

Malmquist, C. P. Depressions in childhood and adolescence, I, *N. Engl. J. Med. 284*: 955–961, 1971; and II, *N. Engl. J. Med. 284*: 887–893, 1971.

Pearce, J. B. The recognition of depressive disorder in children. *J. R. Soc. Med. 71*: 494–500, 1978.

McConville, B. J., Boag, L. C., and Purohit, A. P. Three types of childhood depression. *Can. Psychiat. Assoc. J. 18*: 133–138, 1973.

Poznanski, E., Krahenbuhl, V., and Zrull, J. Childhood depression: A longitudinal perspective. *J. Am. Acad. Child Psychiat. 15*: 491–501, 1976.

Rutter, M., and Graham, P. The reliability and validity of the psychiatric assessment of the child: 1) Interview with the child. *Br. J. Psychiat. 114*: 563–579, 1968.

Rutter, M., Graham, P., Chadwick, O., and Yule, W. Adolescent turmoil: Fact or fiction. *J. Child Psychol. Psychiat. 17*: 35–56, 1976a.

Rutter, M., Tizard, J., Yule, W., Graham, P., and Whitmore, K. Isle of Wight studies, 1964–1974. *Psychol. Med. 6*: 313–332, 1976b.

Shaffer, D. Suicide in childhood and early adolescence. *J. Child Psychol. Psychiat. 15*: 275–291, 1974.

Weinberg, W. A., Rutman, J., Sullivan, L., Penick, E. C., and Dietz, S. G. Depression in children referred to an educational diagnostic center. *J. Pediat. 83*: 1065–1072, 1973.

Welner, Z., Welner, A., McCrary, M. A., and Leonard, M. A. Psychopathology in children of inpatients with depression: A controlled study. *J. Nerv. Ment. Dis. 164*: 408–413, 1977.

The Pathophysiology of Inflammation

JOHN V. HURLEY
Reader in Pathology
Department of Pathology
University of Melbourne
Parkville, Victoria, Australia

When men or animals are injured, a characteristic series of changes follows in the damaged area. This response of living tissues to injury is known as inflammation. There is nothing abnormal about inflammation. The injurious stimulus is abnormal, but the reaction it evokes is the only one that the tissues are capable of producing in the particular circumstances of that type of injury.

The response to injury is not short-lived, as for example the response of striated muscle to stimulation of its motor nerve, but may last for hours or even for days. In its first few hours the reaction is largely independent of the nature of the noxious agent, the response being very similar after widely diverse types of injury. Once this initial reaction has developed, subsequent changes within the damaged tissues depend upon the nature, severity, and duration of action of the injurious agent. It is convenient to describe first the early stages of inflammation and to follow this with an account of the possible later courses of the reaction.

THE PHENOMENA OF THE INITIAL RESPONSE TO INJURY

The complex changes that take place in the first few hours after injury can be appreciated best by study of living transparent tissues. Their essential features were described more than 100 years ago by Addison, Waller, and Cohnheim, and subsequent studies with more elaborate techniques have added little to their findings.

The early changes after injury involve three processes:

·1. *Changes in the caliber of and flow in small blood vessels.* After a brief and inconstant arteriolar constriction, there is sustained dilatation of all small blood vessels within the injured area. At first blood flow through the dilated vessels is rapid, but, as edema develops, the flow rate decreases progressively, and in some areas complete arrest of flow, or stasis, may develop. Stasis may be permanent and result in death of the affected vessel, but in many instances blood flow recommences and ultimately returns to normal.

2. *Increase in the permeability of small blood vessels and the formation of inflammatory exudate.* Two processes contribute to the formation of inflammatory exudate. The walls of small blood vessels in most tissues are freely permeable to water and small solute molecules, but almost completely impermeable to large molecules like plasma proteins. Active vasodilatation as occurs in acute inflammation increases the hydrostatic pressure within the microcirculation. This disturbs the hydrostatic–osmotic balance across the vascular wall and results in net loss of fluid from blood into extravascular tissues. However, the increased intravascular hydrostatic pressure does not increase protein leakage from the microcirculation, and will not account for the high protein content of inflammatory exudate. Cohnheim recognized this and considered that injury must cause some "molecular change" in the wall of small blood vessels. Nearly 100 years later Majno and Palade showed that the basis of protein leakage induced by agents such as histamine is the formation of temporary and reversible gaps in vascular endothelium. Subsequent work has shown that gap formation in normally continuous vascular endothelium is the invariable basis of leakage of plasma proteins into areas of inflammation. With mild and simple types of in-

jury the gaps are produced by active retraction of endothelial cells away from their neighbors, the movement being caused by activation of a contractile protein that is present in endothelial cell cytoplasm. In more severe injuries some gaps arise in the same way, but others are due to destruction of part of the endothelial lining of the leaking vessel. Once gaps have formed in endothelium, the underlying basement membrane forms no effective barrier to the escape of protein molecules, and the hydrostatic pressure within the vessel forces plasma out through the gap into extravascular tissues. The protein content of inflammatory exudate depends upon the relative magnitudes of these two processes, but is always less than that of plasma. Hence any protein that has escaped cannot reenter the blood by diffusion, but must be returned via the lymphatic system. This results in an increase in both the volume and protein content of lymph draining from the area of injury.

3. *Escape of leucocytes from circulating blood into extravascular tissues.* Soon after injury leucocytes within venules in the damaged area can be seen to strike the vascular wall and adhere to it, so that within a short time the inner aspect of many venules becomes covered with a layer of oscillating, adherent white blood corpuscles. The cells that adhere are mostly neutrophil polymorphnuclears together with some eosinophils and monocytes. Lymphocytes are not involved. Leucocytic sticking has been shown to be due to a change in the endothelium that lines the affected vessels, but the nature of this change is not understood.

Many of the adherent cells subsequently pass through the venular wall by active amoeboid movement and move about in the adjacent extravascular tissues. It is believed that both the emigration and subsequent movement of leucocytes occur under the influence of chemical concentration gradients, a process known as chemotaxis. Recent electron microscope studies have confirmed the long held belief that leucocytes emigrate through the junctions between endothelial cells and not through endothelial cell cytoplasm.

THE LATER COURSE OF THE REACTION

Resolution

After injury that is short-lived or is rapidly and successfully overcome by the body's defense mechanisms, the early inflammatory changes may resolve completely or subside leaving a variable quantity of scar tissue within the injured area.

Complete resolution can occur only if the damaging agent does not cause areas of dead tissue above a certain critical size. In most tissues single cells or a small group of cells can be killed, their remains removed, and the defect filled in by division of neighboring cells of the same kind. However, local defects in tissue more than a few cells in size become filled with newly formed scar tissue by processes described below.

Resolution involves subsidence of vascular changes such as vasodilatation and increased permeability, and removal of all abnormal material from the extravascular spaces of the area of injury. As vasodilatation subsides, the hydrostatic–osmotic balance across the wall of small blood vessels returns to its resting state. As a result much of the fluid of the inflammatory exudate is reabsorbed into the venous end of the capillaries. The rest of the fluid and all the protein of the exudate are removed via lymphatics. Lymphatic capillaries have a thinner wall than blood capillaries, and the junctions between their endothelial cells are of simpler form. Some junctions are either normally open or open after physiological stimuli, so that there is no effective barrier to the passage of proteins from the extravascular space into terminal lymphatics. Fine fibrils join the outer aspect of the endothelium of terminal lymphatics to adjacent connective tissue structures. When tissues swell because of accumulation of inflammatory exudate, these fibrils exert an outward pull on the lymphatic wall, so that lymphatics in areas of inflammation become widely distended. Once fluid has entered terminal lymphatics, its passage centrally occurs by the combined action of lymphatic valves and of pressure from surrounding tissues, especially striated muscle. Active contraction of smooth muscle present in the wall of collecting lymphatics aids lymphatic flow.

When emigration of polymorphs ceases in areas of resolving inflammation, most polymorphs disappear within 24 or 48 hours. Some migrate away via lymphatics or tissue spaces, but most die locally, disintegrate, and liberate their lysomal granules and cytoplasmic enzymes into the tissue spaces. These enzymes aid in the digestion of adjacent dead tissue cells; the more polymorphs there are present, the more rapidly does digestion of dead tissues take place. As polymorphs disappear, they are replaced by a population of large mononuclear cells called macrophages. The origin of macrophages was in dispute for a long time, but in recent years it has been shown that they are emigrated, transformed blood monocytes. Macrophages are both long-lived and highly phagocytic. When dead tissues produce material that cannot be broken down by enzymes released from dying polymorphs, it is ingested by macrophages. Inside these cells it may either be digested or remain sequestered and unaltered for long periods. A good example of the latter is the carbon particles used in tattooing, which can be seen within the cytoplasm of macrophages many years after tattooing.

Suppuration

If the injurious stimulus persists and is of a type that evokes massive emigration of polymorphs, the inflammation will not resolve but proceeds to suppuration (pus formation). Pus may form diffusely through loose tissues or in body cavities, or be localized into discrete collections known as abscesses. The common cause of suppuration is invasion of tissues by certain microorganisms, the most important of which are staphylococci, some types of streptococci, and *E. coli* and related bacilli. Abscesses develop as follows. Organisms start to multiply soon after their introduction into tissues and liberate increasing quantities of toxin, which damage neighboring cells. An acute inflammatory reaction is evoked, starting soon after inoculation and increasing in intensity as the number of microorganisms increases. If enough toxin forms, cells in the central part of the lesion die. Many extravascular polymorphs die as well, either by reaching the end of their life span or by the action of bacterial toxins. Enzymes liberated from dead polymorphs liquefy and break down the dead cells, and 48 hours after inoculation a ragged cavity filled with pus is present within an area of acutely inflamed tissue. Pus consists of dead and living polymorphs, dead and living microorganisms, and the debris of dead cells suspended in inflammatory exudate. Subsequent changes in the abscess are the result of two simultaneous processes. Proliferation of microorganisms continues, more polymorphs enter the injured area, more tissue cells and polymorphs are destroyed, and as a result the size of the abscess increases progressively. At the same time repair processes begin in surrounding tissues, and a layer of newly formed connective tissue starts to form around the abscess and separate it from adjacent, still inflamed, tissues. Inflammation in the surrounding area subsides as the barrier of new tissue is formed, but polymorphs continue to escape in large numbers from vessels within the new tissue, and migrate inward to add to the amount of pus present in the abscess.

Repair

Like the initial response to injury, repair is a stereotyped process, and the same changes are seen in such diverse circumstances as the walling off of an abscess, the filling in of a defect produced by resorption of a sterile area of dead tissue, and the healing of an open wound. In man and higher animals local defects in tissue are not replaced by tissue of the type that has been lost, but instead by newly formed connective tissue, known as scar tissue. Its main constituents are small blood vessels and lymphatics, connective tissue cells, ground substance, and collagen and elastic fibers. Newly formed vessels arise from the endothelium of existing vessels as outgrowths or sprouts that join one another to form thin-walled vascular loops, oriented at right angles to the base of a wound or the cavity of an abscess. This early scar tissue is called granulation tissue. Its vessels later rearrange themselves and change in structure to become a mature type of microcirculation. New connective tissue cells, known as fibroblasts, arise by mitosis of cells situated in the connective tissues surrounding the wound. The fibroblasts migrate into the tissue defect where they synthesize and secrete into extravascular tissues the proteins of connective tissue ground substance and fibers. Both new blood vessels and lymphatics and new connective tissue cells are of purely local origin—cells derived from the blood have been shown to play no part in their formation. Proliferation of endothelial cells and fibroblasts begins within a day or so of injury, but formation of the new connective tissue fibers, which are required to give strength to the new tissue, does not start until 5 to 7 days later.

Chronic Inflammation

If the injurious stimulus persists but does not evoke massive polymorph emigration, the initial reaction may be succeeded by a long-lasting (chronic) nonsuppurative response. Many types of injury, physical, chemical, and microorganismal, cause this type of response. Chronic inflammation is not stereotyped like the acute reaction to injury, and its characteristics vary widely in different types of injury. It is neither possible nor necessary to describe these variations in detail. However, all chronic inflammation shares certain common features: accumulation of cells is much more prominent than formation of inflammatory exudate, continued destruction of tissue and inflammation proceed at the same time as attempted repair, and the cellular reaction is pleomorphic, many different types of cell being present in the inflamed tissues. The characteristic cell of chronic inflammation is the macrophage and its derivatives, epithelioid cells and giant cells. The naked-eye appearance of chronic inflammation is also variable— it may appear as an ulcer, a diffuse fibrosis of the wall of an organ, or a localized inflammatory lump (granuloma).

MECHANISMS OF ACUTE INFLAMMATION

The stereotyped response seen in the first few hours after different types of injury, suggests that injurious stimuli may not act directly on small blood vessels and leucocytes, but instead may produce their effects indirectly via substances liberated from injured tissues. It is widely believed that such endogenous mediators are responsible for many aspects of the inflammatory response. A large number of substances are known to be present in injured tissues in concentrations that can induce vasodilatation, increased vascular permeability, or chemotactic effects on various types of leucocyte. Potent mediators have been shown to be liberated from mast cells, from antigen-stimulated lymphocytes, from polymorphs, and from various components of the blood coagulation, fibrinolytic, and complement systems of blood plasma. The problem, which is still unsolved, is to determine which, if any, of an embarrassingly large list of mediators is concerned in any particular type of injury.

To add further complexity to the problem, it has been shown that in many types of increased vascular permeability no mediator at all is involved, the leakage being due to direct injury to the wall of small blood vessels within the injured area. It is clear that inflammation should not be regarded as a single mechanism, but involves a number of distinct, yet interrelated processes, which can contribute in varying degree to the response to any particular type of injury. Much more work in both experimental pathology and pharmacology is needed before it will be possible to change the course of the inflammatory response by the administration of drugs with a specific action on one or more mediator systems.

THE FUNCTION OF THE INFLAMMATORY REACTION

What is the purpose of the complex series of events that constitute the inflammatory reaction? Inflammation brings two elements to the site of injury— leucocytes and blood plasma. As Metchnikoff first pointed out 100 years ago, the migration of wandering cells to an area of injury is the constant and characteristic reaction of all types of animal from water fleas to man. The primary function of the migrating cells is phagocytosis—the engulfment and if possible the digestion of living or dead foreign material. In higher animals the cells that migrate in this way are blood leucocytes. Polymorphs and macrophages are powerful phagocytes, and in recent years the ways in which these cells destroy ingested microorganisms have been worked out in considerable detail. Phagocytosis is of great importance in the protection of higher animals from bacterial invasion, and individuals lacking polymorphs or monocytes are prone to frequent and often fatal infections. Polymorphs have a second function in areas of sterile inflammation—lysosomal enzymes derived from living or dead polymorphs break down dead tissues into soluble fragments which can be removed via lymphatics; the insoluble residues are engulfed by macrophages.

The purpose of escape of blood plasma into an area of injury is more complex. In bacterial infections the exuded plasma brings specific and nonspecific antibacterial substances to the injured area. Some of these humoral factors act directly against microorganisms, for example, antitoxins, whereas others act in cooperation with phagocytic cells as nonspecific or as immune opsonins. The subject of the specific or immune response to foreign proteins (antigens) is of immense importance in infections and some other types of injury. It is the function of another system of cells found in both blood and tissues, the lymphocytes. The topic is far too large to discuss in the present chapter.

What role does inflammatory exudate play in noninfective inflammation? Some of its actions are simple, for example, the washing away or dilution of noxious chemical irritants, but its most important role is probably indirect.

Recent work has shown that many of the endogenous mediators of the inflammatory response, especially the factors responsible for chemotactic attraction of polymorphs and monocytes, arise by interaction of components of the plasma complement system. Work in recent years suggests that the most important role of the leakage of plasma into an area of sterile injury is to permit activation of the complement system in the escaped plasma, which in turn attracts polymorphs and monocytes to the injured area.

Very little is known of the control of the later stages of the reaction to injury, healing, and scar tissue formation. Deficiencies in one or more elements essential for healing may delay the process, but no specific accelerators of the processes of repair are known.

References

Hurley, J. V. *Acute Inflammation.* Edinburgh and London: Churchill-Livingstone, 1972.

Lepow, I. H., and Ward, P. A. *Inflammation. Mechanisms and Controls.* New York: Academic Press, 1972.

Ryan, G. B., and Majno, G. Acute inflammation—a review. *Am. J. Pathol., 86*: 185, 1977. (Up-to-date list of references, especially re chemical mediators.)

Environmental Pollutants and Bone Remodeling

C. ANDERSON, M.D., M.R.C.Path., F.C.A.P., F.R.C.P.(C).
Department of Pathology
Health Sciences Center
University of Western Ontario
London, Ontario, Canada

Bone remodeling is a concept that relatively few people understand. Perhaps behavior of bone in the adult has been difficult to grasp because early investigators were not interested in spending the amount of effort and time needed to study in detail those alterations that led to the curious anatomical skeletal

The author is a recipient of research grants, Nos. MA6015 and ME6041 from the Medical Research Council of Canada, from the Atkinson Charitable Foundation, and from the University Hospital Research Trust Fund.

changes one occasionally sees gathering dust in medical museums. The situation has been further complicated in the recent past by scientists who have spent enormous amounts of public funds investigating changes occurring in the levels of substances in the blood and attributing these changes directly or indirectly to abnormalities in bone function without actually studying the supposed bone changes occurring in the skeleton concurrently.

THEORY OF BONE REMODELING

The term bone remodeling indicates a function of the skeletal tissues that involves the replacement of those tissues on an ongoing basis after the individual has reached the stage of skeletal maturity. Bone modeling, on the other hand, refers to the function undertaken by skeletal tissues in order to obtain their adult shape and size, which will not be discussed further here. The reader who is interested in furthering his knowledge of bone remodeling is referred to a work by Frost (1974), from which previous references outlining the rationale and the methods for investigating this subject may be traced. Stated succinctly— although by no means exhaustively—bone remodeling is the process by which the skeleton varies its form and selectively replaces its constituents over the years in response to a number of stimuli, be these mechanico/electrical (in the form of piezo-electrical stimulation) or chemical, responding to the body's requirements or excesses of certain minerals and organic substances that form the basis of bone.

The studies on bone that have attracted most of the research endeavors during the past 20 years or so have been of a chemical or physiological nature. Although a significant proportion of these studies have contributed a great deal to the understanding of the mechanisms of calcium and phosphorus metabolism (the two essential elements in the mineral phase of bone), few have focused on the mechanisms through which bone is capable of responding to specific challenges.

The homeostatic control of levels of ionic calcium in tissue fluids that are necessary for the adequate function of cell membranes depends on a number of factors. Those known to date include the integrity of function of the gastrointestinal tract for the adequate absorption of dietary calcium and the integrity of the function of the kidneys in charge of the appropriate retention of calcium from the glomerular filtrate fluid. It has more recently been shown that metabolites of vitamin D (nowadays considered to be a pro-hormone) are necessary for the proper function of both the gastrointestinal tract and the kidneys (to absorb and retain calcium respectively), through the stimulation of the production of calcium binding protein. It is also known that adequate circulating levels of parathyroid hormone are required for the proper metabolism of vitamin D intermediaries in the kidney tubular cell (in conjunction with appropriate intracellular concentrations of phosphate), and that calcitonin, a hormone produced by the "C" cells of the human thyroid exerts a conservative action with regard to the removal of calcium from the skeleton. When a conflict arises between the maintenance of adequate levels of calcium in body fluids and skeletal integrity, bone—the major reservoir of calcium in the body—is sacrificed in order to provide the required calcium. But bone can do this because it is endowed with the cellular mechanism through which it can respond to these requirements.

Human adult bone consists of a cortical (compact) and a cancellous (trabecular) moiety (Figure 1). This bone is constantly replacing itself on various surfaces (envelopes) in a particular cycle which is characteristic for each bone and each

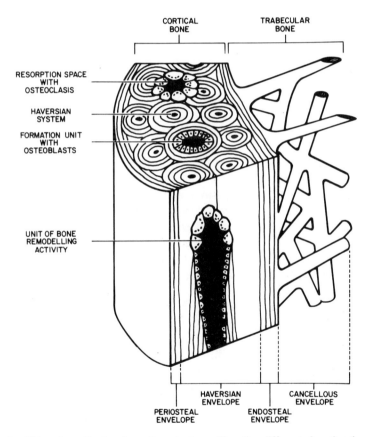

FIG. 1. This schematic drawing attempts to outline the different functional areas of bone. The unit of bone remodeling activity proceeds in cortical bone in an upward direction, the osteoclastic bone resorption being followed by osteoblastic bone formation, thus replacing bone in a lamellar fashion.

site on the same bone. When bone is resting, its surfaces are lined by a layer of flattened mesenchymal cells. When a particular site of bone is stimulated, some of these mesenchymal cells will become activated and transform into osteoclasts. These cells possess the capacity of removing a given quantity of bone in a given time period. Once bone resorption has taken place, mesenchymal cells transform into osteoblasts whose function it is to lay down new bone to suit the new demands of the skeletal site. The osteoblasts fill in the gap previously created by the osteoclasts by forming organic bone matrix and later mineralizing it. These osteoblasts produce a predetermined quantity of bone in a predetermined period of time, and as they do so, they become embedded in their own product and transform into osteocytes retaining fine connections (canaliculi) with their adjoining sister cells. As the reader may appreciate, resorption and formation of a volume of bone takes place within a certain period of time, which is known as sigma and varies for each species. The speed at which this takes place, that is, the number of mesenchymal cells activated in a given volume of bone and the amount of bone that is resorbed and replaced, is frequently referred to as bone turnover rate.

The speed and amount of bone that is remodeled can be measured. There are today on the market fairly nontoxic substances like the tetracycline antibiotics and 2,4 Bis,N,N[1], di carboxy-methyl amino-methyl fluorescein (to name a few) that when administered intramuscularly in adequate solvents will deposit in bone alongside the site where bone is being mineralized at the time of injection. Two injections of any of these substances can be administered at a known time interval (e.g., 14 days), and anything formed between these two "labels" can be identified as having occurred during a specific period of time. Following the last injection, a standardized portion of bone is removed and, when adequately processed, studied with the assistance of an ultraviolet light microscope. The labels will be seen to fluoresce in the tissue. By means of calibrated grids on the ocular lens of the microscope, the tissue and all its characteristics (surface areas, number of elements, lengths of margins, distances between labels, and width of structures) can be measured and expressed in numbers. The rationale and methodology for carrying out measurements through the use of the microscope may be obtained from Weibel and Elias (1967). Although the different bone envelopes may remodel at different speeds within a similar site, the measurements of parameters of haversian bone constitute the most practical envelope of bone to use because of the natural geometrical architecture of cortical bone vis-à-vis the random nature and properties of cancellous bone.

If the results of studies carried out on experimental animals are to be extrapolated to man, then an experimental animal showing sufficient comparable cortical structure to that of man should be used. We have found the dog to be quite satisfactory in this respect. Various measurements are taken on the chosen sample of bone. These include the total surface area of bone examined, the cortical area of bone, and the ratio between the two; the number, width, circumference, and percent of osteoid seams taking a fluorescent label; the mean thickness of completed haversian systems and certain derived calculations such as the activation frequency, the mean appositional rate, the radial closure rate, the osteon formation time, the bone formation rate, and the ratio of resorption to formation. All these measurements and more are explained in the work of Frost (1974). As is always the case when statistical analysis of biological observations is envisaged, the research worker should perform his measurements on a number of sections of each bone sample (e.g., ten) and also have sufficient numbers of experimental animals for his analysis to meet the statistical requirements. It is also important to bear in mind that bone remodeling activity in experimental animals, as in man, varies with age, so that the age-related variations in each parameter should be known.

ENVIRONMENTAL POLLUTANTS

Throughout life man is exposed to a diversity of elements that may adversely influence the status of his health and well-being. This exposure may be acute and/or massive, giving rise to situations recognized medically as instances of intoxication, or they may be chronic, of a minimal dose, producing biological alterations due to their cumulative effects or producing effects long after exposure to that minimal dose is ended. These elements may be present as a result of naturally occurring physical or chemical phenomena in the environment, or they may be present as a result of the presence of man in the environment per se. Although the history of man's industrial activity goes back several millenia, it is only within the past hundred years, as a result of the Industrial Revolution of the nineteenth century and the technological advances of the twentieth century, that the history and hazards resulting from that industrial activity and the effects on health of waste and other by-products have been recognized for their environmental significance. The industrial pollutants influence not only man but numerous other species of life that co-inhabit this planet.

The lay public is aware of the articles on this topic that appear in the media from time to time and the fairly recent institution of governmental agencies whose role it is to study the effects of industry on the environment, to monitor the quality of air, water, and food to which man is exposed, and to propose legislation to force industry to meet certain safety standards. The interested reader is referred to a recent publication by Wallbot (1973) in which more detailed information on the health effects of environmental pollutants will be found, for it is impossible in an article like this to discuss in depth the sources and mechanisms of action, the health effects and other special situations arising from the exposure of man to numerous environmental pollutants. This is particularly so because the aim of this article is to point out the scant information that still exists concerning the effects of environmental pollutants on bone remodeling. Most of the studies on environmental pollutants and bone concern themselves with the fact that a specific pollutant is a "bone seeker" (i.e., is deposited in greater quantities in bone than in other tissues) or with the fact that exposure to a pollutant produces a gross abnormality, a radiologically observable difference, a variation in the ash content or observable cellular abnormalities in the bones of experimental animals (or humans exposed to these same elements) and not in control subjects.

When I became interested in this subject a few years ago, I realized that only a few studies on bone remodeling had been published in the medical and veterinary literature in relation to the toxic effects of high doses of fluoride. It was evident also from epidemiological studies that complications arising from states in man in which there was a decreased or abnormal skeletal mass (which could be attributed to long-term alterations in bone remodeling activity) were more frequent in urban than in rural populations and also more frequent in industrialized than in nonindustrialized communities. Also of note was the fact that a previous publication had described a number of patients in whom bone remodeling activity was reduced to practically zero without there being an obvious attributable cause. Further perusal of the medical and veterinary literature revealed that as skeletal integrity is closely tied to the adequate function of other body systems, one would have to consider whether the effects of particular substances on bone were mediated directly on bone or were an indirect consequence of malfunction of another system (vide supra). Part of the literature on environmental pollutants deals with the action of specific substances in cell culture systems in the artificial situation of the laboratory. If the findings of these in vitro experiments were to be attributable to an in vivo situation, it could be envisaged that bone remodeling—a cell-mediated activity—could also be influenced by these same substances. So the question posed was that if certain environmental pollutants interfered with the function of organs such as the small intestine or the kidneys, would it not be possible that these same pollutants affected bone remodeling primarily before they exerted a secondary action on bone through malfunction of other systems? This possibility merited testing experimentally.

As in the previously mentioned reference on environmental pollutants, lead, fluoride, and strontium 90 were elements known to deposit in bone and to produce demonstrable abnormalities in structure and composition. Lead, arsenic, fluoride, zinc, and vanadium are known to affect the small intestine, while mercury and cadmium are known to affect the kidneys. It was known that these pollutants exerted an effect on tissues in dose-related fashion and that individuals living in areas where there were high concentrations of these pollutants had higher levels of them in their tissues. There existed then a number of environmental pollutants that theoretically could influence bone remodeling. Of recent and more practical importance is the report that aluminum may play a significant role in the production of abnormalities of bone remodeling in patients who are continuously exposed to dialyzing machines. Of all the elements mentioned only a few have been investigated in order to find out whether they exert a primary effect on bone remodeling activity.

EFFECTS OF ENVIRONMENTAL POLLUTANTS ON BONE REMODELING

The study of the effects of environmental pollutants on bone remodeling activity is delicate, costly, and demanding of meticulous attention to detail. In the first place an experimental animal with a bone remodeling pattern similar to man's should preferably be employed. The animals should not have previously been exposed to environmental pollutants, and the normal age-related variations of the bone remodeling activity should be known. It is also advantageous to know as much as possible about the normal biochemical, hematological, gastrointestinal, renal, and parathyroid parameters of the animal. For all these reasons I have found the pure-bred standardized research beagle purchased from a reliable breeding laboratory to be the most adequate experimental animal.

Ongoing studies in this department have dealt with the determination of alterations in bone remodeling parameters produced in dogs by chronic low doses of lead and nitrilotriacetic acid, substances that are known to deposit in bone; and cadium and zinc, substances that are known to produce alterations in the kidney and intestine. During the duration of the experiments complete biochemical and hematological profiles are carried out, together with estimations of blood and tissue concentrations of the elements under investigation, as well as determinations of levels of parathyroid hormones and vitamin D metabolites. Indirect assessments of gastrointestinal and renal functions are performed. Bone remodeling parameters are measured on haversian bone before and after periods of exposure, the experimental results being compared to untreated controls and to the data obtained from the determination of similar parameters for the untreated age-matched dog population. Most of the results have been submitted for publication at present, but as can be seen from Danylchuk (1978), both cadmium and lead produce a marked decrease in bone remodeling activity without there being evidence of dysfunction of other organs that participate in bone physiology. Nitrilotriacetic acid produces minimal defects on bone mineralization by acting directly on bone, while zinc produces no effect at all on bone organs. Thus we have applied a multidisciplinary approach to the physiology of bone and the possible direct effects of environmental pollutants.

THE FUTURE

Major emphasis on the health effects of environmental pollutants is at present being diverted toward the possible effects of these pollutants in cancer causation. Cancer, is after degenerative vascular disease, the major cause of death in industrialized communities.

Complications arising from abnormalities in both skeletal structure and function occur most frequently in the aged population. Industrialized communities, where the complications are most numerous, show a proportional increase of their aged population. Because skeletal complications in the elderly are slow to repair and place a heavy burden on patient care-related activities, they depend on a relatively large proportion of hospital budgetary health costs. Thus in the future the costs of treatment of these patients may increase as a result of pollutants that are being released into the environment at the present time.

There is also a need for increased investigation of the effects of various environmental pollutants on bone remodeling because the end result is a decrease in the quality of life (pain, immobility, fractures) and the corresponding demand on health care costs.

The surface of this topic has barely been scratched. Much more research is needed in order to avoid or minimize these problems.

References

Danylchuk, K. D. The effects of environmental pollutants on bone remodelling. Ph.D. thesis, University of Western Ontario, London, Ontario, 1978.

Frost, H. M. *Bone Modelling and Skeletal Modelling Errors.* Orthop. Lecture Series IV. Springfield, Illinois: Charles C. Thomas, 1974.

Wallbot, G. L. *Health Effects of Environmental Pollutants.* St. Louis: C. V. Mosby, 1973.

Weibel, E., and Elias, H. Quantitative methods in morphology. *Proceedings of the Symposium on Quantitative Methods in Morphology. Eighth International Congress of Anatomists.* Berlin: Springer-Verlag, 1967.

Infectious Hepatitis

Y. E. COSSART, M.B., B.S., B.Sc., D.C.P., F.R.C.Path.
Department of Bacteriology
University of Sydney

and

E. J. WILLS, M.D., B.S., B.Sc. (Med.), D.C.P.
Department of Pathology
Royal Prince Alfred Hospital

The term infectious or viral hepatitis is usually restricted to an acute infection that produces its clinical effects through diffuse involvement of the liver paren-chymal cells. Traditionally, infection by known viruses such as infectious mono-nucleosis, glandular fever, and yellow fever, or bacteria including spirochetes, is excluded. Because of different clinical patterns two groups were described, "in-fectious hepatitis" proper, in which there was frequently a history of prior con-tact with a jaundiced patient, a relatively short incubation period, and resolution to normality; and "serum hepatitis," in which there was a history of previous blood transfusion or injections, a longer incubation period, and frequently a less benign course. Over the last ten years it has become evident that the long-held presumption that these diseases were caused by two different viruses (now called hepatitis A and B) was indeed warranted, and although the agents cannot yet be cultivated in vitro, a great deal is becoming known about their nature. Recently, a third group referred to as "non-A, non-B hepatitis" has been recognized, which will probably prove to be caused by more than one virus.

CLINICAL FEATURES

All three agents produce a similar acute illness. Malaise, anorexia, and vague abdominal symptoms precede the appearance of jaundice by several days. Some patients with hepatitis B experience a prodromal rash or arthritis which may give a clue to the etiology. The serum transaminase levels reflect the extent of liver damage and may be quite elevated in anicteric cases. Thus, in addition to their value in charting the course of the individual acute case, transaminase esti-mations are widely used in epidemiological studies and have revealed many sub-clinical infections. Fatal hepatocellular failure occurs in less than 1% of patients, but is more common in older subjects and individuals with protein undernutrition. Chronic liver damage develops after acute infection in a small proportion of cases. Although recovery is followed by life-long immunity to the infecting agent, there is no cross protection or increased susceptibility to the other two viruses.

LIVER PATHOLOGY

Regardless of which infectious hepatitis virus is responsible, the histological changes in the liver during the acute phase are identical. Furthermore, drugs such as amine oxidase inhibitors or the anesthetic agent halothane may also rarely produce a similar picture. The normal trabecular pattern becomes mosaiclike from the swelling of parenchymal cells, which, in extreme form, leads to "balloon degeneration" of some cells. At the same time, other cells show shrinkage with eosinophilic cytoplasmic condensation and nuclear karyorrhexis to produce acidophilic (Councilman) bodies, which lie free in the sinusoids or are phagocytosed by Kupffer cells. Necrosis is spotty, and lost hepatocytes are replaced by mononuclear inflammatory cells with occasional neutrophils and eosinophils. A similar infiltrate occupies the portal tracts. Phagocytosis of degenerate material by Kupffer cells and portal tract macrophages produces ceroid pigmentation.

Electron microscopy has established that the swelling and pallor of parenchymal cells is due to dilatation of the endoplasmic reticulum and accumulation of flocculent material within the distended cisternae, whereas acidophilic degeneration is associated with closely packed altered organelles in a dense cytoplasmic matrix. Mitochondria show nonspecific abnormalities, and autophagic activity is increased.

Except in the cholestatic form of hepatitis, bile pigment is not prominent by light microscopy, but at the fine structural level cytoplasmic pigment deposits are evident in many cells, and the bile canaliculi may show cholestatic changes. Microvilli along the space of Disse may also be altered, so that there is probably defective transport at both the sinusoidal and the biliary poles of the liver cell.

In the average case, recovery is associated with regeneration of hepatocytes along the essentially unaltered reticulin framework. However, cases with "bridging" necrosis between adjacent portal tracts, central veins, or both are less likely to recover fully. Kupffer cells and portal tract macrophages retain their phagocytosed pigment, while the inflammatory infiltrate, particularly in portal tracts, may persist for six months or more before resolving. At the other extreme, occasional patients develop massive hepatic necrosis with isolated islands of parenchymal cells separated by debris containing pigment-laden macrophages and inflammatory cells. Should the patient survive, complete resolution may follow, or nodular regeneration of parenchymal cells and fibrous scarring may produce a macronodular cirrhosis.

Occasionally there develops a recurrent relapsing form of the disease associated with focal intralobular necrosis (chronic lobular hepatitis). Infectious hepatitis may also progress to chronic active hepatitis, but its overall importance in this entity is uncertain because of the lack of evidence of previous viral hepatitis or, indeed, any other antecedent factor, in the majority of cases. Here the histological pattern is usually that of chronic aggressive hepatitis, characterized by portal tract inflammation that extends into the parenchymal, causing piecemeal necrosis or "nibbling away" and the formation of interlobular septa, with ultimate progression to cirrhosis.

Although convincing virus particles have not been identified in liver biopsies in the other forms, the parenchymal cell nuclei in hepatitis B may contain spherical particles of approximately 23 nm diameter that have been identified by immunoelectron microscopy as the core antigen; occasionally they may be present in sufficient numbers to produce a "sanded" appearance in conventional histological sections. Likewise, small tubular inclusions associated with hepatitis B surface antigen may be seen within the endoplasmic reticulum and, for reasons that are unclear, may be demonstrated at the light microscopic level by certain connective tissue stains, notably Shikata's modified orcein method. Cells with cytoplasmic antigen often have a "ground glass" appearance in hematoxylin-eosin stained sections, but it is nonspecific, since it is associated merely with proliferation of the smooth-surfaced endoplasmic reticulum. Both the nuclear and cytoplasmic antigens can be demonstrated by immunofluorescence, but the problems associated with antiserum preparation preclude this from becoming a routine technique. It is worth emphasizing that although hepatitis B antigens can be demonstrated in liver specimens from cases with chronic hepatitis or asymptomatic carriers, they are not usually seen in the acute case. Furthermore, from a practical point of view, these methods are less useful than the detection of hepatitis B antigen in the blood.

HEPATITIS A

Hepatitis A is the best understood of the hepatitis viruses. It can be transmitted experimentally to man, chimpanzees, and some species of marmosets by oral administration or parenteral injection of either serum or fecal extracts from acute cases. The incubation period is from 2 to 4 weeks, and the agent may be recovered from the feces for about a week before, and a few days after the serum transaminase levels begin to rise. The virus particles are spherical, 27 nm in diameter, of specific gravity 1.34 g/cm^3, and contain RNA. These features together with the presence of similar particles in the cytoplasm of liver cells of acutely infected marmosets, are characteristic of an enterovirus. The epidemiology of hepatitis A is also typical of an enterovirus with spread by the fecal/oral route. The main reservoir of infection is in young children. As with poliomyelitis the symptoms in infants are often so mild that they escape notice unless the agent is transmitted to older members of the household, but even among adults there are many subclinical or anicteric infections. For these reasons the isolation of patients with clinical hepatitis has little effect on the prevalence of the disease in the community even though almost half of the affected subjects can point to the source of their infection as a household contact with a jaundiced person.

Hepatitis A is endemic in situations such as residential institutions for mentally defective persons and underdeveloped countries where it is difficult to prevent fecal pollution of water supplies and foodstuffs. Although a general improvement in sanitation reduces the incidence of hepatitis A, nevertheless half the population in North America, Western Europe, and Australia have been infected before they reach adult life, so that immunoglobulin pooled from unselected blood donations contains sufficient antibody to protect against the disease. It is thought that, like poliovirus, hepatitis A multiplies initially in the lymphoid cells of the intestinal mucosa and that immunoglobulin protects by neutralizing virus particles in the bloodstream before they reach their "target organ," the liver. This accords with the observation that immunoglobulin protects against symptoms if given within a week of exposure. Passively administered IgG does not reach the lumen of the gut; so the infectivity of the individual is not significantly decreased. Travelers, and the staff of institutions where hepatitis is endemic, can be protected by administering immunoglobulin before exposure, but because the half life of injected IgG is relatively short, repeated doses may be needed.

So far all the samples of 27-nm particles extracted from feces of patients with hepatitis A have been antigenically identical. There is therefore every reason to anticipate that an effective vaccine will be made to combat the disease. Despite the ease with which most enteroviruses multiply in human and primate cell cultures, hepatitis A remains as elusive as ever, and no further progress can be made toward this goal until the virus can be grown in vitro. Diagnostic tests for hepatitis A virus in feces are too elaborate for routine use, and in any case very few particles are detectable by the time the patient develops jaundice. Serum antibody is also present at this stage, and quantitative measurement of a rising titer between acute and convalescent samples of blood or even specific IgM formation is therefore required.

HEPATITIS B

Patients with active hepatitis B infection are readily identified by the presence of hepatitis B surface antigen (HBsAg) in their serum. The antigen is present in large amounts (up to 10 mg/liter) and is of various shapes constructed from antigenically identical subunits. The most numerous are small spheres 20 nm in diameter. Most samples contain tubular forms, also 20 nm in diameter but of quite variable length. Least common, and absent from many specimens, are double-shelled particles, 40 nm in diameter.

Treatment with detergent disrupts the small spheres and tubules as well as stripping the other shell from the double-shelled particles to yield a 27-nm-diameter core of different antigenic structure (hepatitis B core antigen, HBcAg). All three forms of HBsAg have a specific gravity of about 1.20 g/cm^3, which is much too light for infectious nucleic acid-containing icosohedral virus particles. Biochemical studies have been hampered by the difficulty of purifying the particles, but it is agreed that they consist mainly of lipoprotein.

The nature of the hepatits B virus is still unknown. The double-shelled particles, which contain a small amount of DNA as well as DNA-dependent DNA polymerase, are generally most favored, but their structure would place hepatitis B in a "new" group as far as virus classification is concerned. Furthermore, hepatitis B has been transmitted experimentally to chimpanzees by plasma containing no detectable double-shelled particles, so that the conclusion that double-shelled particles are infectious should still be treated with reserve. The presence of HBsAg in serum is, however, a marker of infectivity of the sample, and its persistence in an individual indicates that active infection continues even though the liver function tests may have returned to normal.

The pathogenesis of hepatitis B also remains mysterious, and nothing is known about the virus activity during the very long incubation period, which ranges from three to six months. Since immunosuppressed patients experience mild or subclinical but very persistent hepatitis B infection it is thought that the typical illness results from the combination of virus replication and host response.

The part played by antibodies in producing symptoms and immunity is poorly understood. Anti-HBcAg is present in high titer by the time the patient experiences symptoms, and it persists for months or years after the HBsAg has disappeared from the serum. On the other hand, anti-HBsAg appears weeks or months after the antigen is cleared from the circulation, and is usually present in such low titer that it can only be detected by radioimmunoassay or other highly sensitive technique. Nevertheless it is clear that anti-HBcAg is not protective, whereas the possession of anti-HBsAg indicates immunity. Whether the passive administration of anti-HBsAg prevents infection remains uncertain, since clinical trials of its efficiency in hospital staff accidently inoculated with HBsAg-positive blood have given equivocal results.

Periarteritis and glomerulonephritis are unexpected complications that result from deposition of immune complexes of HBsAg and its antibody.

The availability of simple tests for the presence of HBsAg in serum has permitted extensive studies of the natural history of hepatitis B. The existence of healthy carriers of hepatitis B was quickly confirmed, and the application of

HBsAg screening tests to all blood before transfusion has produced a gratifying decrease in the incidence of post-transfusion hepatitis B. It became evident that the clinical distinction between hepatitis A and B was inadequate, since there was general inability to detect HBsAg in over half the patients with hepatitis following blood transfusion, while at least 20% of sporadic cases of hepatitis in adults proved to be caused by hepatitis B. It seems likely that this "natural" transmission of hepatitis B occurs by inapparent inoculation of very small amounts of blood by, for instance, shared razors or brushes. As little as 0.00004 ml of serum has been shown to transmit hepatitis B when inoculated experimentally into volunteers. Venereal transmission also occurs, and about a quarter of the spouses of patients with acute hepatitis B become infected.

The carrier rate in healthy adults varies from about one per thousand in, for example, Western Europe, North America, and Australia, to about one per hundred in Southern Europe, Japan, and India, while it is higher still in some Middle Eastern, African, and Pacific Island communities In countries where the carrier rate is high, it is also common to find HBsAg in sera of patients with chronic liver disease. Transmission from carriers to their infants is commonly observed in the Far East, but rare in other countries.

It is not at all clear whether the geographical variations in the natural history of hepatitis B are due to genetic differences, to social and cultural factors, or to the nature of hepatitis B virus itself.

Support for the latter concept comes from studies of the antigenic structure of HBsAg. Although all samples react with antisera against the "common antigen" *a*, they may be subgrouped according to the presence of one or the other of the minor antigens *d* or *y*. Further subdivision is accomplished by the presence of the *w* or *r* determinant. Despite technical problems with subtyping, these subdivisions have been shown to breed true on transmission from one person to another and to have marked geographical distribution. The *adw* type prevails in carriers in Northern Europe, North America, and Australia, *adr* in the Far East, and *ayw* in para-Mediterranean and African countries. An unrelated antigen, *e* antigen, is sometimes present in the serum of HBsAg-positive persons, particularly those with chronic liver disease, and is located in the outer shell of the 40-nm particles. The *e* antigen reacts with antibody in the sera of other HBsAg-positive individuals, characteristically those who are healthy carriers. Serial studies have shown that *e* antigen is regularly present at the onset of acute hepatitis B and that it is later succeeded by anti-*e*, which is also transient. The value of *e* antigen as a marker of virulence or infectivity of individual samples of HBsAg is not yet established.

Social factors such as rising levels of narcotics abuse and sexual promiscuity are associated with an increasing prevalence of hepatitis B in Western countries. Hepatitis B has become the most important nosocomial infection in hospitals. The introduction of intensive methods of treatment for large numbers of immunosuppressed patients may easily create a reservoir unless stringent precautions are taken to identify and isolate carrier patients before admission.

Some measure of control can be attained by careful technique, but this tends to break down in emergencies. Similarly person-to-person spread cannot be prevented in households of carriers or, indeed, whole communities with a high prevalence of hepatitis B. Several attempts have been made to produce a vaccine by purifying the small spherical HBsAg particles from serum and treating them with formalin to eliminate infectivity. Unfortunately, these preparations are very poorly antigenic and have not succeeded in the field.

HEPATITIS NON-B NON-A

There was general surprise when it was found that laboratory tests for both hepatitis B and hepatitis A were negative in many cases of post-transfusion hepatitis. In such cases the incubation period is about 60 to 90 days, and healthy donors appear to remain infectious for months or years.

Recently this agent has been transmitted to chimpanzees by inoculation of blood from both cases and carriers. Examination of the infective samples by electron microscopy has revealed small spherical viruslike particles. Little is known about the properties of the agent, and it is as yet uncertain whether it should be classified as an enterovirus or a parvovirus. The natural history of the infection is also unknown, but a proportion of patients with sporadic hepatitis also fail to give positive reactions in serological tests for both hepatitis A and hepatitis B, so those cases are probably also due to this third agent. It remains to be seen whether its positive identification will reveal still other unidentified hepatitis viruses.

References

Histopathology
Scheuer, P. J. *Liver Biopsy Interpretation* (2nd ed.). Bailliere Tindall, 1973.

Technical Methods
Viral hepatitis and tests for the Australian (Hepatitis Associated) antigen and antibody. *Bull. W. H. O. 42*: 957–992, 1970.

Review of Experimental Transmission and Epidemiology
Viral hepatitis. MacCallum, F. O., ed. *Br. Med. Bull. 28,* No. 2, 1972.

Control and Natural History
Cossart, Y. E. *Virus Hepatitis and its Control.* Bailliere Tindall, 1978.

Latest Development
Symposium on hepatitis, San Francisco, March, 1978. Report of Proceedings.

Salt, Kidney, and Hypertension

PETER S. CHAN, Ph.D.
Cardiovascular Department
Medical Research Division
American Cyanamid Co.
Lederle Labs.
Pearl River, New York

It has been estimated by the American Heart Association that more than 24 million people, or one in six adults, in the United States alone have hypertension.

Because of the lack of symptoms in the early stages of the disease, of the 24 million people with hypertension, over 40% do not know they have it, and only about 12.5% of the total are under adequate treatment. Epidemiologic studies in various other countries also demonstrate that only about 10 to 15% of those suffering from the disease receive adequate treatment.

In the last 15 years, numerous studies have proved beyond doubt that hypertension is the single most important identifiable factor contributing to other cardiovascular diseases such as stroke, myocardial infarction, heart and kidney failure, and atherosclerosis. These cardiovascular diseases claim more lives in the United States than all other causes of death combined, and were estimated to cost the United States about $26.7 billion in 1977.

There are at least three landmark studies reported on the seriousness of hypertension and the beneficial effects of treatment. They are:

1. The Society of Actuaries (Life Insurance Institute) Study, which indicated that hypertension could decrease life expectancy up to 16 years.
2. The Framingham Study, which showed that people with hypertension have a two to four times higher risk of getting strokes and myocardial infarction and a five times higher risk of incurring congestive heart failure.
3. The Veterans Administration Cooperative Studies, which demonstrated that adequately treated hypertensive patients had much less cardiovascular morbidity and mortality.

What causes human essential hypertension is unsettled at the present time. Undoubtedly multiple causes can lead to hypertension. That is why Page's mosaic theory of hypertension, which was proposed several decades ago, is still viable. The mosaic theory shows that vascular caliber, elasticity, reactivity, blood viscosity, blood volume, cardiac output, and chemical and neural factors are all important in causing hypertension. As we understand it now, many of these changes may be the result as well as causes of hypertension. Hypertension may result from hereditary, renal, neurogenic, environmental, psychological, and endocrine factors acting singly or in combination. Although essential hypertension, which accounts for more than 90% of all cases, has always been interpreted as having an unknown etiology, there is a strong hereditary predisposition to the development of human hypertension. Offspring of parents both of whom have essential hypertension often develop severe hypertension. Identical twins who live in different locations have very similar blood pressures. If hypertension occurs to one of the twins, it will usually occur to the other one. At least five strains of rats, namely the New Zealand (Smirk), the Japanese (Okamoto), the Italian (Milan), the German (Münster), and the Israeli (Hebrew Univ.) spontaneously hypertensive rats, have been successfully bred from regular strains. This strongly supports the notion that heredity is an important determining factor in hypertension. The incidence of human hypertension is intimately related to salt intake. Salt cannot induce hypertension universally in animals or humans if the kidney is able to handle the excretion; so the kidney is important in the initiation and maintenance of hypertension. Even though baroreceptor resetting, central nervous system regulation, autonomic nervous system outflow, cardiac drive, hormonal imbalance, blood vessel reactivity and compliance, and other factors may also be important (primarily or secondarily) in the cause and maintenance of elevated blood pressure, still heredity, salt, and the kidney are stronger components. The kidney must be involved if any hypertension is to be maintained for a prolonged period.

SALT AND HYPERTENSION

Epidemiologic studies have shown that the prevalence of hypertension is directly proportional to salt intake. People who averaged 4 g (Alaskan Eskimos), 7 g (Marshall Islanders), 10 g (northern Americans), 14 g (southern Japanese), and 26 g (northern Japanese) salt intake daily had close to 0, 8, 9, 20, and 39% of hypertension respectively. On the other hand, some people can ingest a large amount of salt but maintain blood pressure within the normotensive limit. This is interpreted as showing a low genetic predisposition to hypertension in this population, and that their kidneys are able to excrete the excess salt.

In a moderately high salt intake population, the blood pressure increases slowly and steadily with age. In a low salt intake population in primitive villages in inland Africa and South America, hypertension is rare, and blood pressure does not increase with age. However, in many coastal villages in Africa where salt intake of the villagers is higher, hypertension is more common, and blood pressure rises with advancing age just as in the Western world.

A strain of rats (Dahl "S" rats) has been bred to produce offspring that are very susceptible to salt-induced hypertension, resembling most cases of human essential hypertension. In this strain, it is very easy to produce frank hypertension by feeding 6 to 8% sodium chloride in the diet. If these rats are fed low sodium chloride, their blood pressure is quite normal when they are young and only slightly higher than normal in adulthood. Hypertension occurs in these rats only when extracellular fluid (ECF) volume or blood volume is increased. If the increased volume is prevented by concomitant administration of a diuretic which increases the salt and water excretion by the kidney, hypertension does not occur.

More than 70 years ago, salt intake was implicated in the pathogenesis of human hypertension. The utility of Kempner's rice diet for the treatment of hypertension was attributed to its low salt content. Salt intake restriction had been effective in the treatment of hypertension long before the advent of the orally active diuretics. Failure to lower the blood pressure by the diet method was attributed to poor compliance. Many studies indicated that the ability to lower arterial blood pressure by dieting is largely due to decreased salt intake rather than a decrease in caloric intake. At present, diuretics alone can control about 50 to 70% of all human essential hypertension, and high salt intake can completely negate the blood pressure–lowing effect of diuretics.

Sodium chloride and water are increased in hypertensive arteries. This may partly explain the increased peripheral resistance resulting from enhanced vasoconstriction in response to vasoactive agents in this condition.

KIDNEY AND HYPERTENSION

The common observation that people ingesting the same amount of salt have different blood pressure levels is attributed to differences in heredity and kidney function. Current concepts indicate that some people with a high genetic susceptibility for hypertension require very slight environmental factors, such as salt intake, neurogenic, psychological, endocrine, and kidney malfunction, to develop hypertension. However, people with low genetic susceptibility will still develop hypertension if environmental factors such as salt intake and kidney malfunction are overwhelming and persist for a prolonged period. Hence, the kidney plays an important role in guarding against the development of hypertension. As the arterial blood pressure increases by any means, the urine output and salt excretion by the kidneys increase until the blood pressure falls back to a lower level. If the blood pressure decreases, the kidneys retain water and salt to maintain the blood volume and return the arterial blood pressure to normal. Recent evidence shows that high salt intake in man without an increase in extracellular fluid or blood volume will not increase the arterial blood pressure; and hypertension will develop only if the extracellular fluid volume is allowed to expand, as it usually will if there is no intervention to prevent it. When effective extracellular volume increases, blood volume increases. Increased blood volume causes an increase in cardiac output, which in turn increases total peripheral resistance; and finally the arterial blood pressure increases. Guyton called this the "cascade" effect, and he estimated that only minute increases in extracellular fluid volume could cause a marked elevation of arterial blood pressure once the full "cascade" effect had occurred.

It has been demonstrated that the baroreceptor reflex, renin–angiotensin, aldosterone, and adrenergic nervous systems are important for acute minute-to-minute control of blood pressure but may make a limited contribution in its long-term control, unless they indirectly influence the kidney functions to reset at a new level. Primary nonrenal lesions in the body can cause hypertension as mentioned above. For example, excess aldosterone as in aldosteronism, excess epinephrine and norepinephrine as in pheochromocytoma, and excess renin as in renal hypertension all can cause sodium and water retention. Overactivity of the nervous system, particularly the renal nerves, can also cause sodium and water retention. Chronic sodium and water retention can eventually lead to expansion of blood and extracellular fluid volume, and finally lead to hypertension. If these primary nonrenal factors fail to involve the kidneys, only transient hypertension will occur, since the kidney will be able to excrete the excess sodium and water because of pressure diuresis and return the arterial blood pressure to normal. But if these primary nonrenal abnormalities are able to involve the kidney to reset at a higher blood pressure, then chronic hypertension will occur. Therefore, in long-term arterial blood pressure regulation, the salt–blood volume–kidney system is the most important determinant and is the final factor, overriding even the powerful nervous systems.

Tobian and his associates found that at a given inflow perfused pressure, an isolated kidney from rats that were susceptible to salt-induced hypertension excreted less sodium and urine volume than that of rats that were resistant to salt-induced hypertension. These data suggested that the kidney from the hypertensive rat was not able to excrete the sodium and water load unless the blood pressure increased. Such sodium and water retention at the normotensive level causes the effective extracellular volume to expand, which in turn resets the blood pressure to the hypertensive state.

In human studies, when young normotensives were fed 25 g/day of salt for 2 weeks, their blood pressure remained at the same level; but when the same amount of salt was given to young people with mild to borderline hypertension, their blood pressure increased.

The kidneys have long been recognized as playing a pivotal role in hypertension and the normal homeostatic control of blood pressure. The transplant of normotensive kidneys to the Italian (Milan) strain of spontaneously hypertensive rat lowered the elevated arterial blood pressure, and the transplant of hypertensive kidneys to a normotensive rat increased the blood pressure. This finding strongly supports the idea that the kidney contains both hypertensive and hypotensive factors. Kidneys have been shown to contain hypertensive factors such as the renin system and hypotensive factors such as the prostaglandin E_2, prostacyclin, bradykinin, and neutral lipids systems. Renal ischemia and renal arterial stenosis or coarctation are known to produce systemic hypertension. Not only are the kidneys important in maintaining the fluid and electrolyte balance of the body, but also they are believed to keep the vasopressor and vasodepressor components in balance in the homeostatic control of arterial blood pressure. Thus, any deficiency in the vasodepressor mechanism will leave the normal vasopressor mechanism unopposed and will lead to hypertension. Exaggeration of a vasopressor mechanism such as the renin system with a normal vasodepressor mechanism will also lead to hypertension. Prostaglandin E_2 and other prostaglandins are believed to be important modulators in regulating the functions of the kidney with respect to water and sodium balance. At least five different forms of experimental hypertension, namely, deoxycorticosterone-salt hypertension, "post-salt" hypertension, Goldblatt hypertension, "post-Goldblatt" hypertension, and Kyoto spontaneous hypertension are characterized by a deficiency in renal production of prostaglandin due to decreased storage of arachidonic acid, the precursor of prostaglandin, in the renal medulla and papilla of the kidney. Thus, hypertension has been suggested to be caused by the deficiency of intrarenal prostaglandin E_2, and the condition allows the normal vasopressor mechanism to operate unopposed.

A failure of the kidney to maintain water and sodium balance at normal blood pressure will eventually lead to hypertension. In order to excrete the excess sodium, the blood pressure rises above the normal level to produce pressure diuresis. In hypertensive individuals, it takes a higher arterial blood pressure to excrete a given load of water and salt as compared to normotensive individuals.

In Goldblatt renal hypertensive rats and dogs, removal of the clip or the clipped kidney in the early phase of hypertension will return the blood pressure to normal. In the late stage of hypertension, removal of the clip or the clipped kidney may not return the elevated blood pressure to normal. Part of the explanation is that hypertension causes hypertrophy of the arteries and other changes in the arteries and other blood pressure regulating systems, and directly influences the untouched kidney to reset at the higher blood pressure. Other factors than the original one are now maintaining the elevated blood pressure by indirect influence on the untouched kidney.

Pressure diuresis and natriuresis are reset in hypertension. The kidney maintains the hypertension because it needs the higher pressure to maintain the sodium and water output.

The small resistance vessels, including those in the kidneys, respond to the elevated arterial blood pressure by increasing wall thickness and the wall/lumen ratio. This increases the resistance to flow and increases peripheral resistance. The sodium and water content of the renal arteries increase in hypertension, and the arteries increase response to vasoconstrictor agents. The kidney resets to balance water and salt excretion at an elevated arterial blood pressure.

The renal circulation is also influenced structurally and functionally in essential hypertension. Hypertension increases the renal vascular resistance and causes reduction of renal blood flow. When hypertension persists for a long period, the glomerular filtration rate will fall, and renal failure may develop. As a result, permanent hypertension will occur.

The exposure of a normal kidney to increased arterial pressure by any manipulation or means for a prolonged period produces in that kidney an ability to maintain hypertension even when the original causes are removed. As hypertension persists, the renal functions slowly deteriorate.

If a slight increase of mean arterial blood pressure is allowed to persist in man for two years, the kidney is able to adapt to maintain this increment of blood pressure. This process will repeat if any increase of blood pressure is permitted to persist for a long period. Over a period of 10 or 15 years, permanent hypertensions ensues.

Long and continued overactivity of any pressor system may produce irreversible damage to the kidney and cause resetting of the pressure to maintain adequate pressure diuresis and natriuresis. No pressor system will be able to maintain prolonged hypertension unless at the same time it produces vasoconstriction in the kidney with resetting of pressure natriuresis. Without kidney resetting, a rise of pressure will lead to natriuresis and decrease of arterial blood pressure, and hypertension will not occur.

In essential hypertension, there is little retention of sodium and water and the blood volume is near normal, but the kidney functions are abnormal at a given blood pressure level. A common abnormality in hypertension is failure of the kidney to excrete sodium and water at normal levels of arterial blood pressure. Arterial blood pressure rises to the point where sodium and water balance can be maintained.

SUMMARY

In human hypertension, the kidney, genetic make-up, and salt intake are more important than the other pressure-regulating systems in the long-range regulation of blood pressure.

Renal function abnormality in essential hypertension is considered both a cause and a consequence. Any form of hypertension must involve the kidney if the elevation of blood pressure is to be sustained.

Whether a hormonal or a chemical imbalance leads to salt retention through the kidney at normotensive level is not clear. As the present hypothesis goes, the genetic predisposition to hypertension, in addition to salt intake and other factors (e.g., autonomic nervous system hyperactivity, baroreceptor resetting, renin–angiotensin excess, deficiency in renal prostaglandin E_2 production, increased ACTH that leads to overproduction of aldosterone and other mineralo-corticoids causing retention of salt and water and an increase of arterial blood pressure for a prolonged period) will cause the kidney to reset at a higher blood pressure; over a long period of time hypertension will ensue.

The kidney holds the key to the initiation and maintenance of high arterial blood pressure. In long-term blood pressure regulation, it overrides all other regulating systems. Constriction or stenosis of the renal arteries and preglome-rular constriction of the arterioles will reduce the glomerular filtration rate at any given level of arterial blood pressure. A higher blood pressure will be required to excrete any given load of salt when compared to the normal healthy kidney. Drastic reduction of nephrons due to renal diseases such as pyelone-phritis will increase susceptibility to salt-induced hypertension. High salt intake in such an individual will produce hypertension despite the low genetic susceptibility.

It appears that people whose parents or grandparents have had hypertension should take a short-term high-salt-intake test for susceptibility to salt-induced hypertension even though their present arterial blood pressure is not elevated. Low salt intake should start early in life in people with high genetic predisposition to hypertension. As a public health measure, low salt intake (less than 4 g per day) should be advocated to all people regardless of their hereditary susceptibility to hypertension. Processed foods, particularly baby foods, should contain as little salt as possible. It is harmful to expose infants to high salt intake.

Any prolonged elevation of arterial blood pressure, no matter how slight, should be avoided or treated, since it will eventually lead to still higher blood pressure over the years.

New diuretics with improved properties (such as renal vasodilatation, anti-aldosterone, antirenin, and so forth) and with low toxicity are needed. Even though the antihypertensive property of diuretics was discovered clinically in a serendipitous manner, diuretics are considered more rational and physiological for antihypertensive treatment than most other categories of antihypertensive drugs. Anti–renin–angiotensin agents which work to antagonize the vasopressor system of the kidney should hold promise. Renal prostaglandins which restore the vasodepressor system of the kidney to oppose the vasopressor systems are another rational approach for the treatment of hypertension. Better antihypertensive agents in the future will undoubtedly center their actions in the kidney.

How Much Lead is Toxic to Man?

ROBERT A. GOYER
Department of Pathology
University of Western Ontario
London, Ontario, Canada.
N6A 5C1

Health problems due to exposure to lead are certainly not new concerns. The potential toxicity of lead has been noted as far back in history as there are records. The concerns about lead, however, serve as a good example of how a health problem may evolve with progress in industrial activity, and an increasing ability to recognize potential adverse health effects with greater and greater sensitivity. This ability to probe more and more deeply into the biochemical and even molecular activities of a pollutant like lead has resulted in the recognition of effects that may border on the interface between what is clearly an undesirable or adverse effect and a nonharmful, physiological or adaptive response. Since it is clear that lead may have serious toxic effects with excessive exposure, and there is no known biological requirement for lead, it is prudent to avoid pollution with this metal to whatever extent is possible. However, lead is ubiquitous, and everyone has some level of body burden. For these reasons decisions regarding permissible levels of exposure must necessarily involve as much understanding as possible regarding subtle effects, and perhaps some philosophical consideration of what is good and bad or acceptable and nonacceptable in terms of our present-day life style.

I will begin with some historical perspective on the problem. A treatise on toxicilogy and pathology published in 1817 in a translation from French by a Philadelpha physician, Jos. Nancrede, states that: "If we were to judge of the interest excited by any medical subject, by the number of writings to which it has given birth, we could not but regard the poisoning by lead, as the most important to be known of all those that have treated of, up to the present time." Hippocrates had warned about lead colic about 400 B.C., and the French author was quite impressed with the long history and large number of medical writings concerned with the subject of lead toxicity (Orfila, 1817). The number of papers on this topic has risen more or less exponentially since the time, and there are still unknown problems. A recent review by a scientist at the National Research Council of Canada states that the number of papers in the scientific literature concerning health effects of lead has risen steadily, reaching about 4000 papers per year in the last five years.

The story of lead and health effects goes back to the beginning of man's working with metals. Lead is one of the seven metals of antiquity and was important then, as now, because it is abundant, is easy to work with, and has many uses. There was an abundance of lead available to both Greeks and Romans because it was a by-product of silver mining. The silver mines in Asia Minor yielded 600 ounces of silver for every ton of lead—so the lead was used to line aqueducts, to cover keels of ships, and for making small pieces of hardware.

Some of the forms and uses of lead that were perpetuated down through the years and had the potential for causing toxicity are cited by Orfila (1817). White lead carbonate, or ceruse, was used as a make-up powder by ladies. Not only did it make them look pale, but continual use produced an anemia that added to their pallor! The Romans are credited with discovering that lead added to food and beverages prevented spoilage, and the addition of a lead acetate not only made cloudy wine clear but made poor wine quite palatable. Apparently this custom persisted to be nineteenth century as noted in the French treatise.

The modern problems with lead pollution started with the industrial era and the increase in lead smelting beginning in the eighteenth century. The use of lead in gasoline began in the mid-1920s. Currently about 300,000 tons of lead are emitted from auto exhausts in North America each year, but there is hope that this will cease in the near future as gasoline for motor vehicles becomes lead-free.

Lead is present in all parts of our environment—soil, water, and all animal and vegetable life. The largest source of lead for persons in the general population is from food; lead is present in most food items, vegetables, and meats. Daily intake for persons in North America is thought to be about 250 to 300 μg. These figures are based on market-basket surveys (like the cost of living index). About 10% of lead ingested with food by adults is absorbed (about 30 μg), and all but a small retained fraction is excreted in the urine. Unabsorbed lead is excreted in feces. There is little gastrointestinal excretion of lead compared with some other heavy metals such as cadmium and mercury. The amount of urine lead varies greatly so that a large increase in excretion must occur to be clinically significant.

An important aspect of lead metabolism is that we are in positive lead balance from the time of conception until about age 50; that is, we begin to accumulate lead, in utero, from maternal blood and continue to accumulate lead the rest of our lives. Total body content of lead for adults in the general population without excessive or occupational exposure to lead is about 200 mg but may be up to half a gram. Ten percent of absorbed lead is retained; that is, about 3 μg of lead, on the average, is stored in bone or soft tissues each day. Retained lead has an average half life of about 20 years.

In the body, lead can be viewed conceptually as in at least two compartments, a diffusible or transportable one and a fixed or nondiffusible form or compartment. Recent studies using isotopic lead suggest at least four compartments. Blood lead is in equilibrium with lead in other soft tissues and labile fractions of lead in end organs; so blood lead is thought to be the best single measure of the current state of lead exposure. Most blood lead is bound to red blood cells.

Until just a few years ago it was generally accepted that Kehoe's (1961) studies on young adults suggesting a gastrointestinal absorption of 5 to 10% with about a 10% retention was applicable to children as well. However, more recent studies suggest that retention of absorbed lead in the growing infant may be over 30%. With this understanding of the metabolism of lead in infants, we can see why infants and young children might be expected to be considerably more susceptible than adults to adverse health effects when exposed to a particular level of lead.

There are also a number of other factors, most of them dietary, that influence lead absorption. The two most important, particularly in terms of children, are iron and calcium deficiencies. Iron deficiency seems to further increase the gastrointestinal absorption of lead, and nearly all children with increased blood lead levels have some degree of iron deficiency. Calcium deficiency, on the other hand, seems to alter the body distribution of lead, resulting in increases in the soft tissues such as blood, brain, and kidney. There is also an associated increase in retention of absorbed lead. So, in trying to predict what potential adverse health effect a particular level of exposure to lead may have, it is very important to account for dietary deficiencies as well as age. Some recent studies in our laboratory have shown that ascrobic acid may actually increase excretion of lead—so here is one dietary factor that may have a beneficial effect.

With this background I would like now to review the pathological effects of lead on the three major organ systems that account for the majority of observed clinical manifestations of excessive lead exposure, that is, the central nervous system, the hematopoietic system, and the kidneys.

The central nervous system effects of lead are certainly the most important clinically, particularly in terms of young children. The present-day concepts of the pathological effects of lead on the nervous system began with the descriptions by Blackman (1937) of brains from 22 children dying in Baltimore of acute lead poisoning, and has since been confirmed or elaborated on by a number of neuropathologists. Pentschew's (1965) explanation for this rather late description of such an old disease is that "when lead encephalopathy was more common, neuropathology was in its infancy." Added to this is the problem that the nervous system effects of lead on humans have been difficult to duplicate in experimental models. However, from the many descriptions in the literature and from my own experimental studies I suggest that the observed morphologic effects can be summarized as follows: The specific picture one sees in a particular brain is dependent on length of exposure and dose. In those persons with recent or acute exposure the prominent pathologic change is cerebral edema. This is associated with an increase in cerebrospinal fluid pressure, dilatation of capillaries and areterioles, and swelling of endothelial cells. Lead seems to have a direct effect on the neurovascular network, resulting in increased capillary permeability. The basis for the increase in cerebrospinal fluid pressure is less clear. Recent experimental studies have shown that lead is concentrated in choroid plexus. On the one hand this function of the choroid plexus may offer some protection to the brain from the direct action of lead, but experimental studies have shown that active transport in the lead-poisoned choroid plexus is altered so that the normal flux of physiologically important solutes into and out of the brain compartment is interfered with.

A second morphological feature is proliferation of astrocytes and, less commonly, microglial proliferation. Pentschew points out that the astrocyte proliferation is necessarily related to neuronal degeneration but may be a primary toxic reaction. We have shown experimentally that the astrocyte is actually the site of concentration of lead in the brain, and that intranuclear inclusion bodies or lead–protein complexes can occur in astrocytes just as they do in renal tubular cells (Goyer and Rhyne, 1973). The basis for the neuronal injury and necrosis is less certain. There are two possibilities: one is that the lead itself does have a direct toxic effect on neurones; the second is that the injured neurone may be the victim of the altered cellular environment and suffer from hypoxia and other metabolic effects. The most common sites for neuronal loss are cortical gray matter, the hypothalamus, and basal ganglia. These sites correspond more or less with the sites of greatest lead concentration in the brain. There are a few studies making the correlations in humans, but it has been show experimentally that lead is most concentrated in gray matter of brains of lead-toxic dogs with lesser but greatly increased amounts in basal ganglia. A recent brief report from England showed that the greatest focus of lead concentration is the hippocampus. Brain lead concentration, although variable, does show a relationship to abnormal morphologic changes.

A number of clinical forms of peripheral neuropathy have been described as due to lead. The antebrachial type, involving the extensors of the wrists and fingers is probably the most common clinical syndrome, characteristic of the "wrist drop" of painters poisoned with lead-containing paint. It is not seen very often today except perhaps in some heavily contaminated lead industries. The brachial and Duchenne forms are even less common, but are described in older references. The peroneal type is the characteristic foot drop, also seen in lead industry, involving peroneal muscles and sometimes the tibialis anticus. The fifth variety is very rare in man but is of interest because it is a common, almost pathognomonic, clinical feature of lead poisoning in horses, which results in an inspiratory stridor dyspnea called "roaring" by veterinarians. Why lead-induced paralysis is localized to a certain groups of nerves and muscles is not known.

There seems to be some relationship between use of muscles and intensity of the neuropathy.

The pathology of the peripheral neuropathy has been pieced together from both human and experimental studies but it not entirely understood. Lead seems to produce changes in the Schwann cell that can lead to segmented demyelination, but this may be reversible with remyelination. The peripheral neuropathy of lead poisoning, such as wrist drop, is usually reversible, particularly with chelation therapy. But if it persists, with continual lead exposure, particularly for longer than two years, it is probably not reversible.

Now we will consider more broadly the irreversible sequelae of nervous system effects of lead. There have been several studies directed to this question during the past few years, but probably the most important one is that of Perlstein and Attila in Chicago in the 1960s. Their study not only defined irreversible sequelae but drew attention to the problem of low-level or subclinical effects of lead on the nervous system. They correlated various neurological sequelae such as mental retardation, seizures, cerebral palsy, and even optic atrophy with clinical manifestations or symptoms of lead toxicity. This group consisted of 425 Chicago children between the ages of 9 months and 8 years. The cause of lead toxicity in 408 of these children from chewing or eating loose plaster covered with old lead-containing paint from slum clearance projects. The other 17 were intoxicated from inhalation of lead from burning of battery casings. Over 80% of those recovering from encephalopathy, that is, reduced level of consciousness or coma and signs of increased intracranial pressure, had a serious neurologic sequela; the less severe the presenting symptom, the less likely were neurological sequelae. They even suggested that nine children actually experienced mental retardation because of lead exposure, even though they were asymptomatic. This diagnosis was made either from routine study of asymptomatic. This diagnosis was made either from routine study of asymptomatic siblings of children with known lead poisoning, or was an inadvertent or accidental finding in a child with a previous history of excessive lead exposure. The relationship of the mental retardation to lead effect was only conjecture but was based on learning that the children were normal early in life; some had started school and performed well initially, only to deteriorate in intelligence later, and, furthermore, there is a high probability that sibs of lead-toxic children also suffered from excessive exposure to lead. And finally there is a smaller group that developed sequelae of lead poisoning and will require lifelong institutional care. The data when blood lead levels are compared with symptoms and follow-up sequelae strongly suggest, but do not really prove, that the large number of asymptomatic children with blood lead levels between 40 and 80 μg/100 ml are at risk for nervous system effects of lead.

This report was followed by more in-depth studies of children with blood lead levels over 40 μg/dl. One such study found that a group of children with blood lead levels over 40 μg/dl was about 10 I.Q. points lower than a control group as measured by the Standard-Binet test. Another study related hyperactivity to increase in blood lead levels over 40 μg/dl, and yet another study found minor neurological dysfunction in a similar group of children. At present, we know very little about the pathological changes in the CNS that produces so-called subclinical effects. No morphology is available, and experimental models simulating this human problem are difficult to design. One of the pathogenetic mechanisms presently under study by several groups in the United States is an effect of lead on acetylcholine and catacholamine metabolism. It has been found that there is a large decrease in choline incorporation in synaptosomes from brains of lead-treated mice, as well as increased levels of catacholine metabolites, particularly norepinephrine, in brain and urine. Also, it has been reported that an increase in excretion of catacholamines occurs in the urine of children with blood lead levels over 40 μg/ml. The significance of all this is yet unknown, but it is hoped that it will lead to a sensitive biochemical measure of lead effect on the nervous system that will indicate when treatment and prevention of further lead ingestion are indicated.

Now let's briefly consider the effects of lead on the hematopoietic system. Lead causes anemia in two ways; it increases red blood cell fragility producing hemolysis, and it also impairs heme synthesis at, at least, three enzymatic steps. δ-Aminolevulinic acid dehydratase (ALA–D) is probably the enzyme in the heme pathway that is most sensitive to lead. Inhibition of this enzyme results in a block in utilization of δ-aminolevulinic acid and in subsequent decline in heme synthesis. Second, δ-ALA synthetase activity is increased, resulting in increased synthesis of δ-ALA. A third abnormality of heme synthesis in lead intoxication is inhibition of the enzyme ferrochelatase. Ferrochelatase catalyzes the incorporation of the ferrous ion into the porphyrin ring structure. Iron in the form of apoferritin and ferruginous micelles may accumulate in mitochondria of bone marrow reticulocytes from lead-poisoned rats.

Other steps in the biosynthetic pathway of heme may also be abnormal in lead toxicity, but the evidence for this is incomplete. Increase in urinary excretion of coproporphyrin, the degradative product of coproporphyrinogen, is a sensitive reflection of lead toxicity. Metabolism of porphobilinogen to coproporphyrinogen proceeds unimpaired, but increased urinary excretion of both of these metabolites does occur in lead poisoning, and the mechanism is not understood. It has been shown that lead inhibits erythrocytic uroporphyrinogen synthetase but has little effect on the hepatic enzyme. These results suggest that the source of protoporphyrinogen excretion following lead poisoning may be from red blood cells. ALA–D is an extramitochondrial enzyme, and later steps in heme synthesis are intramitochondrial. Coproporphyrinogen transport into the mitochondrial matrix might be impaired in the presence of altered inner membrane permeability and reduction in oxidation and phosphorylation. Interference of lead in heme synthesis also results in increase in protoporphyrin, or as it sometimes is called, "free erythrocyte protoporphyrin" (FEP) in blood. It has been shown that FEP is not really "free" but zinc-chelated protoporphyrin IX. The inhibition of ferrochelase by lead prevents the introduction of iron into protoporphyrin IX to form heme. Both in iron deficiency per se and in lead poisoning, the porphyrin chelates Zn nonenzymatically to form zinc protoporphyrin (ZnPP), which, in turn, becomes incorporated into hemoglobin. Because globin containing ZnPP fluoresces when excited, it may be measured fluorometrically and provides a very sensitive indicator of lead exposure.

The renal effects of lead are only of clinical interest in persons with chronic or long-term exposure to lead as measured in years. There are at least two stages in the development of lead nephropathy. The first stage is an acute reversible effect that has been best documented in children. It consists of morphological and functional changes in proximal renal tubular lining cells. These changes include alterations in mitochondrial structure and function, and the formation of intranuclear inclusion bodies or lead–protein complexes. Recent studies have also shown that the inclusion bodies or nuclear lead–protein complexes are removed from nuclei by chelation therapy so that we believe that soft-tissue lead, that is, lead bound to cell membranes and in the inclusion bodies, represents the most labile and chelatable pool of lead in the body.

The mitochondria from kidneys of persons or experimental animals with lead toxicity show swelling, abnormal arrangement of cristae, and attempts at cleavage or budding. They also have reduced oxidative and phosphorylative abilities. These changes are accompanied by an increase in urinary excretion of amino acids, glucose, and phosphate. Again, these changes are reversible with chelation therapy.

Whether acute lead nephropathy, treated or untreated, influences the development of any form of chronic nephropathy without continuous lead exposure is uncertain. Follow-up studies of children in the United States with documented acute lead poisoning show no evidence of higher incidence of renal diseases as adults, so the evidence is that Stage I lead nephropathy is completely reversible.

Stage II nephropathy can be produced in experimental animals by feeding them a high dosage of lead for more than a year. Similar changes are found in workmen with excessive lead exposure for more than two or three years. The interstitial fibrosis becomes progressively more severe with tubular atrophy and eventually reduced glomerular filtration and renal failure. This process may progress for many years without renal failure occurring; so there may be many extraneous factors that influence the ultimate course of this disorder.

Histologic study of kidneys from workmen with lead nephropathy show interstitial fibrosis, tubular atrophy and dilatation, and some hyperplasia of cells in functioning tubules. These changes are nonspecific, but there are a coupled of points of interest here. First, it is not common to find any inclusion bodies in chronic lead nephropathy, and, second, preliminary studies suggest that renal excretion of lead is less in men with the late stage of lead nephropathy than in persons with only acute changes. And finally, glomerular filtration is usually only slightly reduced in spite of the severe interstitial changes. Glomeruli are either normal or near normal with some thickening of basement membranes and swelling of mesangial cells. In the terminal or end stage they become sclerotic. No immune deposits have been found to glomeruli of persons with chronic lead nephropathy.

Table 1 summarizes these considerations of the pathological effects of lead with some consideration of dose response. Blood lead levels are divided into three ranges—up to 40, 40 to 80, and over 80 $\mu g/dl$ of blood. There is general acceptance, and has been for many years now, that persons, young or old, with blood lead levels over 80 $\mu g/dl$ suffer from lead toxicity. The expression of the toxicity may vary somewhat, depending on age and rate of onset. Children are likely to have clinically evident encephalopathy with ataxis, reduced level of consciousness or even convulsions, coma, and death. Peripheral neuropathy is commonly seen in adults and is often manifested by an ulnar palsy or wrist drop. Children may also develop peripheral neuropathy, and it is sometimes stated that popliteal nerve involvement with foot drop is more common in children than adults; but either may occur.

TABLE 1. Relationship of Blood Lead Levels and Pathological Effects

No Effect?			Adaptive Phase Subclinical Effects	Clinical Toxicity
B-Pb less than 40 $\mu g/dl$			40–60 $\mu g/dl$	80 $\mu g/dl$ and greater
10 20 30			U–ALA	CNS–Encephalopathy
Rural Urban Traffic			G.I. complaints	Peripheral neuropathy
people dwellers police			Fever	Anemia
FEP			CNS effects	Renal effects
Adults				
FEP				
Children				
ALAD				

ALAD = δ-aminolevulinic acid dehydratase. (This is probably the enzyme in the heme pathway that is most sensitive to lead.)

FEP = free erythrocyte protoporphyrin in blood. (Interference of lead in heme synthesis results in increase in protoporphyrin.)

Anemia is not a common effect of lead poisoning in adults. Most children with anemia due to lead exposure also have iron deficiency. Renal effects are only a late stage in the adult. Renal tubular dysfunction is present in children with acute lead encephalopathy, but it is overshadowed by the more important neurological effects.

The area of major interest today is what happens to people, children and workmen, with blood lead levels between 40 and 80 µg/dl. These people are generally well, that is, subjectively well, but an increase in urinary ALA excretion begins when blood lead is about 40 µg/ld. Also, if these people are observed closely, they have frequent nonspecific G.I. complaints, and are prone to infections. Children with blood lead levels over 40 µg/dl also seem to have a number of nonspecific CNS problems, which are difficult to measure. According to studies mentioned earlier, they tend to do poorly in school, have short attention spans, and perhaps are hyperactive.

Since there is no known biologic requirement for lead, and it is clear that with high exposure lead is toxic, at what level of blood lead is there no known adverse effect? People in the general population can be further subdivided by blood lead levels depending on occupation and place of residence. Persons in frequent contact with automobile traffic, that is, garage attendants, highway toll collectors, and even traffic policemen tend to have blood lead levels over 30 µg/dl but usually under 40 µg/dl. Urban residents have a mean blood lead of 25 µg/dl, whereas rural residents have an average blood lead level of about 15 µg/dl; so there is clearly an urban-rural gradient. So what is normal? A geochemist, Clare Patterson at the California Institute of Technology, a few years ago calculated that without industrial activity the "natural" blood lead level of man should be less than 1 µg/dl. In the past three or four years it has been noted that activity of aminolevulinic acid dehydratase, the heme synthesizing enzyme present in red blood cells, is inverse to blood lead levels down to blood lead of about 10 or 15 µg/dl. It is generally agreed that this is a biochemical effect of lead, and the body has a large reserve capacity or activity for this enzyme, so we are able to compensate with no adverse health effect. The FEP or ZnPP test is now becoming widely used as a screening test of lead toxicity, and minimal elevations occur in adults at blood lead levels of about 30 µg/dl and in children at about 20 µg/dl. It must be pointed out that FEP is also increased in iron deficiency so that the frequently observed relationship between iron deficiency and increased blood lead levels may result in disproportionate increases in FEP levels. Again, it is not clear whether minor elevations reflect an adverse health effect of lead or not.

In summary, I have tried to provide an in-depth review of the pathological effects of lead with some consideration of dose-response. As the reader can see, there is still some doubt as to the minimum exposure of lead that will produce an adverse health effect. Our understanding of the pathologic potential of this metal is still not complete.

References

Blackman, S. S. The lesions of lead encephalitis in children. *Bull. Johns Hopkins Hosp. 61*: 1-61, 1937.
Goyer, R. A., and Rhyne, B. C. Pathological effects of lead. *Int. Rev. Exp. Pathol. 12*: 1-77, 1973.
Kehoe, R. A. The metabolism of lead in health and disease. The Harben Lectures, 1960. *J. R. Inst. Publ. Health Hyg. 24*: 81-96, 101-120, 129-143, 177-203, 1961.
NAS–NRC. *Airborne Lead in Perspective.* Washington, D.C.: National Academy of Science, 1972.
Orfila, M. P. *A General System of Toxicology,* abridged and partly translated from the French by J. Nancrede. Philadelphia, 1817.
Patterson, C. C. Contaminated and natural lead environments of man. *Arch. Environ. Health 11*: 344-363, 1965.
Pentschew, A. Morphology and morphogenesis of lead encephalopathy. *Acta Neuropathol. 5*: 133-160, 1965.
Perlstein, M. A., and Attila, R. Neurologic sequelae of plumbism in children. *Clin. Pediat. 5*: 292-298, 1966.
WHO, Environmental Health Criteria 3. *Lead.* Geneva, 1977.

Asbestosis

B. A. WARREN, M.A., M.B., D.Phil., M.R.C.Path.
Professor of Pathology, Health Sciences Center,
University of Western Ontario, London, Canada

THE PROGNOSIS FOR A PATIENT WITH
CARCINOMA OF THE LUNG

The outlook at the present time of the patient who has just been diagnosed as having carcinoma of the lung is dismal. In 1957 in Gifford and Waddington's series of 2156 patients who were suffering from lung cancer, in only 464 was resection possible (21.5%), and 347 (16.09%) survived the operative phase. The five-year survival of the 347 patients was 28%, or slightly under 5% for the whole group. The vast majority of patients present with lung cancer too late in the disease for hope of cure; yet the examination of expectorated sputum after staining by modified Papanicolaou technique is an effective method of establishing the presence of lung cancer (Seydel et al., 1975). The relative accuracy of the procedure for diagnosis varies in different series from 65.2% (Umiker, 1966) to 95% when suspicious, inconclusive, and atypical categories are included.

There are a variety of distinct cell types of primary carcinoma of the lung.

Great clinical importance attaches to the cell type, since both the optimal treatment and prognosis are dependent on the exact cell type (Carr and Mountain, 1974). Eighty to 90% of unselected patients with lung cancer should be diagnosed by techniques short of exploratory thoracotomy, and the first screening test should be a proper sputum examination (Neff, 1974). Most carcinomas of the lung arise in the bronchial epithelium and continuously shed cells that can be found in the sputum. Cytologic examination, therefore, can detect lung cancer early in its development. If the source of cells is localized, the majority of patients with early tumors can be cured (Baker et al., 1974).

Cancer of the lung, bronchus, and trachea was the leading cause for cancer deaths in males in Ontario for the period 1969-1973, being 45 per 100,000 population. The crude five-year survival rate for the period 1938-1958, encompassing review of 2457 cases, was 3.8% (Godden, ed., *Cancer in Ontario, 1975*). There was a progressive increase in the cancer mortaility in Ontario due to lung cancer in the years 1931 to 1960 (52 to 889) (*Cancer Mortality by Age, Sex and Site of Disease, Ontario, 1931-1960*). New cases registered in Ontario cancer treatment centers more recently increased from 12,509 in 1973 to 13,272 in 1974 (Godden, 1975).

Early diagnosis of lung cancer can promise the possibility of surgical cure. More efficient methods of early diagnosis would diminish the wastage of human life due to this disease. It is appropriate to trace through a community any agent that increases the risk of malignant neoplasia.

THE RELATIONSHIP BETWEEN ASBESTOS EXPOSURE AND NEOPLASIA: INDIVIDUALS IN THE POPULATION AT RISK

The association of asbestos exposure with neoplasia has now been studied for nearly two decades (Selikoff et al., 1964, 1965, 1972). Those individuals who have had a prolonged exposure to asbestos (i.e., 20 years or so) have had at least a tenfold risk of developing lung cancer (for review see Millard, 1977). Mesothelioma can arise with shorter exposure times and at an earlier period from the time of exposure. The danger to individuals in direct contact with material is now well known. This group includes miners, crushers, and workers in manufacturing industries that use asbestos fibers. The manufacturers that use asbestos in one form or another are diverse; included are producers of fireman's resistant clothing, fire-resistant cloth, gaskets, washers and seals, brake-linings, paper, plastics, and acoustic tiles, builders, and installers of home insulation. Individuals with secondary or nonoccupational contact are the wives of workers who clean clothing impregnated with fine fibers (or people with homes within one half mile of users of asbestos in industry, such as a shipyard applying asbestos) (Hennigar and Gross, 1977). The need for adequate insulation for offices and houses, subsequent to the increase in oil prices brought about by OPEC action, makes elucidation of the hazards posed by inhaled and ingested asbestos fiber more imperative, since asbestos is used as an insulating material in some instances. In the city environment and in the work environment today there may be many individuals exposed to the hazards of asbestos inhalation over prolonged periods without their knowledge.

Chrysotile is the asbestos mineral fiber that is most used in industry; 90% of the fiber is supplied in this form (Hahn-Weinheimer and Hirner, 1977). The output of the fiber from mines and processing plants has increased enormously from the early output of 50 tons from Thetford, Canada in 1877, to an annual output worldwide of 4.3 million tons in 1975 (Lincoln, 1975, cited by Hahn-Weinheimer and Hirner, 1977).

An overview of the Canadian asbestos problem may be found in a report by Charlebois and Rivest (1978) prepared for the Science Council of Canada Committee on "Hazardous Substances of Man-made Origin." Their views on the nature of the hazard are: (1) inhaled asbestos in relatively high dosage causes fibrosis of the lung; (2) the delay period from exposure to appearance of asbestosis-related diseases is 20 to 30 years; (3) cigarette smoking greatly increases the risk of lung cancer in patients who already have asbestos fibers in their lungs; (4) the period of contact with asbestos required to increase the occurrence of mesotheliomas may be short.

THE EVOLUTION OF A CARCINOMA
OF THE LUNG

Microscopic examination of exfoliated cells allows the diagnosis of cancer in its earlier stages before the appearance of clinical manifestations of invasive disease. The original work on the correlation of exfoliated cells from lesions suspected of being cancers was done by Papanicolaou and Traut (for review of historical background and current status of respiratory tract cytopathology see Johnston and Frable, 1976, and Erozan and Frost, 1974). The concept and the technique were not readily accepted at first, but have been proved and now enjoy wide endorsement as a technique to detect in situ changes in the cervix uteri, before the invasive stage of the cancers have developed (the "Pap" smear).

A cancer of the lung does not suddenly arise in normal bronchial epithelium. There are a number of sequential changes that occur, knowledge of which has been built up over a number of years.

Correlations have been made between the morphology of the exfoliated cells and the stage of disease in the epithelium from which these cells were derived (Figure 1) (Frost, 1969). In the respiratory tract the cells undergo changes that occur as part of the response to injury. Normally, the living cells of the bronchial tree are pseudostratified columnar cells with a tuft of cilia on their luminal

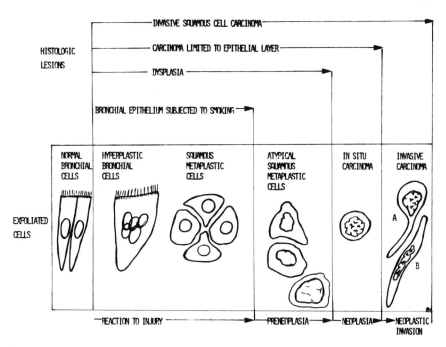

Figure 1. Correlation of the histologic lesions and morphology of the exfoliated cells as repeated prolonged injury progresses to neoplasia (modified from Frost, 1969). In the last column are (A) a "tadpole" cell and (B) a fiber cell. These are morphological forms of malignant cells from a squamous cell carcinoma. (from: B. A. Warren, Basic cytopathology of the respiratory tract Part 1. Medcom Inc., 1979)

surface. These move the mucus produced from the goblet cells toward the upper respiratory tract and the pharynx. Following injury these cilia disappear, and the columnar epithelium undergoes squamous metaplasia; that is, the epithelium is replaced by flat cells.

Further injury results in changes that are recognized by progressively more markedly atypical changes in the nuclei of the cells and a diminution of the cytoplasm surrounding the nucleus. There is an increased nucleocytoplasmic ratio. With repeated insults over a prolonged period, neoplastic transformation of this preneoplastic change occurs, and a carcinoma develops. This carcinoma is at first in situ; that is, it has not invaded the tissues below the normal limitation of the epithelium. This neoplastic transformation may, however, occur in a number of areas within the "field" of action of the injurious agents, i.e., the epithelium of the bronchial tree.

Cytopathological examination of sputa and washings of the bronchial tree of patients can pick up neoplastic transformation at an early stage in the progression of the disease to widespread dissemination. The technique was originally called *exfoliative* cytology, and for a positive diagnosis to be made by the technique the changes must be in the epithelium from which the exfoliated cells in the specimen are derived.

Serial cytopathologic examination of sputa from patients allows the following of pathologic changes in the bronchial tree, and, together with the new methods of fiber-optic bronchoscopy and "brushing" the lesions present in the tree, should open a new phase in both the treatment of the disease and the knowledge of its natural history. For example, there is a critical time interval for the neoplastic transformation of the cells and hence the formation of an in situ carcinoma, and the further progression to *invasion* through the basement membrane. This is a "window of time" when, theoretically, a minor part of a lung with the tumor, which has not yet spread, could be removed surgically with good chance of a permanent cure.

THE DAMAGE BROUGHT ABOUT BY THE
ASBESTOS FIBERS IN THE LUNG:
BIOLOGY OF THE DISEASE PROCESS

There have been a number of experimental studies of the disease processes involved in asbestosis (e.g., Vorwald et al., 1951; Holt et al., 1964; Shin and Firminger, 1973). Chrysotile ($3MgO \cdot 2SiO_2 \cdot 2H_2O$) is a fibrous form of hydrated magnesium silicate. The initial site of reaction in the lung involves the respiratory bronchioles and their alveoli (Hennigar and Gross, 1977), similarly to the reaction site of other dusts. Macrophages that have ingested silica die because the silica particles injure the lysosomal membranes; the interior of the cell is autolyzed by the release of the lysosomal enzymes internally. Material from the dead macrophages is intensely fibrogenic (Hennigar and Gross, 1977). However, a siliceous component is not an essential factor in the development of asbestosis (Vorwald et al., 1951).

Holt et al., (1964) have put forward the following construction of the development of the disease: (1) The asbestos worker inhales a dust with fibers of various lengths of less than about 100 μ. (2) Fibers less than 5 μ in length are immediately taken up by macrophages. If there is a high concentration of these fibers, rapid fibrosis develops, and an acute form of asbestosis occurs (which was seen in the early part of the century). (3) The longer fibers, about 50 μ, become coated with protein and are surrounded, eventually, in the lung substance, with fibrous tissue. After some years these fibers disintegrate, producing large numbers of asbestos fragments, which are ingested by macrophages and give rise to a situation similar to (2). However, chronic inflammation over a period of 15 to 20 years is known to induce neoplastic change. Asbestos-related carcinomas may be squamous or undifferentiated or adenocarcinomatous in type.

The constant movement of the fibers in the lung over a period of many year years would be expected to build up severe fibrotic reaction, together with a low-grade chronic inflammation, and the production of neoplastic change in a similar fashion to the development of scar adenocarcinomata. No satisfactory explanation of the causes of the other types of bronchogenic carcinoma except that of chronic inflammatory change is at present available (Hennigar and Gross, 1977).

ASBESTOS BODIES IN SPUTA AND BRONCHIAL WASHINGS

Methods of preparation of sputa and a quantitative study of the ferruginous-body content of lung tissue have been reported (McDonald, 1975; Rosen et al., 1972). When a person has been exposed to many respirable fibers, "asbestos bodies" are found in his sputum (Figures 2-5). These are also known as ferruginous bodies because iron pigments from red cells are precipitated onto the fiber to produce a drumstick appearance (Figure 2).

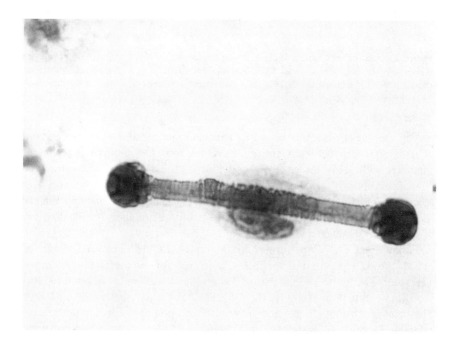

Figure 2. Typical ferruginous or asbestos body of "drumstick" configuration. The nucleus of a macrophage that has partly engulfed the stem of the drumstick is seen. Papanicolaou stained sputum smear X 1500.

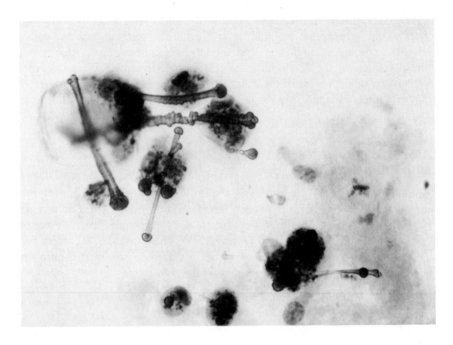

Figure 3. A number of asbestos bodies, which are partly engulfed by "dust" cells or macrophages, are shown. The original fiber becomes encrusted with a golden yellow granular deposit, which is iron-containing. Papanicolaou stained material from right bronchial wash. Filter preparation × 600.

The cytological examination of an adequate number and type of specimens of sputa from productive coughs can, therefore, provide a noninvasive technique whereby, with X-ray evidence of basal fibrosis, the diagnosis of asbestosis can be made. Although ferruginous bodies are not thought to be pathognomonic of asbestosis (Millard, 1977), pulmonary fibrosis, especially of the basal portions of the lungs, and ferruginous bodies would constitute a firm basis for the diagnosis of asbestosis (Hennigar and Gross, 1977).

Farley et al. (1977) performed routine cytopathologic examinations at six-month intervals on sputum specimens from 628 former asbestos workers and 128 control patients. The number of ferruginous bodies in sputa increased as a logarithmic function of the occupational exposure to asbestos in workdays. They concluded that the presence of ferruginous bodies in sputa indicated considerable exposure to asbestos dust, although lack of exposure could not be assumed in their absence. From their work they found that routine cytopathologic procedures were sufficient for the detection of ferruginous bodies in sputa.

Identification of ferruginous bodies as asbestos bodies can be established by

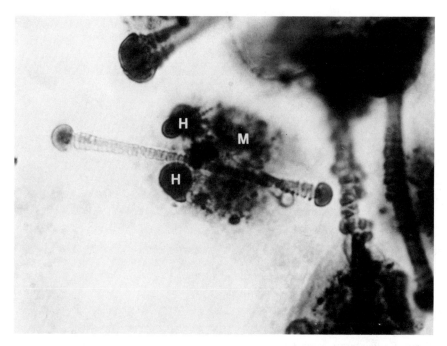

Figure 4. Higher-power view of a "dust" cell or macrophage (M) from Figure 3. The broken-off heads (H) of drumsticks are present, attached to the cell. Papanicolaou stained bronchial wash × 1500.

electron probe X-ray analysis (Chen and Mottet, 1978). By this method chemical components (Si, Mg, Ca, Fe) can be found that are characteristic of asbestos.

Because of the long time frame, it is important now to map the route that asbestos fibers describe through the community and assess the risk of bronchogenic carcinoma due to asbestos fibers occurring in the next 20 years. Monitoring of the changes in known asbestos workers is possible by means of a series of sputa examinations and X-rays at intervals appropriate for the changes present in the cells of their bronchi. Location of sites of breakdown of asbestos granulomata may be achieved by segmental bronchial washings. The identification of segments of the biological course by cytopathology and appropriate mapping of the disease incidence would appear to offer the best estimate of the risk of this disease process.

The use of cytopathology in the investigation of a disease in the patient must be viewed in the context of the biology of the natural history of that disease process. Unfortunately, the natural history of many disease processes, particularly the early development of cancers, is unknown, especially with regard to the time frame involved from the development of a single group of

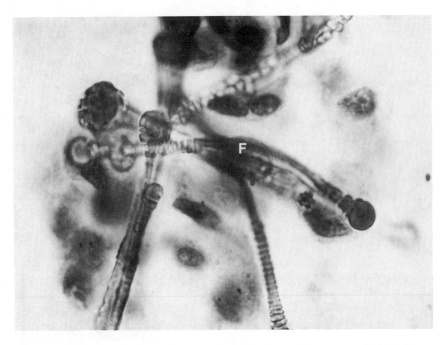

Figure 5. Photomicrograph showing a number of asbestos fibers, some of which (F) are gently curved. Papanicolaou stained sputum preparation × 1500.

cancer cells to disease that causes the individual to seek medical advice. The advantage of cytopathological investigation is that is allows repetitive samples to be taken over a prolonged time, and these samples, in the aggregate, when correlated with other clinical data, can provide information regarding the time intervals between various stages in the progression to malignancy. At the same time the investigation represents a modality of management of the precursor condition for the individual so that early treatment can be instituted if malignant changes develop.

The problem of asbestos fiber inhalation and distribution in the community provides an opportunity for identification of an agent concerned with carcinogenesis, in a discrete morphologic form. A time-frame distribution map of the dispersal of such agents in the community is imperative at a certain stage in the clarification of the relationship of agents in the work-place to disease processes. The approximation of the final analysis of distribution of carcinogens to the real situation depends very much upon the reliability of the initial data, whether it be data from the detection of the disease process or data regarding the death of the diseased patient. In many ways a valuable control would be an independent confirmation of the diagnosis of the disease. Cytopathological investigation

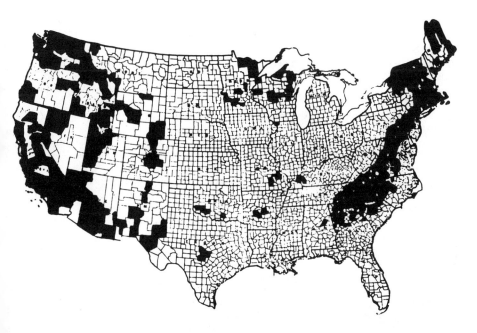

Figure 6. The distribution of quarries by counties and regions that may contain asbestos-bearing formations. (Prepared by the Environmental Defense Fund from data of the Mining Enforcement of Safety Administration.) (See Carter, 1977.) (Reproduced with permission)

can provide this. A starting point for the study of the distribution of the disease process would be the map prepared by the Environmental Defense Fund, which shows the regions that have appropriate mineralogy to produce asbestos-bearing rock (Figure 6). One cannot deny the importance of monitoring the distribution of identifiable carcinogens in the community and the management of high-risk populations, from the point of view of both the best interest of the individual patient and a safe environment.

The support of a grant from the National Cancer Institute of Canada is gratefully acknowledged.

References

Baker, R. R., Marsh, B. R., Frost, J. K., Stitik, F. P., Carter, D., and Lee, J. M. The detection and treatment of early lung cancer. In *Cancer of the Lung,* G. F. Murray, ed. Stration Intercontinental Medical Book Corporation, 1974, p. 39.

Cancer Mortaility by Age, Sex and Site of Disease, Ontario, 1931–1960. Medical Statistics Branch, Ontario Department of Health, 1962.

Carr, D. T., and Mountain, C. F. The staging of lung cancer. *Seminars Oncol. 1*: 229, 1974.

Carter, L. J. Asbestos: Trouble in the air from Maryland Rock Quarry. *Science 197*: 237, 1977.

Charlebois, C. T., and Rivest, F. An overview of the Canadian asbestos problem. *Chem. Can. 30*: 19, 1978.

Chen, W- J., and Mottet, N. K. Malignant mesothelioma with minimal asbestos exposure. *Hum. Pathol. 9*: 253, 1978.

Erozan, Y. S., and Frost, J. K. Cytopathologic diagnosis of lung cancer. *Seminars Oncol. 1*: 191, 1974.

Farley, M. L., Greenberg, S. D., Shuford, E. H., Hurst, G. A., Spivey, C. G., and Christianson, C. S. Ferruginous bodies in sputa of former asbestos workers. *Acta Cytol. 21*: 693, 1977.

Frost, J. K. The cell in health and disease. In *Monographs in Clinical Cytology,* Vol. 2, G. H. Wied, E. von Haam, L. G. Koss, and J. W. Reagan, eds. Baltimore: Williams and Wilkins. 1969.

Gifford, J. H., and Waddington, J. K. B. Review of 464 cases of carcinoma of lung treated by resection. *Br. Med. J. 1*: 723, 1957.

Godden, J. O., ed. *Cancer in Ontario.* The Ontario Treatment and Research Foundation, 1975, pp. 74 and 111.

Hahn-Weinheimer, P., and Hirner, A. Influence of hydrothermal treatment on physical and chemical properties of chrysotile asbestos. *J. Proc. R. Soc. N.S.W. 110*: 99, 1977.

Hennigar, G. R., and Gross, P. Drug and chemical injury-environmental pathology. In *Pathology,* W. A. D. Anderson, and J. M. Kissane, eds. St. Louis: Mosby, 1977, p. 237.

Holt, P. F., Mills, J., and Young, D. K. The early effects of chrysotile asbestos dust on the rat lung. *J. Pathol. Bacteriol. 87*: 15, 1964.

Johnston, W. W., and Frable, W. J. The cytopathology of the respiratory tract. A review. *Am. J. Pathol. 84*: 372, 1976.

Lincoln, B. Asbestos: A world resource. in *3rd Int. Congr. Phys. Chem. Asb. Min. Paper 1*: 1, Quebec, Canada, 1975; cited by Hahn-Weinheimer and Hirner, 1977.

McDonald, J. R. Respiratory tract. Chapter 15 in *A Manual of Cytotechnology,* C. M. Keebler, and J. W. Reagen, eds. Chicago: The American Society of Clinical Pathologists, 1975.

Millard, M. Lung, pleura and mediastinum. Chapter 26 in *Pathology,* W. A. D. Anderson, and J. M. Kissane, eds. St. Louis: C. V. Mosby, 1977, p. 1038.

Neff, T. A. Recent advances in the diagnosis of lung cancer. In *Cancer of the Lung,* G. F. Murray, ed. Stratton Intercontinental Medical Book Corporation, 1974, p. 19.

Rosen, P., Melamed, M., and Savino, A. The ferruginous body content of lung tissue: A quantitative study of eighty-six patients. *Acta Cytol. 16*: 207, 1972.

Selikoff, I. J., Churg, J., and Hammond, E. C. Asbestos exposure and neoplasia. J.A.M.A. 188: *22, 1964.*

Selikoff, I. J., Churg, J., and Hammond, E. C. Reaction between exposure to asbestos and mesothelioma. *N. Engl. J. Med. 272*: 560, 1965.

Selikoff, I. J., Nicholson, W. J., and Langer, A. M. Asbestos air pollution. *Arch. Environ. Health 25*: 1, 1972.

Seydel, H. G., Chait, A., and Gmelich, J. T. *Cancer of the Lung.* New York: Wiley 1975, p. 20.

Shin, M. L., and Firminger, H. I. Acute and chronic effects of intraperitoneal injection of two types of asbestos in rats with a study of the histopathogenesis and ultrastructure of resulting mesotheliomas. *Am. J. Pathol. 70*: 291, 1973.

Umiker, W. O. Relative accuracy of various procedures in the diagnosis of bronchogenic
carcinoma. *J.A.M.A. 195*: 658, 1966.
Vorwald, A. J., Durkan, T. M., and Pratt, P. C. Experimental studies of asbestosis. *A.M.A.
Arch. Ind. Hyg. Occup. Med. 3*: 1, 1951.

Medical Hazards of Underwater Exploration

R. B. PHILP, D.V.M., Ph. D.
Professor, Department of Pharmacology
The University of Western Ontario

The preoccupation of humankind with the depths of the ocean can be traced to
the beginnings of recorded history. It is said that Alexander the Great descended
into the sea in a cask in order to view the wonders of the deep. The Phoenicians
employed divers to cut anchor cables and foul rudder stocks of enemy vessels.
Our reasons for probing the deep have changed but little through the millennia.
We dive for food, profit, exploration, military advantage, to expand our knowledge of our environment, and to enjoy the pure beauty of the underwater world.

Recently, two particular underwater activities have achieved special promi-
nence—recreational and commercial diving. An estimated 2.5 million Americans
have received training and certification as amateur scuba divers, with an equal
number scattered throughout the rest of the world; and it was estimated that by
1980 over 20 million acres of seabed would have been leased for the exploration
for fossil fuel resources. The direct consequence of shrinking world reserves of
oil and natural gas, this exploration has resulted in a rapid expansion of commercial diving. The recreational diver and the commercial diver rest at the extreme ends of the underwater spectrum of physical and mental hazards, but
together they constitute the largest single population that is potentially at risk
from such hazards. Other groups include military divers, divers employed by
governments and institutions, and scientists who utilize diving as a vehicle to
extend their research.

As each succeeding depth barrier has been penetrated by advances in technology, new medical problems have been encountered that demand solution
before divers can safely extend their working capabilities in the ocean. Under-

water medicine is a highly complex and sophisticated specialty that requires not only a comprehensive knowledge of medical science as it relates to the diving situation but also a considerable understanding of the laws of physics.

DECOMPRESSION SICKNESS

Not long after Augustus Siebe developed the first practical diving dress, it became apparent that man could not descend into the sea with impunity. Numerous fatalities and permanent disabilities resulted from the use of his apparatus, and although many novel theories were expounded to explain this, these divers unquestionably suffered from acute decompression sickness (DS). When air is breathed at normal atmospheric pressure (which is equivalent to a column of mercury approximately 760 mm in height), the 20% oxygen (O_2) contained in the air is largely consumed in the metabolic functions of the body. The 80% nitrogen (N_2), however, is an inert gas which does not participate in biochemical reactions; it therefore becomes dissolved in body fluids and tissues until it reaches a state of equilibrium with the surrounding atmosphere. As a diver descends, it is necessary for him to breathe air at increasing pressures in order to offset the weight of the column of water above him. Each 10 meters of depth generates approximately one additional atmosphere of pressure. The equilibration of the diver's body tissues and fluids with this new pressure occurs rather slowly, with the rate varying considerably from tissue to tissue depending on the circulatory supply. Thus, blood equilibrates rapidly, whereas tissues such as body fat, which are poorly supplied with blood vessels, may take a very long time to reach equilibrium. The amount of gas taken up depends not only upon the partial pressure of the inert gas which is being breathed but also upon the solubility of that gas in a particular tissue. The solubility of N_2 in fat is five times its solubility in water. Thus, body fat becomes a significant storage reservoir for N_2.

As the diver begins his ascent, his body will contain a higher concentration of inert gas than that of the air that he is breathing, the degree of difference being dependent upon the length of time that he stayed at his maximum depth. If his rate of ascent exceeds the capacity of blood and lungs to eliminate the excess gas, the difference in partial pressure between the dissolved gas in fluids and tissues and that in the breathing gas will exceed a critical factor, and bubbles will form. If the formation of bubbles is extensive, the signs and symptoms of DS may occur. Bubbles in soft tissues such as muscles, joint capsules, tendons, and so on, may distort nerve endings, producing pain. Interference with normal blood flow by bubbles may deprive areas of the body of essential O_2, thus producing ischemic pain. When joint or muscle pain is the only manifestation of DS, it is referred to as Type 1. If, however, more serious signs and symptoms occur, it is classified as Type 2, which may include general malaise, hypotension, respiratory crisis with coughing and cyanosis, circulatory crisis with retrosternal pain similar to that experienced in a coronary thrombosis, or a neurological crisis with parathesias and/or paraplegia. Visual disturbances and vertigo may also occur. The time to onset varies considerably. Symptoms may commence during the decompression, or they may not be observed for several hours after surfacing. The formation of bubbles in the brain, spinal cord, major nerves, coronary vessels, and other major blood vessels is responsible for the more severe forms of the disease.

The prevention of DS is based upon control of the rate of the diver's ascent to avoid, or at least to minimize, the formation of bubbles. In the early twentieth century Haldane proposed that the pressure could be reduced by one-half without significant risk of bubble formation. Early decompression tables were based on this principle and resulted in a remarkable reduction in the incidence of this disease. It was by no means completely eliminated, however, and as divers progressed to deeper depths, the problem once more became significant. Subsequent theoretical considerations of the rates of uptake and elimination of inert gases like N_2 indicated that significant bubble formation could occur during decompression according to the Haldanian method. Mathematical models of decompression were devised based upon hypothetical body tissues having different saturation half-times ranging from a few minutes to several hours. Since N_2 uptake and elimination proceed in an exponential fashion, it was possible to generate a composite curve representing the rate of N_2 elimination from the whole body. The application of this kind of technology has resulted in further improvement in decompression tables and a subsequent reduction in the incidence of DS; but the advent of the Doppler flow meter, an effective detector of bubbles in blood, has shown that bubble formation occurs in many "safe" decompressions, and DS remains a significant problem.

A great number of variables may influence the susceptibility of an individual to DS. Some of these are well understood, others less so. Such factors as obesity, fatigue, dehydration, recent excessive alcohol consumption, cold stress, and accumulation of carbon dioxide will increase susceptibility; and more recently attention has focused on changes that may be initiated in the blood clotting system by the presence of intravascular bubbles. When a bubble forms in blood, complex circulating proteins such as fibrinogen (the major clotting protein) become oriented at the blood/gas interphase such that water-soluble components of the molecule project into the liquid phase, and fat-soluble components into the gas phase. This physical distortion of the molecule unmasks areas that attract blood platelets, the normal physiological role of which is to protect against blood loss by aggregating in large clumps at sites of vascular injury. They are also primary participants in the formation of a thrombus when aggregation is precipitated within the blood vessel by virtue of damage to the internal lining. When platelets are attracted to the bubble, they aggregate and release components that accelerate the formation of a blood clot. Thus, an intra-vascular bubble may serve as a trigger to produce small platelet thrombi which could then contribute to the pathology of the disease by blocking critical blood vessels. Moreover, bubbles may remain in the vessels long enough to deprive the lining of essential O_2. Cell death may occur, and the lining of the blood vessel may slough off, producing an injury to which platelets may adhere and aggre-gate. Interference with normal microcirculatory flow may result in loss of fluid from the vascular bed and hypovolemic shock.

Treatment of Decompression Sickness

Treatment of DS involves recompression of the afflicted individual, in a medical hyperbaric chamber, to a depth sufficient to compress bubbles and relieve his condition. Slow decompression then ensues at a rate designed to avoid subse-quent formation of bubbles. Toward the end of decompression the patient may breath 100% O_2 in an effort to provide a concentration gradient favoring the rapid elimination of dissolved N_2. Additional therapy may include the intra-venous administration of plasma expanders such as low-molecular-weight dex-tran. This agent has the additional advantage of inhibiting the tendency for platelets to stick together and to other surfaces, and thus may minimize the tendency to form micro-thrombi.

Recently there has been considerable interest in the possibility that drugs that inhibit platelet aggregation might be useful in the treatment or prevention of DS. Such drugs are currently under investigation for the treatment of throm-boembolic disorders, and some, such as aspirin, have shown much promise. Cur-rent research is directed at determining whether these agents might be useful in the therapy or prevention of DS.

DYSBARIC OSTEONECROSIS

This disease, also known as aseptic bone necrosis, was first identified in caisson workers in 1911 and in divers in 1941. In this disease, localized areas in the long bones of the arms and legs die off and are replaced by fibrous tissue. If the lesions are in the shaft of the bone, no serious consequences result. If, however, they occur near the hip or shoulder joints, collapse of the weight-bearing sur-face may lead to severe, arthritic symptoms. This situation has significant medico-legal implications, since it terminates the diver's career. The incidence of lesions detected on X-ray has been variously estimated at 2 to 3% for com-mercial and naval divers, 5% for experimental divers, 30% or more for caisson workers, and 50% or more for Japanese diving fishermen (who have no formal training as divers). The frequency of the condition appears both time- and pressure-dependent. The cause is poorly understood. Recently, careful autopsy of several fatal cases of DS in Japanese fishing divers revealed hemorrhage and thrombosis in the long bones, and similar lesions have been seen in animal experiments. It may be that frequent, temporary blockage of blood flow by bubbles and thrombi may eventually lead to bone death. If this theory is supported by further research, platelet-inhibiting drugs may play a future role in the prevention of osteonecrosis.

INERT GAS NARCOSIS

Not long after the development of effective diving suits it became apparent that man's ability to penetrate the depth was limited by a phenomenon that became known as the "raptures of the deep." It involves the progressive loss of mental capacities and is similar to the onset of the early stages of anesthesia or to alcoholic intoxication. Depending upon the diver and his degree of experience, the signs become subjectively detectable at around 30 meters, increasing as the diver descends. A rule of thumb known as "Martini's Law" holds that beyond 30 meters one additional atmosphere of air pressure is roughly equivalent to the effects of drinking one martini. Like the seasoned drinker, the experienced diver becomes accustomed to working under this handicap, and air dives have been carried out to 100 meters. However, performance testing has shown that significant impairment of mental function occurs at much shallower depths, and the potential danger to the diver should he be faced with a crisis is obvious. The onset of the condition is extremely rapid, and it disappears just as quickly when the diver returns to shallower depths. Laughter, loquacity, light-headedness, and excitement progress to mental confusion, impairment of the time sense, numbness and tingling of the lips and legs, and a characteristic deadpan expression. Divers may fail to perform tasks at depth and report them as having been completed when they return to surface. Stupor, a sense of impending blackout, and manic-depressive behavior may be noted. Unconsciousness may occur at depths in excess of 180 meters. When air is the breathing gas, the condition is referred to as nitrogen narcosis; however, other inert gases are capable of producing similar effects.

The mechanism of inert gas narcosis is poorly understood; however, there is a direct relationship between the oil solubility of the inert gas and its propensity to produce narcosis. Lipid-soluble inert gases adsorb to phospholipid membranes, resulting in an expansion of the membrane surface and increased ion permeability. It is felt that, in the brain, the influx of sodium eventually causes interference with transmission of nerve impulses. Xenon is so narcotic that it has been used successfully as an anesthetic agent at normal atmospheric pressure. Xenon, argon, and nitrogen are the most narcotic of the inert gases.

Nitrogen at high pressure not only produces narcotic effects, but it may modify or significantly alter the pharmacological activity of many centrally acting drugs. With the advent of saturation diving (see below) the possibility that a diver may require medical treatment while living in a hyperbaric chamber has become very real. Presently, our knowledge of the interactions between inert gas narcosis and centrally acting drugs is limited, and considerable work is being directed to improving our understanding of such interactions. Inert gas narcosis is not a treatable condition, and therefore efforts to alleviate the problem must be directed at prevention. To this end operational dives to depths greater than 80 meters usually involve the use of artificial gas mixtures in which a less-narcotic gas has been substituted for N_2. The gas most commonly used for this purpose is helium (He), which has very low oil solubility and does not adsorb to phospholipid membranes, so that its narcotic potential is extremely low. The substitution of He has permitted operational dives to depths of 500 meters or more without the problem of narcosis. Because of the low density of He, however, speech takes on a "Donald Duck" quality, which makes communication difficult and which has necessitated the development of electronic unscramblers.

Helium is found in conjunction with oil and natural gas. It is therefore a finite resource, and current estimates suggest that the world supply of He may become exhausted by 1990. Other gases that may be substituted for He are being sought. Neon appears to be the most likely choice, since it also has a low narcotic potential. Hydrogen has been used, and like neon does not produce the narcotic effect found with N_2. Hydrogen, however, is extremely explosive when O_2 concentration exceeds 4%, a property that makes it less desirable.

HIGH PRESSURE NERVOUS SYNDROME (HPNS)

The requirements of the offshore oil industry dictate that divers must be able to operate effectively at depths of 600 meters or greater, but He/O_2 dives to depths in excess of 200 meters revealed a new physiological hazard. Its symptoms include marked decrement in performance upon reaching depth and gradual improvement with time, unlike the situation with inert gas narcosis. Muscle tremor may occur, and the ability to perform tasks requiring fine muscular control may be impaired. At 500 meters or greater, divers may be able to perform adequately provided that they remain concentrated upon the task at hand; but if their attention should stray, they may lapse into what has been termed micro-sleep. Marked electroencephalographic changes occur during these phases of micro-sleep; and animal experiments have shown that at very high pressures clonic seizures develop. There is a direct relationship between the rate of compression and the depth at which these signs and symptoms commence, suggesting that a large part of the phenomenon is due to the application of pressure itself rather than to any specific effects of He. With very slow rates of compression and frequent stops, experimental dives to depths of 600 meters and more have been achieved without HPNS. These slow rates of compression, however, are not generally practical for operational dives.

Current theory holds that the rapid application of high pressure causes compression of nerve membranes, making the passage of ions more difficult, a phenomenon directly opposite to that of inert gas narcosis. If this theory is correct, then the application of pressure would be expected to reverse anesthesia, since anesthetic agents work by causing increased permeability of nerve membranes to ion penetration. Experimental animals anesthetized with barbiturates have recovered completely when exposed to high pressures of He/O_2. This apparent antagonism between He at high pressure and anesthetics suggested that HPNS might be controllable by the inclusion of a narcotic gas in the breathing mixture. N_2 was the obvious choice, and present evidence suggests that when the inert gas mixture contains one part N_2 for every ten of He, the problems of HPNS can largely be avoided.

OXYGEN TOXICITY

During World War II the Royal Navy developed an O_2 rebreathing apparatus for use by naval divers. Its purpose was to avoid surface detection by preventing the escape of bubbles. The divers breathed O_2 from a bag, and their expired air was circulated through a CO_2-adsorbent material so that the O_2 could be reused. It was quickly discovered that if this apparatus was used at depths much below 10 meters the diver developed muscular twitching, nausea, vomiting, dizziness, tunnel vision, hearing difficulties, and numbness and tingling around the lips. If the diver did not surface shortly after the onset of these early symptoms, grand mal seizures sometimes followed. The convulsant properties of O_2 are by now well documented. When air is breathed at a pressure that attains an O_2 concentration equivalent to 2½ times 100% O_2 at atmospheric pressure, central nervous toxicity becomes a risk. This concentration is achieved at a depth of 140 meters or more. The mechanism of O_2 toxicity is poorly understood, but it has been shown that O_2 is capable of interfering with several essential biochemical processes. High concentrations of O_2 in the brain interefere with the synthesis of gamma aminobutyric acid (GABA), a neurotransmitter in a system that has a modulating effect on brain activity. Suppression of this system produces an increased sensitivity to convulsions. Moreover, GABA has been shown to exert a protective effect against O_2 toxicity in experimental animals. In deep dives involving artificial gas mixtures, it is necessary to control the O_2 concentration carefully within narrow limits. At a depth of 600 meters an O_2 content of 1.62% is equivalent to 100% O_2 at the surface.

Another form of O_2 toxicity involves the respiratory system. When a concentration of 60% or more is breathed on the surface, a progressive deterioration in lung function occurs. This begins with congestion of the alveolar sacs, the formation of small hemorrhages, and finally the collapse and destruction of the alveolar sacs themselves. Interference with the production of surfactant material secreted in the lining of the lungs, which is essential for maintaining normal lung elasticity, may be the cause. Decreased vital capacity, interference with normal O_2 diffusion, and increased airway resistance result. Pulmonary O_2 toxicity is both a time- and a pressure-related phenomenon so that as pressure increases, the time required for the onset of symptoms is shortened. Pulmonary O_2 toxicity may become a limiting factor during saturation diving unless O_2 concentration is carefully controlled.

At a given pressure, the human body becomes fully saturated with inert gas after 24 hours. Further exposure will not result in uptake of more gas; therefore a diver may remain in a hyperbaric chamber for days or weeks without necessitating any longer decompression than that required after 24 hours. Since the equivalent of 60% O_2 at the surface is achieved at a depth of 20 meters, prolonged exposure to this or deeper depths may result in chronic pulmonary O_2 poisoning unless the concentration is reduced appropriately.

BAROTRAUMA

Barotrauma refers to tissue damage that occurs as a result of failure to equalize pressure between a body cavity and the external environment.

Gas Embolism

If a diver holds his breath during the ascent after having breathed compressed gas, the expansion of the gas trapped in the lungs may tear alveolar tissue and rupture blood vessels, allowing gas to enter the pulmonary venous circulation. These gas emboli may return to the heart and thence to the general arterial circulation. Should they occlude the arterial supply to a vital organ, serious consequences may ensue. If gas emboli reach the brain, rapid loss of consciousness usually follows. Blockage of a coronary artery may produce symptoms and signs of a heart attack. Unlike decompression sickness, air embolism is not related to the duration of the dive and may occur even after an ascent of as little as 1 meter. The treatment for air embolism is similar for that of DS. The victim must be transported to a hyperbaric treatment chamber as quickly as possible. The application of pressure drives the gas emboli into solution so that the gas may be eliminated. O_2 breathing is frequently instituted toward the end of the therapeutic decompression in order to maintain adequate oxygenation of the tissues and to facilitate the removal of dissolved nitrogen.

The expansion and rupture of pulmonary alveoli may cause other problems in addition to air embolism. Significant damage to lung tissue may result, mediastinal emphysema may occur (that is, the entry of gas into the area between the lungs), and gas may track upward into the neck region (subcutaneous emphysema). Pneumothorax is a condition in which air enters the pleural cavity and expands during ascent. Expansion of the air will cause collapse of the lung on that side, and the condition may be accompanied by hemorrhage. In general any diver who, on surfacing, displays labored breathing, dry hacking cough, coughing of blood, chest pain, the presence of gas under the skin, or dizziness and fainting should be treated as a medical emergency.

In addition to pulmonary gas embolism, other forms of barotrauma may result from failure to equalize pressure between body cavities and the external environment. During the descent, unless the Valsalva maneuver is performed frequently, external pressure on the eardrum may cause considerable pain (ear squeeze), and there is a risk of rupturing the tympanum if the diver ignores these warning signals. Similarly, sinus squeeze may occur if blockage of the Eustachian tubes prevents equalization of pressure. This may cause severe bleeding from the sinuses. Thoracic squeeze occurs principally in breath-hold diving where compression of the chest occurs during descent. Lung volume will be reduced to 50% at a depth of 10 meters and halved again at 30 meters. Beyond this depth there is a danger that further compression of the lungs may result in some tissue damage, although this is not usually severe unless extreme pressures are encountered. Lung squeeze is not a problem in scuba diving but is theoretically possible if the breath is held during descent.

OTHER UNDERWATER HAZARDS

Numerous marine creatures are capable of inflicting damage on the unwary diver, ranging from the catastrophic bite of a large predatory shark to the minor pain and irritation of a fire-coral burn. Space does not permit a detailed discussion of these hazards. Most can be avoided by applying common sense and respecting the territorial rights of the ocean's inhabitants.

Underwater construction accidents constitute a serious threat to the commercial diver. Of the more than 30 deaths that have occurred in divers on the North Sea oil fields, many fall into this category. An accident that may cause moderate to severe injury on dry land may be fatal at a depth of 200 meters, where rescue is slow and difficult and the supply of breathing gas may be interrupted. Hypothermia is a real threat to the commercial diver, since deep water temperatures may range from 1 to 5°C. Hot-water-heated suits (supplied by an umbilical) are used, and in some cases, preheating of the breathing gas is necessary.

In conclusion, although the list of potential threats to the deep sea diver is lengthy and sobering, adequate training, physical fitness, sound judgment, and practical experience reduce them to an acceptable level, even in sports diving,

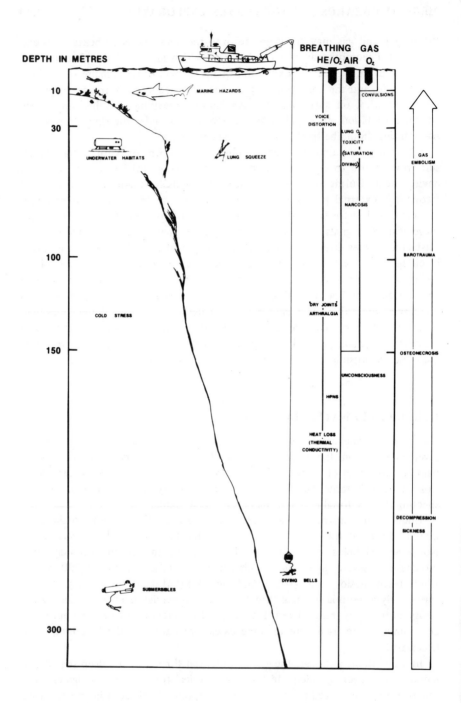

DEPTH IN METRES

BREATHING GAS
HE/O₂ AIR O₂

10   MARINE HAZARDS

30

UNDERWATER HABITATS   LUNG SQUEEZE

VOICE
DISTORTION

LUNG O₂
TOXICITY
(SATURATION
DIVING)

CONVULSIONS

GAS
EMBOLISM

NARCOSIS

100   BAROTRAUMA

COLD   STRESS

DRY JOINTS
ARTHRALGIA

150   OSTEONECROSIS

UNCONSCIOUSNESS

HPNS

HEAT LOSS
(THERMAL
CONDUCTIVITY)

DECOMPRESSION

SICKNESS

SUBMERSIBLES   DIVING BELLS

300

which, overall, has an excellent safety record. "These various hazards discussed above in relation to the deep-sea environment, are illustrated in Fig. 1".

Bibliography

Bennett, P. B., and Elliott, D. H., eds. *The Physiology and Medicine of Diving and Compressed Air Work* (2nd ed.). London: Baillière, Tindall and Cassell, 1975.

Philp, R. B. A review of blood changes associated with compression–decompression: Relationship to decompression sickness. *Undersea Biomed. Res. 1*: 117–150, 1974.

Shilling, C. W., and Beckett, M. W., eds. *National Plan for the Safety and Health of Divers in Their Quest for Subsea Energy.* Bethesda, Maryland: Undersea Med. Soc., 1976.

Strauss, Richard H., ed. *Diving Medicine.* New York: Grune and Stratton, 1976.

The Complete Underwater Diving Manual, compiled and edited by the National Oceanic and Atmospheric Administration and the Office of Marine Resources. New York: David McKay, 1977.

FIG. 1. Medical hazards of diving are shown in relation to depth (Left vertical axis) according to the breathing gas (right vertical axis). Breathing HE/O_2 is associated with distortion of the voice, arthralgia, high-pressure nervous syndrome (HPNS), and hypothermia resulting from the high thermal conductivity of helium. Breathing air may be associated with oxygen damage to the lungs (during saturation diving) and nitrogen narcosis which may result in loss of consciousness at depths in excess of 150 meters. Breathing pure oxygen may result in convulsions and other disturbances of the CNS at relatively shallow depths. The vertical arrow on the right side of the graph summarizes hazards associated with decompression. These are not necessarily related to the depth of the dive.

Medical Problems of Climbing at Extremely High Altitudes

DRUMMOND RENNIE, M. D., F.R.C.P., F.A.C.P.
Deputy Editor
The New England Journal of Medicine
Boston, Massachusetts

I begin by stating what I shall *not* discuss, and why. Long experience in the mountains has taught me what is to practical logic obvious: any member of a mountaineering expedition is liable to any of the ordinary, natural diseases that can occur in the cities and the plains. I have treated an acute attack of gonorrhea that occurred a few days after the patient had arrived, apparently fit, at over 17,000 feet; I have treated acute anxiety in Alaska, acute depression in the Himalayas, and, in Nepal, I had a worrying week trying to get a man with a bleeding duodenal ulcer evacuated by helicopter. Every expedition doctor has his share of stories: pneumonia at 25,000 feet; a bowel obstruction due to worms, two hundred miles from a road; or an epidemic of amebic dysentery on a big face climb. I am not going to talk about such illnesses, though the expedition leader must try to be ready for all of them, simply because they are peculiar neither to mountains nor to altitude, and I cannot compress a textbook of medicine, surgery, pharmacology, and emergency care into one chapter.

The same principle holds for violent trauma: when people go to very high altitudes in mountains they can fall and hurt themselves in every conceivable way from breaking their backs to twisting their ankles. The mortality on big Himalayan expeditions is more than 10%; so problems are certainly more serious and harder to cope with in such remote, high, and hostile terrain. There are numerous textbooks on the treatment of such problems, which also can, and do, occur in Yosemite Valley or even when bouldering at sea level, so I shall not address them here. Similarly, I do not propose to discuss tropical illnesses such as smallpox (which has now vanished), or malaria (which is on the increase), a wide variety of worms, bacillary and amebic dysentery, or giardiasis, because all of these do occur all over the world and are not peculiar to mountains. It is true that the Westerner may meet them for the first time when he is trekking through the forests of northern India toward his mountain, but once more there are several good books for mountaineers that deal with these problems, as well as a large number of standard medical textbooks.* In these texts you will find all the information necessary for first aid and evacuation, how to sterilize water, how to deworm the porters, and what shots to take before you leave in the first place.

Neither shall I deal with the Arctic environment. All other things being equal, the higher one goes, the lower the temperature falls—so that above the snowline, whether it be at sea level in Greenland or at 16,000 feet in parts of Nepal, one has to be prepared for all the hazards of extreme cold such as general loss of body temperature (hypothermia), as well as the specific problems posed by snow-blindness and frostbite. In each case prevention is often easy and effective, whereas treatment is hazardous, problematical, and lengthy. Both prevention and treatment of these conditions are well handled in the books I cite at the end of this chapter.

Of course, all of these illnesses are far harder to deal with in a small, storm-battered tent on a steep, corniced ridge above 20,000 feet than in a comfortable, well-equipped hospital at sea level. In many parts of the world there is absolutely no chance whatsoever for rescue over and beyond that provided by the expedition itself. There are no local climbing rescue associations: it is often forbidden to bring in more than line-of-sight portable radios; it may take well over a week to send out a runner to try to get hold of a helicopter, which itself may not exist, or if it does exist, may not be in a state to fly or may not be able to land and, more importantly, take off with an injured man at a height above 12,000 feet in thick clouds and high winds. All too often care, even in hospital 'centers', is inadequate, ineffectual, and expensive. Any climber who embarks on an expedition to a major Himalayan peak, for example, must accept this one-in-ten chance of being killed; and this risk extends to small expeditions to the lesser Himalayan peaks. All the ordinary risks of climbing are exaggerated by the remoteness and the altitude: the cold is colder, the winds are more powerful, the light is more intense, the distances are greater, and the chances of rescue are smaller. Thus the two vastly experienced British climbers Chris Bonington and Doug Scott, having climbed the 23,900-foot Baintha Brakk (the "Ogre") in the Karakoram in July of 1977, had to make numerous rappels and a six-day descent down an extremely difficult face, Scott having broken both his legs and Bonington having fractured some ribs and severely damaged one hand. Climbers who go to such places must have the automatic, overmastering will to live, or the simplest problem may become a potential killer.

Leaving aside, then, the peculiar difficulties of treatment and evacuation that

---

Medical Care for Mountain Climbers by Peter Steele, published by Heinemann, 1976; *Exploration Medicine,* edited by O. G. Edholm and A. L. Bacharach, published by Wright, Bristol, 1965; and *Medicine for Mountaineering,* 2nd edition, edited by James A. Wilkerson, and published by The Mountaineers, Seattle, Washington, 1975.

surround natural illnesses, trauma, tropical diseases, and the consequence of an Arctic environment in the mountains, we are left with those illnesses that are peculiar to the very high mountains, and which all have lack of oxygen as the precipitating cause. I would emphasize that I am not discussing very sudden ascent as in a balloon or an unpressurized plane (or even in a decompression chamber). I am discussing effects that take more than eight hours and usually one or two days to develop.

Though many millions of people have lived for centuries at or around 4,000 meters (13,100 feet), particularly in the Andean and Tibetan plateaus, it is probable that they have never constituted more than 2% of the world's population. At one time or another living at high altitude may have conferred selective advantages, the Altiplano of the Andes, for example, offering a much easier terrain for cultivation and one much freer from disease, insects, and predators than the nearby Amazonian jungle. This might be one reason why the Inca empire, before the coming of the Spaniards, was so immense (stretching some 4,000 miles in length), so secure, and so advanced.

At every altitude the proportion of oxygen in the air is constant (20.93%), but with increasing altitude the air becomes progressively thinner: in other words, one cubic meter of air at about 18,000 feet contains about half as many molecules of oxygen, and all its other constituents, nitrogen, inert gases, and so on, as one cubic meter of air at sea level. At around 29,000 feet (near the top of Mount Everest), the air is about one third as thick as at sea level. Though there are only 14 "8,000-meter peaks," or peaks higher than 26,250 feet in the world, there are many hundreds of peaks in the Himalayas alone (including the Karakorum and Pamirs) higher than 20,000 feet (6,100 meters); and as governmental restrictions become relaxed and communications become easier, more and more people are making for the high peaks, both in the Himalayan chain and in the Andes, where the highest mountains rise, in Peru and Argentina, to somewhat over 22,000 feet.

When we look at what happens to these lowlanders ascending mountains, it is very important to recognize that there is, as with all physiological functions, tremendous variability between individuals. The reactions on the part of the body to ascent to high altitudes seem to be conditioned by numerous factors, some of which may be genetic, some individual, and some dependent on previous physical training, both at sea level and high altitude. In general high-altitude diseases occur in proportion to the rate of ascent and the height reached. Despite this, however, high-altitude sickness (see below) is common in the Alps of Switzerland and in the Colorado Rockies, where the mountains in general are only 13,000 or 14,000 feet high, and deaths have been recorded in apparently fit young people below 10,000 feet. Other individuals, however, have climbed fairly rapidly and without inconvenience to 18,000 or 20,000 feet, and seem to be relatively resistant, though no one is immune, to the effects of the drop in atmospheric oxygen.

The effects of altitude are far less dependent upon the state of training of the individual than on his own individual make up. The state of fitness is important, of course, in determining whether a climber has the strength and stamina to do the climb, but a very strong and fit climber can still be completely devastated by the effects of altitude. Thus these effects tend to be demonstrated by the same individual in the same way each time he goes to high altitude. Once again I emphasize that these are tendencies and there are numerous exceptions.

ACUTE MOUNTAIN SICKNESS

Since most of us live at or around sea level, and certainly the vast majority of humanity lives below 3,000 feet altitude, I shall not dwell on the particular altitude diseases that occur in people, such as Tibetans and Peruvians of the Altiplano, who have lived all their lives at high altitudes. These diseases are of great theoretical interest to the physiologist and of practical importance to the doctor on the spot but do not really concern us here. Instead we will consider acute mountain sickness (AMS) and its relationship to a number of problems with which it particularly seems to be associated, which only occur on exposure to high altitude, which tend to occur at the same time in relation to ascent as acute mountain sickness, and which make acute mountain sickness far worse. These problems, which may be fatal, are high-altitude cerebral edema (CE) and high-altitude pulmonary edema (HAPE). An important and worrying new observation is that people at high altitude may develop hemorrhages into the backs of their eyes (retinal hemorrhages, RH). Finally, and separate from acute mountain sickness and the other problems already mentioned, there is thrombosis of the big veins of the body, particularly in the legs, and pulmonary embolism.

Acute mountain sickness was first described by a Jesuit friar, Father Acosta, in the Andes at the end of the sixteenth century. Acosta attributed it, perceptively enough, to the thinness of the air, but AMS was not really well categorized into its constituent (and potentially fatal) aspects until the British built railroads up to the copper mines in the Andes, and Dr. Ravenhill in 1913 was able to give a description of a disease that occurred whether people struggled up on foot, on mule back, or in the greatest luxury, by train. Typically AMS is a transient illness, and the higher and faster the ascent the worse it is. For a few hours after arrival, say by helicopter at altitudes between 12,000 and 18,000 feet, most people feel rather euphoric. They feel breathless on the slightest exertion, and they realize that their breathing is disordered, but there is little problem provided they keep still. After a period of 8 to 48 hours, however, they begin to get marked disinclination to eat. All the miserable and lethargic climber (now a patient) wants to do is lie down; and when he gets up, he tends to stagger dizzily around—he is "ataxic." Some people feel better on mild exercise—an effect that may be due to a change in their respiration. Symptoms include breathlessness on exertion, fatigue, insomnia, and great lassitude, and occasionally swelling of the face, the hand, and the ankles. Typically, affected climbers just retire morosely into a corner of their tents, neither eating nor drinking, and take no part in the general business of getting their camps in order, cooking, and preparing for the next day's climb. Usually, with rest, these symptoms end spontaneously in 24 to 48 hours and do not recur unless the climber goes up suddenly to a new altitude.

We have found in various on-the-spot surveys that symptoms of AMS appear in about half of all hikers trekking along an easy route at around 14,000 feet. Most people take some aspirin-like drug for the most common and often worst symptom, headache. The best treatment is to delay one or two days, to climb high but to sleep low, and, if no improvement occurs, to go down to lower altitudes. Some people will never become acclimatized even to moderate altitudes (for example, 14,000 feet), but they are a distinct minority.

The cause of AMS is entirely unknown. Its signs and symptoms (e.g., headaches, dizziness, nausea), are not helpful, since each has hundreds of causes and so is entirely unspecific. Nevertheless an old theory seems to be gaining ground once more. It is possible that the lack of oxygen affects many body cells enough to cause them to swell a little with fluid. This swelling is not very important except in the brain, since the brain is housed in a rigid box, the skull, and there is, of course, no room for the swelling. The particularly vulnerable brain cells seem to be those in the specific centers controlling appetite, vomiting, balance, and sleep. Thus, though the function of the stomach itself may not be upset, vomiting may be a prominent symptom, probably caused by happenings in the brain. An analagous situation is known to occur, for example, with expanding brain tumors. This theory of AMS is entirely unproved as yet but is, nonetheless, very attractive, and much evidence supports it. It is especially attractive because a rare but fatal complication of AMS is true brain swelling or cerebral edema (CE).

CEREBRAL EDEMA

There are many causes of CE, but one of the oddest and certainly least explained types of CE is that which occurs at high altitude. One can only diagnose CE of whatever cause clinically by showing that the nerve at the back of the eye (the optic nerve) is swollen forward or, at surgery, by showing that the brain itself is under high pressure and bulges out when the skull incision is made. The climber's companion sees his friend's moroseness proceed to irrationality, irritability, severe ataxia with a tendency to fall into snow drifts, or a total inability to stand up, and finally an unresponsive coma—the whole process taking but a few hours to progress. He will not respond to verbal commands or even to being moved, but merely lies there breathing stertorously, totally oblivious of his surroundings. Though the danger is extreme, companions often think he is merely "exhausted" or "wants to sleep," and they leave him alone. If exhaustion really is the cause, he will rapidly tell them so. The climber would have been brought down to lower altitudes well before this time had a good "buddy system" been in operation—brought down when he could still walk with help. If he is comatose, he should be given oxygen (in the unlikely event that it is available), but at all costs he should be brought down to lower altitudes, even though this is an extremely difficult and often dangerous procedure involving and imperiling the entire expedition, if it is to be achieved at high altitudes on the new hard routes being climbed in the 1970s. I have seen people deeply unconscious at 13,500 feet who were dragged down on stretchers made out of skis and sleeping bags and at 11,000 feet were sitting up and demanding to know what was happening to them, and were generally displaying considerable annoyance toward their then-exhausted rescuers.

Specific drugs for cerebral edema are few, poorly tested, and ineffective. It is probably a good idea to give a steroid, betamethazone, intravenously and, of course, oxygen. Again, rapid descent is essential whether or not there is oxygen to give. The various osmotically active infusions that are administered by neurologists to shrink the brain in the cerebral edema that occurs during or after operations on the brain are scarcely practical in the mountains and have certainly not been tried out properly in such circumstances, so no proper answer can be given on their use.

RETINAL HEMORRHAGES

The small vessels of the brain in people who have died of high-altitude CE tend to be blocked, and multiple little hemorrhages are seen in the brain substance. Whether they are associated with the hemorrhages that are also seen in the eyes of healthy and unhealthy climbers is not known. About ten years ago we published papers to show that small hemorrhages appearing in the retina of the eye were quite common in people who had been climbing slowly to a height of over 17,000 feet or who had been flown up to that height without any intervening acclimatization. Since then we and others have published numerous papers to show that such hemorrhages are common at about 17,000 feet but decline very rapidly in incidence below that altitude. They probably occur in a third to a half of climbers above 19,000 to 20,000 feet but only in about 4% of people climbing at 14,000 feet. They seem to cause symptoms when they occur at that tiny part of the eye called the macula, the part of the retina concerned with the center of the field of vision, where central incoming rays of light are focused to the retina by the lens, because this is the part of the retina able to cope with detailed distinctions. Since the vast majority of retinal substance has to do with the detection of gross movements and shadows in the periphery of the field of vision, most of the hemorrhages are unnoticed by the climbers, and no one yet knows whether their presence is an indication that the climber should stay where he is, go on climbing, or immediately come to lower altitudes. My colleagues and I have proved their association with acute mountain sickness, but all of us have seen such hemorrhages in extremely fit people who have acclimatized well and have had no mountain sickness at all. Whether they are associated with sudden severe isometric exertion (as in weight lifters at sea level or in technical climbers at any altitude) is unknown.

HIGH-ALTITUDE PULMONARY EDEMA

Much more common as a fatal or really serious complication of AMS is high-altitude pulmonary edema (HAPE). Pulmonary edema at sea level is a very common medical emergency with dozens of causes, all of them producing a flooding of the spongelike tissues and air spaces of the lung with fluid. As a result the lungs cannot be aerated, and so the blood flowing through the pulmonary (lung) vessels cannot be oxygenated. A very great deal of work has been done to try to elucidate the cause of this serious climbing complication since its first description in the United States in 1960, even though, like cerebral edema, it had been recorded back in 1913 by Ravenhill. HAPE is known to be associated with an extraordinary brisk and reflex contraction of the pulmonary arteries that causes the pressure on the right side of the heart to be increased. (The right ventricle pumps blood through the lungs; the left ventricle sends it on through the rest of the body.) These arteries themselves may leak a little; but it is also known that there is no heart failure in these people, nor has anyone been able to demonstrate any increased pressure in the capillaries (the smallest vessels) of the lungs, any increase in exudation of fluid from these capillaries, any increase in the pressure in the veins of the lung, or any abnormality in the left side of the heart that might cause blood to back up into the lungs, as occurs in the very common condition left ventricular heart failure. Despite intensive investigation, then, the cause is unknown.

What are the symptoms of HAPE? Usually there is increased and unnatural breathlessness. This is tricky to judge because everybody is breathless at very high altitudes, but most people on an expedition tend to know each other and their limits, and they should keep an eye open to see that their companions are not breathless and exhausted beyond what might reasonably be expected. If a companion is coughing a great deal, and particularly if he is coughing up frothy or blood-stained sputum, then it is likely that he is developing pulmonary edema. The fellow climber should then put his ear against the "patient's" chest, at the back. If he hears a little crackling sound—not a wheezing but a gentle crackling or bubbling (called crepitations or rales)—then there is pulmonary edema; and if he is blue (hard to see in multicolored tents) and sick and unable to look after himself properly, he should be brought down to lower altitudes immediately. The urgency of this action cannot be overemphasized because time and time again one hears of people who were able to look after themselves despite the symptoms of AMS and all the symptoms and signs of HAPE, but who only a few hours later were dead. They could have been saved by being frog-marched down the mountain two or three thousand feet.

As with acute mountain sickness, it pays to go up mountains slowly, enjoying the experience as much as possible. It pays to spend extra nights at camps to become better acclimatized, and if there is any sign of high-altitude pulmonary edema, it is essential to bring the climber down to a lower altitude immediately before he becomes a stretcher case and therefore extremely difficult, if not impossible, to evacuate.

Drug prophylaxis should, in general, be avoided. The only drug that seems of any use in acetazolamide (diamox), which produces a very slight increase in urine output with an increased acidity of the blood and a decreased formation of cerebrospinal fluid around the brain. It probably works best at night when it stimulates breathing and, in susceptible people, prevents them from becoming very low in oxygen when asleep. It is useful to take diamox for up to two days before and for two days after ascent by air to a high altitude in an emergency, but I am personally very much against taking drugs when one is going up in a planned fashion, under one's own steam, slowly. Using common sense is at least as effective as drugs and probably a great deal more so. In addition none of the toxic effects of the drugs is met with in this way. For full-blown pulmonary edema a strong diuretic such as furosemide given by mouth (or, if you have a doctor handy, into the vein) is usually pretty effective. Oxygen is suprisingly ineffective, and even if you have oxygen handy, immediate descent is vital.

In summary, AMS, HAPE, and CE can best be avoided by carefully planning one's ascent to include days and, in particular, nights spent reasonably low in order to become acclimatized. The "buddy system" is essential, and at the least sign of trouble the affected climber should be brought down to a lower camp. Nobody likes doing this. Climbers hate to lose hard-gained height, and there are the inevitable idiots who think that to suffer AMS somehow reflects upon their masculinity. Yet a great many lives and a great deal of agony to everybody concerned could be saved in this way. Prophylactic drugs should only be used in an emergency, and oxygen should always be given if it is at hand, but *never* as a substitute for descent.

THROMBOSIS IN VEINS

The last problem, deep-vein thrombosis and pulmonary embolism, is in a different catagory. It generally occurs in people who have been above 19,000 to 20,000 feet for some weeks. Their blood has been getting thicker and thicker as part of the adaptive process, and when they become stormbound and sedentary in tents, one of the veins in their legs may form a clot, so viscous has the blood become.

When this happens the climber is in some danger of having part of the clot break off, sweep through the main veins up through the heart and into the lungs to block off a major pulmonary artery, and so obstruct much, if not all, of the circulation and even kill the climber. This has been reported several times. Less severe obstruction may cause very severe breathlessness with coughing up of blood and total incapacity because a large part of the lung now becomes useless for respiration, since blood no longer flows through it, and gas exchange consequently cannot occur at a time (at extreme altitude) when it is even more essential than usual that the lungs be working extremely efficiently.

This state of affairs can only be avoided by keeping climbers at high altitudes for as short a period as possible. If somebody gets a deep-vein thrombosis, which is heralded by swelling and pain in the leg, particularly in the calf, then he should be brought down to low altitude immediately and the leg kept still and bound up with bandages. If a pulmonary embolus has occurred, he should be evacuated immediately. However, at this stage there is very little one can do, since the anticoagulant or blood-thinning therapies that one would use in a hospital in this country are completely out of the question under the circumstances of the mountain because they require elaborate and repeated checking of the degree of anticoagulation achieved, if they are to be effective on the one hand and if bleeding is to be avoided on the other.

An excellent description of the appalling problems presented by a severely ill man with a pulmonary embolus is given by Houston and Bates in their book *K 2: The Savage Mountain.** This account emphasizes that under circumstances of very high altitude on difficult and dangerous routes with high winds, avalanches, and difficult ice, evacuation of a sick man for whatever cause is a major undertaking and extremely hazardous for every single member of the expedition, and prophylaxis and early action are of the essence if the lives of the victim and of all his rescuers are to be saved.

*Houston, Charles and Robert Bates, *K 2: The Savage Mountain.* London: Collins, 1955.

Human Aging : General Characteristics and Research Strategies

JOHN W. ROWE, M.D.
Beth Israel Hospital, Harvard Medical School,
Boston Massachusetts

> *The attainment of old age is easy and only the inquiry about it difficult and so much the rather, because it is corrupted with false opinions and vaine reports.*
>
> —Francis Bacon

Individuals over 85 years of age represent the most rapidly growing segment of our population. Since 1900 those over 65 years have increased from 4% to the present level of 10% of the population, an increase that will accelerate in the near future. The average age of adult medical patients in our large urban hospitals now approaches 70 years. The rapid growth of our elderly population is important not only for the medical community, but in many aspects of American life, including architecture, urban planning, sociology, economics, and politics. The purpose of this presentation is to introduce the reader to the general characteristics of normal human aging and to discuss the special problems facing the clinical gerontologist, and the research designs at his disposal. Emphasis will be on the physiologic aspects of aging, although the major points are relevant to other areas of gerontologic inquiry.

Aging may be broadly defined as changes occurring over time and, as such, includes all phases of the life cycle including growth and development as well as senescence. Changes that occur after adulthood, including the middle and late years, are the particular province of the gerontologist.

Increasing age after adulthood is associated with an exponential increase in mortality rate, which is preceded by a similar exponential increase in the presence of pathologic changes. These changes have stimulated controversy regarding whether aging should be considered a disease state and, if not, about what the relation is of normal aging to disease-related changes.[1] There is now general agreement that increasing age is accompanied by inevitable physiologic changes that represent normal aging and are separable from the effects of disease states which become increasingly prevalent with age. These age-related changes are the substrate onto which the effects of specific diseases are grafted. These changed have clinical importance to the physician since they influence the presentation of illness, its response to treatment, and the complications that ensue.

The clinical gerontologist is faced with certain special obstacles not faced by students of aging in laboratory animals or isolated organ or cell systems. These special problems derive from characteristics of the experimental animal—man.[2] Man's long life span makes collection of true longitudinal data over the entire life span a slow and costly endeavor. In addition, many research subjects outlive the investigator! One major source of confusion is man's diversity—genetic, dietary, environmental, educational, social, and economic. These factors can all introduce physiologic changes over time that are not reflective of true biological aging. This situation differs vastly from the control exerted by laboratory investigators over such variables.

Review of the physiologic changes in man with advancing age allows development of several principles of clinical gerontology which, short of an encyclopedic collection of all the physiologica data, permit a logical approach to the changes. The first consideration that emerges is that of the phases of the normal life span. The early phase of growth and development, in which rapid increases in many functions occur, generally continues into early adulthood, peaking in the late twenties or early thirties. In those variables that do change with age after adulthood, the change generally begins immediately at the end of the growth and development phase and is generally linear into old age. Two important points thus emerge: first, there is no pleasant "plateau" of the middle years in which we stay in our prime for 20 to 30 years, and, second, the loss of function of most variables that do change with age is linear into the eighth and ninth decade and does not increase as we become older. Thus, the rate of aging does not change in most cases, and an 80-year-old is aging only as fast as a 30-year-old. The 80-year-old is more aged than his younger counterpart, having accumulated more of the changes secondary to age, but he is not losing function at a more rapid rate.

Another important characteristic of age-related changes is their *variability*. There are several different sources of variability, including changes within individuals from organ to organ, and changes from individual to individual in a given population. Such functions as cardiac output, glomerular filtration rate, and carbohydrate tolerance change rather dramatically, whereas others such as nerve conduction velocity and hematocrit undergo no significant change into the eighth or ninth decade. Of major importance is variability within the individual. If an apparently healthy 60-year-old is found on serial prospective measurements to have a cardiac output that is falling at a certain rate, perhaps at the rate average for his age group, this information is of no value in predicting the rate at which his kidneys, thyroid, sympathetic nervous system, or any other organ is changing with time. This apparent failure of various organs to be synchronized in their age-related changes rules against the presence of a basic biological clock. At present one cannot construct a variable termed "functional age" that predicts performance on a physiologic or psychologic test better than the individual chronological age.[3] Also, the variability in human aging from individual to individual is great. In any study of a variable that changes very abruptly with age in a large, healthy population, the variance is always large, and one can easily identify apparently healthy 40-year-olds who perform at the same level as the average 80-year-old. Likewise, many 80-year-olds can be found who perform like the average 40-year-old.

One fairly superficial and simple way of dissecting disease effects from the influence of normal aging is inevitability of the age changes. Although a change may vary from individual to individual in its age of onset or the rate of loss of function, some loss of function should be demonstrable in all subjects. Aging is a universal phenomenon, whereas many disease states, which occur with increasing prevalence as age advances, influence only a small portion of the elderly population. Evaluation of the presence of a change secondary to a disease state or some other non-age-related factor in an elderly cohort would often show two populations: one with the effect and one population with no evidence of the effect. The utility of this approach in determining whether a change is likely or not to be related to age can be seen in the example of mental failure, or organic brain syndrome of the Alzheimer type, as it is presently termed. This loss of mental function with advancing age is thought by many individuals to be characteristic of aging itself; but when populations are studied in detail, it is shown that the prevalence of dementia is no greater than 10% among the elderly. Thus, the presence of an intact intellect in the absence of mental failure is consistent with normal aging and is in fact the rule rather than the exception. This would indicate that the mental failure cannot be considered a normal consequence of aging, but more properly represents a disease that has increasing prevalence in advanced years. This can be contrasted with the menopause, which although variable in its age of onset, is universally present in aged women and thus is more likely to represent a result of normal aging.

Gerontologists have long been concerned with the appropriate methods for differentiating the physiologic consequences of aging from those of concomitant disease or cohort-related changes. Since age is known to have an important influence on an increasing number of physiologic and biochemical variables, and since the detection of a disease depends on the determination that a patient differs from the "normal" for the patient's age, it becomes of primary importance to define clearly the influence of clinically relevant variables. Such "normative data," as they are called by gerontologists, have been used clinically for many years. For example, spirometric measurements of pulmonary function are commonly expressed as percent of expected for age and body size. Similarly, stress or exercise tests, which are employed to evaluate the presence or absence of ischemic heart disease, often use age-adjusted criteria for the maximum heart rate to be achieved during the exercise.

The development of reliable normative data for clinical use has been hampered by the failure in many studies to adequately "clean up" the study population so that in the older age groups only healthy individuals are studied. Far too often, elderly individuals who are the residents of chronic care facilities, nursing homes, or even acute care hospitals, have been used for the study of "normal aging." For example, an individual with pneumonia who has no evidence of obvious clinical renal disease might be included in the study of the influence of age on renal function. Obviously, individuals in such debilitated states are suboptimal for a study that hopes to define normative changes to be used widely in clinical practice. Under ideal conditions subjects should be limited to those individuals who are living in the community, on no medications, and without evidence on detailed testing of any acute or chronic illness. Failure to carefully exclude diseased individuals in gerontologic studies results in a helpless confusion of age- and disease-related changes.

CROSS-SECTIONAL AND LONGITUDINAL STUDIES

Two general study designs are available to the clinical gerontologist. In cross-sectional studies, groups of various ages are observed, and age-related differences are sought. In longitudinal studies, serial prospective measurements are obtained on one group of subjects at specified intervals, and the slopes for these variables, or age-related changes, are determined. Most longitudinal studies concurrently follow subjects in several age cohorts throughout the adult age range, so that slopes for different age groups can be compared.

Cross-sectional studies are generally easily performed and much less expensive and time-consuming than longitudinal studies. However, they must be interpreted with caution, since there are several ways in which they may not reflect true age-related changes.[4]

In interpreting cross-sectional studies, it is important to remember that elderly subjects, especially octogenarians, represent a biased sample of biologically superior survivors from a cohort that has already experienced a 75 to 80% mortality. If the variable under study is related to survival, either as a risk factor or because of a protective effect, a cross-sectional study will seem to show age-related differences that do not exist. This effect, termed selective mortality, is shown in Figure 1, which depicts the influence of age on the blood concentration of "factor X," a risk factor that is found at widely varying levels in the population but does not change with age. Since X is related to survival, a group with a very high level has a shortened life span, and, a group with a low level will have a normal life span. In a cross-sectional study, values for the 30- and 40-

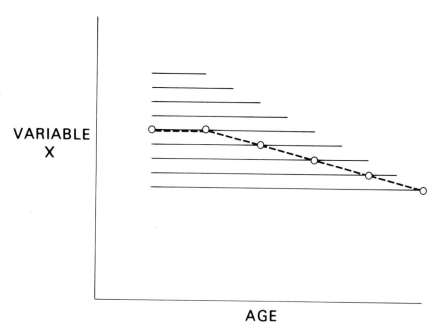

VARIABLE X (y-axis label)

AGE (x-axis label)

Fig. 1. Influence of selective mortality on age trands in cross-sectional data. The X denotes a risk factor associated with mortality. The circles represent mean cross-sectional values and show an apparent decline in X with age, which results from a progressive loss of subjects with high X levels in older age groups. The horizontal lines show that the level of X is not influenced by age.

year-olds are similar. The 50-year-old cohort, however, has lost its members with the highest values, and the variance is less with a lower mean value. This trend continues with advancing age, and the cross-sectional results wrongly suggest that factor X declines with age. This serious methodologic obstacle can be avoided with use of a prospective, longitudinal study design, in which each subject is followed over time, and the rate of change of each variable is calculated for each age cohort followed. When this methodology is applied to the study of factor X, no age effect is found (Figure 1).

An effect similar to that of selective mortality may be introduced in cross-sectional studies by any cause of differential follow-up that is related to the level of the variable under study, such as illness or change in geographic location. In addition, secular changes (that is, changes in the population with regard to the variable) may introduce error into age trends based on cross-sectional observations. Figure 2 shows cross-sectional and longitudinal data from a study on the impact of age on weight.[5] Whereas the cross-sectional data, based on a single examination, indicate a decline in weight with age, the longitudinal data, based

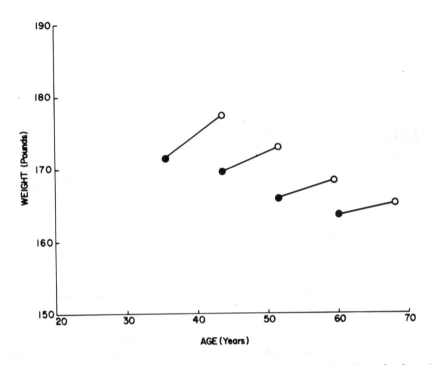

Fig. 2. Influence of age on weight viewed in two different ways (based on the data of Gordon and Shurtleff[5]). The solid circles denote mean weights for age cohorts at a single measurement. These cross-sectional data indicate an apparent age-related decline in weight. The open circles denote weights predicted by longitudinal analysis of data from five measurements and demonstrate that weight increases with age. This effect is most prominent in the youngest cohort and decreases progressively in older age groups.

on five examinations over a period of 18 years, suggest a different trend. The 35-year-old subjects are increasing weight rapidly and heading for a weight, 8 years after their initial examination, that is clearly higher than that of the 43-year-olds. Since the analysis only includes subjects who survived at least 18 years after the first examination, neither selective mortality nor differential follow-up is responsible for this effect. The longitudinal data (horizontal lines) show that the entire population is changing with regard to weight and that the tendency to gain weight decreases with progressively older cohorts.

Despite their advantages over cross-sectional studies, longitudinal studies may have major drawbacks, including the need to study a stable population over long periods and a particular sensitivity to changes in methodology. Subtle changes in laboratory techniques over several years may introduce "laboratory drifts" that are difficult to separate from age-related changes. An example is the "aging" of a sphyngomanometer. Another possible source of error is that subjects who return at regular intervals may become increasingly familiar with the testing environment. This "learning effect," also termed a "stress" or "first-visit" effect, is evident in the blood-pressure data in Table 1. Both systolic and diastolic blood pressure fell between visits 1 and 2 and between visits 2 and 3; thereafter, they increased with succeeding measurements. To avoid this effect in calculation of age trends, it was necessary to exclude the first two measurements from the analyses.

TABLE 1. Stress Effect in Longitudinal Studies

Exam #	BLOOD PRESSURE (MM/Hg)	
	Systolic	Diastolic
1	133.2	84.6
2	129.6	82.4
3	128.2	81.5
4	130.1	82.6
5	131.9	83.2
6	133.9	84.3
7	135.2	85.1

Data are for entire study population of the Framingham Study. Exams are at two-year intervals. To exclude the impact of differential follow-up, analysis includes only subjects present for all examinations.

The major elements in the design of a longitudinal study are the size of the samples, the frequency of measurements, and the duration of the study. Clearly, a variable that changes dramatically with age and is easily measured accurately need only be tested infrequently and for relatively few serial measurements before age-related changes are well defined. On the other hand, variables that change slowly with age and are difficult to measure accurately require frequent observations over a long period.

References

Finch, C. E., The regulation of physiologic changes during mammalian aging. *Q. Rev. Biol.* *51*: 49–83, 1976.

Andres, R. Physiological factors of aging significant to the clinician. *J. Am. Geriat. Soc. 17*: 274–277, 1969.

Costa, P. T., and McCrae, R. R. Functional age: A conceptual and empirical critique. *Proceedings of Research Conference on the Epidemiology of Aging,* National Institute on Aging, Bethesda, Maryland, March 28–29, 1977, in press.

Rowe, J. W. Clinical research on aging: Strategies and directions. *297*: 1332–1336, 1977.

Gordon, T. and Shurtleff, D. Means at each examination and inter-examination variation of specified characteristics: Framingham Study, exam 1 to exam 10, *The Framingham Study: An Epidemiological Investigation of Cardiovascular Disease* (DHEW Publication No. (NIH) 74–478), W. B. Kannel and T. Gordon, eds. Washington, D.C.: U.S. Government Printing Office, 1973.

Nutritional Alteration in Aging and Immune Reactivity: Application of the Rate-Limit Concept

M. A. LANE and E. J. YUNIS
Division of Immunogenetics
Sidney Farber Cancer Institute
Harvard Medical School
Boston, Massachusetts

Aging is a natural process that occurs as a consequence of development, growth, and maturation. As yet, in man, there are no methods to reverse this process. Were this process not accompanied by disease states that affect the quality of life in later years, there would be no reason to study aging other than scientific curiosity. Because disease states tend to accompany the process of aging, there is a strong need to study mechanisms involved in aging, with the ultimate goal of improving the general health of aging populations. Evidence in human and animal populations indicates that inherited attributes control life span and the potential for longevity. Studies in mice have provided evidence that the development of age-associated diseases and the causative factors of aging are controlled by separate processes in the body, dependent upon the functional integrity of the lymphocytes and specific inherited attributes.

Profound deficiencies of T cell function occur with aging. These deficiencies could be the consequence of a genetically programmed failure of thymic function. T cell–mediated immunity is important in tumor immunity, in the host defense against infection, in the preservation of self-tolerance, and in general regulation of the level of immune responsiveness; therefore, the genetically programmed failure of thymic function plays a major role in the pathogenesis of autoimmunity, aging, and age-related diseases. Burnet has presented a genetic interpretation of aging that combines the stochastic random error theory with genetic programming. The apparently random accumulation of error in most cell types results from genetically determined degrees of error-proneness in DNA polymerases and other enzymes that are responsible for the fidelity with which the macromolecular pattern primarily of DNA is replicated, or reconstituted after damage and repair. In mice, a rather clear-cut picture has emerged, indicating that longevity is under the influence of inherited factors that are susceptible to dietary and environmental manipulation.

EFFECTS OF NUTRITIONAL AND DIETARY
MANIPULATION ON THE IMMUNE SYSTEM

Nutritional deprivation has historically been associated with increased susceptibility to infection. In addition, many studies on the relationship of nutritional
deprivation and the expression of disease have indicated that some diseases seem
to be favored by nutritional deprivation, whereas others, like experimental
cancer, seem to be less frequent and less rapidly progressive when protein or
protein–calorie intake is deficient. Jose et al. observed that although Australian
aboriginal children have much acquired heart disease, they rarely express clinical
rheumatic fever. These authors studied the cell-mediated and humoral immune
responses in aboriginal children and noted that although certain apparent cell-
mediated responses seemed to be intact, capacity to produce antibodies to certain antigens was depressed. Afef et al. observed that severe protein–calorie
malnutrition from birth resulted in the appearance of kwashiorkor as early as
6 to 7 months of age. Kwashiorkor in these children was accompanied by hypo-
gammaglobulinemia and deficiencies of both cellular and humoral immune
functions. Smythe et al. found, however, that kwashiorkor in South African children is accompanied by severe cell-mediated immunodeficiency, while immunoglobulin levels are maintained or increased. Protein–calorie malnutrition in
children has also been associated with severe deficiency in T cell numbers and
functions.

We have previously shown, using two short-lived strains of mice, DBA/2f
and (NZBXNZW)F_1, that dietary restriction involving either calorie intake
reduction or calorie intake reduction combined with protein restriction dramatically prolongs life (Table 1). In these early studies it became clear to us that the
dietary influences on immune function were profound. Autoimmune processes
were significantly delayed, whereas strains free of autoimmune reactivity demonstrated lowered immune responsiveness which persisted later in life. In these
studies, we speculated that the effects produced were functional at the level of
cell regulatory mechanisms, i.e., suppressor and helper cell systems, and possibly
also in processes involving handling of antigen–antibody complexes.

Experimental studies on the influence of chronic moderate protein deprivation carried out in our laboratories showed that this form of nutritional deprivation in mice and rats could dramatically depress production of antibodies
while either increasing or leaving intact classical cell-mediated immune responses, including responses to plant lectins, defenses against certain viruses,
rejection of skin allografts, and development of killer cell function against allogeneic or syngeneic tumor cells. Moderate dietary restriction of certain essential
amino acids likewise depressed humoral immunity functions while leaving cell-
mediated immunity intact or increased, whereas more extreme chronic amino
acid restriction produced deficiencies of both cell-mediated and humoral im-

TABLE 1. Survival of (NZBXNZW)F Males and Females Placed as Weanlings on the Following Diets

DIET I 20 CALORIES 22% PROTEIN 5% CORN OIL			DIET II 10 CALORIES 22% PROTEIN 5% CORN OIL		
Sex	SURVIVAL, DAYS		Sex	SURVIVAL, DAYS	
F	150	490	F	240	420
	150	522		315	420
	310	600		350	450
	325	650		380	450
	360	650		402	530
	400	650		402	560
M	275	450	M	90	410
	276	475		100	425
	276	475		330	426
	430	540		335	430
	432	540		350	475
	439	560		400	500

DIET III 20 CALORIES 6% PROTEIN 5% CORN OIL			DIET IV 10 CALORIES 6% PROTEIN 5% CORN OIL		
Sex	SURVIVAL, DAYS		Sex	SURVIVAL, DAYS	
F	150	650	F	125	500
	310	650		175	500
	490	660		390	500
	490	665		450	525
	500	671		470	525
	500	671		475	600
M	340	650	M	400	475
	650	650		410	520
	650	650		410	650
	650	650		440	650
	650	650		450	650
	650	650		450	650

mune functions. Dietary manipulation, therefore, can produce varying effects on the immune system. The effects seen appear to be selective in different diets for alteration of different types of immune reactivity. As many cell types are involved in the production of immune reactivity, we suggest that alteration of immune responsiveness in dietary manipulation occurs at the cellular level in the immune system and introduces a control mechanism that affects cell division.

THE EFFECT OF NUTRIENT REDUCTION ON
SINGLE CELLS—THE RATE-LIMIT THEORY

First, put very simply, a rate-limit is a factor that imposes constraints upon a function, limiting either the occurrence of the function or the number of times a function can occur in a given time period. Let us consider briefly the significance of essential nutrient deficiency at the single cell level. Obviously, total starvation of the cell for an essential nutrient stops cell growth. If, however, nutrients that commonly allow cell growth are supplied at very low concentrations, the cell completes its division cycle and stops in a G_1 resting phase. The time needed to complete a division cycle remains the same, but in the presence of limited nutrients, fewer division cycles in a given time are completed. If a cell is pre-programmed to complete a finite number of divisions in its lifetime, a rate-limiting step capable of controlling frequency of divisions, could, in the absence of other factors, prolong the life of the cell.

Dietary manipulation by protein restriction, single essential amino acid intake reduction, or caloric intake reduction, constitutes an application of the rate-limiting effect at the whole animal level, affecting cell systems undergoing division at the time the dietary manipulation is instituted. If a diet is begun in a mouse at 3 weeks of age, most cell systems will fall under the rate-limit regulation, slowing down absolute maturation. If the same diet regime is begun at 12 weeks of age, after the animal has completed its developmental growth cycle, only cells of the epithelium, the reproductive system, and the erythropoetic and immune systems will be dividing.

Cells of the immune system have finite populational life spans: cell death in the immunocompetent animal is compensated for by maturation of precursor cells, making relative levels of effector and regulator cells in the population somewhat constant. Unfortunately, exact population life spans for effector cells, suppressor cells, and helper cells are not presently known. Cooperation of several cell types is involved in the production of immune responsiveness, beginning with antigen presentation and T cell processing and ending, in normal situations, with feedback T-cell regulated suppression. Cell division is involved in most phases of this responsiveness. A treatment such as nutrient reduction can impose a restriction on the number of cell divisions accomplished in a given time period. Functions performed by cells with longer population lives will be affected less rapidly than those performed by cells with shorter population lives. Cells that must undergo several divisions to accomplish their function in antigen responsiveness may be compromised more than cell types whose responsiveness does not involve division. Close observation of the cell systems most disturbed by the rate-limiting aspect of dietary manipulation will tell us several things: (1) Systems that involve cell division prior to influencing of reactivity will be placed at a disadvantage when limited nutrients are available. (2) Cell systems in which activity is preceded by reorganization rather than division will function normally unless a building block is rate-limited in protein turnover. (3) Stem cells of rapidly dividing cell populations will be conserved if cell division rate is restricted, resulting in lower reactivity levels which persist later in life. (4) regulatory feedback systems will be differentially affected, depending upon whether function is accomplished by division or maturation, and disturbances in coordinated functions will be seen. (5) Short-term observation will measure change in populations with short population lives, but alteration in long-lived populations will be seen only after long observation periods.

Diets that induce chronic protein deprivation (CPD) depress function of the B cell antibody response, while enhancing many aspects of the T cell system. It is significant that mice chronically deprived of protein (8% for 8 weeks) showed a 30% loss of total body weight and a marked decrease in total body protein, including albumin and α_1, α_2, and gammaglobulins. Hematocrit was also decreased. B cell function is depressed because the body lacks essential amino acids needed for the manufacture of protein, including immunoglobulins; but it is not eliminated. Animals suffering from CPD are capable, for example, of near-normal production of specific antibody to the *Brucella abortus* antigen, a response that requires little or no interaction with the T cell helper subsystem.

Chronic protein deprivation, however, does seem to bring about a failure of T and B cell cooperation. There is, for example, a significant reduction in antibody formation against sheep red blood cells in mice, an immune reaction known to require cooperation between B cells and T-helper cells.

Evidence of generalized T cell enhancement is seen in a significantly increased graft versus host reaction in (C3H $\times$ C57BL)F_1 neonatal mice injected with parental C3H cells. Skin allograft rejections are accelerated at all except the most extreme levels of CPD, a phenomenon that is abrogated by thymectomy. One notes a very marked enhancement of spleen cell proliferative response to the plant lectin PHA after CPD, and an increased capacity to resist pseudorabies virus infection. In contrast, there is a lowered resistance to inoculation of streptococci Group A type 6 bacteria. In our experiments the secondary response of T killer cells was maintained at varying levels of CPD (11%, 8%, 5%) and at one-half normal calorie intake; only at the 3% casein level was T killer cell function eliminated.

An important aspect of improved tumor immunity observed in animals on low protein diets is the concomitant depression of B cell–derived blocking factors which can interfere with the lysis of the tumor cells by T cell killer cells. In terms of function, T cell immunity, including the T cell–mediated surveillance mechanism for elimination of malignant and virus-infected cells, becomes vastly more effective because of the absence of inhibition by the serum blocking factors. A depression of the blocking factor has been noted with 11% casein intake, and elimination of production is noted at 6%, 5%, and 3%. The combination of protein restriction and calorie intake reduction in dietary manipulation is even more effective in depressing formation of blocking antibody.

Disturbances of immune function persist even after animals having experienced prolonged malnutrition in their neonatal stage are returned to a proper diet. Dr. Galal Aref in Egypt found that infants exposed from birth to extreme malnourishment (including deprivation of protein, vitamins, calories, and fat) showed evidence of kwashiorkor or severe marasmus by the time they were 7 months old. Those restored to a normal diet continued to show disturbed immune function 6 months to a year later.

Newly weaned animals fed low protein (6%) and low protein–low calorie (6% protein, one-half amount of normal caloric intake) for 2 weeks and then restored to a normal diet, all showed 5 weeks later a decreased number of T cells, depressed T killer cell activity, and decreased production of hemagglutinating antibody (B cell function). Eight weeks later the T killer cell function was still depressed, but hemagglutinating antibody response was back to normal in the low protein group, and almost back to normal in the low protein–low calorie group; not until 12 weeks later were all functions in the low protein group returned to normal. In the low protein–low calorie group, T killer cell activity was still depressed at 12 weeks, and the actual number of T cells was down, although B cell functions had returned to normal.

From these experiments, it can be seen that nutritional deprivation can alter a variety of parameters in immune reactivity. Reduced protein intake interferes with T-helper activity and T–B cell cooperation, yet enhances allograft rejection. With this diet, increased viral resistance and decreased bacterial resistance are observed. T cell killer activity is maintained on a low protein diet; yet when caloric intake reduction is combined with a reduced protein diet, T-killer activity is depressed. Some inhibition of blocking factor production is observed in reduced protein diets, T-killer activity is depressed. Some inhibition of blocking factor production is observed in reduced protein diets, but it becomes more dramatic if combined with caloric intake reduction.

In each of these parameters of immune reactivity, application of the rate-limiting factor can be observed. A reduction in the number of cell divisions occurring in a given time can produce a deficit in cell populations needed to heighten or facilitate a response. Insufficient numbers of cells present at critical periods of cellular interaction can cause decreased responsiveness. Absence of sufficient numbers of suppressor cells may produce a prolonged period of immune responsiveness, while decrease in proteins and amino acids essential necessary for antibody production can result in decreased specific antibody level. As more information is acquired with regard to immune cell population lives, modes of activation, and processes of interaction, diets may be applied selectively to decrease unwanted hyperresponsiveness as is found in autoimmune states, or enhance cytotoxic responses which might be beneficial in tumor prevention. Rapidly dividing cells capable of affecting immune responses can be effectively rate-limited to preserve their numbers for prolonged reactivity or to allow a desired response to escape normal regulatory mechanisms.

The state of the use of dietary manipulation in prolongation of life, retardation of autoimmune reactivity, and delay of tumor production is now approaching its maturity. As a technique to accomplish these functions, its effectiveness has been proved. The next step is to explore the mechanisms involved. To fully understand what occurs during dietary manipulation, attention must now be paid to which systems in the body are most affected by dietary manipulation and to the interplay of these systems. For immunologists, many intriguing questions remain to be answered. It will be most useful in the future to apply the rate-limit concept in terms of effects on cell division, populational replacement and phase-shifting of regulatory cell systems by dietary manipulations that are beneficial to the host in alleviating age-associated problems in immune reactivity.

Selected References

Burnet, F. M. An immunologic approach to aging. *Lancet 2*: 358–360, 1971.

Cantor, H., and Boyse, E. A. Functional subclasses of T-lymphocytes bearing different Ly antigens. II Cooperation between subclasses of Ly+ cells. *J. Exp. Med. 141*: 1390–1399, 1975.

Good, R. A., Jose, D., Cooper, W. C., Fernandes, G., Kramer, T., and Yunis, E. J. The influence of nutrition on antibody production and cellular immune responses in man, mice and guinea pigs. In *Proceedings of the Kroc Foundation Conference—Malnutrition and Immunity*. New York: Raven Press, 1976.

Schneider, E. L. In vivo versus in vitro cellular aging. In *Birth Defects*. Original Article Series, Vol. XIV, No. 1. New York: Alan R. Liss, Inc., 1978.

Yunis, E. J., ed. Symposium on immunopathology of aging. *Fed. Proc. 33:* 2017, 1974.

The Pathology of the Aging Brain

M. J. BALL, M.D., F.R.C.P. (C)
Associate Professor of Neuropathology
University of Western Ontario
London, Canada
Director, Neuropathology Research Laboratory
University Hospital
Fellow, Canadian Geriatrics Research Society

Although the expected life span, particularly for people in Western societies, has been rising dramatically in the last several years, a common condition known in medical circles as *dementia* and variously referred to (frequently incorrectly) as "chronic organic brain syndrome," "senility," "senescence," "senile psychosis," "senile delirium," or "chronic confusional state," continues to baffle biomedical investigators while posing enormous problems for many of our health care agencies and especially our psychiatric and geriatric institutions.

Such patients manifest varying degrees of impairment of memory; disorientation; impairment of all intellectual functions such as comprehension, calculation, knowledge, and learning; impaired judgment; and lability and shallowness of affect. In the earlier phases of this relentless process, a person has less interest in goals, less incentive to stick to a task, trouble concentrating, and difficulty screening out unimportant environmental stimuli. His achievement of personal ambitions and fulfillment of social responsibilities gradually become less important; he becomes increasingly self-absorbed; and his anxiety increases, often with marked irritability. He complains specifically of loss of memory for recent events, often coupled with insistence that his memories for past events remain crystal clear. As the condition worsens, he ignores appropriate dress and personal cleanliness, there is progressive flattening of affect, his orientation in time and space are faulty, and he easily becomes lost. Eventually there is a total ablation of both recent and remote memory. He is totally apathetic, with blunting of all feelings, and in the terminal stages paralysis, mutism, incontinence of both bladder and bowel, stupor, and coma appear.

This constellation of signs and symptoms, best referred to as dementia, has been surrounded for many years by ill-founded speculations about its etiology and its frequency. One of the favorite notions of both physicians and the general public is that dementia is due to cerebral vessel disease. Much of the medical literature is replete with the synonymous use of "arteriosclerotic cerebral vascular disease" for dementia and, in the lay vernacular, "hardening of the arteries." Recent studies both of a clinical nature[1] and of a pathological type[2] have confirmed that narrowing of the cerebral arterial tree by the process known as atherosclerosis can account for the problem in only about 8 to 12% of all patients admitted to the hospital with dementia as their main complaint. In more than two-thirds of them, instead, the correct diagnosis is *Alzheimer's disease*—the most common form of memory loss in the elderly, named after the neuropathologist who first described the brain changes in this disorder.

The enormous prevalence of Alzheimer's disease in North America is to date still not apparent from the usual sources of medical statistics, since regrettably the condition may not even be listed in the hundreds of "certifiable" causes of death. Too often, the death certificate states merely that such a patient died from "bronchopneumonia," "heart failure," or some other incidental terminal event. By extrapolation from European studies, it has been estimated[3] that 65% of all American senior citizens suffering from dementia have Alzheimer's disease; that there are at least 600,000 cases at any one time (and possibly as many as 1,200,000 if milder forms are also included); that the incidence may be 14 times greater than that of multiple sclerosis; and that at least 100,000 deaths are directly attributable to this condition every year in the United States. The senile variety of Alzheimer's dementia may in fact be the fourth or fifth most common cause of death in America![4] Moreover, this condition carries the definite threat of a "malignant" outcome. The life expectancy of patients just diagnosed as having Alzheimer's disease drops from an anticipated figure for nondemented men of similar age of 8.7 years or for mentally normal women of 10.9 years down to only 2.6 years in demented men or just over 3 years for demented women.[4]

Because many of the changes observed in the brains of such people both with the naked eye and under the microscope—the diminishing brain weight, the shrinkage or atrophy of the cerebral gray mantle known as the cortex, the cellular changes known as senile plaques, and neurofibrillary tangles—are also seen in brains of mentally normal old people, a stubbornly persistent myth has circulated that "organic brain syndrome" is merely an inevitable physiological consequence of getting older. This misconception is finally being put to rest by careful investigations in several neuropathology laboratories in England,[2] the United States, and Canada, wherein it is becoming increasingly clear that there is a very definite *quantitative* difference between the lesions in brains of mentally normal older people and those suffering with Alzheimer's dementia.

The electron microscope has permitted examination of some of these cellular abnormalities at very high magnifications. The *senile plaque* (Figure 1) appears to be a focus of degenerative changes in the ends of several nerve cells occurring in a spherical configuration, endings of both axons and dendrites—together known as neurites, hence the synonym "neuritic plaque."[5] The abnormalities

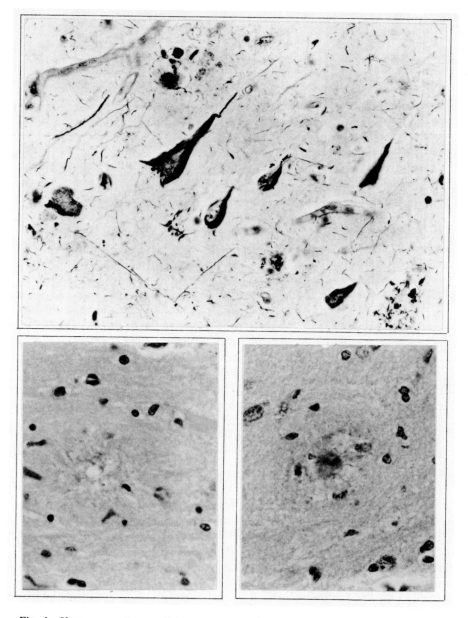

Fig. 1. Upper: several pyramidal neurones contain neurofibrillary tangles of Alzheimer (silver stain, × 400). Lower left: senile plaque (hematoxylin-eosin stain, × 400). Lower right: senile plaque showing central amyloid core (periodic acid-Shiff stain, × 400).

in these neuritic endings interfere with the synaptic contact points between many neurones. The periphery of a senile plaque is composed of reactive glial cells, the supporting framework population of the cerebral parenchyma. Frequently the center contains an abnormal protein substance, known as *amyloid,* also felt to be a secondary reactive change to the degenerating neurites. Some recent evidence suggests the amyloid core is composed of immune complexes deposited from the bloodstream. The *neurofibrillary tangle of Alzheimer* (Figure 1) is felt to be a coarse, fibrillar aggregation of microfilamentous protein material, having a very close chemical similarity to the neurofilaments normally present in nerve cells, but possibly arranged in an abnormally twisted configuration of "paired helical filaments."[6]

The density of senile plaques in the cortex of demented patients has been shown to be much greater than in the gray matter of mentally normal older subjects,[2] and in our laboratory the same distinction has been shown for the density of nerve cells with neurofibrillary tangles in the cortex of people with Alzheimer's disease as compared to normal aged controls.[7]

The cause of organic dementia of the Alzheimer type is still an intriguing mystery. However, one of the most popular hypotheses is that a "slow" viral infection of the central nervous system may produce these changes.[8] A much less common type of dementia, known as Creutzfeldt-Jakob disease, with a more rapid course and usually fatal within a few months, serves as a model for this theory, since that condition has already been proved to be a transmissible form of encephalopathy. Although brain material from patients with Creutzfeldt-Jakob disease injected into experimental animals will consistently produce an almost identical, spongiform degeneration of their central nervous systems, the precise agent in such material has never been isolated. Unfortunately, identical experiments with material from classical cases of Alzheimer's disease have so far not shown any similar capacity for transmissibility of the causative agent. The observation that certain families are unusually predisposed to Alzheimer's disease and other so-called degenerative neurological conditions raises the possibility of a genetic susceptibility to such "slow" viral agents.

The toxic metal aluminum has also been postulated as a cause of Alzheimer's dementia.[9] In human brain tissues the concentrations of aluminum have been found in multiple samples to correlate fairly closely with the degree of neurofibrillary change seen microscopically. The observation of high aluminum levels in brain tissue from both normal and demented older people may, on the other hand, prove merely to be an age-related phenomenon.

Neurochemists analyzing cerebral cortex from subjects with organic dementia are reporting a striking reduction in the activity of choline acetyltransferase, an important enzyme in the production of the neurotransmitter acetylcholine.[10] Data on the topographic distribution of histological changes within the hippocampus, a crucial relay center in the limbic system subserving memory function, also have suggested that specific neurochemical pathways in the cerebral cortex may be preferentially afflicted in Alzheimer's disease.[11] It is unfortunately not clear whether such chemical alterations are primary events or merely secondary phenomena. The therapeutic implications for replacement of missing enzymes or substrates are, of course, enormous.

While the precise pathophysiological mechanism underlying Alzheimer's dementia is still not understood, the fact that chronic organic brain disease is no longer a neglected backwater of neuropsychiatry augurs well for the future.[1] The investigation of such disorders as diseases rather than as some inevitable concomitant of aging is an encouraging harbinger of eventual prevention or cure.

References

1. Wells, C. E. Chronic brain disease: An overview. *Am. J. Psychiat. 135*: 1-12, 1978.
2. Tomlinson, B. E., and Henderson, G. Some quantitative cerebral findings in normal and demented old people. In *Neurobiology of Ageing,* R. D. Terry and S. Gershon, eds. New York: Raven Press, 1976, pp. 183-204.
3. Terry, R. D. Dementia—a brief and selective review. *Arch. Neurol. 33*: 1-4, 1976.
4. Katzman, R. The prevalence and malignancy of Alzheimer's disease: A major killer. *Arch. Neurol. 33*: 217-218, 1976.
5. Terry, R. D., and Wisniewski, H. The ultrastructure of the neurofibrillary tangle and the senile plaque. In *Alzheimer's Disease and Related Conditions,* G. E. W. Wolstenholme and M. O'Connor, eds. London: J. and A. Churchill, 1970, pp. 145-183.
6. Wisniewski, H. M., Narang, H. K., and Terry, R. D. Neurofibrillary tangles of paired helical filaments. *J. Neurol. Sci. 27*: 173-181, 1976.
7. Ball, M. J. Neuronal loss, neurofibrillary tangles and granulovacuolar degeneration in the hippocampus with ageing and dementia. *Acta Neuropathol. (Berl.) 37*: 111-118, 1977.
8. Roos, R. P., and Johnson, R. T. Viruses and dementia. in *Dementia,* C. E. Wells, ed. Philadelphia: Davis, 1977, pp. 93-112.
9. Crapper, D. R., Krishnan, S. S., and Dalton, A. J. Brain aluminum distribution in Alzheimer's disease and experimental neurofibrillary degeneration. *Science 180*: 511-513, 1973.
10. Editorial. Cholinergic involvement in senile dementia. *Lancet 1*: 408, 1977.
11. Ball, M. J. Histotopography of cellular changes in Alzheimer's disease. In *Senile Dementia: A Biomedical Approach,* K. Nandy, ed. New York: Elsevier-North Holland, 1978 (in press).

III
DISEASES OF THE
BLOOD VESSELS

Interaction of Fibrin with Blood Platelets and Other Cells

MARIA BENEDETTA DONATI
GIOVANNI DE GAETANO
Istituto di Ricerche Farmacologiche "Mario Negri"

FIBRIN FORMATION AND DISSOLUTION

Before reviewing the interactions of fibrin with blood platelets and other cells and their possible implications in human physiology and pathology, let us attempt briefly to describe the processes leading to the formation and dissolution of fibrin. Fibrin is an insoluble substance derived from the enzymatic activity of thrombin on a soluble circulating protein, fibrinogen. Thrombin does not circulate in the blood as such but as its precursor prothrombin (factor II). Activation of prothrombin to thrombin is triggered by another enzyme, called activated factor X (Xa), the product of activation of factor X. This zymogen occupies a key position in the cascade of reactions leading to fibrin formation (Figure 1). It may be activated through at least three pathways: an "intrinsic" one (involving factors XII, XI, IX, and VIII, in the presence of prekallikrein and kininogen), an "extrinsic" one (involving tissue factors and factor VII), and a "direct" one, which may be triggered by platelets, tumor cells, and possibly other cells.

Once formed, fibrin is usually stabilized by a transpeptidase (factor XIII) and then removed by a proteolytic process leading to activation of the inactive plasminogen into the lytic enzyme plasmin. This process is called fibrinolysis and involves activators and inhibitors present in plasma, within the vascular walls, and in many tissues. Fibrin formation and dissolution may occur both in vitro and in vivo.

In contrast, retraction of fibrin clots possibly only takes place in vitro; the significance and clinical relevance—if any—of this phenomenon are still obscure. For many years it was considered simply a laboratory parameter of fibrin-platelet interaction and of platelet function (for example, clot retraction is much disturbed in platelet-rich clots from patients with the severe, congenital bleeding disorder known as Glanzmann's thrombasthenia; see also below).

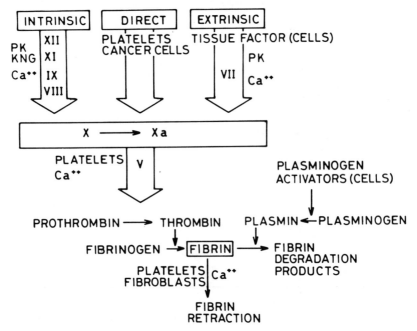

FIG. 1. A scheme of the coagulation of fibrinolysis systems, PK = prekallikrein, Coagulation factors are indicated by the corresponding roman numeral.

INTERACTIONS OF FIBRIN WITH BLOOD PLATELETS

Blood platelets may interact with fibrin and its formation in several ways:

1. Platelet membrane offers a catalytic surface on which interactions between clotting factors are greatly facilitated. This property is usually referred to as platelet factor 3 activity and is mainly linked to the phospholipid composition of the plasma membrane. Platelet factor 3 becomes available when platelets are activated by foreign surfaces or by contact with other platelets (aggregation). It is largely independent of the platelet release reaction.

2. As already mentioned, platelets can *directly* activate coagulation factor X, a property enhanced by endotoxin or by hyperlipidic diets. The biochemical basis of this activity is still unknown.

3. Platelets may also contribute to fibrin formation through other properties documented in well-defined experimental systems in vitro, the clinical significance of which must still be defined:

a. Platelets stimulated by ADP may activate factor XII, thus promoting the contact phase of blood coagulation (contact product forming activity).

b. Platelets stimulated by collagen may activate factor XI, thus bypassing the initial step of factor XII activation (collagen-induced coagulant activity).

c. Platelets catalyze the formation of activated factor X (intrinsic factor Xa forming activity). This activity is different from that mentioned in paragraph 2, since it requires the presence of factors XIa, VIII, and IX.

d. Platelet membrane provides factor V activity.

e. Platelets are able to protect factor XIa from inactivation by its natural inhibitor anti-XIa.

f. During the release reaction platelets discharge a heparin-neutralizing activity (known as platelet factor 4) which could protect factor Xa from inactivation by its natural inhibitor anti-Xa, this inhibitor being strongly potentiated by trace amounts of heparin.

g. Intact platelet membrane also provides antithrombin activity, apparently different from the antithrombin activities in plasma.

4. Platelets induce fibrin clot retraction (see preceding section) and promote clot tensile strength (measured in a pharmacological bath for isolated organs or in a thrombelastograph). Platelets are also able to interact with polymerizing fibrin formed by different clotting enzymes (thrombin, reptilase, ancrod) and may affect fibrin polymerization itself. Platelet adherence to polymerizing fibrin may result in the construction of links between platelets and fibrin in hemostatic plugs and thrombi. Unlike the interaction of platelets with polymerizing fibrin, clot retraction requires metabolic energy. In addition, platelets have to be stimulated to retract fibrin clots. Platelets retract clots formed by thrombin, but they do not retract clots formed by thrombinlike enzymes such as batroxobin (reptilase) or ancrod, although the association of platelets with different types of fibrin seems to be very similar. Platelets stimulated by ADP, adrenaline, collagen, or thrombin retract clots formed with thrombinlike enzymes. Primary aggregation inhibitors, such as prostaglandin E_1, inhibit retraction of reptilase fibrin in the presence of ADP or collagen, whereas inhibitors such as aspirin, which prevent platelet release but not primary aggregation, are ineffective. The clot retraction mechanism(s) therefore seems to be related to the first phases of the platelet adhesion—aggregation reaction. These mechanisms also show many striking analogies with the mechanisms controlling smooth muscle contraction. Extensive morphological changes have been described in platelets inducing fibrin retraction, and it has been suggested that clot retraction may depend on formation and retraction of large pseudopods. However, several observations indicate that the mechanism(s) by which stimulated platelets induce fibrin retraction may be much more complex.

Platelets play a crucial role in formation of the hemostatic plug and in the pathogenesis of thromboembolism. Primary hemostatic plugs are formed almost entirely of platelet aggregates, but they become unstable if fibrin formation is impaired. Platelets contribute in many ways to fibrin formation and structure; therefore, their role goes far beyond events of primary hemostasis. Thrombin—both the product and the catalyst of the clotting cascade—acts in turn as a potent stimulator of platelets, thus favoring their contribution to fibrin formation and their interaction with evolving or polymerized fibrin. On one hand, bleeding in congenital or acquired afibrinogenemia may be due to the lack of stability and consolidation of platelet plugs devoid of fibrin; on the other hand, platelet aggregates in vivo may contribute to the propagation of thrombi, since aggregates interact more extensively with polymerizing fibrin.

INTERACTIONS OF FIBRIN WITH CELLS
OTHER THAN PLATELETS

The participation of fibrin in a number of biological processes such as inflammation, tissue repair, immunological reactions, and cancer metastasis indicates that it may interact in vivo with other cells besides platelets, such as fibroblasts, macrophages, and tumor cells.

Red Cells

The ability of red cells to adhere to polymerizing fibrin has been evaluated and compared to that of platelets. Under well-defined experimental conditions, 70 to 90% of platelets and 5 to 8% of red cells were deposited on fibrin evolving on a rotating bar. Platelet aggregation induced by ADP and thrombin or agglutination of red cells by isoagglutinins increased the rate and degree of association of cells with fibrin. Nonspecific trapping of cells or cell aggregates into the fibrin net appears to be the mechanism of the red cells–fibrin interplay.

The pathophysiological significance of this interaction remains to be established. Red cells have long been considered important in hemostatic plug formation. However, so far the availability of ADP from disrupted erythrocytes has mainly been considered in this context. The observation that anemic subjects with a normal platelet count may have disturbed hemostasis could partially support the hypothesis that a limited number of red cells trapped in fibrin impair formation of the hemostatic plug. On the other hand, it has recently been suggested that intravascular red cell aggregation, which may occur when the fibrinogen concentration is high and the blood flow reduced, might increase the rate of propagation of the thrombus.

Leucocytes

Polymorphonuclear leucocytes can interact with fibrin through a number of activities. First, they can contribute to fibrin formation: when appropriately stimulated, in vitro or in vivo, they make available a procoagulant material (called tissue factor) which can activate blood clotting through the extrinsic pathway (Figure 1). From electron microscopic evidence in canine jugular veins it appears that leucocytes interact with evolving fibrin and serve as a mechanism for anchoring fibrin strands to the venous wall. The development of leucocyte tissue factor activity in response to chemotactic stimuli might be of major importance in the pathogenesis of some forms of postoperative venous thrombosis which occur when the endothelial walls are intact.

Leucocytes are also a source of proteolytic and fibrinolytic activity. They release neutral pH proteases which degrade fibrinogen and fibrin, yielding split products different from those produced by plasmin.

Selective enhancement of leucocyte fibrinolytic activity has been proposed as the mechanism whereby salicylates act as fibrinolytic agents in man. The production of proteases and plasminogen-dependent fibrinolytic activity, as well as of procoagulant activity, is greater in leukemic cells than in their normal counterparts.

Macrophages

Macrophages are peculiar migratory cells that, upon activation, acquire a number of new enzymatic and phagocytic activities. Alveolar macrophages from guinea pigs bind fibrinogen and fibrin, whereas, in the same immunofluorescence staining system, lymphocytes, granulocytes, and erythrocytes do not show "fibrinogen staining." In a fashion similar to platelets, macrophages show a peculiar affinity for soluble fibrin and fibrin/fibrinogen complexes when compared with fibrinogen or fibrin degradation products. The fibrin binding sites on the macrophage surface are trypsin-resistant, and binding is calcium-dependent. The presence of fibrin on the macrophage surface has been considered responsible for the swelling and induration of delayed hypersensitivity skin reactions in humans and laboratory animals. Macrophage binding to evolving fibrin may be a host defense mechanism whereby the reticuloendothelial system removes fibrin from blood, thus preventing it from contributing to thrombosis. Increased production and release of a protein that converts the inactive precursor (plasminogen) into the active fibrinolytic enzyme (plasmin) has been reported in activated macrophages, and in other actively migrating cells such as those from ovarian follicles shortly before ovulation. This activity has been considered important in the development of the cell's migratory capacity, since it would prevent actin cable formation, a prerequisite for anchorage-dependent growth.

Fibroblasts

Fibroblasts are the cells with which fibrin most likely comes into contact when it is deposited at extravascular sites (during inflammatory processes, tissue damage and repair, immunological reactions). In inflammatory processes the newly formed fibrin possibly guides fibroblast migration and provides the matrix along which new connective tissue is laid down. This supposed sequence of events is backed to some extent by pathological findings of fibrin deposits in immunological disorders such as glomerulonephritis and rheumatoid arthritis. In vitro evidence suggests that fibroblasts interact with fibrin in a rather complex manner:

- a. Similarly to platelets and macrophages, fibroblasts adhere to polymerizing fibrin.
- b. Fibroblasts induce retraction of fibrin clots (in the absence of platelets).
- c. Fibroblasts promote fibrin formation through the production of a pro-coagulant activity, mainly triggered by cell adhesion.
- d. Fibroblasts favor fibrin stabilization through a transpeptidase activity similar to platelet factor XIII.
- e. Fibroblasts can promote fibrin dissolution through the availability of plasminogen activator activity.

Human and animal fibroblasts have been seen on electron microscopy to adhere to polymerizing fibrin (not to fibrinogen or fully polymerized fibrin) and to be trapped within the fibrin net. Moreover, the manner in which they cause retraction of fibrin formed by the action of thrombin is in many ways similar to clot retraction promoted by platelets. Fibroblasts contain contractile proteins that are responsible for their motility and contraction. These contractile proteins, like thrombosthenin in platelets, may be involved in fibrin retraction induced by the cells. As a result of different stimuli, fibroblasts can in fact develop morphological, biochemical, and pharmacological properties similar to those of smooth muscle cells (myofibroblasts), with which they have a common embryological origin. Microfilament formation in fibroblasts appears to be a fairly generalized cell adaptational process, which probably plays an important role in tissue repair or regeneration. Connective tissue diseases such as Dupuytren's or Ledderhose's syndromes (fibromatosis of, respectively, the palmar or plantar aponeurosis) could be due to abnormally increased fibroblast contractility. The capacity to induce fibrin clot retraction may therefore be considered a functional counterpart of the morphological finding of microfibrillar systems developing in different cells under appropriate stimulation. In this context, it is interesting to note that skin fibroblasts from patients with abnormal wound healing are unable to induce fibrin clot retraction in vitro; this ability is also lost in aged cells even though they become progressively larger and thus have larger reaction surfaces.

Fibroblast capacity for duplication in vitro is well defined in time and inversely proportional to the age of the donor. In other words, the behavior of the fibroblasts in vitro reflects the history of the subject from whom they are derived. It is suggested that during senescence fibroblasts lose their receptors for fibrin, and it is known that they lose HL-A antigens. During aging in vivo, a change in the interaction between connective tissue fibroblasts and fibrin could contribute to the decreased tissue repair capacity seen in elderly people. At the moment we do not know whether decreased ability of fibroblasts to retract fibrin, and it is known that they lose HLA antigens. During aging in vivo, a greatly increases with age.

The procoagulant activity provided by fibroblasts is thromboplastin-like and can trigger the extrinsic clotting pathway (Figure 1). This cell function could play an important role in the pathogenesis of some vascular diseases. Tissue factor antigen has been found in very high concentrations in atheromatous plaques, surrounding cholesterol crystals. Thus, in atherosclerosis, activation of clotting mechanisms might not only follow rupture of the plaque, but also minimal damage of surrounding fibroblasts. Abnormal increase of this activity has indeed been documented in two genetically distinct disorders, progeria and Werner's syndrome, characterized by early appearance of atherosclerotic lesions, premature aging, increased thrombotic risk, and premature death.

Cancer Cells

Many of the steps leading to cancer cell dissemination and implantation in distant organs (detachment from the primary tumor, local invasion and penetration into capillaries, transport in blood or lymph, reentry and lodgment in target tissues, invasion, and growth), appear to involve intravascular or extravascular fibrin. First, fibrin formation may be favored by procoagulants produced by cancer cells. Mainly tissue factor activity has been shown in tumor and leukemic cells (in both human and experimental malignancies). More recently, a serine protease, directly able to activate factor X, was found in human and animal tumor cells. Some cancer cells thus appear to share whith normal platelets a particular coagulant activity (factor X activating activity) which could represent a "new" alternative cellular pathway for initiation of clotting (Figure 1). It is not yet known whether the nature or degree of production of procoagulant activity by cancer cells represents a marker of malignancy or is of any importance in cancer cell growth and dissemination. As a result of this activity or of a less specific inflammatory reaction, fibrin can be deposited at the tumor periphery, thus providing a structure along which cancer cells may grow. Based on this theoretical sequence of events, treatment with anticoagulants has been attempted in tumor-bearing animals and (to a lesser extent) in cancer patients. However, both the suitability of the models used and interpretation of the results so far have been questioned. Therefore no definitive conclusions can be drawn from these studies.

Cancer cells have fibrinolytic activity, mainly plasminogen activator activity, generally to a higher degree than their normal counterparts. The presence of or increase in plasminogen activator activity in fibroblasts has been proposed as a phenotypic indicator of oncogenic transformation. Fibrinolytic activity, together with proteolytic (mainly collagenase) activities associated with malignant cells, may contribute to cohesive failure in solid tumors, resulting in easier release of cancer cells into the bloodstream. In some experimental and clinical conditions, treatment with antifibrinolytic agents has proved effective in limiting the metastatic process.

Invasiveness and loss of growth control in transformed cells is probably mediated by changes in the cell surface components, including loss of the capacity to interact with fibrin. In fact, fibroblasts transformed by various means, like old cells, are unable in vitro to induce retraction of fibrin clots; the loss of this activity has recently been proposed as a marker of oncogenic transformation in fibroblasts from patients with lung cancer.

CONCLUSION

It is striking how cells with different biochemical and functional characteristics have common pathways of interaction with fibrin; namely, the capacity to promote fibrin formation by release of procoagulants, to adhere to forming fibrin, and to lyse formed fibrin. These appear to be the steps of a cellular reaction mechanism to various stimuli which can operate in conditions such as formation of the hemostatic plug, cellular responses to immune stimuli, fibroblast activity in tissue repair, or cancer cell detachment from a primary or metastatic nodule.

ACKNOWLEDGMENTS

Part of the authors' work referred to in this survey was supported by Grant NIH PHRB-1-RO1, CA 12764-01, National Cancer Institute, National Institutes of Health, Bethesda, Maryland, U.S.A. Judith Baggott helped prepare the manuscript.

References

de Gaetano, G., and Garattini, S., eds. *Platelets. A Multidisciplinary Approach,* New York: Raven Press, 1978.

Donati, M. B., Poggi, A., Mussoni, L., de Gaetano, G., and Garattini, S. Hemostasis and experimental cancer dissemination. In *Cancer Invasion and Metastasis: Biologic Mechanisms and Therapy,* S. B. Day et al., eds. New York: Raven Press, 1977, pp. 151–160.

Niewiarowski, S., Stewart, G. J., Nath, N., Tai Sha, A., and Lieberman, G. E. ADP, thrombin, and *bothrops atrox* thrombin like enzyme in platelet-dependent fibrin retraction. *Am. J. Physiol. 229*: 737-745, 1975.

Semeraro, N., and Vermylen, J. Evidence that washed human platelets possess factor X activator activity. *Br. J. Haematol. 36*: 107-115, 1977.

Warren, B. A. Tumor metastasis and thrombosis. *Thromb. Diath. Haemorrh. Suppl. 59*: 139-156, 1974.

Hemodynamic Effects of Arterial Stenosis

J. KEITH FARRAR, Ph.D.
Departments of Clinical Neurological Sciences and Biophysics
University of Western Ontario

During the past ten years there has been a great deal of clinical and experimental investigation into the alterations in blood flow caused by the presence of a stenosis (narrowing) in a major artery. Such reductions of the arterial lumen can produce local hemodynamic disturbances as well as more distant effects due to a restriction of blood flow. Atherosclerotic narrowing of the arteries is one of the most common problems in the circulatory system; so most of the work presented will refer to this type of stenosis. The general principles however, apply equally to any type of narrowing. Prior to a discussion of recent experimentation in this field, I will review briefly some of the basic concepts regarding flow in arteries and through constrictions.

HEMODYNAMIC CONSIDERATIONS

As fluid passes from a tube of large diameter into one of smaller diameter, it must be accelerated to a higher velocity in order to maintain the same volume flow rate in the narrow channel. Similarly, as the fluid exits the stenosis at high velocity, it must be decelerated upon reentry into the larger channel. This acceleration/deceleration produces marked changes in the velocity profile. At the entrance to the stenosis, the slow-moving streamlines near the wall are forced toward the center of the channel and accelerated, while viscous forces tend to retard the rate of acceleration of the central core. The normally parabolic velocity profile in the input channel becomes flattened in the stenosis with high fluid velocity near the wall as well as in the central core. In the diverging portion of the stenosis, the high velocity (low pressure) stream exits into a region of lower velocity (higher pressure), resulting in a pressure gradient opposite to the direction of flow. This gradient combined with wall friction retards movement of fluid near the wall, while the central core decelerates but continues to move downstream. If this adverse pressure gradient becomes large enough, fluid adjacent to the wall immediately distal to the stenosis may move in a reverse direction, producing a separation region of slow-moving fluid. The region of separation becomes larger as the degree of stenosis and/or exit velocity is increased, resulting in turbulent eddies and the formation of vortices. At this stage, flow at the exit of the stenosis becomes a turbulent jet.

The shearing stress on the endothelial surface of an artery is proportional to the velocity gradient at the wall.[1] Shear stress will be increased at the entrance of a stenosis because of the high velocities occurring near the wall. In the region of flow separation distal to a stenosis, shear stress will be zero at the point of separation and reattachment, and will be relatively small between these two points because of the low fluid velocity.

Turbulence may develop either within or distal to the stenosis because of the relatively high fluid velocities and the inherent instability of divergent flow. (The fluid must decelerate and diverge to fill the larger vessel.) Turbulence will be associated with an increased loss of energy and the production of vibrations in the vessel wall.[2]

There is a loss of energy when the fluid is accelerated at the entrance (contraction loss), a viscous (frictional) energy loss as the fluid flows through the stenosed segment, and a third loss as the fluid is decelerated in the expanded area distal to the stenosis (expansion loss).[3] The transfer of lateral pressure energy to kinetic energy (acceleration) is fairly efficient, and thus the contraction loss will be much smaller than the other two. The viscous energy loss is primarily the result of friction forces that develop between the moving fluid and the wall boundary. The amount of energy lost will be directly proportional to the kinetic energy of the fluid and to the length of the stenosis, and inversely proportional to the diameter. Most of the increased kinetic energy involved in carrying the flow through the stenosis is lost at the sudden expansion by the formation and maintenance of vortices and in providing the viscous drag required to decelerate the flow. This expansion loss will be proportional to the degree of area expansion and to the square of the velocity (kinetic energy). The total energy loss caused by a stenosis can be represented by a summation of the above three losses, the net effect being a reduction in pressure distal to the stenosis. The major factors determining the magnitude of the pressure loss are the flow velocity and the ratio of cross-sectional areas. The length and shape of the stenosis and the viscosity of the fluid influence this loss to a lesser degree.

The above discussion is based to a large extent on observations made under conditions of steady (nonpusatile) flow. In the real situation, the flow velocity and velocity profile will change considerably during the cardiac cycle. Periods of laminar unidirectional flow, separated laminar flow, and turbulent flow may all occur in the distal segment at different phases of the cardiac cycle, depending on the input velocity and the severity of the stenosis.

POSTSTENOTIC DILATATION

The arterial lumen immediately distal to a stenosis is frequently found to be dilated. Poststenotic dilatations have been reported with virtually all types of stenoses including atherosclerotic lesions. Turbulence in the poststenotic segment has been found to be a necessary condition for this type of dilatation to occur.[2] The turbulence produces vibrations in the vessel wall which may be heard as a murmur (called a "bruit"). Experimental studies have demonstrated that poststenotic dilatation will result when a moderate stenosis is accompanied by distal turbulence (bruit), but that no dilatation occurs when a minimal or extreme stenosis is present without turbulence. Vibration of the vessel wall appears to be a key factor. Roach and associates have shown that when isolated human arteries are subjected to low frequency vibrations (30–300 Hz), the distensibility of the arterial wall increases, and the vessel dilates. Arteries from experimental animals showed a similar increase in distensibility in poststenotic segments. This led them to postulate that the vibrations resulting from turbulence may alter the linkages between elastic fibers in the vessel wall, thus increasing the distensibility. Other workers have suggested that the increased drag forces produced by flow disturbances initiate a local relaxation of arterial smooth muscle in the poststenotic segment, resulting in dilatation.

The damage done to the arterial wall appears to be reversible. If the bruit (turbulence) disappears either by removal of the stenosis or by a reduction in flow velocity, the dilatation also disappears within 24 hours. Poststenotic dilatation may result in an increased reduction of pressure distal to the stenosis, since the degree of area expansion is effectively increased.

ENDOTHELIAL DAMAGE AND THROMBUS FORMATION

One of the most serious complications of arterial stenosis is damage to the vessel endothelium and thrombus formation resulting from variations in shear stress. Patel et al.[1] have recently reviewed the literature concerning the responses of the vessel wall to hemodynamic stress. The majority of recent research in this area has been focused on clarifying the role of hemodynamics in atherogenesis. Particular attention has been devoted to the study of endothelial damage induced by increased shear stress and the subsequent tissue repair processes set in motion.

The velocity of flow increases at the entrance of a stenosis, and the velocity profile is markedly flattened. This creates a region of very high shear stress. If the shear stress at the wall exceeds a critical value (approx. 375 dynes/cm^2), the surface begins to deteriorate histologically, leading to a loss of endothelial cells and deposition of fibrin. Prolonged exposure to high shear stress has been shown to result in erosion of the cellular components and basement membrane and subsequent deposition of fibrin and blood elements on the eroded surface. This has the effect of perpetuating the atherosclerotic process through re-injury as well as creating a potential source of emboli.

Flow in the region of separation is relatively stagnant, which would encourage interactions at the vessel wall; and platelets are known to accumulate in this region. This has led some authors to suggest that platelets may become activated when passing through the regions of high shear at the entrance of the stenosis and subsequently be trapped in the region of flow separation. These platelets could then react with the vessel wall, resulting in an increase in permeability to lipids, and so on. This is an ideal site for thrombus formation, since both stagnant flow and the presence of activated platelets will enhance coagulation. Turbulence in the region distal to a stenosis may also be capable of producing endothelial damage equal to or greater than that caused by high shear stress. This damage presumably results from high frequency stress components associated with turbulence.

It is clear that the flow disturbances at a stenosis will act to enhance the development of further atherosclerosis through endothelial damage and will provide a breeding ground for future emboli.

REDUCTION OF TISSUE PERFUSION PRESSURE

It is well known that at some point in the development of an arterial stenosis, the degree of narrowing becomes sufficient to interfere with blood flow to the tissue normally supplied by that artery. Substantial reductions in cross-sectional area of the lumen may occur without significant decreases in distal pressure. Reductions in pressure do occur, of course, but are relatively minor under "resting" flow conditions, and are difficult to detect accurately. However, beyond a certain degree of constriction, even small further reductions in lumen area are accompanied by increasingly large and seemingly disproportionate reductions in pressure. These observations have led to the concept of a "critical" arterial stenosis beyond which marked reductions in pressure and flow will occur. This concept is somewhat misleading in that it implies that a stenosis may be classified as significant or not significant based solely on the knowledge of the cross-sectional area. This is certainly not the case, since the pressure drop across a stenosis also depends on the velocity of flow, fluid viscosity, and the length and shape of the stenosis and on the presence and efficiency of collateral circulation.[3,4] Of these additional factors, the most important are velocity of flow and collateral circulation.

Many studies have demonstrated that if the flow rate through a stenosis is doubled, the pressure drop occurring across the stenosis will increase by a factor of three to four (recall that the pressure loss is proportional to the kinetic energy). Therefore a stenosis that produces only minor pressure drops under resting conditions may be quite important during exercise when flow demands may increase to five to ten times the resting levels. Collateral circulation may also significantly influence the pressure drop occurring across a stenosis. In the previous discussions, we have considered only the flow/pressure relationships through an isolated vessel. In the real situation, there are alternative collateral channels through which flow and pressure may be transmitted to the distal arterial segment. This becomes obvious in the case of complete occlusion where the pressure and flow distal to the occlusion are provided solely through collateral pathways. In general, the collateral channels are comprised of small arteries and arterioles with a high resistance to flow. Because of this, their importance as alternative sources of flow and pressure is restricted to situations in which a large pressure drop has already been created by the stenosis. This is discussed in more detail below.

As the input pressure to a vascular bed is reduced, the peripheral arterioles will dilate, thus reducing their resistance to flow. This tends to maintain flow at a relatively constant level. When the arterioles become maximally dilated, further reductions in input pressure result in parallel reductions in tissue blood flow. Therefore, an arterial stenosis will reduce tissue perfusion only when the pressure drop caused by the stenosis exceeds the dilatatory capacity of the distal vessels. In other words, tissue blood flow will remain constant until the increase in resistance caused by the stenosis exceeds the decrease in resistance provided by dilatation of the distal vessels.

In most instances, a stenosis will not produce a reduction in tissue blood flow under resting conditions. Collateral channels tend to minimize the effective increase in arterial resistance (decrease in perfusion pressure) by providing an alternate route for flow. The distal arterioles are then able to compensate through dilatation. The problem arises when there is an increased demand for flow. Normally, when tissue metabolism increases, the arterioles dilate, thus reducing their resistance to flow; and, since perfusion pressure is high, the flow increases to meet the demand. In the presence of a stenosis, however, this process is much less efficient. The pressure available for tissue perfusion is reduced even at rest so that the maximum possible increase in flow will be less than normal. Furthermore, the arterioles will be dilated to compensate for the stenosis, and therefore the degree to which they can respond to a superimposed dilatatory stimulus (increased metabolism) will be impaired. And finally, as flow through the stenosis and collaterals begins to increase, the pressure drop also increases, resulting in a further reduction in tissue perfusion pressure. The end result is that the net increase in flow will be less than that required by the tissue, and ischemia will develop. As the degree of stenosis increases, the situation progressively worsens, and eventually, with very severe or multiple stenoses, the distal arterioles will be unable to compensate, even at rest, because of severely reduced tissue perfusion pressure.

A special case in which the collateral channels are very efficient occurs in the arterial supply to the brain. There are four major input vessels, and all four channels are joined to one another at the base of the brain (the Circle of Willis). Any one of these vessels may be completely occluded with only minor reductions in pressure occurring in the distal segment (20-30%). Flow increases in the other three channels to compensate for the loss of flow in the fourth. This collateral compensation becomes less efficient if the remaining vessels are also diseased. In other locations, both within the brain and elsewhere, the collateral channels are generally very small although there is good evidence to suggest that they are capable of increasing in size over a prolonged period of time. The pressure reductions are much more severe than those noted above, however, and ischemia is more likely to occur.

SIGNIFICANCE AND TREATMENT OF STENOSES

The presence of a stenosis in a major artery will result in a wide variety of hemodynamic disturbances. The effects of these disturbances may be divided roughly into two categories. The primary or local effects of an arterial stenosis would include the following: (1) damage to the elastic components of the wall, resulting in increased distensibility (poststenotic dilatation); (2) damage to the endothelium, activation of platelets, and production of areas of relatively stagnant blood flow, resulting in enhanced development of further narrowing (atherosclerosis) and the creation of potential sources of emboli; and (3) reduction of pressure distal to the stenosis, resulting in an increased reliance on collateral circulation. The secondary or distant effects, and in fact the reasons that most patients ultimately seek medical treatment, are both the result of reduced blood flow, produced by different mechamisms: (1) tissue ischemia resulting from an embolic occlusion of one or more distal vessels; and (2) tissue ischemia either at rest or during periods of increased metabolic demand, resulting from an inadequate tissue perfusion pressure.

The relative importance of the above two causes of ischemia depends to a large extent on the location of the stenosis. Cerebral ischemia resulting from a stenosis in the carotid artery is most often caused by embolic occlusion and less frequently due to a reduction in tissue perfusion pressure. There are two reasons for this. First, blood flow in the brain is relatively constant at all times, and large increases in flow (greater than 100%) rarely, if ever, occur. Therefore, variations in pressure reduction resulting from flow velocity fluctuations would not be expected. Second, the extensive collateral blood supply at this level of the circulation tends to minimize any reductions in pressure that do occur. Thus, in terms of tissue perfusion pressure, this is an extremely stable system, and embolic occlusion becomes the major cause of tissue ischemia. In other parts of the body (e.g., the legs), ischemia is most often the result of inadequate perfusion pressure. In these areas, flow demands may increase tenfold or more, leading to large pressure losses both in the stenosis and in the small, high-resistance collateral channels.

The treatment of an arterial stenosis, to be truly effective, must reduce the combined resistance of the stenosis plus its collaterals, or, in the case of the arteries in the neck, must reduce or remove the source of emboli. Thus there has been an almost exponential growth in the incidence of vascular surgery in recent years. The aim of these operations is to restore the blood flow (and/or the ability to meet increased demands for blood flow during exercise) or to remove a lesion that is producing emboli. There are a variety of surgical techniques used for this purpose.[5] Although there are many variations, the two major types of procedure involve either the removal of the stenosis or the insertion of an alternate route for blood flow which bypasses the stenosis. The first of these will reduce the resistance of the stenosis directly, whereas the second techniques reduces the resistance of the collateral circulation. Another method of treatment that is beneficial in reducing the risk of emboli is the administration of pharmacological agents that inhibit platelet activity. This is particularly useful when the source of emboli is uncertain or when the lesion is inoperable.

CONCLUDING REMARKS

It should be stressed that our knowledge of arterial stenosis and associated hemodynamic disturbances in man is limited to a very large extent to those changes that occur with severe narrowing. With few exceptions, the treatment of these disorders is also restricted to those patients in which tissue ischemia has already occurred. In patients with stroke, the brain is often damaged irreparably by the initial insult, and restoration of flow will do little more than reduce the risk of further ischemia from the same source. Similarly, the treatment of stenoses in other areas often results in a relief from the symptoms with very limited functional improvement. It is hoped that in the near future, we will be able to detect and treat an arterial stenosis before tissue ischemia develops. This will clearly involve improvements in our ability to detect and recognize alterations in hemodynamic parameters such as the velocity profile at a much earlier stage in the development of a stenosis.

References

Patel, D. J., Vaishnav, R. N., Gow, B. S., and Kot, P. A. Hemodynamics. *Ann. Rev. Physiol.* *36:* 125–154, 1974.

Roach, M. R. Poststenotic dilatation in arteries. In *Cardiovascular Fluid Dynamics,* Vol. 2, D. H. Bergel, ed. New York: Academic Press, 1972.

Berguer, R., and Hwang, N. H. C. Critical arterial stenosis: A theoretical and experimental solution. *Ann. Surg. 180:* 39–50, 1974.

Strandness, D. E. Flow dynamics in circulatory pathophysiology. In *Cardiovascular Flow Dynamics and Measurements,* N. H. C. Hwang and N. A. Normann, eds. Baltimore: University Park Press, 1977.

Noon, G. P. Flow-related problems in cardiovascular surgery. In *Cardiovascular Flow Dynamics and Measurements,* N. H. C. Hwang and N. A. Normann, eds. Baltimore: University Park Press, 1977.

Cardiac Assist Devices: Update on Current Uses and Future Prospects

HOOSHANG BOLOOKI, M.D.
Professor of Surgery
University of Miami School of Medicine
Attending Cardiac Surgeon
Jackson Memorial Hospital and the
Miami Veterans Administration Hospital

Cardiac or circulatory assist devices have been applied clinically since 1958. Until recently, their application was limited to patients with acute severe left ventricular dysfunction. Since 1972, a few patients with lesser degrees of cardiac dysfunction have received this type of treatment with satisfactory results.

PHYSIOLOGICAL BACKGROUND

The principle of circulatory assist considers that the left ventricle is acutely unable to pump a sufficient amount of blood to meet the metabolic demand of the tissues in spite of receiving a large volume (preload). Consequently, cardiac dilatation ensues, which results in an elevation of left ventricular resting tension and an increase in myocardial oxygen consumption.[1] As such, it is assumed that, if some of this volume is diverted from the left or the right side of the heart into a secondary pumping system (auxiliary pump) and returned to the circulation with or without oxygenation, it would be possible to allow the heart to work at its maximum efficiency supplemented by the assist delivered by the auxiliary circuit (cardiac assist device). The concept of disability of the left ventricle to pump sufficient blood volume per beat in spite of receiving a large volume of blood led to the utilization of the standard cardiopulmonary bypass in 1958 and left heart bypass with or without implantable devices in 1962 in patients with cardiogenic shock or acute left ventricular failure following cardiac surgery.

By the addition of a cardiac assist device to the circulatory system, the two pumping mechanisms, the patient's heart and the auxiliary pump, placed either in series (as in left heart bypass) or in parallel (as in right heart bypass), were to maintain tissue perfusion while sufficient time was given for the myocardium to heal and regain its contractility to an extent compatible with life. For a number of reasons, however, but primarily because of extensive damage to the myocardium in these patients, survival in the initial patients was low in spite of availability of manpower and equipment required for application of such a circulatory assist system.

In terms of the Starling hypothesis for cardiac function as a pump, left ventricular failure occurs at the time when in spite of a large volume of blood within the left ventricle (maximum fiber length), the heart is unable to produce sufficient cardiac output. This mechanism leads to a shift in the left ventricular function curve to the right and downward. But instead of removing the excess volume from the left or the right ventricle, by addition of an auxiliary pump it is possible to oxygenate the blood and return it to the patient in a continuous or in a pulsatile form during the cardiac cycle.

PRESENTLY USED CIRCULATORY ASSIST DEVICES

The most widely used circulatory assist device at the present time is the intra-aortic balloon pump.[1] This system, which was utilized clinically in 1967 and was studied further by the Myocardial Infarction Shock Unit of the Massachusetts General Hospital in 1970, is currently used in the day-to-day practice of cardiology and cardiac surgery across the country. The concept was initially introduced by Moulopoulos, was revised by Kantrowitz, and was perfected by the Massachusetts General Hospital team.

The intra-aortic balloon pump (Figure 1) is employed by insertion of a balloon catheter of size 7F through one of the femoral arteries, over a vascular graft 10 mm in diameter, into the descending thoracic aorta. The balloon catheter has at its end a long, sausage-shaped Polyurethane® balloon of one or up to

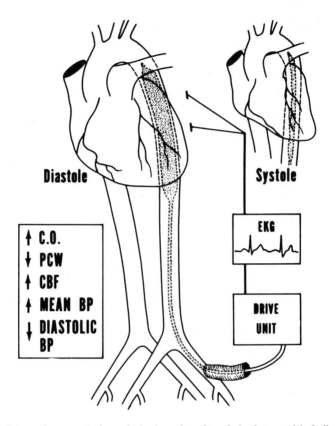

FIG. 1. Schematic presentation of the insertion site of the intra-aoritic balloon pump. Balloon inflates during cardiac diastole and deflates systole (inset). The hemodynamic effects of the intra-aortic balloon pump are shown in the lower inset. EKG = electrocardiogram; CO = cardiac output; PCW = pulmonary capillary wedge pressure; CBF = coronary blood flow; BP = systemic blood pressure.

three segments. The balloon is pulsated (inflation and deflation) using a gas (CO_2 or helium) synchronized with the cardiac cycle by a computer console setup. Since cardiac systole follows the electrocardiographic R wave of the QRS complex, the balloon is pulsated so that inflation occurs immediately after systole and deflation procedes upstroke of the aortic pressure wave form.[2] By exact timing of the balloon, systolic unloading is produced, and left ventricular afterload is decreased sufficiently to enhance the cardiac output by approximately 10 to 15%. Balloon counterpulsation produces an increase in diastolic blood pressure and a decrease in systolic aortic pressure. Balloon location in the descending thoracic aorta allows disposition of a volume of blood equal to the volume of the gas that enters the balloon in the course of cardiac diastole. The balloon also produces a relative vacuum within the column of blood in the descending thoracic aorta during balloon deflation, resulting in a rapid decrease in diastolic aortic pressure. The blood displaced from the aorta is replaced by blood from the left ventricle during ejection.[1]

The clinical indications for the intra-aortic balloon pump are limited to situations where acute left ventricular failure has occurred, usually because of myocardial infarction or ischemia. The major indication for the use of the intra-aortic balloon pump is acute left ventricular failure at the completion of the open heart operation in patients undergoing myocardial revascularization or cardiac valve replacement. The survival rate with this modality of therapy in post-open heart surgery cardiac failure varies between 54 and 60%. The intra-aortic balloon pump is also used in patients with cardiogenic shock, where its use alone or in combination with cardiac surgery has produced an overall survival rate of approximately 48%. The latter indication has been mostly defined after continuous hemodynamic monitoring with a Swan-Ganz catheter and calculation of cardiac output and pulmonary capillary wedge pressure. Patients who present clinically with cardiogenic shock due to acute myocardial infarction (exhibiting a systolic blood pressure of less than 80 mm Hg, tachycardia, evidence of low tissue perfusion) and a cardiac index of less than 2 liters/min/m^2 and a pulmonary capillary wedge pressure of greater than 18 mm Hg are candidates for support with this device.[3] The satisfactory results obtained with balloon counterpulsation in patients with cardiogenic shock are also attributed to judicious use of newer pressor agents (dopamine) and afterload reduction with intravenous nitroglycerine or sodium nitroprusside in the setting of an intensive care unit. The most recent indications for the use of the intra-aortic balloon pump have been in patients who have preinfarction syndrome complicated by electrocardiographic changes and chest pain, or patients who have ventricular dysrhythmia not manageable with drug treatment. A few patients with malignant rhythm disturbances have responded favorably to the intra-aortic balloon pump followed by cardiac catheterization studies to define the coronary anatomy, and myocardial revascularization when necessary. The intra-aortic balloon pump also is utilized in patients who develop acute myocardial infarction in the course of general surgical procedures, or those patients who have a borderline cardiac function and require a major general surgical operation. We have been successful in such patients with the utilization of this device and have carried out the surgical operation with balloon support intra- and postoperatively. In patients who develop an acute myocardial infarction complicated by a low output syndrome after surgical procedures, the intra-aortic balloon pump has been a useful adjunct therapy. The intra-aortic balloon pump has not been effective in reversing the clinical course of patients with septic or hemorrhagic shock.

CARDIOPULMONARY BYPASS SYSTEM

Cardiopulmonary bypass (Figure 2) has been used as an assist device since early stages of cardiac surgery. Use of this device as an assist system is indicated in patients with acute pulmonary emboli resulting in rapid cardiac failure and in patients with ventricular fibrillation unresponsive to drug therapy. In a few patients with malignant hyperthermia (seen in the course of general anesthesia) cardiopulmonary bypass has been used to decrease the body temperature. This device is also helpful in kyperkalemic states (serum K^+ higher than 7 mEq/liter) when ventricular fibrillation has ensued and is unresponsive to other methods of therapy. The drawbacks of this method are: circulatory assist with a linear (non-pulsatile) pressure, cell destruction, and coagulopathy when duration of bypass exceeds three hours.

MEMBRANE OXYGENATORS

This system has been most commonly used in patients who require a circulatory assist for a respiratory distress syndrome and poor oxygenation. The patient is attached to the system in a mode similar to that used for cardiopulmonary bypass. Cannulation for blood return from the patient is from the femoral vein, and the femoral artery is used for arterial inflow to the patient (Figure 2). During the standard cardiac surgical procedures, for the purpose of cardiopulmonary bypass, a bubble oxygenator is utilized (Figure 2). The setup with a membrane oxygenator simply replaces the bubble oxygenator with a polyurethane membrane which allows oxygenation of the blood for a long period of time (up to seven days) with minimal heparinization. In this fashion sufficient time is alloted for the lung to recover from its parenchymal disease. In a number of studies, use of this device in adult respiratory syndrome has been associated with patient survival after many days of respiratory support. Membrane oxygenators also are utilized instead of the bubble oxygenators in patients undergoing cardiac surgery. As compared with bubble oxygenators, circulatory support with a membrane oxygenator (or membrane lung) is associated with minimal blood cell destruction and platelet aggregation. Thus, intrapulmonary, cerebral, and intra-vascular microemboli are prevented. Membrane oxygenators also allow a longer period of cardiopulmonary bypass without any coagulation problems. These oxygenators, however, have not become universally accepted because of the need for a reservoir in the cardiopulmonary bypass system. Normally, the bubble oxygenator itself serves as a reservoir where a large volume of blood is reserved and can be returned to the patient in emergency situations. With a membrane oxygenator, however, there is only a small reservoir in the system (unless an additional reservoir is added) so that if an emergency situation arises, it is impossible to return a large volume of blood to the patient rapidly. This

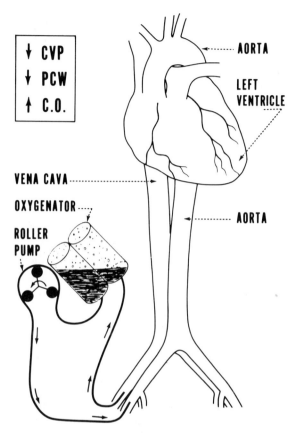

FIG. 2. Schematic presentation of the method of application of standard cardiopulmonary bypass via the femoral artery and vein as an assist method. For standard cardiopulmonary bypass, a bubble oxygenator is used. For prolonged assist, a membrane oxygenator is utilized. CVP = central venous pressure. Other abbreviations as in Figure 1.

drawback, however, is considered minimal by many cardiac surgeons, since numerous improvements in the cardiopulmonary bypass system are associated with the use of membrane oxygenators.

LEFT HEART BYPASS

This system was initially utilized in patients with cardiogenic shock because most of these patients were showing a high left ventricular end-diastolic pressure or left atrial pressure.[2] Because of inability of the left ventricle to pump forward a sufficient volume and because of its dilatation due to an increased preload, Dennis and associates advocated a left heart bypass system. They advanced a cannula into the left atrium through the internal jugular vein in a number of patients with cardiogenic shock and were able to assist their patients in this fashion. The cannula removed blood from the left atrium and delivered it into a regular roller pump. Blood was then returned to the patient without need for oxygenation. Along the same line DeBakey developed a left heart assist system that could be implanted in the patient's chest by means of two grafts, one connected to the left atrium and the other to the aorta. With a hydraulic system, driving the Polyurethane® membrane portion of the left heart assist system, blood could be extracted from the left atrium and returned into the thoracic aorta in synchrony with the cardiac cycle. Clinical application of this system produced a number of survivors, but it required a second operation for removal of the device after patient survival.

Connolly and Wakabayashi utilized a nonheparinized left heart bypass system where a heparin-coated cannula could be advanced into the left atrium via the jugular vein and with tubings that also were heparin-coated. The blood could be removed from the left atrium and returned to the aorta via the femoral artery, thus avoiding problems with anticoagulation. With this system, these investigators were successful a number of times. However, the left heart bypass system never actually gained clinical acceptance because of its inability to improve the cardiac function appreciably and because of excessive blood trauma. This assist system does not increas coronary blood flow and does not improve the blood pressure, although adequate cardiac output is maintained. The number of survivors with the use of this device has been small, and the utilization of the system has required a great deal of manpower and expertise.

Most recently Litwak has used a simplified method of left heart bypass in patients unable to be weaned from cardiopulmonary bypass at the completion of open heart surgery.[2] In the Litwak system (Figure 3) the blood is taken from the left atrium directly with a cannula that is sutured to the left atrium. Blood is returned to a roller pump and then returned to the ascending aorta via a cannula that again is sutured to the aorta. Both of these cannulae are brought out of the chest cavity at the completion of the operation, and the chest is closed. At the completion of the assist period an obtrerator is threaded into each cannula, and the cannulae are obliterated, thus avoiding the necessity of returning the patient to the operating room. With the Litwak system, a 33% survival rate was achieved in a group of 14 patients. This system has been infrequently used clinically.

PARTIAL LEFT VENTRICULAR ASSIST DEVICES

The partial left ventricular assist devices are a series of circulatory assist devices that are attached directly to the left ventricle and are pneumatically actuated. Blood is removed from the left ventricle and is returned to the aorta (Figure 4). In a system devised by Drs. Norman and Bernhard, the blood is removed from

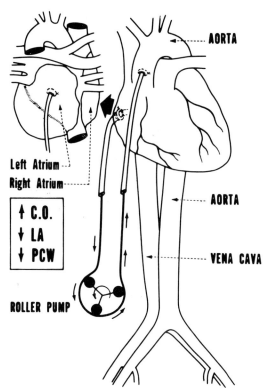

AORTA

Left Atrium

Right Atrium

↑ C.O.
↓ LA
↓ PCW

AORTA

VENA CAVA

ROLLER PUMP

FIG. 3. Schematic presentation of the Litwak left heart bypass system. The outflow catheter is in the left atrium (inset), and the inflow catheter in the ascending thoracic aorta. Both catheters have been brought out of the chest wall. LA = left atrium. Other abbreviations as in Figure 1.

the left ventricular cavity via a large cannula that is placed in the apex of the left ventricle and is returned to a housing case that contains two Polyurethane® membranes through which the blood is passed, and then is returned to the abdominal aorta (Norman)[4] or the ascending aorta (Bernhard). An air tubing is connected to the assist device, which is brought into the chest wall or to the abdominal cavity, with attachment to the pump housing. Air is delivered on a sequential basis to the pump housing, producing counterpulsation between the assist device and the left ventricle. Therefore, during cardiac systole blood is removed from the left ventricle and is delivered into the pump. During diastole the membranes are squeezed by the air in the pump casing, and the blood is returned to the aorta. Two valves, one attached to the inflow cannula from the left ventricular cavity and another to the outflow graft which is connected to the aorta, produce one-way blood flow. This system has been utilized by Dr. Norman in a number of patients, and a similar system has been used by Dr.

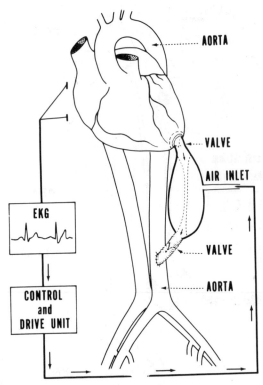

FIG. 4. Schematic drawing of the setup for the partial left heart bypass, abdominal left ventricular assist device (ALVAD). The pneumatically driven device is implanted in the abdominal cavity with the inflow to the device attached to the apex of the left ventricle and the outflow of the device to the abdominal aorta. There are two one-way valves in the inlet and outlet of the device. Abbreviations as in Figure 1.

Pierce at Hershey, Pennsylvania with one successful instance[5] and by Dr. Bernhard in a number of patients with two survivors.

Much of the effort at the present time is directed to improving the efficacy of this equipment as compared with the intra-aortic balloon pump. This equipment increases the coronary blood flow because of its counterpulsation effect and also because of decreased diastolic blood pressure. It increases the cardiac output to approximately two to three times more than that achieved by an intra-aortic balloon counterpulsation. This system can be utilized only in patients who are unable to respond to the intra-aortic balloon pump before the left ventricular failure has reached an irreversible stage. At the present time the clinical experiments with this device are limited to those patients who are moribund, and hence the number of survivors is small. An extensive amount of physiological data, however, has been gathered showing that this device is capable of maintaining circulation when the patient's left ventricle is almost unable to produce any cardiac output. The procedural demand for use of this device is a major one, and removal of the device afterward requires an operation, either through the thoracic cavity for the Bernhard system or through the abdominal wall for the Norman system.

FUTURE CONSIDERATIONS

Much of the difficulty with the circulatory assist devices has been related to the extensive operative procedure required on a patient who is unable to produce sufficient cardiac output to maintain his body metabolism. These operations are actually gross and deviate from the fine surgical technique and minimal invasion of the tissues that is required in patients who are extremely ill. Because of this and because of the requirement for a great deal of research manpower and financial aid, many of these systems have failed to gain clinical acceptance.

The intra-aortic balloon pump has been the only device to date to require minimal risk and minimal surgery. Morever, this equipment has allowed simplicity of function, minimal manpower, easy introduction and removal, and a minimal need for hemodynamic monitoring prior to or during its utilization. The cost benefit of this equipment has been acceptable, and because it can be used with minimal need for highly skilled personnel, it has become an important adjunct in the care of patients with acute cardiogenic shock or those who are unable to be weaned from cardiopulmonary bypass at the completion of cardiac surgery. This system is presently being utilized in most cardiac surgery centers across the country and in many small community hospitals. The equipment is portable, and patients can remain on this device for many days (our record is 45 days) without any particular problems.

It is obvious, however, that no more than one-half of the patients with cardiogenic shock or with left ventricular failure after cardiac surgery respond to cardiac assist with an intra-aortic balloon pump. Therefore, there is a need for another advanced type of cardiac assist device which can perhaps salvage some of those patients who are salvageable eventually but do not respond to balloon pumping. To salvage this group some of the medical centers have used partial left ventricular assist devices or cardiac transplantation. Transplantation has been reserved mostly for those patients who have chronic left ventricular failure. For acute left ventricular failure, the scientific community has yet to find a solution better than balloon pumping. Since the development of an artificial heart is long overdue, and because the physiologic difficulty with development of biocompatible material and satisfactory driving systems has been excessive, any new ideas are welcome in this area of medical science.

Part of the difficulty in development of an artificial heart or an adequate circulatory assist system at the present time, is unavailability of sufficient patient material that can utilize this type of device. Cardiac surgery as a source of this patient material has advanced to such an extent that the patients dying in the course of surgery, overall, number less than 5%. Cardiogenic shock, another indication for the treatment, develops in less than 5% of patients with acute transmural myocardial infarction. Therefore, advancement in cardiac therapy and cardiac surgery has produced, happily, only a small number of patients who are not benefited by these methods of management. It is only the far advanced patient, who does not respond to standard therapy, who requires elaborate circulatory assist devices. Hence, the research in this area is limited to that group of patients who are moribund and cannot be salvaged by any other means—and rightly so because the patients with less extensive disease should not be subjected to this type of experiment. The utilization of an intra-aortic balloon pump, needed by approximately 10% of our patients in 1973-1976, at the present time is required by less than 5% of these patients, of whom one-half are saved by the intra-aortic balloon pump.[1] The patient who is not responsive to the intra-aortic balloon pump, however, usually has had a prolonged period of cardiopulmonary bypass already and is not a satisfactory candidate for any further circulatory assist therapy. As a result, the number of patients available for the latter type of intervention is extremely small.

References

Bolooki, H., ed. *Clinical Application of Intra-aortic Balloon Pump.* Mt. Kisco, New York: Futura Publishing, 1977.
Bregman, D. Mechanical support of the failing heart. *Current Problems in Surgery,* 13, No. 12. Chicago: Yearbook Medical Publishers, December 1976.
Mundth, E. D. Assisted circulation. In *Surgery of the Chest,* J. H. Gibbon, Jr., ed. Philadelphia: Saunders, 1976, pp. 1394-1415.
Norman, J. C., Molokhia, F. A., Harmison, L. T., et al., An implantable nuclear-fueled circulatory support system. I. Systems analysis of conception, design, fabrication and initial *in vivo* testing. *Ann. Surg. 176:* 492, 1972.
Pierce, W. S., Donachy, J. H., Landis, D. L., et al. Prolonged mechanical support of the left ventricle. *Circulation 58, Suppl. I:* 133, 1978.

The Experimental Approach to Atheroembolic Stroke

B. J. JEYNES, Ph.D.
Department of Pathology
University of Western Ontario
London, Ontario, Canada

Stroke, the apoplexy of former days, is a debilitating or fatal affliction that results from the death of brain parenchymal cells. The observable character and quality of the damage depend upon which brain cells are rendered permanently inoperable. In referring to stroke, it is understood that the cell death is due to inadequate or deprived cerebral blood perfusion rather than to cell death associated with, for example, a tumor, trauma, or foreign body. This decreased regional perfusion can result from one of two general occurrences: either hemorrhage (usually related to vascular wall deficiencies such as aneurysm or atherosclerosis) or occlusion (frequently related to the phenomenon of thrombosis or embolism).

This paper will deal with an occlusive event that contributes significantly to stroke development, atheroembolism. It is important at the outset to distinguish between atheroembolism, which is the embolization of atheromatous material derived from a mature atherosclerotic plaque, and thromboembolism, which is the embolization of thrombus material, whether it is associated with atherosclerotic plaques or with other vascular wall disorders. The latter is a distinct and well recognized phenomenon. However, because thrombosis is also a complication of atherosclerosis and is frequently related to the endothelial surface over atherosclerotic plaques, the term atheroembolism is too often interpreted as meaning thromboembolism. As we shall see, the system reaction to the two materials is separate and distinct. (By system reaction I mean the mechanisms by which the blood and the vessel wall and flow of blood maintain the integrity and fluidity of the blood.)

The process of atheroembolism results from the ulceration of the contents of a mature atherosclerotic plaque into the bloodstream, and is classified as one of the four complications of atherosclerosis (Haust and Moore, 1972), the others being calcification, thrombosis, and hemorrhage. In the brain the phenomenon is clinically associated, as are other forms of embolism, with both permanent and transient manifestations. The former are represented by complete strokes and the latter by events such as TIA's (transient ischemic attacks) and occurrences

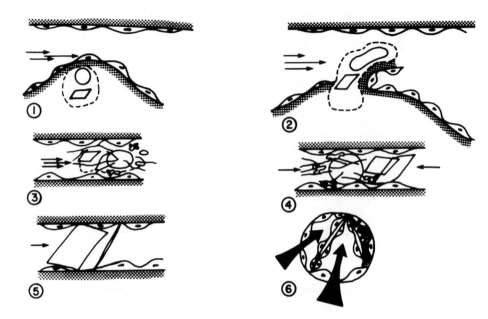

FIG. 1. Schematic illustration of sequence of events in embolization by atheromatous material. The development of the atheromatous plaque results in the formation of an elevated ridge which projects into the main axial stream of the blood flowing through the vessel (1). Within the mature atheromatous plaque there are crystalline and noncrystalline materials (indicated by a rhombid and a circle). Ulceration of the surface of the elevated plaque (2) probably occurs as a result of shear force parameters of the axial stream. The contents of the plaque are released into the blood flowing over the ulcerated area. Blood reacts to the released material (3), a reaction that particularly involves the noncrystalline material and is characterized by a thrombogenic response. There is also the start of an inflammatory reaction. Impaction of this combined embolus of atheromatous material and the reaction of the blood to it occurs in a vessel downstream from the site of the ulceration (4). Following these reactions, instituted after impaction, clearance of all material except the crystals may ensue (5). Reaction by surviving endothelial cells over and around the crystals and associated connective tissue elements can result in reestablishing functional flow through the impacted area but with reduced total vessel lumen (6).

of amaurosis fugax (fleeting blindness). Most frequently the emboli arise from the carotid bifurcation in the neck. Another frequent site of embolization is the union point of the two vertebral arteries where they form the basilar artery. Other sites can and do ulcerate, less frequently but in some cases no less devastatingly.

Generally, atheroembolism produces decreased vascular perfusion by blocking, partially or totally, smaller downstream vessels. The limit of the resulting ischemia/infarction is dependent upon five basic factors: (1) the amount of material ulcerated; (2) the blood reaction to the ulcerated material; (3) the availability and extent of collateral circulation; (4) the effectiveness of the reticuloendothelial system (RES) in removing the reactants and their by-products; and (5) the survival of the vessel wall at the sites of impaction and occlusion. Currently, our understanding of these factors, independently and synergistically, is at best rudimentary.

WHAT EXPERIMENTS HAVE TOLD US

To begin with, there are but nine publications that present experimental data about atheroembolism. Only two of them deal with cerebral atheroembolism. This paucity is partially due to the fact that it was not until the mid 1940s that the phenomenon of atheroembolism was seriously considered to be associated with organ infarction. Two other problems seem manifest regarding the scarcity of research in this area: first, many observers have been preoccupied with describing only the morphology of the occlusive lesions (this is particuarly evident in clinical case reports); and second, it did not, until recently, seem to be of interest to the scientific community to investigate the mechanisms by which these occlusions developed and either persisted or dissipated.

The basic question at the crux of the experimental work is this: How does ulceration of atheromatous material bring about sufficient vascular occlusion to cause infarction? Although the particular focus of this discussion is stroke, data produced in other organ systems are equally pertinent because many of the cellular and biochemical interactions are common throughout the vascular system. All of the experiments have consisted of injecting either heterogeneous human atheromatous material or pure cholesterol into the vascular system of an animal model, usually the rabbit. Pure cholesterol was injected because it was, and still is, considered by some to be the most important embolizing component in the plaque material.

Both the amounts and concentrations of material injected have varied, so that it is difficult to come to any quantitative conclusions regarding the effect of discrete amounts. There is, however, some evidence to support the idea that the quantity of material ulcerated may play a role in terms of overcoming the ability of the body to cope adequately with ulcerative events. In recent work in this laboratory, injections of relatively large quantities of homogenized liver into rabbit carotid systems were unable to kill the animals at levels that exceeded twice the ascertained dose for injected human atheromatous material. This would suggest that, independent of the mass of the material ulcerated, there is some other component to the mechanism that kills the animal, by which permanent occlusion is made possible. This of course does not exclude a variably significant synergistic contribution by the mass parameter. Its importance was demonstrated by Warren and Lytton (1976) when they showed that there was a "loading limit" of atheromatous material injected into rabbit lower limb arteries, beyond which the development of a retrograde thrombus back into the aorta would kill the animal. Below the threshold limit, the animals survived and seemed capable of coping with the material. A limit of approximately 50 mg has been established in this laboratory for rabbits weighing between 2 and 3 kg when atheromatous material is injected into the common carotid artery. This model is currently being used to examine some of the other factors involved in athero-embolic stroke, particularly blood reaction to the components of the material.

Regardless of the organ studied there is a remarkable consistency in the literature reports describing the kinds of arterial lesions produced, the reactions to the materials, both during and after the production of the lesion, and the time-sequence of the events. Generally the reports detail the following scenario: ulceration, blood reaction to the ulcerated material, impaction, clearing of non-crystalline material, organization around the crystals, and reestablishment of endothelialized channels (Warren and Vales, 1975). During atherogenesis the maturing atheromatous plaque accumulates numerous components in various physical states, including crystals of cholesterol and its esters and numerous other noncrystalline entities. The precise identification of the noncrystalline materials is not known entirely. Perhaps best known are the lipids. Harland et al. (1973) listed 17 types of lipid. Of the remaining material, there is no detailed biochemical description available. What is available in consistent morphological description of the material, a list that includes myelin figures, various cellular organelles and debris, membranes, and "amorphous material."

Although we take about the process of ulceration rather casually, it is still somewhat of a mystery. Aside from trauma and iatrogenic incidents, most re-searchers feel that the cause of plaque ulceration is the shear force of blood flowing over the lesion. What is unclear is whether it is a high or a low shear force that precipitates the stripping of the covering endothelial surface over-lying the atherosclerotic plaque. Experimental evidence has been presented for both. This area of biophysical research is still being pursued for a more definitive response to the question. Another consideration concerns the possible effects of introducing *human* atheromatous material into *animal* models. Might this not compromise results by contributing to a system response via the coagulation or platelet mechanisms? The answer is probably, but not significantly, at least not on morphological grounds. Experimentally produced lesions are very similar to those described in the clinical literature, especially when similar organ systems are compared. It may be that at the biochemical or physiological level there are effects with respect to immunological contributions to the activation and char-acter of a system response to embolizing atheromatous material, but no such effects have been demonstrated. However, this possibility may be worth bearing in mind when considering the blood and vascular reactions to the embolizing materials.

There are two quite separate reactions to embolizing plaque material. One is the response to the presence of the crystals of cholesterol and its esters, and the other the response to the remaining material. Common to both, however, is an early inflammatory reaction, evidenced especially by the presence of numerous eosinophils, as well as other polymorphonuclear leucocytes. The resultant panarteritis is not definitely explicable, but is believed to occur either in response to damaged endothelial cells (Warren and Vales, 1973) or in response to the presence of certain lipids known to be present in atherosclerotic plaques and demonstrated to be inflammatory. These include particularly 26-hydroxycholesterol and cholestane $3\beta,5a,6\beta$ (Harland et al., 1973). The reaction to the crystals (either by themselves or together with other reactions) is multifaceted. It includes smooth muscle cell migration to the site of impaction, connective tissue proliferation, macrophage ingestion (which is size-dependent), a giant cell reaction, and the reestablishment of endothelial-lined channels. The reaction to other lipid material is unclear except for the inflammatory response evoked by some lipid entities, and the observations by two researchers that the lipids do not appear to be thrombogenic. The reaction to the nonlipid component of the plaque material seems to be essentially to activate the reticulo-endothelial system (RES). There is, evidence from our work, that there is a thrombogenic element in the nonlipid portion of the ulcerating atheromatous material. Perhaps it is this thrombogenic response that is critical in determining the ability of the system to cope with this kind of insult. Further, it may also be the reaction most amenable to clinical control.

The description that follows is a detailed composite of the data in the literature on the cellular sequence of events during atheroembolism. Figure 1 summarizes the description.

At the time of ulceration the contents of the mature atherosclerotic plaque are emptied into the bloodstream. Once in the blood this material reacts with the blood contents, not only attracting reticuloendothelial and polymorphonuclear cells, but also initiating a thrombogenic response; and fibrin and platelet aggregates accumulate in and around the material, particularly with the noncrystalline, and most likely with the nonlipid material. An atherothromboembolus is thus formed. The material continues to embolize until it reaches an artery whose caliber is too small to allow the bolus to pass. At this point a whole new set of reactions begins to take place. At the site of impaction there may or may not be damage and/or death to the surrounding endothelial cells. The survival of the endothelium is critical. If there is damage, there may be an augmentation of the inflammatory response, further aggravating the panarteritis associated with the early stages of the overall reaction. Further, there may be a decreased ability to complete the process of organization. After approximately 24 hours the noncrystalline material, and very small crystal fragments, are removed by the actions of the fibrinolytic and RE systems, and the inflammatory response subsides gradually from this point on. Only the large crystals remain. From their time of impaction they are believed to evoke the following sequence of events. The impaction of the crystalline material, acting either synergistically with other components or alone, triggers the migration of smooth muscle cells to the site of occlusion. These cells produce collagen and other connective tissue elements around the crystals. By this time histiocytes, which were attracted to the crystals earlier have probably fused to form the giant cells seen near the surface of the crystals. A thinly layered substance on the surface of the crystals can sometimes be seen, which has been described as osmophilic. It may be important with respect to cellular response to the presence of the crystals. During these early stages of organization, the endothelial cells begin to replicate, eventually covering the crystals and their associated connective tissue cells and elements. Of course if the endothelium did not survive, this latter reaction would not occur, and further organization would be halted. Ultimately the crystals are sequestered from the flow of blood, which is reestablished by the formation of endothelial lined vascular channels between and around the isolated crystals. Although minute partial dissolution of the crystals has been described, removal of whole large crystals in this manner would be severely prolonged. Others have observed the crystals partially extended through the vessel wall. This is thought to be a result of a vasoconstrictive response of the wall to the stimulus of impaction.

It is these last few stages that are most frequently described in the case history literature, and it is the presence of the accular spaces that many consider essential for proving that the blocking of an occluded vessel suspected of causing an infact was precipitated by an atheroembolic accident, since these spaces are remnant evidence of the presence of crystals.

There are, of course, numerous variations in this train of events. If occlusion occurred suddenly in a large artery, the acute loss of blood to an organ, or a large portion of it, such as the brain, could be fatal. End artery occlusion would also be more difficult for the system to cope with, owing to a lack of collateral circulation, as would arteries in which large thrombi formed around the material impeding access of the RES to the material, which would normally be more readily cleared away. In these cases the organ being supplied by the affected artery would develop a complete or partial infarction.

FUTURE CONSIDERATIONS

From the data presented here it can be seen that there is a plethora of unanswered questions. Three general matters are of great immediate interest. The first is an understanding of the balances involved in returning vessels to a functional patent state after an atheroembolic incident. To name only a few, one must consider the antithetical functions of (a) the fibrinolytic system, the serum anticoagulation factors, the antiplatelet-aggregating substances such as PGI_2

(formerly PGX or prostacyclin), and the RES, on the one hand, versus (b) the coagulation and platelet pathways and platelet aggregating substances such as collagen and TxA_2 (thromboxane A_2), on the other. The time restriction is also important. The time intervals during which cells can survive without nutrients or without removal of their waste products in these circumstances are unknown. Our understanding of their synergistic interactions is almost nonexistent.

The second priority is to understand the reactions just mentioned as they relate to the embolizing material as a whole and to separate components of it. We know that as a whole the material is inflammatory. We suspect that lipids are nonthrombogenic, and that elements of the nonlipid component, to an unknown extent, are thrombogenic. It may be that the fulcrum point of the balancing factors rest with the *final* volume or mass of the bolus. This in turn may be directly related to the extent and rate of the thrombogenic reaction to one or more components of the embolizing material. If this thrombogenicity can be controlled, perhaps the resultant balance will favor vessel patency and hence survival of the involved organ. Efforts are currently under way to identify the thrombogenic components of atheroma.

The third major priority is to relate the known data to methods of clinical control. This knowledge can be applied at various stages of the embolic event. For example, control of blood pressure may alter the susceptibility of the endothelial cells to ulceration. The use of anticoagulants such as heparin or anti-platelet-function drugs such as aspirin, imidazole, or EG626 may reduce the thrombogenic reaction in the pathogenesis of occlusion. Finally, if the thrombogenic element can be identified, then perhaps it may be amenable to dietary or pharmaceutical control, and reduce the effect of the thrombotic contribution toward the development of a threatening and unmanageable atheroembolus.

References

Harland, W. A., Smith, A. G., and Gilbert, J. D. Tissue reaction to atheroma lipids. *J. Pathol. 111:* 247–254, 1973.

Haust, M. D., and Moore, R. H. In *The Pathogenesis of Atherosclerosis,* R. W. Wissler and J. C. Geer, eds. Baltimore: Williams and Wilkins, 1972.

Warren, B. A., and Lytton, D. G. The effects and morphology of atheroembolism in limb arteries: An experimental study. *Pathology 8:* 231-245, 1976.

Warren, B. A., and Vales, O. The ultrastructure of the stages of atheroembolic occlusion of renal arteries. *Br. J. Exp. Pathol. 54:* 469-477, 1973.

Warren, B. A., and Vales, O. Electron microscopy of the sequence of events in the athero-embolic occlusion of cerebral arteries in an animal model. *Br. J. Exp. Pathol. 56:* 205–215, 1975.

Noninvasive Diagnosis of Vascular Diseases: Principles and Applications

BRUCE S. CUTLER, M.D.
Associate Professor of Surgery
University of Massachusetts Medical Center
Worcester, Massachusetts

Angiography remains the ultimate diagnostic technique for the assessment of peripheral vascular disease. However, the sophisticated and invasive nature of arteriography has restricted its application to hospitalized patients who are being seriously considered for surgical therapy. For the practicing clinician wishing to screen a patient in his office for deep venous thrombosis, or to objectively assess the progress of a patient with a superficial femoral artery occlusion, angiography is of limited value. Noninvasive diagnostic methods have been developed to provide objective information at low cost, without risk for the outpatient with peripheral vascular disease. As yet, no standard noninvasive test comparable to the electrocardiogram has emerged; instead, there has been a proliferation of noninvasive instrumentation. This chapter will review a selected number of noninvasive techniques which have been shown to be of value to the practicing clinician in assessing common problems in patients with peripheral vascular disease.

OCCLUSIVE ARTERIAL DISEASE

The ultrasonic Doppler velocity meter is the instrument most widely used to study peripheral vascular disease. The probe of the instrument contains both a transmitting and a receiving crystal. The transmitting crystal emits an ultrasonic signal in the range of 5 to 10 MHz which can penetrate several centimeters of soft tissue. If the ultrasonic signal strikes blood in motion, the beam is reflected from the red cells to the receiving crystal. If the blood is moving toward the probe, an apparent increase in frequency is produced—the Doppler effect. If the blood is moving away from the probe, there is an apparent decrease in frequency. The frequency shift is proportional to the velocity of the red cells (Figure 1). In many ultrasonic Dopplers the shift in frequency is converted to an audible signal which tells the physician that the instrument is positioned over a vessel containing blood in motion. With minimal training, one can easily distinguish

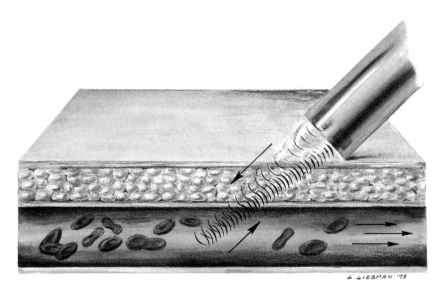

L·LIEBMAN '73

Fig. 1. Portable ultrasonic velocity meter. An ultrasonic signal is emitted from a piezo-electric crystal located in the Doppler probe. The signal is reflected from a moving stream of blood back to a second receiving crystal. If the blood is moving toward the probe, an apparent increase in frequency is produced—the Doppler effect.

the staccato sound of unobstructed arterial flow from the slow crescendo–de-crescendo of collateral flow around an arterial obstruction. Venous blood flow has a characteristic "wind in the trees" sound. Several moderately priced pocket-sized ultrasonic Dopplers are commercially available. The clinician can readily use the pocket Doppler for the tests described in this section to gain objective information about his patient with arterial occlusive disease.

The presence of arterial occlusive disease can be suspected when diminished or absent peripheral pulses are detected on physical examination. However, precise evaluation of pulses may be hampered by obesity or edema. The ultra-sonic Doppler makes possible the determination of blood pressure in the lower extremities by detecting the presence of blood flow even when a peripheral pulse is not palpable.

Ankle/Arm Index

A standard 12-cm blood pressure cuff is placed circumferentially around the ankle and inflated above brachial systolic pressure. As the clinician listens over the posterior tibial or dorsalis pedis pulse locations, the cuff is slowly deflated. The point at which arterial blood flow is detected is the ankle systolic pressure.

By dividing the ankle pressure by the brachial arterial pressure, one obtains the ankle/arm index. Since the normal ankle pressure is usually slightly higher than the brachial pressure, the normal ankle/arm index is > 1.0. Ankle/arm indices < 1.0 can only occur because of proximal arterial stenosis or occlusion. The ankle/arm index is a simple office or bedside determination which can often rule in or out the presence of occlusive disease. Ankle/arm indices that are less than normal but > 0.5 usually mean occlusive disease at a single level. Values < 0.5 are seen in patients with multilevel disease. An index < 0.25 is usually seen in patients who are severely symptomatic with rest pain or tissue necrosis.

The ankle/arm index may help in the management of the patient with occlusive disease. For example, an index < 0.5 correlates with a poor prognosis for the healing of ischemic ulcerations. The ankle/arm index can be used to assess the patency of an arterial reconstruction. Frequently, tibial occlusive disease precludes the palpation of peripheral pulses postoperatively; however, if the ankle/arm index is substantially improved from its preoperative value, the graft is patent. The ankle/arm index is a useful objective means to follow the development of collateral circulation in patients with iliac or femoral artery occlusions who are being managed conservatively.

Segmental Doppler Pressures

Measurements of pressures at more than one level can provide information regarding the site of arterial occlusion. Blood pressure cuffs are placed around the proximal thigh, calf, and ankle and the pressures recorded while flow is detected with the ultrasonic Doppler at the ankle level (Figure 2). In this manner, *segmental pressures* at the common femoral, popliteal, and tibial level can be estimated. If the brachial artery pressure is assumed to be equal to central aortic pressure, then gradients across the iliac, femoral, and popliteal vessels can be determined. Since variations in cuff placement and fit will produce small artifactual pressure differences, a gradient of at least 10 mm Hg is necessary to be considered abnormal. For example, a difference of 40 mm Hg in pressure between the brachial artery and the thigh pressure would be indicative of significant aortoiliac occlusive disease. Similarly, a gradient between thigh and calf readings is seen in patients with superficial femoral artery occlusion or stenosis. Diabetic persons frequently have extensive calcification of arterial walls which may make the vessels incompressible and thereby interfere with the measurement of segmental Doppler pressures. Pressures as high as 300 mm Hg may not obliterate the Doppler signal at the ankle. Segmental Doppler pressures may be used to predict the success of major amputations. A thigh pressure > 50 mm Hg has been associated with a 90% success rate in the healing of below-knee amputations.

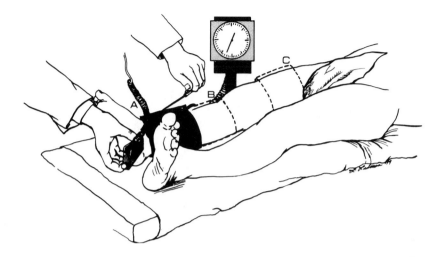

Fig. 2. Segmental Doppler pressures. Blood pressure cuffs are placed around the proximal thigh, calf, and ankle and the pressures recorded while flow is detected with the ultrasonic Doppler at the ankle level.

Exercise Testing

Patients with intermittent claudication are notoriously inaccurate in estimating the distance that they can walk. An objective assessment of the severity and location of the claudication is helpful in selecting patients for surgery and in following the course of those who will be managed nonoperatively. Exercise testing in the vascular laboratory is attractive because it dynamically tests the activity that produces the patient's symptoms. It also permits one simultaneously to assess the myocardial response to exercise in patients who may be candidates for surgical reconstruction.

Prior to exercise, segmental Doppler pressures are obtained. The patient then walks on the treadmill at a standard speed of 2 mph on a 12% grade. Simultaneous ECG monitoring is important because of the frequent association of coronary artery disease with peripheral vascular disease. Even with the low levels of exercise performed by patients with claudication, 30% will develop ECG evidence of myocardial ischemia during treadmill testing. This information frequently helps in planning the management of the patient with claudication. During exercise the patient is asked to report the onset of claudication, its location, and severity. After the patient has exercised maximally, he lies down, and the ankle/arm index is measured immediately and thereafter at five-minute intervals until it returns to pre-exercise levels (Figure 3).

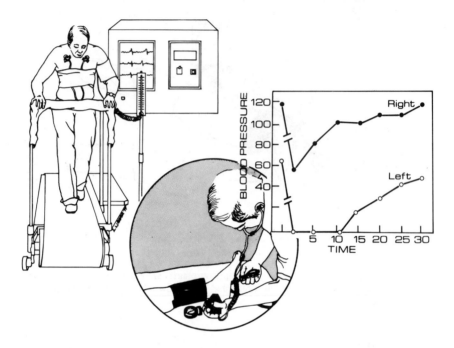

Fig. 3. Treadmill exercise testing. Ankle/arm indices are obtained prior to exercise (center). The patient then walks the maximum distance on the treadmill at 2 mph, 12% grade with simultaneous ECG monitoring (left). The ankle/arm index is repeated at 5-minute intervals and plotted. A drop in the ankle/arm index to zero following maximal exercise suggests severe multilevel occlusive disease (right).

If there is a significant proximal arterial stenosis, the decrease in peripheral resistance produced by exercise will result in an increased gradient across the stenosis. The net effect is a drop in the ankle/arm index. In patients with severe proximal occlusive disease or multilevel disease, the ankle/arm index post exercise may drop to 0 mm Hg and may remain unmeasurable for 10 or more minutes. Post-exercise ankle/arm indices correlate well with the degree of collateral circulation. The greater the drop in the post-exercise ankle/arm index and the longer the delay in return to pre-exercise levels, the poorer the collateral circulation.

Exercise testing is a reliable way to distinguish a variety of types of leg pain that mimic claudication. Arterial occlusive disease is the only source of lower extremity pain that will produce a drop in ankle/arm index following exercise. Occasionally, a patient will complain of claudication and have what seem to be normal pedal pulses on physical evaluation and a normal ankle/arm index at rest by Doppler testing. In such cases a mild degree of stenosis may exist that causes an insignificant pressure drop and permits pulsatile flow at rest. With exercise the pressure gradient increases dramatically, the distal pulses disappear, and the ankle/arm index falls.

Physical assessment of the arterial circulation of the lower extremities can be hampered by obesity, edema, trauma, hypotension, vasoconstriction, and so on. Determination of the ankle/arm index and segmental Doppler pressures can easily provide objective information under these circumstances. Exercise testing, if performed under standardized conditions, probably provides the best means of evaluating the degree of disability, assessing improvement after surgery, and following the progress of those patients being managed conservatively.

VENOUS DISEASE

Deep venous thrombosis is a frequent diagnosis, particularly among hospitalized patients; however, the diagnosis made on clinical grounds alone is only about 50% reliable. Although venography will accurately establish the presence of venous obstruction, for reasons of cost and patient discomfort it is not a satisfactory screening test. Nor is it helpful in distinguishing phlebitis from other causes of lower extremity pain which is a frequent office or outpatient dilemma.

Several noninvasive tests have been developed to detect deep venous thrombosis. Because of the portability of the equipment, low cost, and patient acceptance they have become satisfactory screening techniques for deep venous thrombosis and in some situations have decreased the necessity for the diagnostic venogram.

The Ultrasonic Doppler

In experienced hands, the ultrasonic Doppler has an accuracy of 95% in diagnosing deep venous thrombosis. The pocket Doppler can be used to make the diagnosis at the bedside even in the presence of orthopedic appliances. The primary drawback is that some experience in interpreting venous signals is necessary to obtain high levels of accuracy. Nonetheless, even the occasional user can considerably improve his clinical diagnostic accuracy with the ultrasonic Doppler.

To assess the deep venous patency in the lower extremity the Doppler probe is first used to locate the common femoral artery. The probe is then moved medially until the venous signal is maximal. The normal venous velocity signal varies with respiration and has a quality similar to wind rustling leaves. The patient then performs a Valsalva maneuver, which arrests venous return, and the velocity signal disappears. Release of the Valsalva should cause an abrupt augmentation of the venous signal. Iliofemoral thrombosis diminishes or abolishes the post-Valsalva velocity signal. A second maneuver is used to assess patency of the femoral vein. While listening over the common femoral vein at the inguinal level, the examiner first compresses the medial thigh, then the popliteal fossa, and finally the calf. Compression of each of these areas should cause an augmentation in the venous signal if the deep venous system is patent. Patency of the popliteal vein can be assessed in a similar manner by placing the probe over the popliteal vein and compressing the calf. Last, the patency of the posterior tibial vein is evaluated. Normally, calf compression causes no augmentation in the venous signal unless valvular incompetency exists. Release of calf compression should cause marked augmentation in the venous signal unless deep venous thrombosis is present.

The Doppler method for detecting deep venous thrombosis is a rapid, relatively simple bedside procedure, but yields less objective information than other techniques. The method is relatively insensitive to calf thrombi or to partially occlusive clots in larger vessels. False-positive results can occur as a result of venous compression by the transducer itself, vasopasm, or examining an elevated limb drained of its venous reservoir.

Impedance Plethysmography

Impedance plethysmography is 95% accurate in detecting deep venous thrombosis. Although the method is more cumbersome than the ultrasonic Doppler, the results are more objective.

Impedance plethysmography is performed by inflating a pneumatic tourniquet above venous pressure at the midthigh level, causing a pooling of blood in the distal limb. Sudden release of the tourniquet causes an abrupt augmentation of venous outflow from the normal extremity. In the presence of deep venous thrombosis, the blood must "percolate" more slowly through small collateral vessels, and venous outflow is considerably slower. Since blood is a good conductor of electricity, changes in venous volume may be detected by changes in electrical resistance or impedance. By simultaneously measuring electrical impedance around the proximal calf at the time the thigh tourniquet is released, one can electrically determine the rate of venous outflow. In the presence of a deep venous obstruction the rate of venous outflow is reduced, producing a decreased rate of fall in impedance. The slope of the impedance curve for the first three seconds following cuff release is plotted on a scoring graph to establish the statistical likelihood of a deep venous thrombosis (Figure 4).

Impedance plethysmography is relatively insensitive to calf thrombi. It may also fail to detect a partially occlusive thrombus in a major vein. Any physiological factor that interferes with venous outflow, such as elevated central venous pressure or external compression by a tumor, may yield a false-positive result.

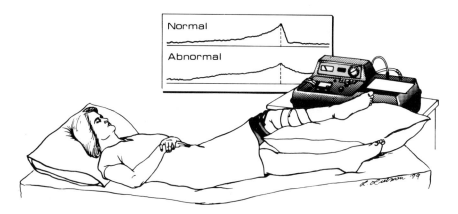

Fig. 4. Impedance plethysmography. Release of a venous tourniquet causes an abrupt augmentation of venous outflow from the normal extremity and a rapid fall in impedance (inset). In deep venous thrombosis, venous outflow is impaired, and the fall in impedance is slower (inset).

EXTRACRANIAL ARTERIAL OCCLUSIVE DISEASE

Occlusive disease of the carotid bifurcation is a well recognized cause of stroke. Early detection of such lesions, either when they are asymptomatic or when they only produce transient symptoms, has been a major interest of cardiovascular research. The goal of noninvasive extracranial assessment is to reliably detect hemodynamically significant degrees of carotid stenosis and to have some means of identifying ulcerated lesions which may be the source of cerebral emboli. The technique should also be simple to perform and relatively inexpensive so that it may be used to screen large numbers of patients. No single technique to date can satisfy all these criteria.

Periorbital Doppler Examination

The external carotid artery is an important source of collateral circualtion when the internal carotid artery is stenotic or occluded. The ophthalmic artery is a branch of the internal carotid and communicates with the external carotid circulation via supraorbital, infraorbital, and lateral nasal branches. Normally, the blood flows *toward* the extracranial circulation in the periorbital arteries, but when the internal carotid artery is stenotic or occluded, the blood flow in the periorbital vessels is reversed. The flow reversal may be detected with a directional Doppler (Figure 5). Hemodynamically significant carotid stenosis may be detected with an accuracy of 90%.

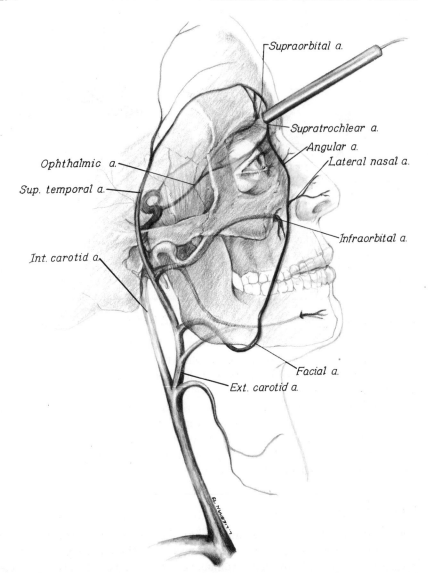

Fig. 5. Periorbital Doppler examination. Normally, blood flows toward the extracranial circulation in the periorbital arteries, but when the internal carotid artery is stenotic or occluded, the blood flow in these vessels is reversed. This reversal may be detected with a directional Doppler.

The flow probe is positioned over the supraorbital artery in the supraorbital notch. The probe must be held lightly to avoid compression of the artery. After the direction of flow is determined in the supraorbital artery, a similar technique is used to evaluate the direction of flow in the frontal and lateral nasal arteries. Additional confirmation that the external carotid is providing significant collateral flow may be obtained by compression studies. If the superficial temporal artery anterior to the ear is compressed, there should be a decrease or an obliteration of the Doppler signal over the supraorbital artery. In the presence of normal, antegrade flow, compression of the superficial temporal artery will usually cause no change in the velocity signal or only slight sugmentation.

Hemodynamically insignificant ulcerated plaques, which can be the source of embolic transient ischemic attacks, will not be detected by periorbital Doppler examination. Also, occlusive disease of the ophthalmic artery or intracranial portions of the carotid cannot be distinguished from disease at the bifurcation. Nonetheless, in experienced hands reliable results can be obtained at reasonable cost by this technique.

Ocular Plethysmography

The presence of a hemodynamically significant stenosis of the internal carotid artery will produce a small time delay in the transmission of the arterial pulse via the ophthalmic artery to the globe of the eye. Ocular plethysmography compares the arrival times of each ocular pulse with each other and with that of the external carotid artery sampled at the ear. An eye cup similar to a contact lens is placed on the surface of both anesthetized eyes and connected via a saline-filled tube to two pressure transducers. A second set of transducers sample pressure changes from each ear lobe. Pulses from both eyes and ears are recorded simultaneously. In addition, an electronically generated differential pulse is used to magnify the small time delays seen with intermediate degrees of carotid stenosis (Figure 6).

When the results of this technique are compared with arteriography, an accuracy as high as 90% in detecting hemodynamically significant lesions has been reported for this method. Ocular plethysmography cannot distinguish occlusive disease occurring in the intracranial portions of the carotid artery from stenosis at the carotid bifurcation. Nor can it detect an ulcerated plaque unless it is hemodynamically significant. Since ocular plethysmography relies on comparison of ocular pulse arrival times between the two eyes, balanced degrees of stenosis in both internal carotid arteries will yield a normal-appearing ocular plethysmogram. This is one of the most troublesome sources of false-negative results.

Ocular plethysmography is well accepted by patients, is moderate in cost, and

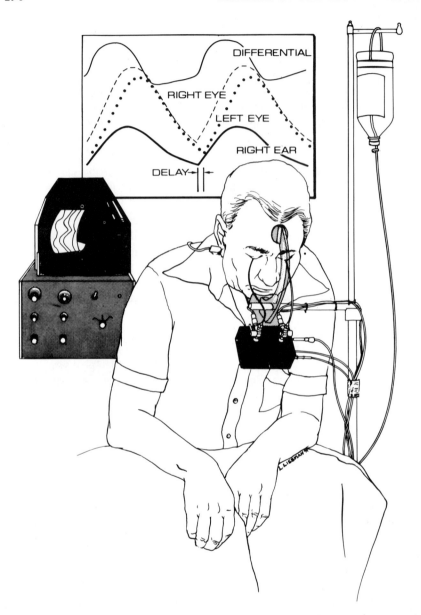

Fig. 6. Ocular plethysmography. This method compares the arrival times of each ocular pulse with each other and with that of the external carotid artery sampled at the ear. An eye cup similar to a contact lens is placed on the surface of both anesthetized eyes, and connected via a saline-filled tube to two pressure transducers. The resultant pulse waves are recorded for visual comparison. In addition, an electronically generated differential pulse is used to magnify the small time delays seen with intermediate degrees of stenosis (insert).

yields objective data. It is a useful means of following the progression of disease in asymptomatic patients.

Pulsed Doppler Imaging

The etiology of 50% or more of transient ischemic attacks is thought to be embolic, arising from ulcerated atherosclerotic plaques at the carotid bifurcation. Unless these ulcerations are associated with significant degrees of stenosis, they are undetectable by either the Doppler or ocular plethysmography. Several imaging techniques are currently being developed, of which the pulsed ultrasound appears to be the most promising means of evaluating the anatomy of the carotid bifurcation.

The pulsed Doppler emits short periodic bursts of ultrasound. The receiving crystal is time-gated to receive the reflected signal at varying intervals after the transmitted pulse. By varying the time delay and using several gates, the instrument will simultaneously detect flow from multiple points along the ultrasonic pathway. The Doppler probe is held in a mechanical sensing arm that records the position of the probe on a storage oscilloscope. The probe is then scanned across the skin surface. Each time the ultrasonic beam detects blood flow, a spot is generated on the storage oscilloscope. By careful scanning of the entire surface overlying the vessel, an ultrasonic "arteriogram" can be generated. A permanent copy of the image can then be recorded on Polaroid film. The pulsed Doppler can produce transverse as well as longitudinal cross-sectional views (Figure 7).

When compared to conventional arteriography, Doppler imaging has an accuracy of approximately 85%. Ultrasonic arteriography is an attractive adjunct to periorbital studies or ocular plethysmography, since neither of the latter two can differentiate between a near-total occlusion which is operable and a total occlusion which is inoperable. The ultrasonic Doppler can make this distinction reliably. One of the major sources of false-negative results in ocular plethysmography is the presence of balanced bilateral disease, a situation that can be readily identified by Doppler imaging.

One of the technical factors limiting the usefulness of Doppler imaging is the presence of calcium in the arterial wall, which reflects the ultrasonic signal and causes a shadow of the subjacent lumen. Calcification has been reported to significantly interfere with pulsed Doppler imaging in 5 to 25% of patients.

The resolving power of a pulsed Doppler is currently 1.0 to 1.5 mm, which limits its usefulness in detecting small ulcerated plaques. The instrument is costly and only semiportable; it is sufficiently sophisticated that its use will probably be restricted to larger medical centers with a specialized interest in extracranial arterial occlusive disease. The periorbital Doppler probably provides the most reliable screening test for office or clinic use at the present time.

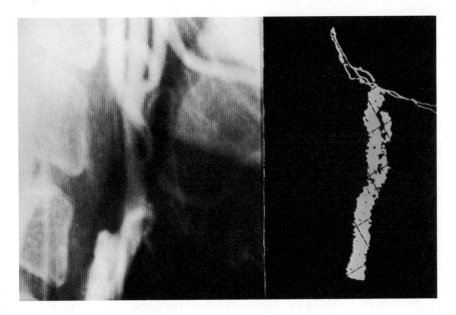

Fig. 7. Pulsed Doppler imaging. Lateral arteriogram (left) of carotid bifurcation showing total occlusion of internal carotid artery. Ultrasonic "arteriogram" (right) of the same patient. (Courtesy Waleed Hajjar.)

Bibliography

Barnes, R. W. et al. Noninvasive ultrasonic carotid angiography: Prospective validation by contrast arteriography. *Surgery 80*: 328–335, 1976.

Bernstein, E. F., ed. *Noninvasive Diagnostic Techniques in Vascular Disease.* St Louis: Mosby, 1978.

Cutler, B. S., et al. Assessment of operative risk by ECG stress testing in patients with peripheral vascular disease. *Am. J. Surg.,* 137. 484–490. 1979.

Dean, R. H., and Yao, J. S. T. Hemodynamic measurements in peripheral vascular disease. Monograph. *Curr. Probl. Surg.,* August 1976.

Rutherford, R. B., ed. *Vascular Surgery.* Philadelphia: Saunders, 1977.

Nature of the Clinico-Pathological Problem Encountered in Surgical Approach To Ischemic Heart Disease

STACEY B. DAY, M.D., Ph.D., D.Sc.
Sloan Kettering Institute For Cancer Research
New York, New York

Coronary artery surgery for ischemic heart disease again faces charges of lack of proper methods of evaluation and absence of scientific evidence for the efficacy of the operation. Again a medical generation argues a question that was posed at least two generations ago. It is doubtful that the case evidence for either of the adversary forces has changed much over the last 20 years, save perhaps that vastly increased numbers of patients are now candidates for operation. Indeed, with advances of contemporary sophisticated cardiac technologies, coronary artery bypass operation ought now to be safer, and assessment of operability of coronary artery disease ought to be more easily evaluated, by coronary arteriography, left ventriculography, and cardiohemodynamic assessment of left ventricular function.

The subjective nature of angina pectoris and ischemic heart disease, as well as patient anxiety and demand for treatment and relief of pain, must be considered against this evidence.

SUBJECTIVE NATURE OF ISCHEMIC HEART DISEASE

The subjective nature of patient reporting and personal attitudes and the difficulty in making reliable self-assessments of coronary heart disease are well established. Strategies such as counting the number of nitroglycerine tablets required per day, or relating the pain only to one reference area of the chest to the exclusion of all other possible referral points of the body, only add to difficulties of patient evaluation. Table 1 presents findings at analysis of test studies of a pharmacological compound suggested to have useful coronary vasodilating and "coronary-flow increasing" potential. The compound tested had been proved "successful" outside of the United States.

A statistically controlled double-blind cross-over study was devised so that observer bias could be eliminated as far as possible. In these clinical studies placebo treatment was included. Since the technic was double-blind, neither the patient, the clinician, nor the investigator was aware of the actual treatment

TABLE 1.   Sample testimonial reporting of patients studied in this controlled
double blind cross-over study.

	Period	Placebo or Test Drug	Subjective Report of Patient
Pt. LB	1	Placebo	Marked improvement
	2	Placebo	No comment
	3	Test drug	Much improved
	4	Placebo	Much better
	5	Placebo	Increase of angina pain
	6	Placebo	No comment
	7	Test drug	No pain 4 days
	8	Test drug	Going out of town
	9	Test drug	No pain at all
	10	Placebo	More pain
	11	Test drug	No comment
	12	Test drug	Rash
Pt. HB	1	Test drug	No comment
	2	Test drug	No comment
	3	Test drug	No pain all week
	4	Placebo	Feels much better
	5	Placebo	Europe
	6	Placebo	Few pains
	7	Test drug	No pain
	8	Test drug	"Thinks it's the real thing"
	9	Test drug	Feels fine
	10	Placebo	Fine
	11	Placebo	Felt improved
	12	Placebo	Felt better
Pt. CW	1	Placebo	Light angina, same frequency
	2	Placebo	More pains
	3	Placebo	Chest pains more severe
	4	Test drug	More nitroglycerine needed
	5	Test drug	Daily nausea in A.M.
	6	Test drug	No change
	7	Placebo	Same
	8	Placebo	Same chest pain
	9	Placebo	Still frequent and severe angina
	10	Test drug	Pain slightly better
	11	Test drug	Angina unchanged
	12	Test drug	Angina, no change

prescribed for any one patient at any given time over a 12-week test period. It was not known at which exchange points in time active agents were substituted for placebo, or vice versa. Since the research investigator was "blind" and could not know the treatment received by any patient in the study before its conclusion, it is reasonable to consider this methodology as scientifically sound and philosophically honest. At the end of each patient 12-week test period, codes identifying placebo or active agent given to the patient at each phase of the study were revealed, and analysis of clinical and scientific results was made.

Before admission to the test study, each patient had undergone a 3-month titration phase using the active drug. This pre-examination trial was designed to evaluate the maximum dose of active drug tolerated by the patient, and to determine any adverse drug reaction (skin rash, nausea, vomiting, vertigo, etc.). Patients with such adverse reactions were not admitted to the test study. To avoid the possibility of pharmacological "carry over" of active drug, a period of at least 1 month (1–3 months) was obliged, during which the test medication was omitted from the patient's therapeutic regimen. The double-blind test program was not undertaken until this metabolic clearing phase had been completed.

After study, results for evaluation included clinical case histories, standard clinical measurements (blood pressure, pulse rate, cardiac index), recording of the number of nitroglycerine tablets required daily to counter acute attacks of angina pectoris, routine EKG's and in many cases serial exercise EKG studies.

Of 68 patients with coronary heart disease admitted for evaluation, 18 failed to complete the 12-week test program because of *side reactions* and 13 simply dropped out of the program. Four deaths were recorded during the study. Of 33 patients who completed the entire double-blind study, as well as the pretrial titration evaluation, it appeared to this observer that 26 unequivocally showed no real improvement over placebo therapy; 7 appeared to show some possible improvement.

Setting aside from present discussion physiological and clinical parameters, it became clear that few patients, in such a controlled study, are capable of differentiating at which periods they are receiving active drug or placebo. Subjective reporting of symptomatology may bear little relationship to test drug activity or to presumed pharmacological affects that may accurately relate the patient's observations to test drug use. Table 1 demonstrates the testimonial nature of patient report in this disease.[2]

Ideally not only should surgical operations be evaluated by methodologies as stringent as just described, but selection of candidates for surgical operation should take into account previous medical history insofar as it relates to relief of symptomatology and varying therapeutic regimens. While it is not possible to undertake surgical double-blind methodologies, present surgical techniques make it possible to refine selection of candidates for coronary bypass surgery. Reliable objective determination of the anatomy of the coronary circulation is now a common procedure. There are, however, important precautionary physiological concepts to be borne in mind, which make good interpretation by such techniques by no means a simple or an absolute promise for predictable clinical outcome in a given case.

ARTERIOGRAPHIC EVALUATION OF CORONARY ARTERIES

On rare occasions severe coronary artery pathology may be discovered as an incidental finding during the course of general investigations. Figure 1 illustrates

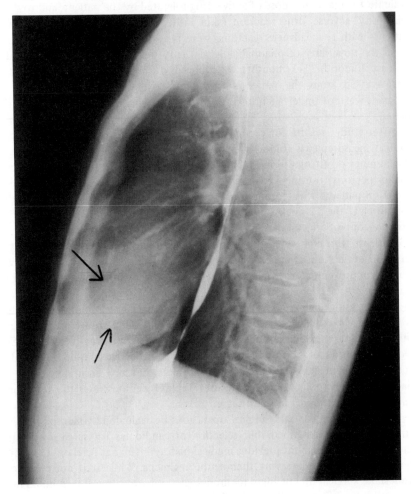

FIG. 1. Incidental finding in human patient of calcified coronary arteries.

severely calcified coronary arteries in a patient undergoing surgical evaluation for gastrointestinal disease. Figures 2 and 3 show comparatively normal coronary arteries in patients undergoing noncoronary cardiac evaluation. These demonstrations are of interest because they were made by *retrograde aortography*

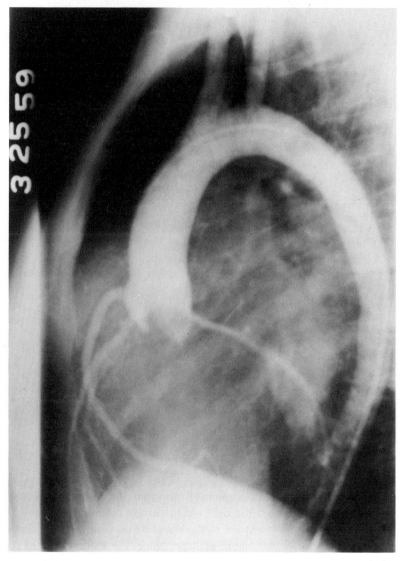

FIG. 2. Normal coronary arteries in human patient. Study performed by retrograde aortography prior to development of cine-coronangiography.

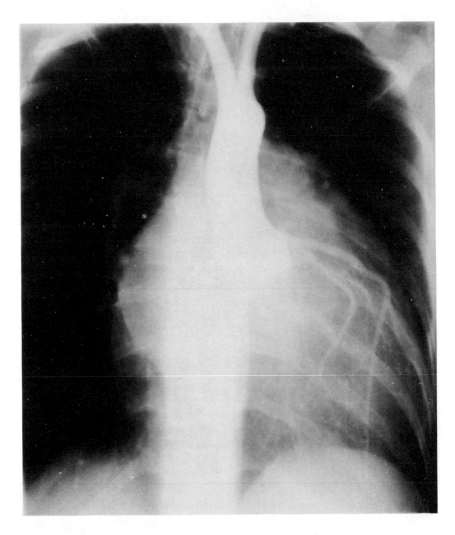

FIG 3. Normal coronary arteries in patient evaluated by retrograde aortography during work-up of +1 M.S. (mitral stenosis).

before the introduction of cine-coronary angiography. In this early procedure a catheter was inserted through the right brachial artery and positioned above the aortic valves. Injection of contrast medium was made during systole. Present coronary angiography permits more accurate delineation and location of coronary disease by superior and more reliable technology. On occasion this methodology may demonstrate intercoronary collateral vessels that may redistribute blood to the myocardium.

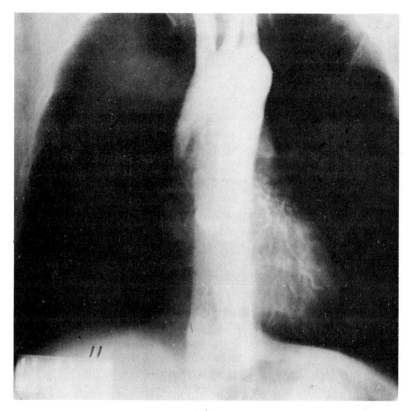

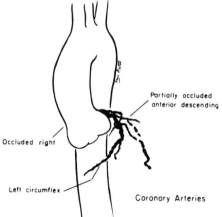

FIG. 4. Preoperative coronary angiogram. Note the complete absence of contrast dye in the area of the heart supplied by the right coronary artery. The diagram schematically interprets the coronary arteriographic findings.

Notwithstanding these refined techniques, objective evaluation of the clinical patient may still be hazardous. Figures 5, 6, and 7 are instructive in this respect.

Consider the case illustrated in Figure 5. Coronary arteriography was performed on a 61-year-old married white female, who 10 months prior to hospital admission, had experienced the onset of crushing chest pain. Shortly afterward she complained of increasing fatigue and consulted her LMD, who diagnosed an acute myocardial infarction and hospitalized her. The present study was done 10 months after her initial attack. There is marked evidence for severe atherosclerotic disease. The left anterior descending coronary artery is occluded shortly after the bifurcation of the main left coronary artery. The right main coronary artery appears to be large but somewhat irregular. The circumflex coronary artery is patent but tortuous and narrow. Some days after admission the patient died, and postmortem autopsy examination was performed. Figures 6 and 7 demonstrate the actual critically severe degree of disease present. This pathology is exceptionally well demonstrated in the semiserial microphotographic sections of the principal coronary arteries, as described in accompanying legends. Important lessons may be drawn from this case. Eighteen years ago I wrote, and certainly the truth is the same today when increasingly larger numbers of patients are clamoring for surgery,

If the past is indeed prologue to the future, both physicians and surgeons may well study with profit the correlations presented here of antemortem preoperative coronary arteriographic findings and postmortem necropsy anatomical findings of the coronary arteries in these same patients. The degree of disease which the surgeon is confronted with indicates the unreality of the physician's understanding of the miracle he anticipates will take place. It is clear from such cases that if surgery is ever to succeed the physician must turn his patients over for treatment long before the degree of pathology encountered in these cases has already determined the final outcome of the patient in terms of his days left to live.

DISCUSSION

Hopes preferred of surgeons should not obscure impartial appraisal of the difficulties to be encountered even in the best hands, and with the most modern of surgical techniques. It is clear that for optimum success the patient should be sent to the surgeon before there are irreversible advanced changes in the coronary vascular tree. But what is this point in time? And how do we determine it for each and every patient? Taken to extension, does "early enough" signify approval of prophylactic surgery or merit surgery even before the disease has set in? Clearly few responsible clinicians would warrant that point of view. Further, in face of the complex physiology and pharmacology involved in ischemic heart

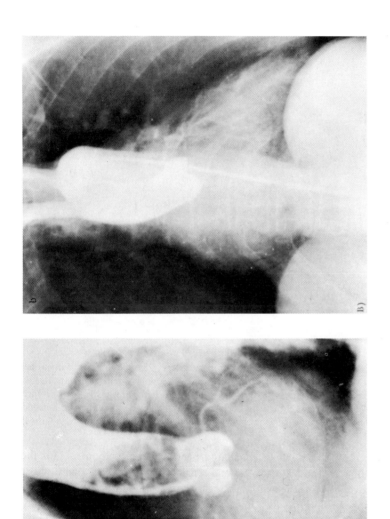

FIG. 5. (a) Objective evaluation of coronary arteries by preoperative coronary arteriography. Accompanying serial sections of these arteries at postmortem autopsy examination revealed a degree of disease far in advance of that suggested here. (b) Evidence for severe disease in the right coronary artery (unfilled) is more evident here than in the preceding lateral film (a). In both views these preoperative coronary arteriograms should be compared with the pathological sections of the same coronary arteries taken at post mortem. (Figs 6.7.).

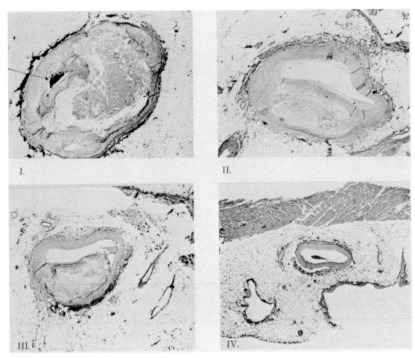

FIG. 6.

FIGS. 6 and 7. I. Left anterior descending coronary artery, 95% reduction of lumen. See arrow. Other areas are artifacts during preparation of section. 8 mm segment. II. Left anterior descending coronary artery. 8–20 mm segment. III. Left anterior descending coronary artery. 21–25 mm segment. Partially occluded with plaque. IV. Left anterior descending coronary artery. 29–34 mm segment open. V. Main stem. Right coronary artery. Grossly

disease, is it certain that such incapacitated hearts as eventually arrive for the surgeon's mending are (not) already beyond repair? May the myocardial vascular bed respond favorably to renewed increased coronary blood flow? What are the vascular resistance changes to this renewed blood flow, and how are they manifested? Can small-bore resistance vessels adjust promptly? How do they so adjust? Are collateral vascular beds and supportive channels that may have sustained the heart, and that undoubtedly developed slowly over time, capable of functioning under the new status quo? What is the nature of the underlying circulatory hemodynamic change in the overall myocardial vascular bed? How will these changes be reflected in the postsurgical patient?

And perhaps finally, and conceivably of most critical importance, whatever the nature of the surgery performed, is it not, even under the most favorable of circumstances, but a *palliative recourse.*[1]? Surgery does not cure the metabolic

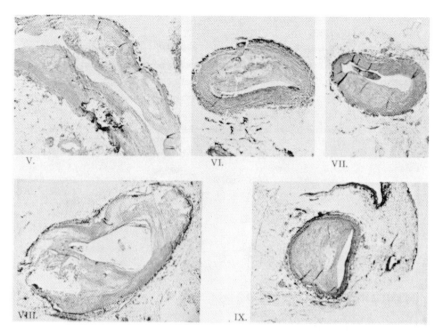

FIG. 7.

narrowed lumen. VI. Right coronary artery. 8-11 mm segment. Occlusion by atherosclerotic plaque. VII. Right coronary artery. 25-32 mm segment. VIII. Main stem. Left coronary artery. Section taken at 4 mm segment. Calcified and very atherosclerotic. Central lumen only patent. Other areas are artifacts in preparation. IX. Left circumflex coronary artery. 2-10 mm segment. These nine illustrations demonstrate semiserial sections as taken at autopsy examination. The extreme nature of disease is evident. All photomicrographs have been taken at the same magnification. All measurements are taken from the point of origin of the vessel.

process that is responsible for the pathology of the disease. Surgery cannot *cure* atherosclerotic heart disease. Moreover, as has been demonstrated in this writing, even good-quality coronary angiograms may not precisely reflect the total disease in the coronary tree. What imperative promises that the morbid process will not continue *distal* to the point of surgical anastomosis of the bypass graft? Even though cine-coronary angiography has permitted remarkable improvement in selection of surgical candidates, the nature of coronary artery disease should never be underestimated. At best a palliative procedure calls for scrupulous and careful patient selection. In irresponsible hands, in poorly selected patients, post-surgical results are likely to be poor. The truth is that there is probably no single medical field extant, at the present time, in which trust and confidence as a basis of the interrelationship between physician and surgeon are more needed. Rather than barking at each other's dilemma, or posturing with adverse hostility, if the surgical procedure is to be performed at all, it is not unreasonable to expect that such a controversial therapy be undertaken by groups or teams in which both physicians and surgeons are equally responsible, and in which both are fully participatory, ethically and practically, in the care of the patient.

References

Day, Stacey B. The surgical treatment of ischemic heart disease: An experimental and clinical study with an account of the coronary and intercoronary circulation in man and animals. The Moynihan Prize Essay of the Association of Surgeons of Great Britain and Ireland, 1960.

Day, Stacey, B. A double-blind clinical trial of the use of a pharmaceutical compound in angina pectoris. Test of its physiological properties and its effect on the exercise EKG of 50 patients with advanced ischemic heart disease. Closed report submitted for Evaluation by F.D.A. 1968. (New drug application study.)

Coronary Artery Bypass: Facts, Controversies, and the Future

ELDRED D. MUNDTH, M.D.
Professor of Surgery
Chairman Dept. of Cardiothoracic Surgery
Hahnemann Medical College and Hospital
230 N. Broad St.
Philadelphia, PA. 19102.

Since the earliest clinical experience with coronary artery bypass in 1967, there have been an estimated 400,000 such procedures performed, with a steady increase annually in the number of cases done. It is estimated that over 80,000 coronary bypass procedures were done in this country in 1977, and it has been projected that it soon may become the most common elective surgical procedure performed.

Although the incidence of coronary artery occlusive disease (CAD) continues to be extremely high and the complications of ischemic heart disease (IHD) are the leading cause of death, the annual death rate from IHD has been slowly declining. This undoubtedly reflects both an improvement in medical manage-ment of ischemic heart disease and the influence of surgical treatment of its complications. The relative extent to which the natural history of the disease is modified by either surgical or medical therapy remains controversial.[1-3]

It is generally accepted that symptomatic relief of angina is markedly im-proved after coronary artery bypass (CAB).[1-3] Significant improvement in func-tional status can be expected in 90 to 95% of patients undergoing myocardial revascularization, and complete relief of symptoms in 75%.[1-4] The improvement in functional status has been well corroborated with more objective forms of evaluation, including improved graded exercise tolerance, improvement in myo-cardial perfusion by radionucleide scanning techniques, improved (nonischemic) response to atrial pacing, and decrease in myocardial lactate production. The duration of symptomatic improvement following CAB is continually being evalu-ated, but the initial excellent functional results are unquestionably tempered by time, primarily on the basis of progression of coronary atherosclerosis. Nonethe-less, long-term (>5 years) symptomatic improvement and bypass graft patency have been encouraging in the great majority of patients.[5,6]

AREAS OF UNCERTAINTY AND CONTROVERSY

Effect of CAB Surgery on Life Expectancy and on the Incidence of Subsequent Myocardial Infarction

Despite the large number of patients who have undergone myocardial revascu-larization for IHD over the past 10 years, there is still considerable controversy relative to the effect of surgery on the incidence of subsequent myocardial in-farction and mortality as compared to current medical management.[1-3] The reason for the uncertainty despite the large clinical experience is the relative lack of prospective randomized clinical trials. To date, approximately 1300 patients in various cooperative studies have been randomized to either medical or surgical therapy and followed up to a period of 3 years. In these studies, there has been no statistically significant improvement in the incidence of myocardial infarction or survival in operated patients compared to medically treated patients with comparable disease at an average follow-up period of approximately 3 years.[1] On the basis of these particular studies, coronary bypass has not been recom-mended for prevention of mycardial infarction or to improve survival in IHD. However, other, nonrandomized studies comparing medical to surgical therapy have indicated both improved survival and a lesser incidence of subsequent myo-cardial infarction in patients undergoing CAB surgery.[4] Thus, there has been substantial criticism of the available prospective randomized studies, involving: (1) inadequate numbers of patients from any single institution with extensive

experience contributing to higher operative mortality and incidence of perioperative infarction, (2) relatively low graft patency rates, (3) the question of
completeness of revascularization, and (4) exclusion of patients with main left
coronary artery disease, unstable angina, or myocardial infarction in the previous 6 months.

As a corollary, an apparently valid criticism of previous nonrandomized series
comparing survival of surgical versus medically treated patients is related to the
fact that the survival of medically treated patients in these studies was significantly less than current survival figures.[1] Obviously, to gain meaningful data
comparing surgical and medical therapy, it will be essential for any study to have
available optimal medical *and* surgical therapy. It is also essential that the studies
be carried out for a sufficient follow-up period of at least 5 years to achieve a
meaningful comparison relative to the natural history of the disease.

Although subject to the criticism of a nonrandomized prospective study, the
best available results from current medical and surgical series may be compared
(Table 1). Assuming that the patient population is relatively comparable in terms
of anatomic extent of disease, it would appear that patient survival may be improved by *optimal* coronary bypass surgery. Optimal CAB surgery infers an
overall low operative mortality ($\leq 3\%$), low incidence of perioperative myocardial infarction ($\leq 5\%$), acceptable graft patency rates at 1-year follow-up ($\geq 75\%$
of all grafts patent), and complete revascularization. Although data concerning
the incidence of late mycardial infarction are less extensive, the more successful
surgical series in terms of the factors enumerated above have reported a relatively low incidence of subsequent infarction in the range of 1 to 3% per year.
In current surgical practice, these figures are regularly attained by major institutions with highly experienced medical-surgical groups. Unquestionably, prospective randomized studies having the benefit of both optimal medical and surgical
therapy are needed to definitively resolve the controversy.

Effect of Myocardial Revascularization on Left Ventricular Function

The seemingly contradictory reports of the effect of myocardial revascularization
on left ventricular function,[1] varying from enthusiastic reports of marked
improvement to pessimistic reports that the existence of significant left ventricular function is a contraindication to surgery, reflect the relative imprecision of
preoperative diagnostic methods in evaluating the pathophysiology of abnormal
left ventricular function. With currently available diagnostic modalities, it is
difficult to identify potentially reversible myocardial dysfunction on the basis
of myocardial ischemia compared to irreversible dysfunction secondary to extensive segmental or diffuse patchy fibrosis. Radionucleide myocardial scanning
techniques and semiquantitative segmental ventricular wall contractility studies
in response to pharmacologic intervention have been increasingly helpful but,

TABLE 1. Comparison of Long-Term Survival with Optimal Medical vs. Surgical Therapy of Coronary Artery Disease

Study	Treatment	Type of Study	No. Patients in Study	Time Interval in Years of Cumulative Survival Study	Actuarial Annual Mortality Rate	Projected* or Real† 5-Year Cumulative Survival
VA coop.[1]	Medical	Randomized	354	4	4.3%	78.5%*
Sheldon[2]	Surgical	Nonrand.	741	7	1.8%	89.4%†
Hall et a.[3]	Surgical	Nonrand.	846	5	2.3%	88.2%†
Tyras et al.[4]	Surgical	Nonrand.	1541	5	1.4%	92.8%†

1. Read, R. C., Murphy, M. L., Hultgren, H. N., and Takaro, T. Survival of men treated for chronic stable angina pectoris. A cooperative randomized study. *J. Thorac. Cardiovasc. Surg. 75*: 1, 1978.

2. Sheldon, W. C. Effect of bypass graft on survival: A six to ten year follow-up study of 741 patients. Presented at the First Decade of Bypass Surgery for Coronary Artery Disease. An International Symposium. Sept. 1977, Cleveland Clinic, Ohio.

3. Hall, R. J., Garcia, E., Mathur, V. S., et al. Long-term, follow-up after coronary artery bypass. Presented at the First Decade of Bypass Graft Surgery for Coronary Artery Disease. An International Symposium. Sept. 1977, Cleveland Clinic, Ohio.

4. Tyras, D. H., Barner, H. B., Kaiser, G. C., et al. Long-term benefits of Myocardial revascularization. *Am. J. Cardiol. 41*: 357, 1978.

313

as yet, are not sufficiently precise to be definitive. In those instances where myocardial ischemia has been identified in association with ventricular wall hypokinesia, appropriate CAB surgery has proved effective in significantly improving both segmental and overall left ventricular function. In those instances where revascularization surgery has been successful in improving left ventricular function, physiologic and anatomic corroboration has been demonstrated by ventriculographic documentation of improved segmental wall contractility and left ventricular ejection fraction, by evidence of improved myocardial perfusion angiographically, and by myocardial perfusion scanning techniques. Failure of improvement in functional status and survival has been relatively universal where extensive fibrosis has been present in the absence of documented myocardial ischemia or a specific mechanical defect such as left ventricular aneurysm, mitral regurgitation, or associated valvular disease.

On the basis of currently available data, coronary artery bypass surgery may be indicated in carefully selected patients with significant left ventricular functional impairment, meeting any of the following general selection criteria:

1. Associated angina indicative of potentially reversible myocardial ischemia.
2. Positive rest or stress thallium myocardial perfusion scan indicative of myocardial ischemia.
3. Ejection fraction $\geqslant 0.2$.
4. Dyskinesia involving not more than one or two left ventricular wall segments.
5. Hypokinesia rather than akinesia.
6. Intermittency of episodes of cardiac failure which may be associated with so-called ischemic anginal equivalent.
7. Presence of a significant mechanical defect such as left ventricular aneurysm, mitral regurgitation, or associated valvular disease.
8. Bypassable coronary artery disease.

Effect of Myocardial Revascularization on Progression of Coronary Artery Disease

As is true of all forms of atherosclerosis, coronary artery disease is a progressive degenerative disease involving the coronary arterial wall, eventually leading to significant stenosis or occlusion of major coronary arteries with consequent reduction of coronary blood flow and myocardial ischemia. Coronary artery bypass surgery has the objective of improving myocardial perfusion distal to occlusive disease and, as such, is a palliative procedure that may have little pathophysiologic effect on the intrinsic arterial disease. The question of whether myocardial revascularization has any effect upon the natural history of CAD has been difficult to answer from clinical experience to date. There appears to be a significantly increased propensity for a high-grade proximal stenosis to progress to total occlusion with a patent bypass graft distally, whereas disease distal to the graft anastomosis appears to be unaffected by the graft. However, progression of disease in ungrafted vessels is significant and is commonly the cause of recurrence of angina symptoms in patients with patent grafts. Since few, if any, studies achieve 100% angiographic restudy, the actual incidence of significant progression of CAD is ungrafted and grafted vessels is unknown. Since many of the later restudies are stimulated by recurrence of symptoms, the data often are derived from a preselected patient population, with a probable greater apparent than actual incidence of progression. Unquestionably, progression of disease in both ungrafted and, to a lesser extent, grafted vessels contributes to clinical deterioration with the passage of time after initial successful revascularization and amelioration of symptoms.

In most follow-up angiographic studies after CAB surgery, the greatest rate of occlusion of initially patent bypass grafts occurs in the first year postoperatively. Graft occlusion rates at approximately 1 year postoperatively vary from 5* to 25% in different series, whereas late graft occlusion is much lower. Postoperative angiographic study of graft patency 5 to 7 years after CAB surgery has shown an annual attrition rate of only 2% per year in grafts patent 1 year following surgery.

Effect of Perioperative Myocardial Infarction upon
Short- and Long-Term Results after CAB Surgery

Despite the fact that myocardial revascularization is often undertaken to prevent myocardial infarction, as in unstable angina, there is a significant incidence of perioperative myocardial infarction (PMI) that occurs in association with CAB surgery.[3] The incidence of perioperative infarction varies from 3 to cover 20% as reported in different series. With improved techniques of coronary artery bypass, improved anesthesiology management, more complete revascularization, and improved methods of myocardial preservation during surgery, the incidence of perioperative infarction has been reduced significantly in the past 2 years to substantially less than 10% in most series. Although some studies have show no significant difference in early mortality, the majority of current data demonstrates a significant deleterious effect of PMI on long-term survival and subsequent infarction. A recent study indicated that although there was no difference in the relief of angina at 6 months postoperatively, the incidence of subsequent infarction was three times greater in those who sustained a PMI compared to those who did not. Thus, it appears that the occurrence of PMI has little effect on functional results but has a significant adverse effect upon the incidence of subsequent myocardial infarction and survival.

---

*Five percent occlusion rates pertain primarily to internal mammary to LAD grafts.

Choice of Coronary Bypass Graft Conduit, Graft Patency Rates, and Sequential versus Individual Grafts

Graft failure has been shown to be related not only to poor arterial run-off and technical problems with the construction of the bypass graft but also to the potential for intrinsic changes in the graft itself. Intrinsic changes in the bypass graft can be due to the process of fibrous intimal hyperplasia (FIH) or the occurrence of atherosclerotic disease. The internal mammary conduit (IMA) has been reported to have higher graft patency rates and greater resistance to FIH and atherosclerosis than the saphenous vein graft (SVG) (Figures 1 and 2). The limitations of the IMA graft, however, are significant. They include:

1. Inadequate size (< 1.5 mm diameter).
2. Inadequate pedicle length and size of IMA to reach distal vessels.
3. Only two IMA grafts available in any given patient, many of whom require three, four, five, or occasionally more grafts.
4. Inadequate free flow through the open graft (< 100 ml/min).
5. Occasional existence of proximal subclavian artery disease.
6. Possible total flow capability limitation in larger coronary arteries with large run-off.

Most surgeons use the IMA graft primarily for bypass of a relatively normal distal left anterior descending coronary artery and observe the restrictions noted above; thus comparison of graft patency and operative results to the SVG to a variety of distal arteries is difficult because of the intrinsic selection process in the use of the IMA graft. With these considerations in mind, it is somewhat difficult to interpret data indicating a 1-year graft patency rate of 95% for IMA grafts compared to 80 to 85% patency for SVG. Unquestionably, the IMA conduit is an excellent choice for CAB surgery with the above restrictions in mind.

A pertinent point that has been raised is the fact that anatomic patency of a graft does not assure physiologic adequacy of the bypass, particularly under conditions of stress where coronary blood flow may be required to increase markedly. Previous studies have indicated that peak IMA graft flow capability may be substantially less than that achieved with an SVG to the same vessel. It has been shown that myocardial ischemia can occur even in the presence of a patent graft where the flow capability is less than the demand under conditions of stress. Despite the known limitations of the SVG, it remains widely used with impressive results, particularly in patients with multivessel disease.

The sequential or "snake-graft" using the saphenous vein has had considerable success (Figure 3). Patency rates of sequential grafts have been reported to be at least comparable to individual bypass grafts to a single vessel. The increased total flow through a sequential graft may contribute to increased patency rates, but

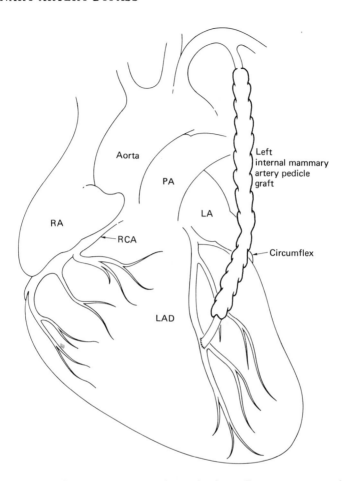

FIG. 1. Left internal mammary artery. Left anterior descending coronary artery bypass.

the potential drawbacks of (1) inadequacy of total graft flow capability in a single graft conduit to multiple arteries under conditions of increased demand, and (2) occlusion of the graft resulting in potential loss of all coronary vessels bypassed, must be considered.

Completeness of Revascularization and the Result of CAB Surgery

Judgment of "completeness" of myocardial revascularization is, at best, ill-defined and subject to inherent bias in interpretation of angiographic studies. Revascularization may be judged relatively incomplete at any time post-operatively by observing either (1) significant stenoses in major coronary arteries

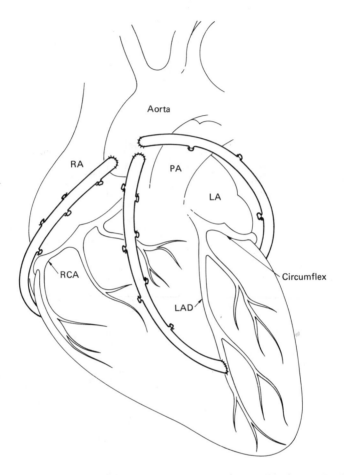

FIG. 2. Triple aorta coronary saphenous vein bypass grafts to the left anterior descending, right and circumflex coronary arteries.

not grafted or (2) occlusion of a bypass graft to a vessel with a significant stenosis. In either case, regional myocardial perfusion may be insufficient, leading to myocardial ischemia.

As a corollary to data indicating that operative mortality is not markedly influenced by the number of coronary bypass grafts constructed, inadequacy of revascularization, i.e., leaving major diseased vessels ungrafted, has been shown to increase operative and early mortality. Similarly, studies of early and late functional results have demonstrated that incompleteness of revascularization at any time postoperatively leads to a significant reduction in symptomatic relief of angina. Study of postoperative left ventricular function has indicated that improvement in segmental ventricular wall contractility and global left ventricular function occurs only when myocardial revascularization is relatively complete.

A recent study of late survival as influenced by graft status and degree of revascularization has indicated that 6-year late survival was 98% for patients with optimal correction as compared to 83% for patients with incomplete correction ($P < 0.02$). The same study also indicated that 6-year late survival was 94% for patients in whom all grafts were patent as compared to 70% in patients whose grafts were all occluded ($P < 0.01$).

In conclusion, it is apparent that early and late survival and functional status are greatly influenced by the completeness of myocardial revascularization and graft status.

Other areas of uncertainty in coronary bypass surgery are (1) the apparently poorer results of revascularization in females with CAD, (2) indications and results of surgery for evolving myocardial infarction and the complications of acute myocardial infarction (3) advisability and results of reoperative CAB surgery, (4) indication for combined versus staged multiple vascular procedures in association with CAB surgery, and (5) indications for surgery based upon location and extent of CAD and the nature of intercoronary collateral circulation.

Unquestionably, the future of CAB surgery will depend upon the continuation of careful study of the natural history of the disease and objective evaluationof the benefits of surgery. Until improved methods of prevention of CAD are developed, it is apparent that effective coronary bypass surgery is the best available mode of treatment for symptomatic ischemic heart disease and, possibly, an effective means of improving survival.

References

McIntosh, H. D., and Garcia, J. A. The first decade of aortocoronary bypass grafting, 1967-1977. A review. *Circulation 57*: 405, 1978.

De Bakey, M. E., and Lawrie, G. M. Aortocoronary artery bypass. Assessment after 13 years. *J.A.M.A. 239*: 837, 1978.

Mundth, E. D., and Austen, W. G. Surgical measures for coronary artery disease. *N. Engl. J. Med. 293*: 13-19, 75-80, 124-130, 1975.

Sheldon, W. C., and Loop, F. D. Direct myocardial revascularization—1976 progress report on the Cleveland Clinic experience. *Cleve. Clin. 43*: 97, 1976.

Mathur, V. S. and Guinn, G. A. Sustained benefit from aortocoronary bypass surgery demonstrated for 5 years: A prospective randomized study. *Circulation 56 (Suppl. III)*: 190, 1977.

Campean, L., Lesperarce, J., Corbara, F., Hermann, J., Cronchin, D., and Bourassa, N. G. Late changes in aortocoronary saphenous vein bypass grafts (5 to 7 years after surgery). *Circulation 56 (Suppl. III)*: 132, 1977.

The Pathology of Cerebral Aneurysms

WILLIAM E. STEHBENS, M.D., D.Phil., F.R.C.P.A., F.R.C. Path.
Professor and Chairman, Department of Pathology
Wellington Clinical School of Medicine
of the University of Otago
Director of the Wellington Cancer and
Medical Research Institute
Wellington, New Zealand

An aneurysm is a localized, persistent pathological dilatation of a blood vessel, usually of an artery. Aneurysms resulting from the yielding of components of the vessel wall are regarded as "true" aneurysms. "False" aneurysms result from the rupture of vessels whether of spontaneous or traumatic origin and feature persistent continuity between the vessel lumen and the extravascular space. The wall of a false aneurysm is formed by pre-existing perivascular tissues bordering the extravasated blood in conjunction with fibrin deposited at the time of extravasation. The wall may ultimately become fibrotic, and an endothelial lining may extend into the inner surface of the false sac. Difficulty was encountered in the past in differentiating between these two types of aneurysm. It is now known that most aneurysms are of the true variety. False sacs are usually due to either traumatic disruption of the parent artery or rupture of an aneurysm with the formation of a false sac as a secondary lobulation of the aneurysm.

There are many types of cerebral aneurysm; and while most have been classified according to their cause, the most common varieties, which will be considered first, have been classified according to shape and size.

FUSIFORM ANEURYSMS

As the name implies, these aneurysmal dilatations are fusiform in shape (Figure 1). They affect the largest arteries at the base of the brain predominantly (internal carotid, basilar, and vertebral arteries), and they then cause pressure symptoms by compressing brain substances or cranial nerves, particularly when associated with tortuosity and displacement of the parent artery. They may contain laminated thrombus in their lumen. Rupture occurs only rarely, but continued enlargement results in a spherical or saccular aneurysm with an afferent and an efferent artery. Such aneurysms are due to degenerative changes in the arterial wall associated with atherosclerosis, the elastic tissue, muscle, and

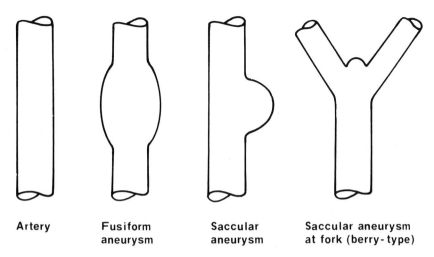

| Artery | Fusiform aneurysm | Saccular aneurysm | Saccular aneurysm at fork (berry-type) |

FIG. 1.   Diagram illustrating types of cerebral aneurysms.

fibrous tissue being damaged or destroyed, and the resultant weakness allows dilatation of the lumen (Stehbens, 1972).

SACCULAR ANEURYSMS

Saccular arterial aneurysms at sites not related to arterial forks are to be seen on the vertebral, basilar, and internal carotid arteries in particular. These saccular aneurysms occur as lateral evaginations (Figure 1) in very atherosclerotic vessels. They enlarge and can cause severe pressure symptoms and signs. They contain laminated thrombus and sometimes calcification in their walls. Rupture is infrequent.

The most common variety of saccular arterial aneurysm in the cerebral circulation is the "berry" type aneurysm, in which the sac forms in the bifurcation of the artery (Figure 1). These aneurysms have been found in up to 7 to 8% of routine autopsies (Stehbens, 1972). They are multiple in approximately one-third of cases. A familial incidence has often been claimed, but there is no statistical evidence to support this allegation. These aneurysms are not common in the young, the peak incidence being at approximately 50 years of age. Very few cases in the first decade, and many of those that are said to be so are of dubious validity. The bulk of the aneurysms manifest themselves between 40 and 70 years of age. There is a slight unexplained predominance in the female in most countries after the age of 40, with a slight predominance in the male under 40 years of age. Most aneurysms of this type found at autopsy are less than 1 cm in their largest diameter. Their walls are often thin, although sometimes atherosclerotic mural plaques are visible with the naked eye. In view of their development relatively late in life and the development of atherosclerosis in the sac wall often of a similar or even a greater degree of severity than that in the parent artery, it has been deduced that atherosclerosis runs a rapid course in the walls of aneurysms. The base of the aneurysm is fairly wide when compared to the diameter of the parent vessel, and few can be regarded as pedunculated despite the fact that they have been likened to berries. Most aneurysms over 1 cm in diameter exhibit evidence of rupture and therefore may contain laminated thrombus. A few aneurysms of 2 or 3 cm in size do not contain thrombus. Small aneurysms only 1 or 2 mm in diameter are detectable at autopsy but are frequently overlooked by angiography. More than one secondary false aneurysm may be attached to the sac giving the aneurysm a multilocular appearance. Calcification, though unusual in these cerebral aneurysms, may occur, and can be demonstrated radiographically. Most berry aneurysms are found on the anterior half of the circle of Willis, and the most frequent site at autopsy is the middle cerebral artery. Radiologists assert that the more usual site is the anterior communicating artery, but angiography misses those on the middle cerebral artery in a significant percentage of cases. Approximately 90 to 95% of all aneurysms will be found either on the first 3 cm of the middle cerebral artery, in the angle formed by one anterior cerebral artery and the anterior communicating artery, on the internal carotid artery at its bifurcation, or at the origin of either the posterior communicating or the anterior choroidal artery from an internal carotid or at the basilar artery bifurcation. Any aneurysm that is of unusual appearance or that occurs at an unusual site, should be suspected as being due to other causes, rather than being of the "berry" type.

The complications arising from cerebral aneurysms are similar to those pertaining to aneurysms at any other site (Stehbens, 1978). Rupture, the most important complication, exacts a high mortality, although a minor leakage can occur subclinically and be found incidentally at autopsy. Recurrent leakage may precede a final massive hemorrhage, and recurrent attacks of subarachnoid hemorrhage provide the important clue to diagnosis.

Hemorrhage into the subarachnoid space may be quite massive. It is usually most pronounced at the base of the brain anteriorly situated between and around the frontal lobes, the Sylvian fissures, and the interpeduncular fossa. It extends to a variable extent over the convexities of the cerebral hemispheres. If the aneurysm is embedded in brain, it may bleed directly through the brain into the ventricular system with blood then leaking into the posterior fossa of the skull, and little blood may be found anteriorly. Massive bleeding into the brain, particularly the frontal and temporal lobes, occurs in 60 to 70% of patients who die of a ruptured cerebral aneurysm. In many instances there is also intraventricular rupture, though in a few instances there is hemorrhage into the ventricles with only minimal cerebral damage. In approximately 15% of patients there is concomitant hemorrhage into the subdural space, but this is usually not severe in degree and is rarely of any clinical significance. A second important complication is ischemic infarction believed to be the result of vascular spasm following rupture of the aneurysm. In approximately 60% of brains at autopsies of patients dying from a ruptured cerebral aneurysm, areas of infarction may be found most often related to the vessel on which the aneurysm lies. The infarction varies considerably in size and is frequently cortical in distribution. The exact pathogenesis of the infarction is obscure.

Embolism from a mural thrombus in an aneurysmal sac may occur in large aneurysms outside the skull, but there is little evidence to suggest that this could be the case with intracranial aneurysms.

Pressure symptoms occur in two ways: First, when the aneurysm ruptures an expanding hematoma can act as a space-occupying lesion producing secondary pressure lesions in the midbrain and pons and in the neighboring brain. Other pressure lesions including intraoccular hemorrhage, uncal herniation, and secondary nerve lesions occur, but are not peculiar to cerebral aneurysms. The second mode of the production of pressure lesions results when the aneurysm grows to a large size and acts as a space-occupying lesion. This is a major though infrequent complication of cerebral aneurysms. Within the skull large sacs containing laminated thrombus have been found up to 9 cm in diameter. Such an occurrence, however, is quite rare. Smaller aneurysms may also produce pressure lesions depending on their location, and a variety of clinical pictures may ensue. The cranial nerve most often involved is the third nerve.

Yet another major complication is multiplicity (33%), and therapy directed to one aneurysm may be followed by rupture of another sac. As many as eight or nine aneurysms have been found in one patient.

In the absence of treatment, approximately two-thirds of patients presenting with their first subarachnoid hemorrhage from aneurysmal rupture can be expected to die within the first year. Most recurrent hemorrhages that follow within a period of only a few weeks prove fatal, and those who survive may be seriously incapacitated as a result of cerebral damage (Stehbens, 1972).

Etiology

This type of aneurysm has long been considered to be either congenital or developmental. Such aneurysms are not congenital, and the hypothesis that they are secondary to some developmental vascular fault or weakness is not based on sound scientific evidence. Factors for consideration are the following:

1. *Arterial Variations.* Anatomical variation of the circle of Willis has been alleged to be more frequent in patients with cerebral aneurysms. There is little to substantiate this supposition that anatomical variations are developmental errors, and their frequency in patients with cerebral aneurysms is not based on

sound scientific information. In the case of aneurysms of the anterior communicating artery, there is frequently a significant shunt of blood from one anterior cerebral artery to the contralateral vessel via the anterior communicating artery. The anterior communicating artery is therefore frequently an arterial fork rather than a single anastomotic vessel as is often depicted in textbooks.

2. *Hypertension.* Hypertension of one cause or another is present in approximately 60% of patients. On theoretical grounds, hypertension is likely to aggravate aneurysms, and some hypertensive patients may have an unruptured aneurysm in association with a primary intracerebral hemorrhage.

3. *Congenital Abnormalities.* It is frequently alleged that congenital abnormalities are unduly prevalent in patients with cerebral aneurysms. In the only statistical analysis the prevalence of congenital abnormalities in a series of 250 subjects with cerebral aneurysms was compared with a control series of 849 subjects and with a series of 351 with primary nonaneurysmal cerebral hemorrhage. Completely at variance with and definitely contrary to the widely held belief, the differences in the prevalence of congenital abnormalities were found to be not statistically significant. Two diseases in particular, however, are not infrequently complicated by cerebral aneurysms, namely, (1) coarctation of the aorta and (2) polycystic disease of the kidneys. Since these are the only two congenital diseases usually associated with longstanding hypertension and severe degenerative changes in the vessels, the association of these two diseases with cerebral aneurysms is probably due to the hypertension. The concurrence of aortic coarctation and cerebral aneurysm may not be encountered so frequently in the future because of the current trend towards correction of the aortic coarctation at an early age.

In recent years patients with large arteriovenous aneurysms of the brain have been found to have an aneurysm on one or the other of the arteries feeding the arteriovenous shunt, and the aneurysm in these cases is in all probability the result of hemodynamic changes. Aneurysmal dilation of the afferent artery is seen in traumatic arteriovenous fistulas and is assuredly due to hemodynamic factors rather than to any association with congenital abnormalities. It is also to be noted that arteriovenous aneurysms of the brain may not in fact be due to a congenital maldevelopment of vessels, but rather due to the persistence and enlargement of small arteriovenous aneurysms caused by trauma.

4. *Atherosclerosis.* Atherosclerosis does not tend to be as severe in the cerebral arteries of these patients as in those with primary intracerebral hemorrhage, though microscopically it can usually be demonstrated in a cerebral artery particularly near the entrance to the aneurysm.

5. *Medial Gaps (Defects) of Forbus.* At the forks of the cerebral arteries it was demonstrated by Forbus (1930) that the media is interrupted by a wedge of adventitial tissue (outer coat) which extends inward to the intima (the inner coat). Forbus referred to such interruptions as medial defects despite the fact

that there is no evidence that they are areas of mechanical weakness. These interruptions of the middle coat are therefore better known as medial interruptions, gaps, or even raphes. The most logical explanation of these medial interruptions is that they constitute raphes or mechanical anchors for the circularly arranged muscle coats of the adjoining surfaces of the two daughter branches, for the muscle pulls at times in almost opposite directions (Stehbens, 1978). It is pertinent that the raphes occur most often in acute angles rather than obtuse angles. These medial interruptions or raphes occur both in the crotch of the arterial fork where cerebral aneurysms of the berry type occur and also at the lateral angle of the arterial fork where aneurysms do not occur. Furthermore though some of these medial interruptions are present at birth, they increase in frequency with age and are also found in both large and small arteries within and outside the cranial cavity, both in man and in other animals. Despite this wide distribution in man and other animals, cerebral aneurysms of the berry type occur predominantly in man. They are infrequent in the arteries supplying the viscera in man, and so far authentic cases of cerebral berry aneurysms have been reported in only three chimpanzees. Thus the distribution of these medial gaps is at variance with the occurrence of cerebral aneurysms in nature, and it is therefore most unlikely that there is any cause-and-effect relationship. Microscopically, examination of very early aneurysms indicates that the medial interruptions (defects) are involved fortuitously, or alternatively they are involved secondarily to early aneurysmal dilatation. It is usually alleged that these medial defects or gaps are areas of weakness through which aneurysms occur. The evidence for this is most unconvincing. The evidence at present strongly suggests that the aneurysms are neither congenital nor based on any demonstrable weakness in the artery wall, but rather that they are acquired degenerative lesions secondary to degenerative changes in the intima and media which normally occur in the arterial wall at sites of branching. These degenerative changes have been attributed to hemodynamic stresses. The yield and hence dilatation can be regarded as a manifestation of loss of tensile strength due to engineering fatigue of the connective tissues of the vessel wall (Stehbens, 1972).

The frequency of cerebral aneurysm of the berry type has been attributed to the unique structural differences in the cerebral arteries which have thinner walls than the extracranial arteries (both the middle and outer coats) and the elastic tissue virtually confined to the internal elastic lamina (the inner coat). There may also be other hemodynamic factors such as a rapid blood flow that is faster than that in the extracranial vessels. Hypothetical weaknesses have been invoked as a cause of cerebral aneurysms, but such suppositions are not worthy of serious scientific consideration, unless some evidence in support of such suppositions is forthcoming. It is of course always difficult to prove a negative, particularly in regard to hypothetical factors for which there is no evidence.

Very small cerebral aneurysms microscopically often contain little in the wall except a very thin layer of fibrous tissue. Some proliferation of musculo-elastic tissue may be observed, simulating the thickening of the inner layer that occurs in the parent arteries. The elastic tissue, however, soon disappears and does not lead to the formation of accessory elastic laminae as occurs in the development of atherosclerosis. This intimal-like thickening continues and ultimately progresses to overt atherosclerosis. Ultrastructurally the changes in the aneurysmal wall are also identical with those occurring in the development of atherosclerosis of the cerebral arteries (Stehbens, 1975a). Experimental studies of flow in glass models of arterial forks with and without berry aneurysms suggest that vortices are formed at the forks of vessels and that these vortices are responsible for the degenerative changes occurring about the fork. These vortices occur at very low velocity rates, and it has been postulated that the aneurysm acts in the capacity of a resonance chamber (Stehbens, 1975b).

ANEURYSMS OF INFLAMMATORY ORIGIN

Bacterial aneurysms are usually referred to as mycotic, but the term mycotic implies a lesion of fungal origin and should be restricted to aneurysms of this nature, for they are occasionally encountered. Most bacterial aneurysms are associated with bacterial endocarditis and less often with severe pulmonary inflammatory lesions or septicemia. Bacterial aneurysms of cerebral arteries occur primarily, although not exclusively, in the second and third decades. Usually the aneurysm is small—less than 1 cm in diameter and peripherally located on the terminal branches of the middle cerebral artery in particular. Bacterial aneurysms are not infrequently multiple and can be demonstrated angiographically. *Streptococcus viridans* is the most common causative organism. The aneurysm is believed to result from the impaction of a septic embolus in a small side branch or at a fork with a resultant acute septic arteritis and dilatation of the arterial wall. Bacterial aneurysm should be suspected in any aneurysm of unusual appearance and particularly those peripherally situated. Antibiotic therapy may control infection but does not necessarily preclude rupture of an already expanded aneurysmal sac. These aneurysms can rupture and produce fatal intracerebral and subarachnoid hemorrhage. Occasionally aneurysms complicate local infections, either due to a meningitis or an acute sphenoidal sinusitis.

Syphilis, once believed to be a common cause of cerebral aneurysm, is now disregarded as a serious factor in the pathogenesis of cerebral aneurysms. Syphilitic cerebral aneurysms are probably extremely rare if they occur at all.

Mucormycosis can occasionally produce an arterial dilatation, though more frequently it causes a mycotic arteritis with superadded thrombosis, hemorrhage, or infarction as the primary complication.

TRAUMATIC ANEURYSMS

Trauma is an occasional cause of cerebral aneurysms. In general a false sac forms when the artery is partially torn or ruptured, and the bleeding is insufficient to cause fatal intracranial hemorrhage. It is possible that the artery may be partially severed and the intact adventitia (outer coat) may then dilate forming a small sac. These aneurysms are quite rare and may be associated with severe head injuries including a fractured skull. Small peripherally placed aneurysms may undergo spontaneous thrombosis, but they may also be responsible for delayed hemorrhage.

DISSECTING ANEURYSMS

Dissecting aneurysms of the cerebral arteries are most rare. A dissecting aneurysm, though usually the result of trauma, may occur spontaneously. The dissection commences when there is a tear of the inner coat. The blood then dissects along a plane of cleavage in the vessel wall and then may rupture either back into the original lumen or externally causing fatal hemorrhage. In the cerebral arteries, the dissection is usually between the inner and middle coat, whereas extracranially it is usually more externally situated.

MILIARY ANEURYSMS

Miliary aneurysms of Charcôt and Bouchard are small microscopic aneurysms perhaps less than 1 mm in diameter and situated on intracerebral arteries (Stehbens, 1972). These small miliary aneurysms are believed to bleed causing fatal intracerebral hemorrhage, the common variety of stroke due to a hemorrhage. These miliary or micro-aneurysms have recently been demonstrated by means of postmortem micro-angiography and are most frequent in hypertensive persons, especially in those over the age of 50 years. They are caused by severe degenerative changes in the intracerebral arteries similar to atherosclerosis. They may leak only a small quantity of blood or undergo spontaneous thrombosis. On these occasions, they may produce minor cerebral disturbances which are known to occasionally precede fatal primary intracerebral hemorrhage.

CONCLUSION

The frequency with which aneurysms involve the intracranial arteries is in contrast with the rarity of aneurysms on extracranial arteries of similar caliber in man. The difference in frequency is no doubt due to the structural differences in the cerebral arteries and possibly also to the higher rate of blood flow. The premature development of atherosclerosis in berry aneurysms suggests that experi-

mental aneurysms will prove to be most useful for the study of abnormal hemodynamics and of the development of atherosclerosis.

References

Forbus, W. D. On the origin of miliary aneurysms of the superficial cerebral arteries. *Bull. Johns Hopkins Hosp. 47*: 239–284, 1930.

Stehbens, William E. *Pathology of the Cerebral Blood Vessels.* St. Louis: C. V. Mosby Co., 1972.

Stehbens, W. E. Ultrastructure of aneurysms. *Arch. Neurol. 32*: 798–807, 1975a.

Stehbens, W. E. Flow in glass models of arterial bifurcations and berry aneurysms at low Reynolds numbers. *Q. J. Exp. Physiol. 60*: 181–192, 1975b.

Stehbens, William E. *Hemodynamics and the Blood Vessel Wall.* Springfield, Illinois: Charles C. Thomas, 1978.

Brain Revascularization:
Extracranial-Intracranial Bypass Grafting

ROBERT M. CROWELL, M.D.
Massachusetts General Hospital and
Harvard Medical School
Boston, Massachusetts

Most strokes are caused by cerebrovascular occlusion with decreased brain blood
flow. Surgical restoration of blood flow is thus a rational approach for the prevention (or even reversal) of ischemic strokes. Indirect brain revascularization by
carotid endarterectomy can benefit many cases,[8] but this approach is of no
value for inaccessible intracranial (or high cervical) occlusive disease. For inaccessible occlusive lesions, direct brain revascularization can be accomplished by
extracranial–intracranial bypass procedures which have become feasible since the
development of microneurosurgery.[15] Results to date are tentative but promising, particularly for superficial temporal to middle cerebral artery (STA-MCA)
bypass. This report reviews the current status of procedures for extracranial-
intracranial bypass; STA-MCA anastomosis is presented in some detail.

PROCEDURES

Long Grafts

For inaccessible occlusions of internal carotid artery (ICA) or MCA, bypass grafting is a logical surgical approach. To provide immediate high volume flow, several authors have advocated interposition of the grafts between common carotid (or external carotid) and cerebral vessels (ICA or MCA branch)[7] (see Figure 1). Grafts of saphenous vein, radial artery, or synthetic materials have been utilized. Early reports have indicated high flow (up to 300 ml/min at surgery), high mortality (up to 30%), and low long-term patency (about 50%). Utilization of cortical MCA branch for the recipient vessel may diminish complications. The possibility of prompt large flow increment makes long grafting desirable, but results to date confine the approach to the developmental stages.

Vertebro-basilar Revascularization

Recently several surgeons have anastomosed the occipital branch of external carotid artery to the posterior inferior cerebellar artery (PICA)[13] (see Figure 2). The method provides augmented collateral circulation for the vertebro-basilar circuit, provided the occlusive process is proximal to PICA take-off. Technical feasibility has been demonstrated, together with flows greater than 100 cc/min, excellent angiographic filling of the posterior circulation, and low morbidity-mortality. Data on long-term patency and stroke rates are not available. Early results are thus encouraging, but indications have not been established.

Superficial Temporal-Middle Cerebral Artery (STA–MCA) Bypass

STA–MCA anastomosis (Figure 3) is the most promising form of direct brain revascularization, and the remainder of this report focuses on this procedure, including personal experience with the method.

In 1967 Donaghy and Yasargil introduced microsurgical STA–MCA bypass in man.[15] Reichman recommended several technical alterations, including a small craniectomy for exposure, utilization of both STA branches for two separate anastomoses, interrupted suture technique, and beveling of STA back toward MCA origin.[10] Chater advocated use of the large angular branch of MCA to enhance flow and patency rates.[1,2] Robertson has recommended linear incision over STA (instead of a scalp flap) to accelerate surgery and preserve STA vasa vasorum.

The role of STA–MCA bypass in preventing (or even reversing) strokes has not yet been fully defined. However, in selected cases, STA–MCA bypass carries

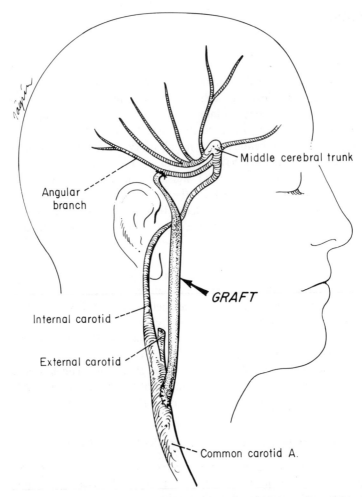

FIG. 1. Long grafts from carotid to an MCA branch can provide immediate and large flow augmentation. Patency and complications have been disappointing thus far, but technical development is under way. (Revised with permission from R. M. Crowell, Direct brain revascularization, Fig. 1-2, p. 3, in H. Schmidek and W. H. Sweet, eds., *Current Techniques in Operative Neurosurgery*, Grune & Stratton, 1977.)

a low risk and appears to diminish the incidence of TIAs and cerebral infarction.[1,2,4,6,9,10,12,14–16] Regional cerebral blood flow (CBF) studies may help characterize indications for the procedure.[11] The best method for defining indications for new therapy is the randomized clinical trial, and a large collaborative study of this type is presently underway.

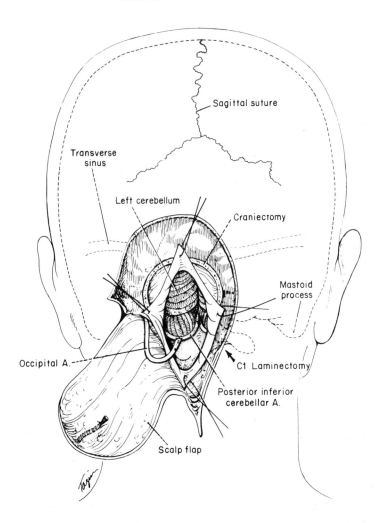

FIG. 2. Vertebro-basilar revascularization can be achieved by anastomosis of the occipital branch of external carotid to posterior inferior cerebellar artery (PICA), a vertebral artery branch. Experience is limited but encouraging. (Revised with permission from R. M. Crowell Direct brain revascularization, Fig. 1-3, p. 2, in H. Schmidek and W. H. Sweets, eds., *Current Techniques in Operative Neurosurgery,* Grune & Stratton, 1977.)

USE OF STA–MCA BYPASS

Since STA–MCA bypass is the most promising and widely used for of cerebral revascularization, the remainder of this report is entirely confined to STA–MCA bypass.

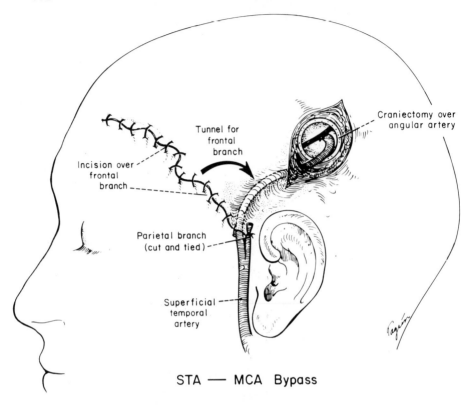

STA — MCA Bypass

FIG. 3. STA–MCA bypass is the most promising and widely used form of direct brain revascularization. An incision over the frontal STA and small craniectomy provide good exposure. The angular branch of MCA gives best flow and patency.

Tentative Indications

In general, STA-MCA bypass is logical therapy for symptomatic cerebral ischemia with obstruction inaccessible to carotid endarterectomy. Several specific clinico-angiography indications have been proposed:

TIAs. Bypass is probably best employed to block the evolution of TIAs into a frank stroke. Thus the best indication is focal TIAs, with hemiparesis, numbness, or aphasia, related to inaccessible ICA or MCA stenosis or occlusion.[1,2,10,12]

Slow Strokes. Bypass may arrest or even reverse the gradual evolution of the occasional stroke which unfolds over days. Limited experience suggests this will probably prove a good indication.[12]

Planned Therapeutic Occlusion. Initial bypass may be needed when carotid (or MCA) occlusion is needed for intracranial aneurysm or during carotid endarterectomy. The indication appears sound, but identification of cases with such feeble collateral as to require revascularization is as yet uncertain.[16]

Progressive Dementia. Multiple cerebrovascular occlusion may rarely lead to generalized hypoperfusion and dementia without infarction. STA-MCA grafting may reverse such syndromes.[9]

Acute Strokes. Some evidence suggests emergency bypass may arrest infarction,[3] but clinical experience thus far has been discouraging.

Contraindications

Fixed deficits are generally not improved through bypass grafting.[2,16] Therefore many patients with ICA occlusion and stable neurologic deficit are not good candidates for surgery, especially when the deficit is severe. When an embolic mechanism is likely, bypass probably will not help. Surgery is hazardous with extreme age or debility, severe cardiopulmonary disease, and uncontrolled diabetes and hypertension. When STA or MCA branches are less than 0.8 mm in diameter, bypass is unlikely to provide substantial flow augmentation.

Preoperative Evaluation

Careful history taking is frequently critical in establishing the indication for bypass; elicitation of a history of TIAs is the most favorable indication for surgery. Physical examination should include a detailed neurological examination and vascular examination, including palpation of STA branches to determine suitability for grafting. Preoperative studies include EKG, serum triglycerides, and serum cholesterol. Frequently cardiac consultation is needed. Computed tomography can identify stable infarctions and unanticipated pathology (e.g., tumor) which may preclude surgery. Transfemoral complete angiography is essential to delineate cerebrovascular occlusions, collateral circulation, and arteries suitable for bypass. CBF studies may prove useful in identifying candidates for surgery.

Operative Technique

Atropine and Droperidol may be given as premedication prior to general anesthesia, which is generally halothane or balanced technique (nitrous oxide, Innovar, and curare). Controlled ventilation is used to maintain pCO_2 at 35 to 40 mm Hg. Precordial EKG and radial arterial blood pressure are monitored continuously on a Tektronix portable oscilliscope. Infusions of colloid, dopamine, or nitroprusside maintain normal blood pressure. Only for particularly lengthy procedures is a Foley catheter inserted (e.g., two grafts or exploration of cervical carotid prior to bypass). Oxacillin is given, 2 g every 6 hours intra-venously, prior to surgery and for 48 hours thereafter.

The patient lies supine, with the head turned away from the operated side. A small roll elevates the shoulder on the side of surgery, and the head is fixed in a three-point head rest. The side of the head is shaved to the midline and well behind the ear.

In addition to the usual craniotomy kit, several microsurgical instruments are essential. We use the Zeiss operating microscope No. 1 with 250-mm objective, 160-mm angled oculars, and 12.5X high-eyepoint eyepieces. The stereoscopic binocular observer tube is attached to the left side of the scope for the surgical assistant. Jeweler's forceps adapted for bipolar coagulation are used for precise hemostasis. Jeweler's forceps and a 5″ iris scissors serve well for preparation of arteries. Temporary clips (Kleinert-Kees) are helpful for atraumatic temporary occlusion. A short blade-breaker and segment of broken razor blade allow accu-rate arterotomies. Fine silastic tubing is a useful stent during suturing. The anastomosis is performed with an 8-inch Barraquer needle holder and 10-0 monofilament nylon suture material on a BV-6 needle (Ethicon).

Linear skin incisions are used to permit (1) rapid STA preparation with preservation of vasa vasorum and (2) satisfactory cortical exposure without a large scalp flap. One or two incisions may be needed (see Figure 3): in all cases the angular artery is exposed by one incision; in some cases the same incision, directly over the parietal branch of STA, may be all that is needed. In most cases, however, the frontal branch of STA is larger, and this is exposed through a separate frontal incision (Figure 3). After superficial skin incision down to fat, the plane superficial to STA is developed with Metzenbaum scissors under the operating microscope. Small scalp flaps are elevated to either side, and a length of STA is exposed, undermined, and mobilized, as side branches are carefully coagulated and cut. Adventitia is left on the 10-cm STA segment except at its end, where extra tissue is carefully removed. The STA tip is beveled appropri-ately, and after checking STA flow, the vessel is irrigated with heparinized saline (Figure 4).

The MCA branch we use is generally the angular,[2] which is usually the largest available. An incision over a point 6½ cm rostral to the external auditory canal will expose this vessel nicely. A craniectomy (or small trephine) is placed over the angular artery, and the dura is incised to reveal the vessel. Under 16X magnifica-tion, the arachnoid over the MCA branch is cut to free up 10 mm of recipient artery. After placement of Kleinert-Kees clips, an arterotomy is made with a razor blade, and an additional small elipse of vessel wall is excised.

To join STA to MCA, we use 12 to 14 interrupted sutures of 10-0 monofila-ment nylon (Figure 4). A small silastic stent tube in the MCA branch facilitates suturing. To maximize MCA filling, the graft is beveled back toward MCA origin. Sutures must accurately include STA atheroma, which can be extensive. Sutures

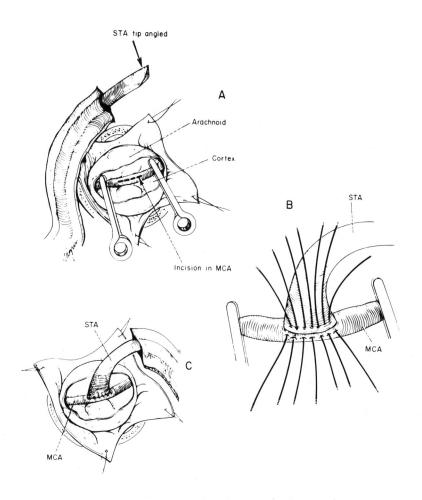

FIG. 4. Technique of STA–MCA bypass: (A) Some adventitia is left on STA which is beveled to maximize the ostium. (B) After craniectomy, the MCA branch is prepared and anastomosis begun. (C) The anastomosis is completed microsurgically with interrupted suture technique. (Revised with permission from R. M. Crowell, Direct brain revascularization, Figs. 1–6 and 1–8, pp. 9 and 11, in H. Schmidek and W. H. Sweet, eds., *Current Techniques in Operative Neurosurgery*, Grune & Stratton, 1977.)

are placed slightly closer together near the corners where leaks are prone to occur. Before the last two stitches are tied, the stent is removed and the STA opened briefly to expel clots and air. When all clips are removed, the suture line is inspected at 25X for large leaks which may require additional sutures. In most cases, mild pressure with a cottonoid encourages adequate hemostasis. Graft flow may be measured with an electromagnetic flowmeter.

The dura is closed loosely and covered with gelfoam. The graft is routed without compression through the craniectomy and the muscle, which is loosely approximated with interrupted sutures. The galea is closed with interrupted silk, the skin with running nylon.

Postoperative Management

For 24 to 48 hours, normal blood pressure is carefully maintained with drugs and arterial catheter. After 48 hours, mobilization begins, and blood pressure is controlled with oral agents. Aspirin (600 mg) and dipyridamole (50 mg) are given twice daily for 6 months to foster graft patency. Angiography is generally performed at 1 week to assess bypass patency.

Complications

Major complications have been infrequently reported; these include postoperative infarction (related to failure of graft or native collateral), intracranial hematoma, meningitis, and cardiopulmonary sequelae. Reported minor complications include transient focal deficits, seizures, wound infections, and scalp edge necrosis.[1,2,4,10,12,16]

Discussion

As at other centers, personal experience with 34 cases of STA-MCA bypass has been encouraging (see Tables 1-3). Graft patency has been 90% (28/31). Complications have been infrequent and largely minor. There were no deaths. Bypass has eliminated TIAs in 16 of 17 cases, and stroke has been rare (2 cases).

Acute strokes treated with bypass have not improved beyond the expected recuperation.[3] Two slow strokes appeared to improve promptly in relation to bypass. One case with dementia was not benefited by surgery. Preliminary bypass permitted carotid endarterectomy or permanent carotid ligation in two of two cases where native collateral seemed inadequate. Follow-up has demonstrated two cerebral infarctions: One patient with multiple intracranial occlusions suffered infarction on the side contralateral to surgery. Another patient suffered a small infarct when her graft, previously open by angiogram, occluded some months after surgery.

TABLE 1. Case Material* (34 Grafts)

Presentation	No. of cases	Angiography	No. of cases
TIAs	17	ICA occl.	10
Acute stroke	5	ICA stem	5
Slow stroke	2	MCA occl.	3
Dementia	1	MCA stem	3
Aneurysm	2	Multiple occl.	9
Other	4	Aneurysm	1

*Patients ranged in age from 39 to 77 years (avg. = 58) and included 23 males and 8 females.

TABLE 2. Results

Flow	Angiography	Clinical outcome
15–190 cc/min (avg. 45)	1 early occlusion 1 late occlusion 28 open 4 ND	TIAs eliminated 16/17 Acute stroke improved 0/5 Slow stroke improved 2/2 Dementia improved 0/1 Aneurysm thrombosed 2/2 Other—no new stroke 4/4

TABLE 3. Complications

	No. of cases
Death	0
Stroke	
Contralateral side, 2 weeks postoperatively	1
With late graft occlusion by atheroma	1
Minor	
Transient deficit	2
Seizure	2
Scalp edge necrosis	3
Scalp infection	1

Case Report

A case report serves to illustrate this experience:

R. M., a 36-year-old right-handed truck driver, experienced episodes of numbness and severe weakness of the right face, arm, and leg. The spells lasted from 1 to 10 minutes, were never accompanied by dysphasia, and occurred daily during the week prior to admission. The patient smoked over one pack of cigarettes per day. His mother had died at 51 of myocardial infarction.

Examination showed BP 160/80 with normal neurologic function. A study of CBF (xenon inhalation) was normal. Serum cholesterol was 224 mg%, with serum triglycerides of 242 mg%. Cerebral angiography disclosed a tight stenosis of the left middle cerebral artery (see Figure 5, (a)).

On 12/23/76 the left superficial temporal artery was anastomed to a branch of the middle cerebral artery. The postoperative course was smooth, without further spells over an 18-month follow-up. Angiography showed filling of four branches of MCA via the graft (see Figure 5, (b)). Weight reduction and cessation of smoking were instituted.

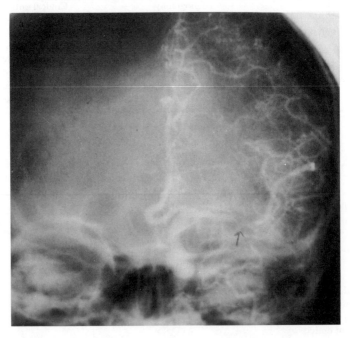

A

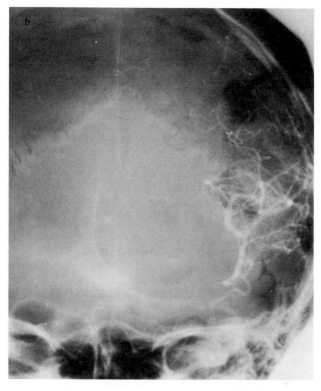

B

FIG. 5. (A) AP left carotid angiogram shows middle cerebral artery stenosis (arrow) in a man with TIAs. (B) After surgery, external carotid angiogram shows the STA–MCA bypass providing extensive additional filling of MCA branches; TIAs have ceased for 18 months.

SUMMARY

STA-MCA bypass probably reduces stroke risk for patients with TIAs and inaccessible occlusions. The procedure may prove valuable for slow strokes, generalized hypoperfusion, and planned therapeutic occlusions. Studies of CBF and metabolism may help select cases for operation. A controlled study of bypass results is underway to evaluate these indications.

Other forms of brain revascularization await evaluation: Occipital-PICA anastomosis can augment vertebro-basilar perfusion, and long grafting may be useful for rapid (even emergency) cerebral revascularization.

Acknowledgments

Dr. M. G. Yasargil taught me STA–MCA bypass. Frank Marcoux and Stuart Fitz-Gibbon carried out the blood flow measurements. Mrs. Edith Tagrin prepared the line drawings. Dr. R. G. Ojemann provided constructive criticism. This work was supported in part by Teacher-Investigator Award NS11011 and grants NS 10828 and NS13165 from the National Institute for Neurological and Communicative Disorders and Stroke.

References

1. Chater, N., Mani, J., and Tonnemacher, K. Superficial temporal artery bypass for cerebrovascular occlusive disease. *Cal. Med. 119*: 9–13, 1973.
2. Chater, N., and Popp, J. Microsurgical vascular bypass for occlusive cerebrovascular disease: Review of 100 cases. *Surg. Neurol. 6*: 115–118, 1976.
3. Crowell, R. M., and Olsson, Y. Effect of extracranial-intracranial vascular bypass graft on experimental acute stroke in dogs. *J. Neurosurg. 38*: 26–31, 1973.
4. Gratzl, O., Schmiedek, P., Spetzler, R., Steinhoff, H., and Marguth, F. Clinical experience with extra-intracranial arterial anastomosis in 65 cases. *J. Neurosurg. 44*: 313–324, 1976.
5. Holbach, K. H., Wassmann, H., Hoheluchter, K. L., and Jain, K. K. Differentiation between reversible and irreversible post-stroke changes in brain tissue: Its relevance for cerebrovascular surgery. *Surg. Neurol. 7*: 325–331, 1977.
6. Lazar, M. L., and Clark, K. Microsurgical cerebral revascularization: Concepts and practice. *Surg. Neurol. 1*: 355–359, 1973.
7. Lougheed, W. M., Marshall, B. M., Hunter, M., Michel, E. R., and Sandwith-Smyth, H. Common carotid to intracranial internal carotid bypass venous graft: Technical note. *J. Neurosurg. 34*: 114–118, 1971.
8. Ojemann, R. G., Crowell, R. M., Fisher C. M., et al. Surgical treatment of extracranial carotid occlusive disease. *Clin. Neurosurg. 22*: 214–263, 1975.
9. Peerless, S. J. Techniques of cerebral revascularization. *Clin. Neurosurg. 23*: 258–269, 1976.
10. Reichman, O. H. Extracranial-intracranial arterial anastomosis. In *Cerebral Vascular Disease: Ninth Conference,* J. P. Whisnant and B. A. Sandok, New York: Grune and Stratton, 1975, pp. 175–185.
11. Schmiedek, P., Gratzl, O., Spetzler, R., et al. Selection of patients for extra-intracranial bypass surgery based on rCBF measurements. *J. Neurosurg. 44*: 303–312, 1976.
12. Sundt, T. M., Jr., Siekert, R. G., Piepgras, D. G., Sharbrough, F. W., and Houser, O. W., Bypass surgery for vascular disaease of the carotid system. *Mayo Clin. Proc. 51*: 677–692, 1976.
13. Sundt, T. M., Jr., and Piepgras, D. G. Occipital to posterior inferior cerebellar artery bypass surgery. *J. Neurosurg. 48*: 916–928, 1978.
14. Tew, J. M., Jr. Reconstructive intracranial vascular surgery for prevention of stroke. *Clin. Neurosurg. 22*: 264–280, 1975.
15. Yasargil, M. G., Krayenbühl, H. A., and Jacobson, J. H., H. Microneurosurgical arterial reconstruction. *Surgery 67*: 221–233, 1970.
16. Yasargil, M. G., and Yonekawa, Y. Results of microsurgical extra-intracranial arterial bypass in the treatment of cerebral ischemia. *Neurosurgery 1*: 22–24, 1977.

The Current Status of Blood Vessel Grafts and Indications for Use

WILLIAM M. ABBOTT, M.D.
RAPHAEL WALDEN, M.D.
*From the Department of Surgery, Harvard Medical School
and the General Surgical Services, Massachusetts General
Hospital, Boston, Massachusetts*

The replacement of a diseased blood vessel with a normal one or some analogue has been the goal of surgeons and physicians since ancient time. Although some early success occurred in the first part of the twentieth century, it was only in 1952 when Dubost in France first reported successfully replacing a segment of abdominal aorta with an aortic homograft that the modern era of vascular grafting began. Although much knowledge and experience have been gathered since, the materials currently used for replacement of arteries are still imperfect in design and concept. This brief review will attempt to highlight certain aspects of vascular grafting, including what is presently known about the ideals in replacement grafts on theoretical grounds. The review will also show how these grounds are supported by experimental and clinical information to aid the surgeon in making a rational selection of available grafting materials. Finally, the review will attempt to touch upon future possibilities for these grafting materials.

Various types of grafting materials have been tried clinically since the 1950s. These include arterial homografts, venous allografts, heterografts (mainly bovine carotid artery), and collagen tubes created in the patient's subcutaneous tissue (Sparks mandril). Various polymers such as Vinyon-N, nylon, Teflon, Orlon, and Dacron have also been tested for grafting possibilities. After initial enthusiasm, most of these substances failed as grafting materials because of high rates of occlusion, aneurysm formation, and rupture. The contemporary materials used are autogenous vein, human umbilical cord vein, and several types of Dacron and Teflon. These will be reviewed in detail.

THEORETICAL ASPECTS

The precise characteristics of a graft necessary to achieve perfect results as an arterial substitute are not known. There has been considerable investigation, and our general understanding is improving. Yet the imperfect results associated with blood vessel grafting are clearly related, at least in part, to graft design. Careful examination of the life-table patency curves of vessel grafts reveals several distinct slopes to such curves, implying a number of biologic events. In the early phases, the causes are clearly technical, that is, those usually occurring in the first 24 hours. Hemodynamic events can also be implicated at this point and represent a second phase of causative events. In this phase, graft failure results owing to an existing adverse combination of variables between graft-related factors and local host hemodynamic factors. This usually persists for several weeks. A third phase, during which yet another group of grafts fail, exists during the first one to two years. Although atherosclerotic disease progression may be involved to some extent, chronic changes occurring in the grafts themselves are responsible for many of these failures. The last cause, and one which has been probably overly implicated in graft failure, is atherosclerotic disease progression. Because atherosclerosis is a rather slowly progressive disease in most patients, it seems unlikely that all graft failures can be explained by this. On the other hand, atherosclerosis may be augmented by adverse hemodynamics generated by imperfectly designed grafts. It is therefore very important that theoretic aspects of blood vessel grafts be elucidated.

Basic Properties of the Normal Artery

The various factors that enable proper blood flow through an artery should be studied before analogues to replace it are considered.

1. *Visco-Elastic Properties—Compliance.* The mechanical properties of normal vessels have long been ignored in consideration of the desirable attributes of a vascular graft. Normal artery is visco-elastic, a quality that is essential in the vessel's physiologic function—in mechanical terms, its compliance. Compliance is important, since it is a key determinant in the efficient transmission of pulsatile energy from the central pumping source to the periphery. Compliance is also a major factor governing the impedance of a blood vessel or a blood vessel bed, that is, the resistance to pulsatile flow. Normal artery is very compliant, whereas with age and the advent of arterial disease an artery tends to lose compliance. Over the course of time, normal arteries may become totally incompliant because of wall calcification. Yet, by and large, these vessels remain patent; hence compliance is obviously not the only parameter of the normal artery to be considered.

2. *Flow Surface Thrombo-resistance.* Another important parameter of the normal artery is the physico-chemical properties governing the relative thrombo-resistance or thrombogenicity of the vessel's surface when exposed to blood. Physical interactions at the interface between surface and blood are related to surface-free energy, which is measured as critical surface tension using the technique of multiple contact angle determinations. A critical surface tension ranging from 20 to 30 dyne/cm is thought to be most biocompatible with blood, and the ideal zone is between 24 and 26 dyne/cm. Above and below this zone, surfaces

are relatively thrombogenic and react with blood to stimulate clot formation. The surface chemical composition of the biocompatible surface, as determined by measurements of multiple attenuated infrared reflection spectroscopy, show that it is predominated by glycoproteinaceous materials. It is important to realize, however, that the so-called thrombo-resistant surface can be achieved in several ways. The endothelial cell-lined surfaces of arteries and veins, the internal elastic lamina, and the basement membranes of some vessels all possess these characteristics.

3. *Endothelial Cell Properties.* One additional important feature of the normal blood vessel is the presence of a physiologically functioning endothelial cell layer. Not only do endothelial cells possess the necessary physico-chemical characteristics of thrombo-resistance, but they have additional features that keep them from accumulating thrombus. Studies of endothelial cells in culture have shown them to have anti-platelet factor-3 and soluble clotting factor VIII antigen. Both arteries and veins also have fibrinolytic activator activity. How these function is not exactly known, but clearly the endothelial cells possess characteristics over and above those mentioned previously, so that an intact vessel may have blood in it totally static for a long period and, if undisturbed, may not undergo thrombosis.

4. *Hemodynamic Factors.* Hemodynamic factors are also necessary to the normal situation. It is quite clear that the above-mentioned normal characteristics of the vessel interact with hemodynamic factors, and a critical balance between adverse variables and salutory hemodynamics is what is responsible for keeping the vessel patent. Volume flow is an obvious simple hemodynamic parameter, and for arteries there is some evidence to suggest that it is pulsatile rather than steady flow that is important in the prevention of thrombus. Flow also generates shear forces that, within certain ranges, may prevent thrombus accumulation but without causing the damage known to occur when high shearing forces act upon the endothelium. Some investigators suggest that high-frequency vessel wall motion, or resonance, which has been observed in visco-elastic conduits, also contributes to the prevention of thrombus formation. It is not known which hemodynamic factors may contribute to thrombus formation or prevention or exactly how they may do so. It is clear that hemodynamics and flow are important ingredients, especially if there is any deviation from the normal characteristics of the vessel. The interaction between the three major factors influencing patency or occlusion in a blood vessel is illustrated in Figure 1.

Thrombo-reactivity

It will be helpful before considering vascular grafts to develop the concept of thrombo-reactivity. When any conduit is exposed to blood, it enters a state

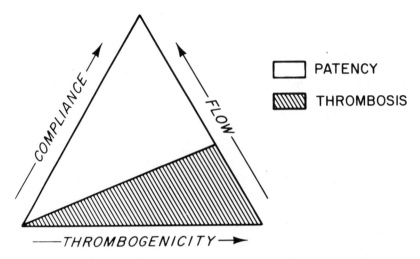

FIG. 1. Illustration of the interaction between the major factors influencing patency or thrombosis of a blood vessel.

defined by us as "thrombo-reactive." This state may be described in terms of degree and duration, which, in turn, are determined by the interaction between the mechanical properties of the vessel wall, the physico-chemical characteristics of the intimal surface, and the presence of endothelial cells. Deterioration of any of these factors may increase the thrombo-reactivity to a threshhold level that will lead to initiation of clotting. That threshold depends upon the flow conditions; that is, the greater the flow, the higher the threshold. In favorable circumstances, adaptive and regenerative mechanisms will tend to reduce the level of and shorten the period of thrombo-reactivity. The graft thereby stabilizes, as exemplified in our discussion of autogenous vein grafts.

VASCULAR GRAFTS

The properties and characteristics of the various prototypes of contemporary vascular grafts may now be considered.

Autogenous Veins

The implanted vein begins as a conduit that is less compliant than artery but more closely matches normal artery than many other materials do. Since it is usually grafted into a circulation that is less compliant because of age or disease, the match becomes even closer. Unless the vein has been badly damaged, it retains its compliance over the course of implantation, in spite of the fact that it accomodates to the stresses of the arterial circulation by developing wall thickening and dilating in diameter to a certain extent. With the first exposure to flowing blood, the endothelial layer is partially or completely lost, exposing the underlying basement membrane or subendothelium. Although this layer also possesses the physico-chemical characteristics of long-term thrombo-resistance, the graft is initially "thrombo-reactive," as exhibited by morphologic studies which show that platelets have attached and may undergo some transformation. The factors determining whether they actually undergo release of active substances with initiation of clotting are not known, but as mentioned, flow conditions and other hemodynamic factors are important in determining whether the thrombo-reactive state actually results in gross thrombus formation. At the same time, over the course of days to several weeks, the endothelial layer is reconstituted in vein grafts, thus completely stabilizing the situation and restoring it to a nearly physiologic condition. In some instances, although grafts will "heal" (the term used to describe endothelial cell repopulation), they will also undergo a response of subintimal cellular proliferation to a certain degree. This can reach pathological proportions and has been reported as responsible for vein graft occlusions, especially in the aorto-coronary position. Although all the factors that determine whether or not this assumes pathological proportions are not known, both flow and compliance mismatches have been implicated. But in all probability, vein is such a satisfactory conduit because it basically has good mechanical properties to begin with and has an underlying thrombo-resistant surface. Thus, when vein becomes thrombo-reactive at implantation, it is not of great degree so that it may still retain its patency provided certain critical flow conditions are met. Also, its unstable thrombo-reactive period is limited and has the potential for full re-endothelial reconstitution or healing and thereby complete stabilization.

The satisfactory nature of vein as a conduit is illustrated by the cumulative patency rate of a large series of autogenous saphenous vein bypass grafts for femoropopliteal occlusive disease, as shown in Figure 2. The results with saphenous vein grafting in the medium- to small-vessel circulation are the best reported. The saphenous vein is the grafting material of choice in these locations and has now become the standard against which any new synthetic or other conduit must be compared.

Yet autogenous vein grafts have several serious limitations. Venous grafting is not practical for large vessel replacements. The usual source, the saphenous vein, is not always available, because of disease, previous arterial reconstructions, or unsuitability of size. Also, complications encountered in harvesting it, along with the amount of time spent in doing so, increase the potential for damaging the vein. A totally suitable alternative would be very desirable.

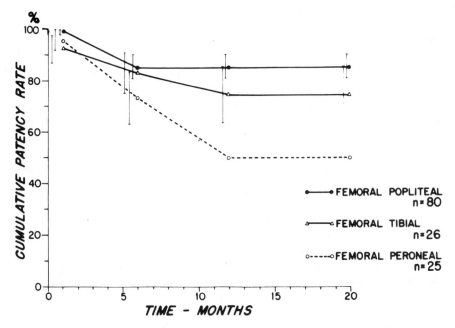

FIG. 2. Cumulative patency rate of autogenous saphenous vein femoropopliteal bypass grafts (233 consecutive cases).

Nonviable Biological Conduit—Human Umbilical Cord Vein Graft

Human umbilical cord vein is the newest alternative to saphenous vein suggested for medium- to small-vessel reconstructions. Umbilical veins are treated by glutaraldehyde fixation, mechanically strengthened with a Dacron mesh coating, and stored in ethanol. Not a great deal is known about such conduits, although what we do know suggests that they behave more like viable grafts than do the synthetics. The mechanical properties of human umbilical cord vein prior to implantation closely resemble those of normal vein. The physico-chemical characteristics of the surface also resemble those of native vessels. Morphologically these vessels have at least what appear to be some retained endothelial cells, by scanning electron microscopy. Although relatively thrombo-resistant, the basement membrane of this graft is what is primarily exposed. After implantation, however, less is known. Short-term studies suggest that the mechanical properties are retained, but the healing and stabilization potential of the graft with repopulation of endothelial cell integrity is not known. It is encouraging, however, that the unstable period of thrombo-reactivity does seem finite. Although it is not yet widely available because of FDA investigational guidelines, there is a great deal of initial enthusiasm for this graft. Early implantation results are encouraging, as illustrated in Figure 3. Yet the experience with this material must still be presumed to be early, as it is two years at the minimum, if not three, before any new grafting material can be accepted with confidence.

Synthetic Conduits

Synthetic vascular grafts have the great advantage of availability in multiple sizes and shapes. They are easily sterilized and stored at room temperature for immediate access and use. Their cost is relatively low. As mentioned, many polymers have been tried, but Dacron and Teflon have evolved into the present are as the basic material of choice.

Dacron

Different techniques are used in the manufacture of polymeric fiber tubes, ending with a woven or knitted textile construction. The grafts are porous in order to provide (theoretically) the possibilities of fibrous tissue ingrowth and stabilization of the flow surface. Porosity is controlled by size of thread (denier) and

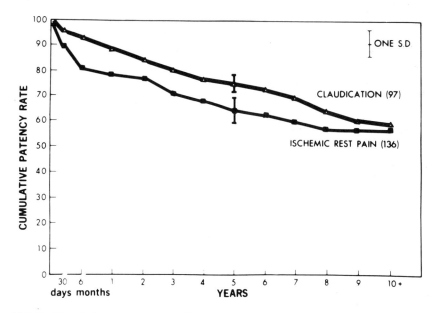

FIG. 3. Cumulative patency rates of human umbilical cord vein bypass grafts to popliteal, tibial, and peroneal arteries (131 cases).

tightness of the weave or knit (needles per inch). Recent knitted fabric tubes have veloured yarns on the internal or the external surface, or sometimes both, in order to promote tissue incorporation. Crimping is included in the graft's configuration to provide greater flexibility. Woven grafts are less compliant and bend poorly. They are less porous, with resultant diminished fibrous ingrowth and poorer healing potential. Hemostasis at the time of operation is less of a problem. The tensile properties of the material and its low propensity for degradation in biological systems make Dacron suitable for use as a vascular substitute. However, the mechanical properties of Dacron (as with other existing prosthetic conduits) are not satisfactory. It is basically incompliant even when knitted, and with implantation, accompanied by fibrous tissue reaction, becomes even less so.

Synthetic conduits possess flow surfaces that, in native form, are not in the thrombo-resistant zone. Dacron grafts, for example, have a critical tension surface of 45 dyne/cm and obviously do not have endothelial cells. The initial event occurring when any material is exposed to flowing blood is the deposition of a thin proteinaceous film in an attempt to "passivate" the surface. In the case of Dacron (and Teflon), however, neither of these passivated films quite falls into the necessary thrombo-resistant zone. Therefore these grafts, because of mechanical and surface properties, are more thrombo-reactive than the previously mentioned veins.

Although porosity, which was mentioned above, was incorporated into graft design to stimulate fibrous ingrowth, with its attendant need for "preclotting" by forcing clotting blood through the interstices porosity, it may be a fortuitous help to the satisfactory function of some of these grafts. The reason is that totally polymerized fibrin is thrombo-resistant chemically. Even so, during the unstable period, the synthetic graft is probably more thrombo-reactive, as mentioned above, so that flow conditions are even more critical. This is one clear explanation of why larger-diameter, high-flow systems such as the aorta will accept synthetic prostheses much more readily than the medium- to small-caliber circulations.

It was hoped that the porosity would allow fibrous tissue ingrowth with eventual true healing by endothelial cell repopulation. In man, however, such healing is, at best, incomplete, with most re-endothelialization being seen at the proximal and distal end of grafts growing in from the native vessels with only patchy re-endothelialization in the middle. Thus, most synthetic prostheses studied have only partial stabilization of the surface. Although the remainder of the surface may be in the thrombo-resistant zone chemically, it remains somewhat thrombo-reactive because it only possesses a passivated fibrin layer. Hence, these grafts are always in dynamic equilibrium, and if enough adverse changes occur, such as with reduction in flow, a decreasing compliance, or damage to the surface, this dynamic equilibrium could be disturbed, allowing clotting to occur.

In other words, synthetic prostheses that remain patent always do so in some-what tenous condition. In large vessel applications, however, the results of Dacron grafting are quite excellent, mainly for aneurysm replacement. In re-placements for occlusive diseases, the results are also quite good. Brewster and Darling recently reported cumulative patency rates of 98.7% after one year and 91.2% after five years for aorto-femoral grafts of knitted Dacron.

Teflon

Teflon is also manufactured in the form of woven or knitted material. Its tensile properties seem to be slightly better than those of Dacron, but it is as incom-pliant. It possesses a critical surface tension of 18 dyne/cm. Following implanta-tion, it develops a surface that is capable of taking up lipid and develops occlusive processes showing histologic resemblance to atheromata. Other events occurring following implantation are generally similar to those described for Dacron.

Expanded Teflon (PTFE)

A new synthetic material has also recently become available in which the knitted or woven textile manufacturing principles are not used. This is expanded micro-porous polytetrafluoroethylene, or Teflon. This material possesses the same thrombogenic critical surface tension of 18 and presumably accumulates a thrombogenic passivated layer of above 30 similar to standard Teflon grafts. The mechanical properties of PTFE are also not very satisfactory, and compliance testing of these grafts reveals them to be among the most rigid. There is a re-portedly large clinical experience, although hard data regarding the success of the material are scant. Early reports, however, are enthusiastic, and for the short term, expanded polytetrafluoroethylene constitutes an exciting potential alternative when the saphenous vein is unavailable. Perhaps the best data about PTFE come from the combined experience of the members of the New England Society for Vascular Surgery. In a recent objective report from this source using actuarial methods, the results for distal leg reconstruction are not very satisfac-tory, with an overall cumulative patency rate of 54.4% at between 9 and 12 months. Interestingly, most of the failures occurred in the first 30 days during the presumed "unstable" period.

RECOMMENDATIONS FOR USE

Large Vessels

Dacron remains the material of choice for large vessel grafting. It seems reason-able to reserve the use of woven materials for grafts that are going to remain straight or have a minimum of curvature. They would thus be applicable for arterial replacements that are going to remain entirely in the abdomen or the thorax. They are applicable to the cardiac surgeon, replacing segments of thoracic aorta where hemostasis is definitely a problem. They would also be applicable to resection and grafting of abdominal aortic aneurysms and especially of ruptured abdominal aortic aneurysms, where, again, hemostasis and blood loss are great factors in the acute survival of the patient. For elective operations involving the abdominal aorta, and especially elective aortic operations for occlusive disease where it is likely that the graft will extend from the abdomen below the inguinal ligament to the femoral artery, knitted Dacron grafts would seem a better choice. The distinct benefits of velour remain to be conclusively proved, but the theoretical evidence supporting it would suggest that this is an advantage. Teflon should probably be reserved for the rare incidences of patient sensitization to the Dacron polymer.

The status of large vessel replacements has evolved satisfactorily over the years, and although some room for improvement exists, the results at present are quite good. Future improvements will probably involve the use of better synthetic polymers as the basic material with better flow surfaces. Attention will also be given to the mechanical properties because of the adverse consequences of differing poorly matched visco-elastic properties at the junction of graft and host circulation.

Medium and Small Vessels

For replacement materials in the medium- to small-vessel reconstructions, we are left with certain hard facts. At the present writing, there is no proven suitable alternative for saphenous vein, if it is unavailable. It would therefore be prudent for surgeons to consider patients needing these medium- or small-vessel reconstructions as to the severity or urgency of the problem. For patients with claudication, for example, it is probably best to use the saphenous vein exclusively and only to perform the operation if saphenous vein is available. There is enough evidence to suggest that a patient with claudication may be made worse by failed reconstruction to make reconstruction with an alternative method indicated only under stringent circumstances. For those patients with more urgent indications for operation, such as in the so-called limb salvage situation, saphenous vein is still the best material, especially in those patients in whom reconstruction will be carried distal to the popliteal artery. When saphenous vein is unavailable and popliteal artery reconstruction is possible, present data do not support a clear-cut choice between the alternatives. On theoretic grounds, the umbilical vein would seem the best choice, especially if tibial vessel reconstruction is needed.

A satisfactory synthetic material for medium- to small-vessel reconstructions is not yet available. Future development will have to take into consideration all the basic characteristics required for a blood vessel substitute:

1. Appropriate visco-elastic properties, mainly to avoid compliance mismatch with the native vessels,
2. Adequate flow surface thrombo-resistance,
3. Capacity for true and total endothelial cell reconstitution,
4. Good tensile strength and low propensity for degradation in biologic systems,
5. Nonantigenicity,
6. Availability in multiple sizes and shapes at relatively low cost with ease of sterilization and storage.

References

Baier, R. E., and Abbott, W. M. *Comparative Biophysical Flow Surface Properties of Contemporary Vascular Grafts.* Symposia Specialists, Inc. Medical Books, in press.

Brewster, D. C., and Darling, R. C. Optimal methods of aorto-iliac reconstruction. *Surgery 84(6)*: 739, 1978.

Dardik, H., and Ibrahim, M. I. Evaluation of Glutaraldehyde-treated human umbilical cord vein as a vascular prosthesis for bypass to the popliteal, tibial, and peroneal arteries. *Surgery 83*: 577, 1978.

Darling, R. C. Autogenous Saphenous vein bypass grafts for femoropopliteal occlusive disease. In *Vascular Grafts,* P. N. Sawyer and M. J. Kaplitt, eds. New York: Appleton-Century-Crofts, 1978, pp. 237–242.

Johnson, W. C. Report on regional experience with PTFE (Gore-Tex and Impra) bypass graft material. Fifth Annual Meeting of the New England Society for Vascular Surgery. *Arch. Surg.,* in press.

IV

CURRENT CLINICAL MANAGEMENT

Gastrointestinal Ulceration in the Burn Patient

EDWARD J. LAW, M.D.
Associate Professor
Department of Surgery
Southern Illinois University
School of Medicine
Springfield, Illinois

The gastrointestinal tract is a frequent target for both primary and secondary disease. Peptic ulcers represent one of the most common and serious nonmalignant diseases involving the gastrointestinal tract. Acute ulcers of sudden onset are found in association with a wide variety of disease processes and stress-causing states. Head trauma, septic states, and a wide varety of other factors have been implicated. One place where such acute ulcers are frequently encountered is in association with burn injuries.

HISTORY

The association between burn patient and ulcers has been recognized for roughly 150 years. It was first noted by Swan in Edinburgh in 1823. In France, in 1832, Dupuytren reported ulcers in the stomach in association with burns. In 1840, William B. Curling, a British surgeon, extensively reviewed ten cases of ulcers of the duodenum in patients with burns. All patients died, and all had severe gastrointestinal hemorrhage. This extensive and excellent review led to Curling's name being attached to problems of this type. The term Curling's ulcer is still sometimes widely used for post-burn duodenal ulcers and sometimes for any type of post-burn ulcer. After the original descriptive work recognizing the problem, relatively little occurred in regard to the management of such ulcers for many years. After the 1900s, as surgery for peptic ulceration became more common, there were reports of attempted operative intervention, occasionally with success. In the majority of cases, however, the combination of an ulcer complication sufficiently severe to require surgery, plus a large burn usually resulted in a fatal outcome. Additional isolated case reports continued to accumulate. Only fairly recently have series of cases been accumulated at any one center, however, with the largest group being those cases reported by Pruitt from Brooke Army Medical Center. Research into the pathogenesis and management of post-burn gastric and duodenal problems has gradually progressed.

ETIOLOGY

The basic cause of post-burn ulceration of the gastrointestinal tract remains unknown. It is felt that the presence of acid is essential to the development of stress ulcers and that the old clinical dictum "No acid, no ulcer" applies. For a number of years attempts to demonstrate increased acid in patients with stress ulcers were essentially unsuccessful. More recent studies appear to indicate that there actually is a relative increase in acid in those patients post burn who have progressed to the development of proven ulcers. It has also been shown that mucous production in the stomach is decreased post burn.

A wide variety of other mechanisms have been postulated as potential causes of this condition. Various theories have laid stress on hemoconcentration post burn. Impairment of the circulation to the mucosa has been demonstrated in a number of animal models and endoscopically in patients. It is of interest that mucosal circulatory changes and post-burn ulcers occur in germ-free mice with much the same frequency that they occur in normal controls.

Hormonal changes are known to occur in the post-burn state. Circulating levels of hormones known to be ulcerogenic, such as cortisol, adrenaline, and noradrenaline, are shown to be elevated. It has not been shown, however, that serum gastrin levels increase in the post-burn period. Burn toxins and neurogenic effects have been considered of importance by other authors.

INCIDENCE

The usual method by which the incidence of post-burn ulcers is determined has involved the tabulation of those ulcers discovered at autopsy and adding to this those patients with recognizable complications of actue ulceration, usually hemorrhage and free perforation. However, it is known that the actual incidence of ulcer disease is higher than this. Studies involving upper gastrointestinal radiography in burn patients, and more recently routine fiberoptic endoscopy, have been carried out. (Figure 1) These studies have shown that the incidence of clinically asymptomatic ulcers is higher than the figures that depend on autopsy material and complications would indicate. Sevitt and others have shown that the incidence of post-burn ulcers in children is higher than that encountered in burned adults. This is the reverse of the situation encountered in regard to peptic ulcer disease generally, where the attack rate in adults is far higher than that in children.

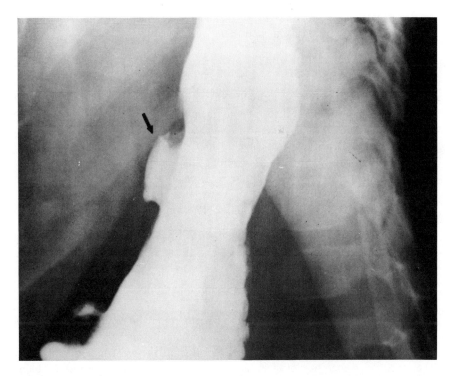

FIG. 1. This upper gastrointestinal series shows a deep penetrating stress ulcer of the lesser curvature of the stomach in a pateint with a 60% third degree burn.

Some case series have used the incidence of severe gastrointestinal hemorrhage as part of their measure of the presence or absence of ulcer disease. However, burn patients may have other problems predisposing them to gastrointestinal hemorrhage so that the figure obtained by this value may be inaccurate. This is especially true because most burn patients have some degree of gastritis. In earlier writings on the subject of stress ulcers post burn, it was found that symptomatic ulcers were uncommon in burns covering less than 20% of the body surface, and that they were also rare in patients with very large burns. However, the relative freedom of patients with very large burns from stress ulcers is now felt to have been a function of the fact that until recently patients with such burns had relatively brief life expectancies after sustaining their injuries. Therefore, the majority did not survive long enough to permit the development of frank ulcer disease. As patients with progressively larger burns have continued to survive, the ulcer incidence in this group of patients has increased. Reports of the ulcer incidence vary, depending on criteria employed for diagnosis. An all-over ulcer incidence of about 20%, as suggested by Moncrief, seems

to be a reasonable estimate of total ulcer incidence. This figure may be subject
to modification by prophylactic and therapeutic measures.

CLINICAL BURN COURSE

It is well documented that virtually all patients with large burns undergo a
transient episode of ileus. The mucous membranes of the gut, if observed in
experimental animals or by fiberoptic endoscopy, are seen to become blanched.
Multiple petechial hemorrhages develop in the lining of the stomach and duodenum. Subsequently, superficial erosions may develop in the mucous membranes. In some instances, the submucosa is penetrated, at which point they are
classified as ulcers. The majority of these erosions and ulcerations however,
remain small and clinically asymptomatic. If examinations of the stools of burn
patients are carried out routinely to check for the presence of blood, however,
small amounts of blood invisible to the naked eye will be detected in 60 to 80%
of all patients with extensive burns. Small, undetected erosions and ulcers are
felt to be the source of the bleeding. The majority of endoscopically visible
lesions in burn patients are otherwise asymptomatic or are associated only with
this subclinical bleeding.

Pain is almost never encountered as a patient complaint, even in patients with
proven ulcers. The typical peptic ulcer symptoms of pain related to meals and
relieved by milk and antacids are not reported in the great majority of cases.
Therefore the recognition of ulcers is relatively difficult unless a serious problem
develops. The most common first symptom reported in burn patients who
develop ulcer problems is hemorrhage. This may be minor, or it may progress to
massive exsanguinating hemorrhage and death. The problem of perforation of
the wall of the stomach or duodenum also occurs, with somewhat lesser frequency. In this case, gastric content escapes into the abdominal cavity and
causes a severe reactive peritonitis. Initially this inflammation is not infected by
bacteria, but relatively soon secondary infection develops, and the patient then
develops a bacterial peritonitis. A still less common problem, occasionally
encountered, is obstruction of the stomach. Non-burn patients with chronic
peptic ulcers may develop scarring of the pyloric outlet with vomiting and
eventually inability to eat. This problem develops very slowly, and this type of
scarring is not encountered in patients with post-burn acute ulcers. However, an
acute ulcer at the pyloric outlet may cause secondary spasm which can be suf-
ficently severe to cause temporary obstruction. The nutritional problems thus
created can be severe.

MANAGEMENT OF COMPLICATIONS

As stated, the most common complication of stress ulcers is hemorrhage. It is
estimated to be roughly five times as common as perforation. Bleeding may first

mainfest itself as vomiting of blood or recovery of blood from the nasogastric tube. In some instances, the passage of bright red blood from the rectum or the development of melena is the first indication of the problem. If bleeding is mild, anemia may be the first indication of difficulty. In this instance, other causes of anemia must be ruled out. If mild gastrointestinal bleeding is diagnosed, a program of conservative management by antacids and frequent feedings should be begun. If severe bleeding is present, the stomach should be emptied of blood and clots using a nasogastric tube, and a regimen of antacid management should be carried out. The nasogastric tube may be left in place, and antacids should be instilled hourly. Aspiration should be carried out at regular intervals. The patient should be progressively increased to a milk or tube feeding regimen as indicated. Since these patients usually have large burns, many will have indications for the use of tube feeding on nutritional grounds. The patient should be typed and cross-matched, and an intravenous line appropriate to the administration of blood should be inserted. Serial hematocrit determinations should be obtained at intervals of four to six hours, and the patient should be closely observed.

it is also desirable that the patient be evaluated for other problems that might compound the problems of a bleeding ulcer. Burn patients may develop bleeding diatheses for a variety of reasons. Such problems are usually secondary to septic states, but medication-related problems may be encountered. It is therefore desirable that a bleeding work-up be obtained at this time.

In many cases, probably the great majority, bleeding episodes are relatively limited in scope and respond well to conservative management. If hemorrhage is significant, work-up at this point is appropriate, and fiberoptic endoscopy should be carried out. If bleeding is severe, the usual additional conservative measures for its control should be tried. Iced saline lavage, intragastric installation of noradrenaline, and angiographic attempts to identify and control bleeding sources should be considered as appropriate.

It should be recognized that nonoperative attempts to control bleeding should not be unduly prolonged. Because the burn patients are usually gravely ill, and because there is often a reluctance to operate through a burn wound, management attempts by conservative means may be continued too long. In general, if an adult's blood loss exceeds three units in 24 hours, surgical intervention should be carried out promptly. Pruitt, and others, from Brooke Army Medical Center have reported 42 operative cases with 15 survivors. Seven of these patients recovered from the operative procedure but expired later of septic or other complications. The operation recommended by this group is subtotal gastrectomy and vagotomy. (Figure 2) They also stress that multiple ulcers are present in a significant number of cases. These should be searched for at the time of surgery. The majority of the Brooke cases were adults. In children, vagotomy and pyloroplasty has been recommended by some authors.

There is great reluctance to operate through a burn wound, and it should be recognized that laporatomy can be performed through eschar. The wound

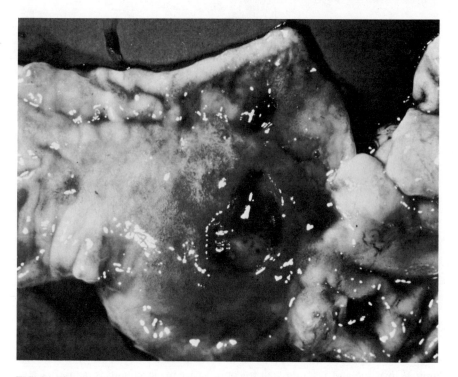

FIG. 2. This specimen includes the resected antrum of the stomach and the duodenum of a burn patient undergoing surgery for stress ulcer. A typical ulcer of the first portion of the duodenum is shown.

edges should be protected as far as possible by drapes, sewed to the wound margins. Subsequently, closure of the abdominal wall should be carried out with wire, and retention sutures are advised. Suture of the eschar should not be done, since this would result in infection. Subcutaneous fat may be loosely closed.

Perforation of post-burn ulcers is occasionally encountered. The incidence of perforation is about one-fifth the incidence of serious hemorrhage. The majority of such perforations are in the anterior wall of the duodenum, although perforations of the stomach are also encountered. When perforation occurs, the patient usually develops abdominal distention and ileus. The typical severe pain and boardlike rigidity of the abdomen commonly encountered in perforated peptic ulcers may be found. However, especially if the abdominal wall is burned, these findings may be masked. The difficulties in making the diagnosis are manifold. The burn patient is usually febrile, and leukocytosis is present; he may suffer from intermittent episodes of ileus and abdominal distention. Physical examination of a burned abdomen is difficult and unrewarding, and appropriate X-ray studies should be made when the clinical suspicion of perforation exists. Once the diagnosis has been made, there should be no hesitation about the decision to perform surgery. If necessary, circulating volume should be reestablished. A large-bore intravenous line should be inserted, and fluids should be given rapidly. Ringer's lactate or plasma may be suitable. If a Foley catheter is not in place, it should be inserted for monitoring urinary output. Intravenous antibiotics should be begun, and as soon as the patient is stable, laporatomy should be performed. The operation of choice usually consists of closure of the perforation, possibly with reenforcement by omentum. If surgery has been performed sufficiently early, a more aggressive operation may be appropriate. Postoperatively, if only simple suture of the perforation has been done, it should be recognized that the conditions leading to the formation of the ulcer are still operational, and, when bowel function has resumed, an antacid regimen should be implemented.

The problem of pylorospasm is occasionally encountered in burn patients. It usually presents as nausea and vomiting with meals. In such cases, several different diagnoses must be considered. Ileus secondary to sepsis is the most frequent cause of post-burn nausea and vomiting. If ileus is not present as demonstrated by the presence of active bowel sounds, fecal impaction should be considered. In the event that neither of these problems is present, the possibility of either a channel ulcer with pylorospasm or superior mesenteric artery compression syndrome should be considered, especially if the vomiting is frequently repeated and unduly prolonged. Occasionally, a patient with a large burn who has lost a great deal of weight will develop superior mesenteric artery compression of the terminal portion of the duodenum. This results in partial or complete obstruction of the third portion of the duodenum. The differential diagnosis of these two problems usually depends on the performance of an upper gastrointestinal series. In the event that duodenal compression syndrome is present, positioning of the patient in a semiupright position for feeding will usually take care of the problem. If a channel ulcer with spasm is the cause of the obstruction, it can usually be resolved by a period of several days of nasogastric suction, possibly with the intermittent installation of antacids through the nasogastric tube. If the patient is unable to eat for a prolonged period because of gastrointestinal problems, malnutrition may become a severe problem. Burn patients routinely enter a hypermetabolic state, and their caloric and protein needs are far greater than normal. Intravenous nutritional support should therefore be considered until oral feedings can be resumed.

PROPHYLAXIS

As indicated, the dictum "No acid, no ulcer" applies to stress ulcers as well as to other forms of ulcer disease. It was recognized clinically in several centers that regular administration of milk by drip on an around-the-clock basis drastically decreased the ulcer incidence post burn. Antacids are also felt to be of benefit. In a series of studies from Brooke Army Medical Center, it was shown that regular administration of antacids greatly decreases the complication rate and the actual incidence of stress ulcers. Therefore, regular prophylactic administration of some form of antacid regimen should be implemented in all hospitalized burn patients.

In recent years, it has also been recognized that many of the burn patients' problems have their genesis in secondary malnutrition. Sepsis is also known to cause stress ulcers. Therefore, it appears likely, although it has not been shown conclusively by experiment, that ulcer problems may be improved by better nutritional support. It is also felt that better control of sepsis will, in some degree, be reflected in a decreased ulcer incidence.

In the past few years Cimetidine has undergone extensive trial in the management of peptic ulcer disease. It appears likely that this drug will have application in the prevention and management of post-burn ulcer disease, but large-scale patient experience is not yet available.

LONG-TERM FOLLOW-UP

In the majority of cases where acute stress ulcers have been diagnosed during the acute burn phase, the problem disappears with healing of the burn. Once the patient is fully recovered, ulcers do not usually persist into the post-burn period. This, of course, does not apply to adults who have preexisting peptic ulcers at the time of their burn injury.

SUMMARY

The post-burn development of gastric and duodenal ulcers is a potentially life-threatening problem that contributes to the morbidity and the mortality of patients with large burns. The underlying cause of post-burn ulcers remains unknown. However, the problem depends on the presence of acid in the stomach; therefore, antacid prophylaxis will significantly reduce the incidence of ulcer disease. Once symptomatic complications have developed, conservative management can be employed to control most of these problems. In the event that uncontrollable hemorrhage does develop, or if free perforation occurs, surgical intervention should be carried out promptly. The mortality rate following these complications is high, but improving.

Further Reading

Czaja, A. J., McAlhany, J. C., Andes, W. A., et al. Acute gastric disease after cutaneous thermal injury. *Arch. Surg. 110*, May 1975.

Day, S. B., MacMillan, B. G., and Altemeier, W. A. *Curling's Ulcer: An Experiment of Nature*. Springfield, Illinois: Charles C. Thomas, 1972.

Einheber, A., Wren, R. E., Porro, R. F., et al. "Curling's ulcer" in the germfree mouse. *Nature 214,* April 1967.

McAlhany, J. C., Czaja, A. J., and Pruitt, B. A. Antacid control of complications from acute gastroduodenal disease after burns. *J. Trauma 16(8):* 645, 1976.

Moncrief, J. A., Switzer, W. E., and Teplitz, C., Curling's ulcer. *J. Trauma 4(4):* 481–494, 1964.

Pruitt, B. A., Foley, F. D., and Moncrief, J. A. Curling's ulcer: A clinical-pathology study of 323 cases. *Ann. Surg. 172(4):* 523–539, 1970.

Sevitt, Simon. Duodenal and gastric ulceration after burning. *Br. J. Surg. 54(1):* 32–41, 1967.

Watson, L. C., and Abston, S. Prevention of upper gastrointestinal hemorrhage in 582 burned children. *Am. J. Surg. 132:* 790–793, 1976.

Classification and Management of Pancreatitis

ANDREW L. WARSHAW, M.D.
Associate Professor of Surgery
Massachusetts General Hospital and
Harvard Medical School
Boston, Massachusetts

Pancreatitis is not a single entity. Inflammation of the pancreas can be acute or chronic, inconsequential or life-threatening, painful locally or disruptive to multiple organ systems. Included within the term pancreatitis are multiple diseases with multiple etiologies, expressions, and therapeutic requirements. Significant advances in knowledge in recent years have nonetheless underscored the limitations of our understanding of these processes.

ETIOLOGY

Table 1 lists antecedent "causes" of pancreatitis. With the exception of direct physical trauma to the pancreas and possibly the direct toxicity of excessive plasma lipids upon the pancreas, the exact pathogenetic relationship between these antecedents and pancreatic inflammation is not known. Explanations such

TABLE 1. Antecedent "Causes" of Pancreatitis

Acute	Chronic
alcohol (?)	alcohol
biliary disease	biliary disease (?)
hypercalcemia	hypercalcemia
hyperlipoproteinemia	hyperlipoproteinemia
trauma	trauma
peptic ulcer	heredity
ischemia	protein malnutrition
viral infection	Asian variety
drugs	
pregnancy	
tumors	
congenital abnormalities	

as obstruction of the pancreatic duct, chemical toxicity, or reflux of bile or duodenal fluids into the pancreas have proved to be simplistic and inadequate.

Activation of trypsin probably begins the process. This proteolytic enzyme can then activate other enzyme systems in the pancreas, including phospholipase A (lecithinase) and elastase. The action of phospholipase A includes catalyzing the conversion of biliary lecithin to lysolecithin which damages pancreatic tissues. Inasmuch as its other potential substrates include pulmonary surfactant and cell membrane phospholipids, release of activated phospholipase A may account for some systemic manifestations of pancreatitis. Elastase destroys the elastic lamina of arteries and veins and, along with other activated proteolytic enzymes, contributes to disruption of vascular integrity and local hemorrhage.

The sequence of pancreatic tissue injury starts with local inflammation, acinar disruption, and escape of activated pancreatic enzymes. Loss of plasma from the damaged pancreatic capillary endothelium causes sludging of the remaining red cells and compression of the capillaries by the swollen surrounding gland, and leads to decreased tissue perfusion, ischemia, and pancreatic necrosis. Release of vasoactive substances such as the kinins and histamine is believed to cause systemic capillary disruption, loss of plasma volume and vascular tone, and shock.

The above considerations apply primarily to acute pancreatitis. As will be discussed below, chronic pancreatitis is probably a different disease entity, and most of its forms develop insidiously by progressive parenchymal destruction and fibrosis.

CLASSIFICATION

The widely used Marseilles classification of pancreatitis, given in Table 2, has its own limitations. For example it is not possible clinically to distinguish between

TABLE 2. Marseilles Classification of Pancreatitis

I. *Acute* (single attack)

II. *Acute recurrent* (multiple attacks, normal pancreatic histology during asymptomatic intervals)

III. *Chronic recurrent* (multiple attacks with asymptomatic intervals, but permanent tissue injury established)

IV. *Chronic persistent* (pain unremitting or very frequent, steatorrhea, or diabetes; also includes asymptomatic variant with pancreatic calcifications or proven fibrosis)

Stage II and Stage III; to do so would require histologic examination of the pancreas. Also, the word "stage" implies the possibility of evolution. Actually the transition of true acute pancreatitis into chronic pancreatitis (Stage I or II going on to stage III or IV) is rare indeed. Biliary pancreatitis almost never becomes chronic, and alcoholic pancreatitis usually shows permanent pathological changes in the pancreas at the time of the first clinical presentation. Table 1 emphasizes the separate sets of causes for acute and chronic pancreatitis and illustrates how little overlap there is. True transition from acute to chronic pancreatitis may occur in some abnormal metabolic states (hyperparathyroidism, hyperlipidemia) and, rarely, in that form of biliary tract disease wherein fibrosis at the orifice of the pancreatic duct propagates the pancreatic injury.

It is practical and useful to classify pancreatitis simply as (a) acute (one or two attacks), (b) recurrent acute (three or more attacks, clinically well in intervals), and (c) chronic (persistent symptoms of pain or signs of diabetes, malabsorption, or pancreatic calcification). It is implicit that within these categories the disease is still not a uniform entity, that "pancreatitis" may be many similar but different diseases.

DIAGNOSIS

The pillar of laboratory diagnosis of acute pancreatitis is an elevated serum amylase. Amylase, however, may also rise in a variety of other diseases involving the intestine, liver, genitourinary tract, lung, and salivary glands, and in metabolic derangements such as diabetic ketoacidosis. Because renal tubular reabsorption of amylase decreases in acute pancreatitis, renal clearance of amylase increases. The amylase/creatinine clearance ratio, based upon this phenomenon, has been found to be a generally reliable index of acute pancreatitis and to differentiate it from other causes of elevated serum amylase.[1] Amylase clearance does not increase in chronic pancreatitis.

Other laboratory tests, such as serum calcium, glucose, and bilirubin, do not add much to differential diagnosis, but may help to indicate the severity of the attack and to prognosticate the likelihood of major complications or death. Major attempts are being made to develop objective criteria for evaluating acute pancreatitis,[2] and for selecting the 5 to 10% of patients who will go on to have the fulminant form of the disease. These criteria will greatly simplify the task of evaluating new approaches to therapy.

Radiographic aids to diagnosis remain limited. Plain roentgenograms of the abdomen may or may not show a "sentinel loop" of intestine, which is non-specific in any case. Upper gastrointestinal barium studies often but not invariably show evidence of pancreatic swelling and inflammation. Ultrasound may show pancreatic edema, but there are too many false positives and negatives to generate confidence. Calcification within the pancreas occurs only in some cases of chronic pancreatitis.

Although new techniques such as analysis of serum isoenzymes of amylase may be more helpful in the future, at present there remain difficulties and uncertainties in our ability to diagnose pancreatitis. These difficulties carry over into problems of treatment.

MANAGEMENT

Acute Pancreatitis

Ninety to 95% of cases of acute pancreatitis subside spontaneously. This is fortunate, for we know no better how to stop the process than we know how it got started. Our treatment is limited to the general approach of resting the pancreas by fasting and nasogastric suction in order to reduce the hormonal stimuli to pancreatic secretion. Drugs such as Trasylol (aprotinin), which inhibits trypsin and other proteolytic enzymes, or glucagon, which inhibits pancreatic secretion, have been ineffective in clinical trials. Antibiotics, intended to reduce the incidence of secondary infections, have had no proven benefit either. For the vast majority of cases, surgery is entirely unnecessary unless the diagnosis is sufficiently in doubt because of severe signs of peritoneal inflammation that exploratory laparotomy is necessary to exclude visceral perforation or infarction.[3] Note that an elevated serum amylase also occurs in these latter circumstances.

Some surgeons have espoused immediate common duct exploration for patients whose pancreatitis is caused by choledocholithiasis, with the aim of mitigating the attack. This philosophy depends upon being able to distinguish patients with stones from those without them. In our experience, this differential diagnosis may be extremely difficult, inasmuch as serum bilirubin and alkaline phosphatase will rise equally whether due to intraluminal biliary obturation or extraluminal compression by edema. The exception is a subgroup of patients with "pseudopancreatitis," who have hyperamylasemia due to an impacted common duct stone, but no significant pancreatic inflammation.[1] Clinically these patients have no major signs of pancreatitis (pancreatic tenderness or mass, volume requirement, hypocalcemia, shock), and chemically the amylase/creatinine clearance ratio is within normal limits despite the increased serum amylase. Especially if the presence of gallstones can be confirmed by ultrasonography, this subgroup of patients can be safely operated upon immediately with the expectation that the pancreas will appear normal and that there is no increased risk of postoperative pancreatitis.

In a small minority of cases—5 to 10%—the process is not self-limited but takes a fulminant course, manifested by major intravascular plasma loss, hypotension, renal failure, profound hypocalcemia, and respiratory failure. The mortality in such patients exceeds 50%, and the major complication rate exceeds 50% in the survivors. Although it is common practice to refer to this form of the disease as hemorrhagic pancreatitis, its hallmark is really pancreatic *necrosis* (Figure 1), probably the result of ischemic injury due to reduced perfusion of the gland. The urgent problem in early management is cardiovascular collapse: the generalized leaky capillary endothelium, volume losses, tachycardia, and hyperdynamic shock. These phenomena are believed to be induced by the vasoactive substances released from the pancreas into peritoneal exudate, and it is increasingly accepted that removal of this toxic ascitic fluid has a profoundly and rapidly beneficial effect on the cardiovascular status of the patient. Technically this can be accomplished by peritoneal lavage using standard percutaneous dialysis techniques; in some cases, however, the toxic fluid may be loculated in the lesser peritoneal sac, so that the dialysis catheter placed anteriorly in the general peritoneal cavity is ineffective. If the

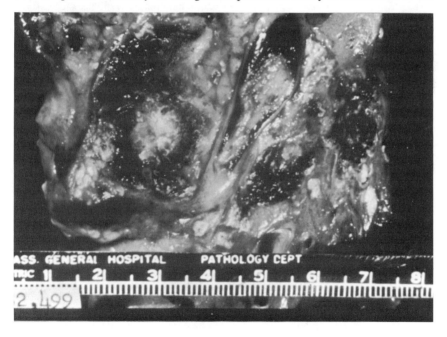

FIG. 1.

patient is not unequivocally improving within a few lavages, the lavage catheters should be replaced operatively in the lesser sac. If laparotomy is to be undertaken, consideration should be given at that time to placing gastrostomy, feeding jejunostomy, and cholecystostomy tubes to anticipate the patient's longer-term problems with ileus, biliary and gastrointestinal obstruction, nutrition, and sepsis.[3]

Lavage therapy for acute fulminant necrotizing pancreatitis should be viewed as an emergency resuscitative maneuver, intended to keep a dying patient alive. If it is successful, as it will be in up to 90% of cases, this group of patients still remains at high risk of subsequent major complications, the sequelae of pancreatic necrosis.[4] If the quantity of tissue necrosis is sufficient to be manifested as increasing pancreatic inflammation, usually seven to ten days after the onset of pancreatitis, surgical debridement is necessary. Other complications of this still-sterile inflammatory process include gastroduodenal obstruction and thrombosis of contiguous blood vessels, leading to infarction of the colon or small intestine. Secondary infection of the necrotic tissue produces a pancreatic abscess, which is almost always fatal unless it is surgically drained. Even with drainage, the mortality of pancreatic abscesses is more than 30%.

Pancreatic pseudocysts are collections of pancreatic secretions that have escaped from damaged pancreas and, unresorbed, have become encapsulated with granulation and fibrous tissue. It is now recognized that many peripancreatic fluid collections formed during acute pancreatitis will be successfully reabsorbed, and that pseudocysts represent the failure of that process. Pseudocysts that persist for more than four to six weeks are unlikely ever to resolve spontaneously and carry excessive risk of complications such as hemorrhage, rupture, or infection. These persisting pseudocysts should be surgically drained, preferably by internal anastomosis to the upper GI tract.[4]

Recurrent Acute Pancreatitis

The management of recurrent attacks of pancreatitis is no different from that of the first attack, but the identification and elimination of causative factors assumes increasing importance. The likely possibilities include toxic drugs (alcohol, estrogens, corticosteroids, azothioprine, sulfonamides), gallstones, metabolic abnormalities (hypercalcemia, Type I or V hyperlipoproteinemia), and anatomic abnormalities (papillitis, congenital abnormalities).

Many of the tests used in searching for these factors must be performed during a quiescent interval between attacks. Cholecystography, for example, is unreliable in the presence of pancreatitis, although ultrasonography can be used at any time to look for gallstones. Underlying hypercalcemia due to hyperparathyroidism may be masked by the depression of serum calcium that occurs during the acute attack. Hyperlipidemia can be considered a treatable antecedent cause, not simply a concomitant feature of the acute phase, only if it persists during the convalescent phase.

The attempt to identify anatomic abnormalities is best delayed until well into convalescence to avoid stimulating recrudescence of the pancreatitis. The form of papillitis that appears to be a legitimate cause of recurrent pancreatitis involves the orifice of the pancreatic duct. The diagnosis is suggested by a positive morphine-prostigmine test (morphine 10 mg IM + prostigmine 1 mg IM → threefold rise in serum amylase over next three hours with reproduction of "pancreatic pain"). Confidence in the diagnosis is strengthened by the demonstration of a tight pancreatic duct orifice during endoscopic retrograde cannulation. Pancreatograms are usually normal nonetheless. Treatment is by transduodenal sphincteroplasty including transampullary septectomy.

Chronic Pancreatitis

The manifestations of chronic pancreatitis range from nothing to constant severe pain, from apparently normal function to endocrine insufficiency (diabetes) or exocrine insufficiency (malabsorption, particularly fat). The pain may be constant, intermittent, or present only during defined attacks (relapses). Medical treatment of the disease consists of providing insulin, oral pancreatic enzymes to aid food digestion, and analgesics. Surgical treatment is directed exclusively at pain relief; despite some claims to the contrary, no surgical procedure can restore the functions of a destroyed pancreas or even prevent further loss of function. Whether and when pain is sufficient to warrant surgery becomes an individual decision influenced by narcotic need, control of alcoholism, and the degree of disruption of the patient's life. Of parallel importance in decision making are the odds that a given surgical procedure will relieve the pain, for not all patients have pathological anatomy that permits successful palliation. Obviously, the better the chances of a good result, the sooner and more enthusiastically will surgery be advised by the physician and accepted by the patient.

There are a number of operations for chronic pancreatitis. The radiographic configuration of the pancreatic and bile ducts, preferably obtained by preoperative peroral endoscopic retrograde cannulation of the ampulla of Vater and injection of contrast medium (ERCP), provides the best means for choosing the operative procedure optimally suited to the individual pathologic anatomy and most likely to be effective. This information is supplemented by examination of the pancreas by ultrasound or CT scanning to detect pseudocysts (Figure 2). As a corollary, it is then possible to predict preoperatively the chances for postoperative pain relief.

Pseudocysts. These extraductal encapsulated collections of pancreatic juice, discussed previously with acute pancreatitis, are actually much more commonly a feature of chronic pancreatitis, in which pain is their major manifestation.

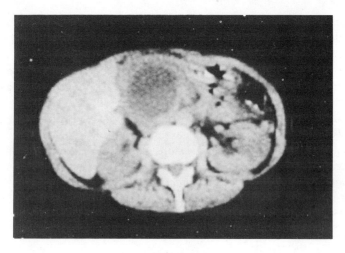

FIG. 2.

Finding a pseudocyst is in effect fortunate because a relatively high rate of pain relief (about 70%) follows surgical drainage by anastomosis to stomach or intestine. Pain persisting after pseudocyst drainage is presumably due to the underlying chronic pancreatitis and may require further therapy. Pain recurring later may be due to a new pseudocyst.

Ductal Dilatation. In contrast to the 3-mm diameter of the normal main pancreatic duct (Figure 3), the duct in some patients with chronic pancreatitis may measure 15 mm or more (Figure 4). It is widely assumed, but never proved, that this dilatation results from obstruction by fibrosis. Partial stenoses at several points may produce a "chain-of-lakes" appearance. Ductal dilatation, offering excellent prospects for pain relief, is treated by lateral pancreatico-jejunostomy (modified Peustow procedure). A long anastomosis is made between a Roux-en-y limb of jejunum and the pancreatic duct, which has been fileted open for as much of its length as possible (Figure 5). Pain is relieved in up to 90% of patients who stop drinking.

Ductal Sclerosis. This form of the disease, characterized by general narrowing of the main pancreatic duct and its branches by fibrosis, does not lend itself to decompressing anastomoses and is more difficult to palliate successfully. The most common treatment is by resection of part or all of the pancreas. Distal (hemi-) pancreatectomy is technically easy but not often effective because the disease is not often confined to the tail of the pancreas. The 95% distal pancreatectomy (Child procedure) is technically difficult, ensures the onset of diabetes, and has been unreliable in giving pain relief. Resection of the head of the pancreas (Whipple procedure) or all of it is a major undertaking not within the scope of all surgeons or all hospitals. Even so, successful pain relief follows

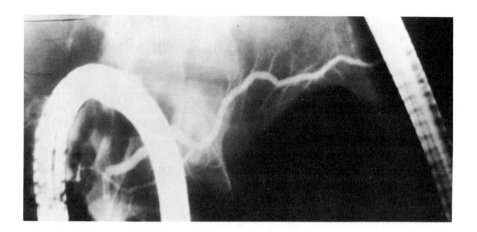

FIG. 3.

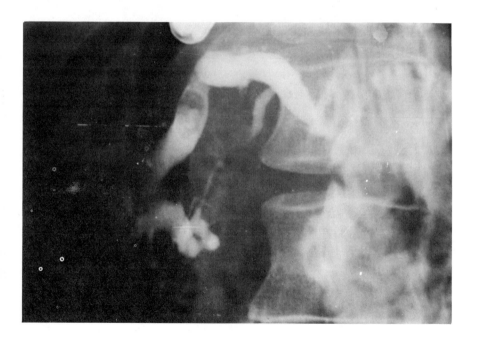

FIG. 4.

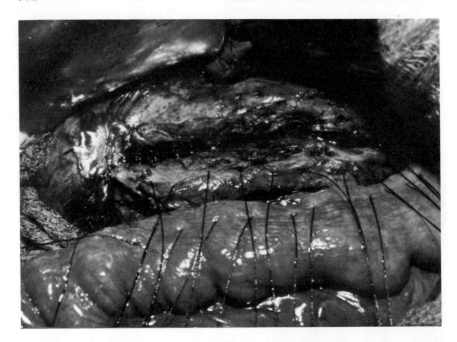

FIG. 5.

in only half of the patients. Attempts are being made to ameliorate the problem of induced (pancreatico-prival) diabetes after total pancreatectomy by harvesting the islet cells from the removed tissue and reinfusing them into the portal vein to plant them in liver. Overall, pancreatic resection in my view has been a disappointing mode of treatment for chronic pancreatitis.

An alternative operation which yields about 50% success at a lower cost is the vagotomy, distal gastrectomy, and gastrojejunostomy. This approach is based upon the principle of permanently "resting" the pancreas (as nasogastric suction is used in acute pancreatitis) by eliminating neural and hormonal stimuli to pancreatic secretion. It is not a panacea but is simple, is minimally destructive, and may be helpful for patients who are troubled enough to take a chance on it.

Common Bile Duct Stenosis. The lower common duct, passing through the head of the pancreas, is at risk of being narrowed by the surrounding inflammation and fibrosis (Figure 6). The stenosis can cause obstructive jaundice (mimicking pancreatic carcinoma), secondary biliary cirrhosis, acute suppurative cholangitis, or chronic low-grade cholangitis and pain. This pain may be indistinguishable from pancreatic pain. Serum alkaline phosphatase elevation is the most consistent, although not specific, laboratory index of the phenomenon. The possibility of intrapancreatic common duct stenosis means that a cholangiogram is mandatory whenever operative treatment of chronic pancreatitis is con-

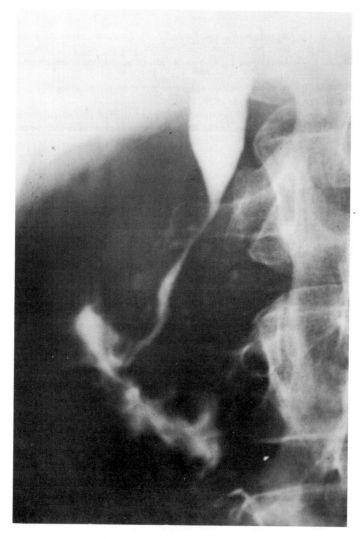

FIG. 6.

templated. Relief of the chronic partial common duct obstruction may in fact be all that is needed to relieve pain in some cases.[5]

References

1. Warshaw, A. L., and Fuller, A. F., Jr. Specificity of increased renal clearance of amylase in diagnosis of acute pancreatis. *N. Engl. J. Med. 292:* 325, 1975.

2. Ranson, J. H. C., Rifkind, K. M., and Turner, J. W. Prognostic signs and nonoperative peritoneal lavage in acute pancreatitis. *Surg. Gynecol. Obstet. 143*: 209, 1976.
3. Warshaw, A. L., Imbembo, A. L., Civetta, J. M., et al. Surgical intervention in acute necrotizing pancreatitis. *Am. J. Surg. 127*: 484, 1974.
4. Warshaw, A. L. Inflammatory masses following acute pancreatitis: Phlegmon pseudocyst, and abscess. *Surg. Clin. N. Am. 54*: 621, 1974.
5. Warshaw, A. L., Schapiro, R. H., Ferrucci, J. T., Jr. et al. Persistent obstructive jaundice, cholangitis, and biliary cirrhosis due to common bile duct stenosis in chronic pancreatis. *Gastroenterology 70*: 562, 1976.

Portal Hypertension—What Is the Best Way to Treat Bleeding from Varices?

KENNETH G. SWAN, M.D.
MACEO M. HOWARD, M.D.
JOYCE M. ROCKO, M.D.
BENJAMIN F. RUSH, JR., M.D.
Departments of Surgery and Medicine
College of Medicine and Dentistry of New Jersey
New Jersey Medical School
Newark, New Jersey

Cirrhosis of the liver is currently the sixth ranking cause of death in the United States, and bleeding from esophageal varices is the leading cause of death from patients who have cirrhosis of the liver.[2]

Although, traditionally, the management of acute bleeding from esophageal varices is a medical, as opposed to a surgical problem, the surgeon is nonetheless frequently called upon to participate in the initial evaluation of the patient who has sustained a life-threatening hemorrhage from bleeding esophageal varices. The management of this condition reflects operative as well as nonoperative considerations. The nonoperative considerations include the use of such traditional techniques as the Sengstaken-Blakemore tube and parenteral vasopressin.

The Sengstaken-Blakemore tube (Figure 1) is a combination of externally

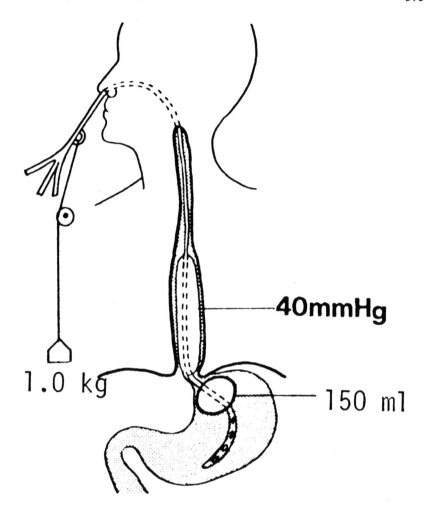

FIG. 1. Sengstaken Blakemore technic.

applied forces that attempts to apply direct pressure upon the esophageal varices, or their collateral circulation, within the proximal portion of the stomach, utilizing balloon tamponade. The latter is most appropriately applied to the proximal stomach, since there are well recognized complications of the utilization of the esophageal balloon. The latter may become necessary should traction upon the gastric balloon fail to arrest bleeding from esophageal varices. This therapeutic failure is recognized by continued bleeding from an additional nasogastric tube placed in the region of the esophagogastric junction (Figure 1), while the gastric balloon is inflated and under tension (1.0 kg).

Use of the esophageal balloon is attended by two important complications: distal esophageal stricture, secondary to prolonged use of the esophageal balloon and pressure necrosis of the esophageal wall, and asphyxiation, secondary to rupture of the gastric balloon, which allows the esophageal balloon to progress rapidly to the oropharynx. The latter hazard relates to the fact that the entire mechanism is usually placed upon 2.2 lb (1 kg, 1 liter of fluid) traction, and the sudden appearance of the esophageal balloon within the oropharynx causes asphyxiation and results in sudden death. This potential complication has led many clinicians to interdict use of the esophageal balloon by literally cutting off the esophageal balloon catheter prior to insertion of the Sengstaken-Blakemore tube. If a Sengstaken-Blakemore tube is to be inserted for the management of acute bleeding from esophageal varices, then the patient should be assigned to an intensive care unit where a nurse, or another allied health professional, is in constant attendance with a surgical scissor available for immediate transection of the esophageal balloon catheter, should the gastric balloon rupture. Likewise, care must be directed to the traction upon the Sengstaken-Blakemore tube in that compression necrosis of the nares can attend the use of this tube, if it is not carefully monitored. Also, esophageal rupture can occur if undue tension is placed upon an inadequately filled ($<$ 150 ml) gastric balloon.

The use of vasopressin (the naturally occurring octapeptide of posterior pituitary gland origin, which is made commercially available, utilizing extraction procedures from bovine and porcine pituitary glands, by the Parke-Davis Company) is based upon the premise that this potent vascular smooth muscle stimulant (vasoconstriction) reduces blood flow through almost all major vascular beds. With regard to the portal venous system, the use of vasopressin is predicated upon its mesenteric arterial constrictor effects which reduce blood flow through the gut and, therefore, through the portal vein and cause commensurate reductions in portal venous pressure. Recent reports indicate that vasopressin, whether administered intra-arterially or intravenously, causes comparable reductions in superior mesenteric blood flow (Figure 2) in the subhuman primate,[3] and, thus, suggest that this agent, at a dose of 10^{-1} units/kg of body weight/min, can be instituted immediately for the control of portal hypertension in portal hypertensive man. Although previous investigation[4] had suggested that this agent could be utilized more efficaciously with the intra-arterial (superior mexenteric artery) route, recent studies have suggested that this is, in fact, not the case, and that even in portal hypertensive man, the agent can be used with minimal side effects when compared to the intra-arterial route, if delivered intravenously to accomplish the same result.[5]

Thus, this agent should be considered in the initial management of a patient who is presumed to be bleeding, based upon endoscopic determination of the

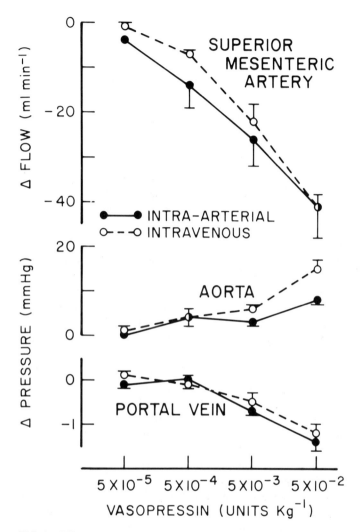

FIG. 2. Effects of vasopressin upon primate mesenteric hemodynamics.

presence of bleeding from esophageal varices and a history of chronic liver disease, whether due to chronic alcoholism, postnecrotic cirrhosis, or other disease states such as schistosomiasis. An easy technique for determining the desired concentration, or dose rate, is to assess the patient's total body weight in kilograms and divide this value by four. The result of this equation (Figure 3) expressed in terms of ampoules (20 units/ampoule at a volume of 1 ml/ampoule) of vasopressin, when diluted by a liter of solute, such as 10% dextrose, provides a

$$\frac{\text{Weight (kg)}}{4} = \text{Number of ampoules (vasopressin)}$$
$$\text{per liter solute*}$$

---

*Delivered I.V./ 1.0 ml/min = 5×11^{-3} units/kg-min

FIG. 3.

concentration that can be delivered at a rate of 1 ml/min, intravenously, to accomplish a relatively safe vasopressor effect of vasopressin (5×10^{-3} units/kg-min.).

Since the effects of vasopressin upon arterial pressure are more subtle than the effects of this agent upon pulse,[6] the clinician utilizing this agent should monitor both parameters, but, more specifically, pulse and electrocardiographic evidence of cardiac arrhythmia to demonstrate possible toxic side effects of vasopressin, particularly in the older age group. If there is significant bradycardia, or significant hypertension, or the presence of arrhythmias, then the patient is sustaining possible toxic effects of vasopressin, and the rate of administration of this drug should be commensurately reduced.

If these measures fail to control the bleeding from esophageal varices, then the possibility exists that utilizing percutaneous transhepatic portographic techniques, the varices themselves can be cannulated, or at least the tributaries of the varices, and appropriate sclerotic agents such as autologous blood clot, powdered gelfoam, and sodium sotradecol can be effectively used to close off the tributaries to these varices or the varices themselves.[7]

Should the above measures fail to control bleeding from esophageal varices, then the surgeon is presented with the problem of whether emergency surgery should be implemented. This decision is, of course, based upon the physical condition of the patient and, in general, a Child's classification[8] C will not tolerate emergency surgery well. The fact that a certain percentage of such patients do survive emergency surgery for control of bleeding from esophageal varices has caused patient selection to appear ambivalent and has led many to search for a more meaningful categorization of such patients and their operative risks. Likewise, a Child's classification A patient bleeding from esophageal varices may not necessarily survive emergency surgery for control of that condition and for similarly unclear reasons. In general, however, emergency surgery should be relegated to those patients who are in relatively good condition with regard to operative risk, namely, Child's classification A andB patients.

At the time of surgery, the question of the operative procedure of choice is primarily a personal one and relates to the use of either the traditional portacaval (Eck fistula) shunt,[9] the mesocaval (Drapanas) shunt,[10] or the more recently introduced distal splenorenal (Warren) shunt.[11] In the hands of its most devout proponent, the emergency portacaval shunt (Figure 4) carries a 50% mortality from the operative procedure, but this has to be balanced against the alleged 80% nonoperative mortality among patients who have been documented to bleed from esophageal varices secondary to portal hypertension and cirrhosis of the liver and who, in fact, are discharged from the hospital after initial cessation of bleeding from the varices and, therefore, fail to return for definitive surgical care. The mesocaval shunt (Figure 5) is a relatively simple procedure compared to the alternate operative procedures to control bleeding from esophageal varices as an emergent procedure and depending upon the experience of the surgeon. The operative mortality is approximately 10%, and the incidence of post-shunt encephalopathy is acceptable (10%).[10] The distal splenorenal shunt (Figure 6) had been reserved as a procedure for the elective management of bleeding from esophageal varices; however, the proponents of this procedure have more recently recommended that it be used in the emergent control of the same condition and have reported a reasonably acceptable success rate with the use of this procedure under these circumstances.[12]

If the initial bleeding episode is brought under control with appropriate nonoperative measures, then the question of elective surgery for the prevention of a future, possibly life-threatening, exsanguinating hemorrhage from esophageal varices is a controversial issue. The question of whether to utilize the standard portacaval shunt, the mesocaval (Drapanas) shunt, or the more recently introduced distal splenorenal (Warren) shunt is unsettled at the present time. The

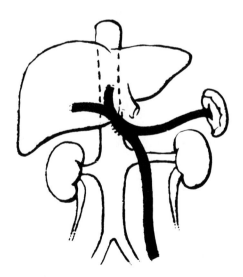

FIG. 4. Side by side portocaval.

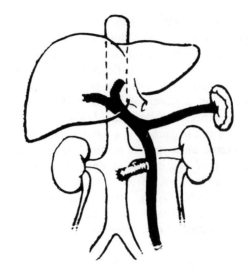

FIG. 5. "H" graftmesocaval.

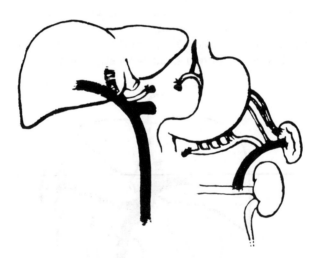

FIG. 6. Distal splenorenal.

dispute as to the procedure of choice may reflect the individual surgeon's experience with and, therefore, facility with any given operative procedure. For
most, the distal splenorenal (Warren) shunt is a more technically formidable
procedure than is the traditional portacaval (Eck fistula) shunt or the mesocaval
(Drapanas) shunt.

In the case of the portacaval shunt, the surgical procedure is aimed at reducing portal venous pressure and presumably, therefore, pressure within esophageal varices by achieving a direct anastomosis between the portal vein and the inferior vena cava. In the case of the mesocaval shunt, the technical considerations are based upon the premise that the superior mesenteric vein can be anastomosed to the inferior vena cava while, at the same time, permitting adequate perfusion of the liver through its portal vein via the contributaries of the latter, namely, the splenic vein and inferior mesenteric vein. The basic premise that supports the use of the distal splenorenal (Warren) shunt is that selective decompression of esophageal varices, by way of the short gastric veins leading to the spleen and the splenic vein leading to the left renal vein, can decompress the varices while, at the same time, maintaining portal venous (superior mesenteric and inferior mesenteric veins) perfusion of the liver, which in fact is dependent upon this source of blood for its basic nutritional sustenance.

The results of all of these procedures are described in terms of (1) prevention of existent or recurrent hemorrhage, (2) preservation of hepatic function, and (3) prevention of hepatic encephalopathy. The proponents of the various operative procedures describe minimal operative mortality when these procedures are used electively and minimal hepatic encephalopathy or deterioration of hepatic function postoperatively. The problem in assessing the results of all of these reports relates to the lack of an adequate and scientifically validated definition of hepatic encephalopathy. To date, there are few hard data to support the use of one operative procedure over the other, with regard to the incidence of hepatic encephalopathy. This statement is based upon the fact that, as yet, there is little available information to define this medical/surgical phenomenon, or to predict its ultimate outcome, let alone its most appropriate clinical management. The optimal surgical procedure, whether utilized electively or as an emergent means of managing exsanguinating hemorrhage from esophageal varices, awaits ultimate definition.

Other considerations in the management of portal hypertension through surgical measures include the use of the peritoneal–jugular venous (LeVeen) shunt[13] for the management of intractible (refractory to nonoperative measures such as salt restriction, diuretic therapy, protein limitation, and alcohol abstinence) ascites. In the hands of some, the LeVeen shunt (Figure 7) not only has been critical to the relief of refractory ascites, but also has minimized the incidence of other complications of cirrhosis of the liver and portal hypertension.[14] Nonetheless, this procedure remains controversial, and its ultimate use awaits further definition of indications, contraindications, and immediate, as well as long-term, results. The use of sclerosing agents administered either operatively through cannulation of the coronary veins or nonoperatively through percutaneous transhepatic cannulation of the portal venous sytem, likewise awaits long-term definition of indications, contraindications, and results before

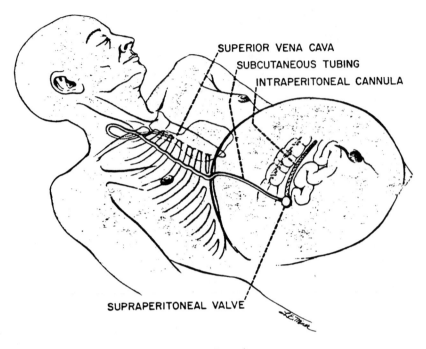

SUPERIOR VENA CAVA
SUBCUTANEOUS TUBING
INTRAPERITONEAL CANNULA

SUPRAPERITONEAL VALVE

FIG. 7. Le Veen shunt.

it can be advocated routinely. Finally, when all else fails, the possibility of hepatic transplantation is always a consideration, but as yet, as in the case of cardiac transplantation, relatively few centers, whether in the United States or abroad, recommend it, based upon successful results of the use of this operative procedure for the management of cirrhosis of the liver and its attendant portal hypertension and associated complications.

References

Report from the Center for Health Statistics. *AMA News,* May 1978.

Snyder, N., Reboucas, G., Conn, M., et al. The effect of esophageal varices on prognosis in cirrhosis. *Gastroenterology 74*: 1163, 1978.

Freedman, A. R., Kerr, J. C., Swan, K. G., et al. Primate mesenteric blood flow: Effects of vasopressin and its route of delivery. *Gastroenterology 74*: 875, 1978.

Baum, S., and Nusbaum, M. The control of gastrointestinal hemorrhage by selective mesenteric arterial infusion of vasopressin. *Radiology 98*: 497, 1971.

Johnson, W. C., Widrich, W. C., Ansell, J. E., et al. Control of bleeding varices by vasopressin: A prospective randomized study. *Ann. Surg. 186*: 369, 1977.

Howard, M. M., Leevy, C. M., Rocko, J. M., et al. Vasopressin and portal venous pressure in portal hypertensive cirrhotic patients. *Gastroenterology 74*: 1162, 1978.

Pereiras, R., Viamonte, M., Hutson, D., et al. Transhepatic obliteration of gastroesophageal varices. *Gastroenterology 70*: 990, 1976.

Childs, C. G., and Turcotte, J. G. Surgery and portal hypertension. In *The Liver and Portal Hypertension,* C. G. Childs, ed. Philadelphia: W. B. Saunders Co., 1964.

Eck, N. V. Kvoprosu O perevyazkie voratnoi veni predvarritelnoye soolshtshenize. *Voyena Med. J. 130*: 2, 1877.

Drapanas, T. Interposition mesocaval shunt for treatment of portal hypertension. *Ann. Surg. 176*: 437, 1967.

Levi, J. U. Present status of the distal splenorenal shunt. 10th Annual Meeting of the Association for Academic Surgery, November 1976.

LeVeen, H., Christoudias, G., Ip, M., et al. Peritoneovenous shunting for ascites. *Ann. Surg. 180*: 580, 1974.

Reinhardt, G. F. Personal communication, 1978.

Inflammatory Bowel Disease

NOEL B. HERSHFIELD, M.D., F.R.C.P. (C)., F.A.C.P.
Associate Professor of Internal Medicine
University of Calgary
Alberta, Canada

This review will discuss ulcerative colitis and Crohn's disease only, since they are the most common forms of inflammatory bowel disease in present-day North American practice. Other disorders mimicking these conditions, such as ischemic colitis, diverticular disease, amoebic dysentry, and so on, will not be discussed. The review will only touch on the most important problems pertaining to these diseases in the writer's opinion, and the reader is advised to consult the many pertinent monographs, books, and journals for detailed information.

The problem of inflammatory bowel disease appears to be increasing. Epidemiological studies are few, and difficult to obtain, since the disease appears to differ in incidence in various parts of the world. The criteria for diagnosis are sometimes not stated. Figures from Baltimore and Oxford suggest an incidence for ulcerative colitis of 5 to 10 per 100,000 of the population. However, most authorities believe the incidence is considerably higher. Whether the problem is really becoming more common or whether it is being discovered more frequently, is not known at present. Geographic differences, however, *do* appear to be important.

The disease appears to affect young productive people although the literature states that ulcerative colitis is a bimodal incidence, in the second and third decades and then in the fifth and sixth decades. We, however, rarely see it over the age of 40 years in this area. Crohn's disease can occur at any age, but again the vast majority of our cases are teen-agers or young adults. We rarely see it in patients over the age of 40, at least in its initial presentation.

Another puzzling feature is the relatively high incidence of Jewish patients in certain studies in the United States, although this preponderance is apparently decreasing. This disease appears to affect middle-class intelligent productive people.

Inflammatory bowel disease consists of two major pathological entities: ulcerative colitis and granulomatous disease of the gastrointestinal tract or Crohn's disease. Ulcerative colitis involves the colon only, with the concept of back-wash ileitis being controversial. Crohn's disease can affect any part of the gastrointestinal tract from mouth to anus, but the terminal ileum and right colon are by far the most common sites of occurrence. A pure form of Crohn's disease of the colon exists and is becoming more frequently recognized. The patients with back-wash ileitis may well have a mixture of the two diseases, but at the present time this concept remains speculative.

The name granulomatous disease of the gastrointestinal tract is a misnomer. Approximately 50% of the cases of Crohn's disease do have granuloma under the microscope. It is preferred therefore, to use the term transmural gut disease when describing Crohn's disease, since the inflammation involves the mucosa, the total wall of the intestines, and the peri-intestinal structures.

The term mucosal colitis is sometimes used for ulcerative colitis although this term is not satisfactory. In the fulminant form of chronic ulcerative colitis transmural inflammation with perforation can occur. Perhaps these features are apropos of these diseases, since they are so enigmatic in most of their other features as well.

The cause of these diseases is unknown despite considerable research carried out since the second decade of this century. No infectious agent, no altered immunological process, no food or drink, and no abnormal mental pattern have been satisfactorily incriminated to explain the cause. The cause or causes are likely multifactorial.

The diseases vary markedly in their intensity. Ulcerative colitis is mainly a benign disease, which usually causes relatively little problem to the patient when properly managed. Nevertheless it can be fulminating and cause death, and can require all the skill of the attending physician. Crohn's disease, on the other hand, is far more debilitating. Almost all the patients with Crohn's colitis have surgery; at least 80% of the patients in my experience with small-intestinal Crohn's disease reach the operating room. In addition, recurrence after Crohn's disease surgery is frequent. Over 70% recur after the first operation and over

50% after the second. Conversely, in ulcerative colitis the establishment of ileostomy is virtually curative.

Recognition of these diseases is important, since early treatment can affect the life style although it is arguable that it does anything to stop the progress of the disease. Since the disease appears to be more common now than at any time previously, our index of suspicion must be extremely high. Anyone with the symptoms outlined below that last longer than 6 weeks, has inflammatory bowel disease until it is proved otherwise.

By far the most common presentation is chronic diarrhea. The association of blood in the diarrhea usually means that the patient has ulcerative colitis, although bloody stools can also occur in Crohn's disease more frequently than one would suspect from reading the literature.

Failure to thrive, especially in infants and children, should alert the physician to the possibility of inflammatory bowel disease. In the adult, rapid weight loss is extremely common, and this is especially true in patients with Crohn's disease.

A common feature of Crohn's disease is abdominal pain (which may be the only presenting symptom). It is not a feature of ulcerative colitis. This isolated symptom has occurred in approximately 15% of our series of over 500 patients in ulcerative colitis.

Fever is seen in ulcerative colitis, but it is usually associated with a severe or fulminant form and is usually accompanied by other hallmarks of the condition (i.e., diarrhea and rectal bleeding). In Crohn's disease, fever without any other symptoms can be the only presenting feature (4% of our cases).

Skin disease, especially erythema nodosum in females, has been quite common in our own series. In the absence of a chest X-ray that suggests sarcoidosis, a gastrointestinal X-ray survey is mandatory.

The presence of perianal disease, either fistula in ano or recurrent rectal abscess, frequently is the signpost of underlying inflammatory bowel disease. It should be stated that in some of these cases the bowel disease may be totally asymptomatic.

Other unusual presentations that should alert the physician to the presence of inflammatory bowel disease are obscure liver disease, hydronephrosis, or recurrent renal calculi, Arthritis, especially ankylosing spondylitis, is frequently associated with these disorders, and if it is present, inflammatory bowel disease should be ruled out.

Among the most common hematological and biochemical abnormalities is anemia, especially iron deficiency anemia, but in Crohn's disease folic acid levels are frequently decreased as well. Rarely one will see vitamin B_{12} deficiency in Crohn's disease of the terminal ileum. In patients who have had resections of the terminal ileum, vitamin B_{12} deficiency is somewhat more common. Elevation of the sedimentation rate and leukocytosis with eosinophilia are common features in Crohn's disease, and we have noted thrombocytosis to be extremely common in the acute presentation. Hypoalbuminemia is almost universal in Crohn's. This is likely due to a protein-losing enteropathy or possibly decreased albumin synthesis due to liver disease. Elevation of alkaline phosphatase is commonly seen as well.

Radiological examination of the gastrointestinal tract is of prime importance in the diagnosis of Crohn's disease. It is less important in the diagnosis of ulcerative colitis.

The diagnostic test in ulcerative colitis is the sigmoidoscopy. In moderately severe or fulminant cases of ulcerative colitis, the barium enema is contraindicated because of the potential lethal complication of perforation. Most authorities agree that once diagnosis is established by sigmoidoscopy, there is no great hurry to X-ray the colon. Radiology of the colon in ulcerative colitis becomes much more important when the disease has been present for many years, because of the increasing incidence of cancer as the disease becomes better established.

Barium enema in ulcerative colitis of course will frequently be normal, especially in mild cases, but if positive can tell the physician about the extent of the disease. Whether or not this will alter the management of the case is controversial. Rectal biopsy can be valuable in cases where the appearance of the rectum is borderline, but is not really necessary in cases where changes of ulcerative colitis are obvious.

Radiology of the gut is essential for the diagnosis of Crohn's disease and also in the follow-up of this chronic disorder. The major mistake in diagnosis is failure to include the small intestine in examinations of the gastrointestinal tract. In any patient with suggestive symptoms of small-intestinal involvement, including diarrhea, weight loss, and periumbilical pain, small bowel X-rays are indicated. Sigmoidoscopy is normal in 50% of the patients with Crohn's disease of the colon, but the procedure should be done routinely, as biopsy in this condition may be extremely helpful in establishing a definite diagnosis.

There are other investigative techniques, but they are generally not necessary, since a barium enema and upper G.I. series and follow-through should be enough to establish the diagnosis. Laparotomy is occasionally required to confirm the diagnosis in a very puzzling case.

The management of these disorders is a life-long process for both the physician and patient. One attempts to control the disease and its complications by the use of both specific and empiric therapy. Frequent hospitalization is common, and controlling the emotional problems resulting from chronic illness requires the utmost skill and patience on the part of the physician.

After the diagnosis is made, a long discussion is held with the patient, and explanation is given in simple terms of the various ramifications of this new and frightening event in his life, with the simplest details. I find most people with these diseases to be intelligent and cooperative. Few fail to ask about the possibilities of cancer, childbirth, and surgery; most are relieved to hear that they do not have a malignancy. I do not quote cancer statistics to patients with ulcerative colitis unless specifically asked.

Follow-up and frequent examinations of the patient by X-ray, endoscopy, and blood studies are stressed. All patients are told to report immediately if they experience any untoward events or downward deviation from their "normal" state. In my opinion, there are very few interdictions in the general management of these individuals.

Diets should be nutritious and free except in patients with chronic Crohn's disease. These patients should not have a bulky diet for fear of precipitating obstruction. Elimination of milk does not appear to play any great role in the treatment, except in patients in whom a history suggests milk intolerance. All patients are told about the theory of milk in the causation of this disease, but are also told that as far as we know, it does not have a major role at the present time.

Control of diarrhea can be a major problem. I have no hesitation in prescribing codeine or anticholinergics in patients with Crohn's disease and mild ulcerative colitis. In severe ulcerative colitis, however, these drugs are contraindicated because of the fear of precipitating a toxic megacolon. In general, reduction of solids for a few days and increase in empiric therapy such as Salazopyrine or corticosteroids will suffice to control most diarrheal attacks. If this is unsuccessful, hospitalization and total gut rest with investigation for new complications may be required.

Replacement of specific deficiencies is a major part of therapy in all these patients. Hematinic substances are valuable in the face of iron loss, folic acid deficiency, or vitamin B_{12} deficiency. Easily assimilable elemental diets are useful in patients who fail to maintain weight and in whom albumin levels are falling. Although these diets may sometimes be unpalatable, patients themselves design methods to try to make them more acceptable. Intramuscular vitamin therapy may be necessary in some patients in whom specific deficiencies are detected.

Sedatives, tranquilizers, and narcotics have been rarely needed according to my experience with these patients.

The empiric therapy of this disease includes Salazopyrine, corticosteroids, and immunosuppressive agents. There is good evidence that suggests Salazopyrine is of great value in mild cases of ulcerative colitis, both in the early attack and also in preventing recurrences. Doses of 2 to 3 g per day seem to suffice. Corticosteroids, on the other hand, should only be used in ulcerative colitis when Salazopyrine fails to control the problem. Corticosteroids can be given intravenously, orally, or rectally, and my personal bias for out-patients is the oral route. Rectal corticosteroids may be valuable in cases of localized ulcerative proctitis.

Long-term corticosteroids tend to be extremely dangerous, and one prefers not to use them. If long-term therapy is required, alternate-day therapy frequently will reduce, but not eliminate, the many complications of steroid usage.

If the patient must be hospitalized, the utilization of blood transfusions and intravenous hyperalimentation has been extremely valuable in management. At the present time a study is being carried out in regard to intravenous hyperalimentation in patients with Crohn's disease. Apparently it does not have any long-term effect on the prognosis of this disorder but certainly can delay surgery, until homeostasis is restored.

Advances in current-day medicine such as intravenous hyperalimentation, antibiotics, and better surgical anesthetic procedures have certainly altered the mortality and morbidity of these diseases, and it is now rare to find one of these patients dying. Statistics given in textbooks and journals should be considered in the light of these advances.

Surgical therapy of these diseases is generally accepted to be the last resort. Emergency surgery is obviously necessary for fulminating ulcerative colitis, and I prefer to wait only 24 to 48 hours before deciding on surgery. This period is utilized to stabilize the patient and to administer blood, intravenous fluid, and corticosteroids and antibiotics, in preparation for a successful operation. In 12 years we have only seen four cases of fulminating ulcerative colitis in our institution among 350 cases of ulcerative colitis, with one death.

The decision for surgery in *chronic* ulcerative colitis is somewhat more difficult to make. If the patient is not responding to sulfonamides and corticosteroids and continues to bleed and lose weight, and has intractable diarrhea, surgery is generally offerred and accepted. The problem we face is what to do in the case of the young person who has had the disease for ten years. The incidence of cancer is of course much higher in these patients, and all patients in this category are offered surgery. Efforts can be made to decide whether surgery is required by the use of sigmoidoscopy or colonoscopy and multiple biopsies. These biopsies are an attempt to detect the so-called early changes of carcinoma. At the present time, however, there is not enough information in the literature or in my own experience for me to comment on this. It is our experience that most people at this stage refuse surgery if they are having few or no symptoms. But it is indeed tragic when one of these people comes back two or three years later with an inoperable cancer. We have had six patients with cancer developing in ulcerative colitis over a 12-year period, and only one of them has survived more than one year after the operation.

Surgery for Crohn's disease is also carried out in our practice only when complications arise. These complications include bowel obstruction, overwhelming bleeding, abscess, or fistula formation, or systemic problems that cannot be controlled by medical therapy. The recurrence rate in Crohn's disease is so excessive that one hestitates to operate until absolutely necessary. It has been said that patients with Crohn's colitis rarely develop the disease in their ileostomy, but this has certainly not been our experience. Every year we see more and more of our patients in whom ileostomies have been performed for colonic Crohn's disease, returning with recurrent disease in the distal part of the terminal ileum. Review of these patients' previous operative records and pathology reveals that they did not have ileal involvement during their initial operation. In our experience with Crohn's colitis, surgery is inevitable. We do not have a case that we have followed longer than three years that has not come to surgery.

In summary, I have tried to outline what I consider to be the major features of ulcerative colitis and Crohn's disease, and because of space limitations, have obviously not covered the total picture. Readers are advised to pursue their interests in more detailed fashion in the literature. It would appear that these diseases are becoming more common, and take up a great deal of the time of a consultant in gastroenterology. Obviously more research is needed so that better forms of treatment and better understanding of the pathophysiology of these diseases can be obtained. At present there does not appear to be much that is favorable on the horizon, and we are unfortunately left at best with inadequate means to control an increasing health problem.

References

Acheson, E. D. The distribution of ulcerative colitis and regional enteritis in vital statistics with particular reference to the Jewish religion. *Gut 1*: 291-293, 1960.

Brooke, Bryan N., ed. *Clinics in Gastroenterology,* Vol. 1, No. 2. Philadelphia: W. B. Saunders Co., May 1972.

Hammer, B., Ashurst, P., and Nash, J. Diseases associated with ulcerative colitis and Crohn's disease. *Gut 9*: 17-21, 1968.

Marshak, R. H., and Wolf, B. S. Roentgen findings in regional enteritis. *Am. J. Roentgenol. 74*: 1000-1014, 1955.

Schofield, P. F. The natural history and treatment of Crohn's disease. *Ann. R. Coll. Surg. Engl. 36*: 3-24, 1965.

Short Bowel Syndrome

M. DAVID TILSON, M.D.
Associate Professor of Surgery
Yale University School of Medicine

A syndrome of malnutrition, steatorrhea, and diarrhea follows massive small bowel resection. Knowledge of the clinical syndrome, pathophysiology, and adaptive mechanisms in this condition has increased rapidly in recent years. Several influences have added impetus to research in this area. First, improvements in pre- and postoperative care have resulted in the survival of increased numbers of patients early after massive intestinal resection. Second, the popularization and widespread use of total parenteral nutrition has enabled an increased numbers of patients early after massive intestinal resection. Second, the popularization and widespread use of total parenteral nutrition has enabled an increased number of patients to survive the more chronic phases of short bowel syndrome. Third, physicians have developed an iatrogenic model of short bowel syndrome in jejunoileal bypass for morbid obesity. All of these influences have increased the apparent incidence of short bowel syndrome and have drawn increased attention to its pathophysiology.

ETIOLOGY

Small bowel resection is performed for a variety of indications. In children, massive volvulus is probably the leading indication. In addition, congenital lesions such as intestinal atresia are uncommon but not rare. In middle-aged patients, repeated operations for complications of regional enteritis and resections for radiation enteritis are the leading causes. In the elderly, massive resection is most often required for intestinal infarction from mesenteric vascular accidents.

PATHOPHYSIOLOGY

The course of the patient is determined by the length and site of the resected intestine as well as by the nature of the underlying disease process.[60] For example, it is not unusual for patients with Crohn's disease and radiation enteritis to undergo resections that leave diseased bowel in situ as the intestinal remnant. These patients offer some of the most difficult problems in management. Because of variations in the length of the human small intestine, it is not possible to predict precisely what the consequences of a specific resection will entail. There are several reports of patients surviving with very small remnants of small bowel and colon. As a general rule, a 50% resection is well tolerated by most patients without significant disability. Indeed, a 70% small bowel resection may be tolerated fairly well if the terminal ileum and ileocecal valve are preserved, since the ileocecal valve appears to be a physiologically significant sphincter. In addition, an intact ileocecal valve may reduce bacterial colonization of the small bowel by colonic organisms, preventing bacterial overgrowth and stagnant loop syndrome as additional complications. If the ileocecal junction is resected along with a major portion of the small bowel, or if greater than a 70% resection is carried out with the sphincter intact, nutrition is likely to be significantly impaired.

The ileum is a more useful remnant than the jejunum for two reasons. First, jejunal peristalsis is more rapid than ileal peristalsis. Thus, transit time is shorter after an ileal resection than after a jejunal resection. Second, because of the regional distribution of important sites for active transport in the ileum, resection of the ileum deprives the patient of specific transport mechanisms for vitamin B_{12} and bile salts. Pernicious anemia eventually appears after a delay of two to five years, when body stores of B_{12} are exhausted. The effects of the loss of active bile salt absorption are more immediate.

Dietary fat is largely absorbed by the jejunum. However, absorption depends on the solubilization of the products of lipolysis by bile salts, which deliver these fats to the brush border as a micellar solution for absorption. The bile salts themselves are selectively absorbed by the ileum and returned by the enterohepatic circulation to the liver. The process by which the ileum recovers the bile salts from the chyme for the enterohepatic circulation is so efficient that only a low level of synthesis of new bile salts by the liver is required daily. However, after ileal resection more bile salts are lost in the stool than the liver can make up with its maximum rate of synthesis. Thus, the bile salt pool is depleted. Depletion results in failure of the solubilization phase of fat absorption. Steatorrhea then occurs, although the usual site of fat absorption in the jejunum remains undisturbed.

In the intact gastrointestinal tract, the colon plays an important role in the conservation of water and electrolytes. There is evidence that the small bowel is able to compensate to some extent for loss of the colon, since the water loss from a fresh ileostomy is two or three times as great as the output from a functionally mature ileostomy after a few months. However, after loss of the small bowel with an intact colon, another pathophysiological mechanism comes into play. Fatty acids and bile salts have been found to stimulate secretion of sodium and water by the colonic mucosa. After resection of the ileum, the bile salts which are not reabsorbed and returned to the liver through the enterohepatic circulation pass into the colon and stimulate secretion. Fatty acids which are malabsorbed in the small bowel have a similar effect. This stimulation of colonic secretion may result in watery diarrhea with large losses of fluid and electrolytes. The phenomenon has been referred to as the "castor oil effect" of ileal resection, since castor oil is a poorly absorbed triglyceride of ricinoleic acid with similar secretory effects on the colon.

Deficiencies in the absorption of proteins and sugars are more difficult to document in short bowel syndrome for several reasons. First, the methods for stool analysis and balance studies are tedious. Second, the transport sites for sugars and proteins are more widely distributed than the specific ileal transport sites for bile salts. The disaccharidases and peptidases that accomplish the last phases of sugar and protein digestion in the intestinal brush border generally have a proximal distribution in the gastrointestinal tract. However, after resection of the jejunum, the ileum will be able to absorb these nutrients efficiently after a period of time.

Gastric hypersecretion is common in the early postoperative period after massive small bowel resection, although it tends to decrease with time. Resection of the small intestine removes the source of potent humoral inhibitors of gastric secretion. Historically, the humoral inhibitor effect of the small bowel on the stomach was referred to as an activity of "enterogastrone." More recently, it has been established that a number of small bowel hormones (CCK, secretin, gastric inhibitory polypeptide [GIP], vasoactive inhibitory polypeptide [VIP]) have potent inhibitory effects on the stomach. There is some evidence that resection of the small intestine removes an important site for remote regulation of gastrin release. Since gastric hypersecretion is greater after small bowel resection than after intestinal bypass, it is likely that bypassed intestine continues to play a role in the prevention of hypergastrinemia.[3,45] Gastric hypersecretion tends to be greater after proximal than after distal intestinal resections.

There are several effects of this outpouring of acid juice into the small intestine. First, inactivation of lipase and trypsin may occur because of the low intraluminal pH in the proximal small intestine. Impairment of lipolysis interferes with another stage of fat digestion and absorption in addition to the mechanisms already outlined. Second, the high solute load of excess gastric juice may exceed the transport capacity of the intestinal remnant, and diarrhea can also be accentuated by this means. The effect is particularly pronounced after massive resections, since the amount of hypersecretion appears to be proportional to the extent of the resection. Third, the proximal intestinal mucosa may be injured by the acid delivered to it, and absorption of all nutrients may be impaired.

The absorption of several vitamins and minerals is also likely to be impaired. When there is significant steatorrhea, calcium absorption is usually abnormal, since the free fatty acids can form insoluble soaps with calcium. Osteomalacia with bone and back pain appears in many patients with short bowel syndrome. Magnesium depletion is also common. Urinary stones of calcium oxalate are common because of an increase in oxalate absorption from the colon. This condition, which is termed intestinal hyperoxaluira, it also related to the excess binding of calcium to free fatty acids as soaps.[9] When there is insufficient calcium in the intestinal contents to keep the oxalate relatively insoluble, increased oxalate absorption results. Anemias are also common. Early in the postoperative course, anemia is usually due to blood loss or iron deficiency. Later in the postoperative course, megaloblastic anemias related to folate or B_{12} absorption occur. Finally, steatorrhea tends to reduce the absorption of the fat-soluble vitamins: A, E, D, and K. An abnormal prothrombin time results from deficiency of vitamin K.

INTESTINAL ADAPTATION

After resection of a significant length of small bowel in man, adaptive responses occur which increase the mass and functional capacity of the intestinal remnant. The clinician has an intuitive grasp of this phenomenon in patients. Diarrhea gradually improves, and nutritional status stabilizes. The adaptive phenomenon is also evident after small bowel bypass for obesity, since the rate of weight loss tends to decrease and eventually to plateau. Recent studies also suggest gradual growth of the intestinal villi in man during the first year after small bowel bypass[20] Over the same time frame, improvement in the absorption of fat, carbohydrate, and protein has been documented after massive resection in man.[57] Similar adaptive responses occur in the ileum after resection of the colon.[5,34,59] These changes probably account for the gradual decrease in ileostomy output after total colectomy until a stable state is reached.

Intestinal adaptation has been extensively studied in experimental animals, and the time course for villus hypertrophy is particularly rapid in the rat by comparison to the slow process in man. Indeed, we have found evidence of increased proliferation in the crypt cells as early as the first postoperative day in the rat colon after small bowel resection,[52] a finding that has been confirmed by other observations of very early hyperplasia.[36,38] Adaptive growth is especially conspicuous in the rat ileum, where the villi rapidly double in length, and compensatory hypertrophy is essentially full-blown within two weeks. Since there is no evidence that the absolute number of villi increases,[19] the process in conceptually akin to compensatory hypertrophy of the kidney. The villus is the functional unit of the mucosa as the nephron is of the kidney.[22] These units hypertrophy in size at the level of functional organization, through the process of hyperplasia at the cellular level, while the total number of units remains constant. Finally, recent evidence suggests that the whole gastrointestinal tract participates in the adaptive response, although not all of the changes observed may be beneficial. For example, an increased parietal cell mass develops and may persist for months, perhaps as a result of the trophic effects of gastrin.[58]

The response in terms of the ultimate villus height reached with full compensatory hypertrophy appears to be quite precisely adjusted. Hanson and coworkers have recently reported stepwise increments in the response in direct proportion to the exact percentage of intestinal mass resected.[23]

The mechanisms initiating compensatory hypertrophy have been studied and debated extensively. The reader is referred to an excellent recent review by Williamson for details that are not covered in the following brief discussion.[56] This discussion is based largely on conclusions drawn from the rat, since it is the most widely studied species.

Nutrients in the lumen of the gut are important not only for normal adaptive responses but also for maintenance of normal intestinal mass. For example, atrophy of the gut occurs when oral intake is limited and nutrition is carried out by total parenteral means.[13,28] Indeed, formula diets may cause some atrophy by comparison to solid diets for reasons that are quite unclear. It is not presently known whether the trophic effect of food is due to direct utilization of the nutrients to meet the metabolic needs of the absorptive cells or to indirect effects related to the release of enteric hormones which have a trophic effect on the proliferative cells. There is evidence that both mechanisms are important, and several hormones may actually be involved in the integrated response. For example, low doses of supplemental gastrin restore and maintain normal intestinal mass in animals receiving total parenteral nutrition.[29] However, compensatory hypertrophy cannnot be explained by gastrin alone, since it occurs normally in short gut preparations with simultaneous total gastrectomy and no measurable serum gastrin.[51,40] Similarly, CCK and secretin restore the adaptive response in parenterally nourished animals,[26] which may be related to the stimulation of pancreatobiliary secretions as discussed below rather than to a direct trophic effect of these hormones on the crypt cells. Efforts have been made to identify specific nutrient molecules that reverse the atrophy of TPN when given intraluminally, and interestingly it has also been found that contact of nutrients with the mucosa has indirect trophic effects on mucosa remote from the site of administration.[12,44]

At one time it was believed that changes in the intraluminal nutrition of the mucosa after partial resection accounted for the process of compensatory hypertrophy more or less completely.[10] In its simplest form the theory of intraluminal nutrition may be explicated as the "downstream" hypothesis. There is a linear gradient of villus length in the rat: duodenal villi are the longest, jejunal villi are intermediate, and ileal villi are the shortest. If the ileum is transposed to the jejunal position, its villi hypertrophy just as if the jejunum had been resected. The jejunal villi in the ileal position may (or may not) shrink to the size of normal ileal villi. This fundamental observation suggests that whatever segment receives the maximum concentration of nutritional stimulation will grow. Thus, the model of jejunal resection with ileal growth was considered to be akin to the response after transposition. In brief, after jejunectomy the ileum gets the food. However, this model has fallen short of explaining all of the observations at hand. First, the ileum has been found to hypertrophy after colectomy.[59] Hypertrophy "upstream" from the site of resection cannot be satisfactorily explained by analogy to transposition. Similarly, the jejunum also hypertrophies upstream from the site of an ileal resection.[4] It is possible that an increased intake of food after a distal resection might initiate hypertrophy in a proximal remnant, but balance studies have not been able to establish increased nutrient intake after partial resections of the colon.[34] Pair feeding may also prevent the full response after partial small bowel resection, but it does not eliminate the response after colectomy.[34] Similarly, TPN with no oral intake blunts the adaptive response; but, again, it does not appear to eliminate it.[32] Finally, ileal hypertrophy has been documented in neonates with intestinal atresia, when there is "no hole" through which intraluminal nutrients could reach the distal mucosa.[47]

A close cousin to the intraluminal theory is the view that pancreatobiliary secretions play a pivotal role.[1] Whenever the ampulla of Vater is transplanted in the gastrointestinal tract, hypertrophy develops in its new environs. Recent studies have indicated that topical bile salts alone will elicit a response.[43] Also, bile salts are relatively more important than the pancreatic secretions, although both are required for the maximum and sustained adaptive response.[54] However, other studies have indicated the proximity to pancreatobiliary secretions is not an entirely sufficient explanation for growth, since limited hypertrophy will occur even when these secretions are diverted to the colon.[50,18] Furthermore, the response to small bowel resection is always greater than the response to bypass,[55] when the same test segment receives the pancreatobiliary effluent.

Another line of evidence relevant to both "downstream" theories derives from studies of bypassed intestinal segments. In general, when a segment is bypassed as a Thiry-Vella loop and exteriorized to the skin, it will atrophy. This phenomenon has been documented repeatedly in several species.[21,30,35,42] However, when a closed distal bypassed loop empties by peristalsis into the residual gastrointestinal tract, it either hypertrophies or remains relatively stable.[11,15-17,46,53] This difference in behavior of bypassed loops has led to different conclusions about possible humoral mechanisms in compensatory hypertrophy. For example, the author concluded that a humoral stimulus might be present, when he observed modest hypertrophy in an intra-abdominal segment of defunctionalized ileum (although the functioning remnant had greater hypertrophy, underscoring the importance of the lumen influences).[46] Others have concluded that no humoral effects were evident on examining Thiry-Vella fistulas exteriorized to skin.[6,21,30,42] After reaching the later conclusion, Clarke carried out further experiments perfusing the loops with nonnutritive distilled water.[7] On finding a restoration of the proliferative response, he concluded that there was evidence for both lumen and systemic factors. Others have also attempted "feeding the bypass" with nutrient solutions with varying results and conclusions. Finally, two separate groups have now succeeded in demonstrating a possible humoral effect in an exteriorized loop with appropriate controls.[14,24]

A theory of humoral control for compensatory hypertrophy of the gut was first proposed by Loran and Carbone in 1968.[33] Most evidence over the years suggesting a systemic stimulus has been largely circumstantial.[48] However, evidence for a circulating factor has recently been found in experiments with direct vascular parabiosis[31] and with autografts of intestinal mucosa.[49] Many hormones will no doubt be investigated in the future for "enterotrophic" effects, and a comprehensive theory of compensatory hypertrophy will probably evolve as an integrated concept of interrelated lumen and systemic influences.

For the practical purposes of the surgeon, the basic work reviewed here indicates the following general conclusions: first, the gut remnant is likely to adapt if a patient can be maintained in a relatively normal nutritional state; and second, provision of nutrients both to the gut lumen and to the patient by parenteral means appears to facilitate this process.

CLINICAL COURSE AND TREATMENT

Because of gradual adaptation, the clinical course of a patient after massive resection goes through several stages.[41]

Stage I is characterized by an initial period of massive diarrhea requiring careful replacement of major fluid and electrolyte losses. Diarrhea exceeds 2 to 2½ liters each day. Feeding is by total parenteral means. This stage usually lasts from one to three months. All electrolytes should be monitored closely during this phase, including calcium, phosphate, magnesium, and zinc.

Stage II is a period of adaptation during which oral intake is gradually initiated and increased. This stage may last for a few months to over a year, and it is usually a time of great frustration for the patient and his physician. The patient may gradually lose weight and have little appetitie, despite maximum efforts at nutritional support. Osteomalacia and anemia may appear during this time.

In *Stage III,* maximum adaptation is achieved, and a relatively normal home existence is regained. Some patients never reach this stage of oral nutrition, but encouraging progress has been made in making the transition to life at home with continuing parenteral nutrition.[27]

The emphasis of treatment depends on the clinical stage of recovery. During Stage I, when diarrhea exceeds seven to eight bowel movements per day or more than 2½ liters of fluid per day, any attempt to begin oral feedings is unwise.

Intravenous fluids only should be used during the early postoperative period, and total parenteral nutrition should be instituted as soon as septic complications are controlled. The most effective medication for diarrhea in the early phase is codeine. Antacids and Cimetidine should be used to control gastric hypersecretion. It is unusual for a surgical procedure to be required for the control of gastric hypersecretion. Indeed, if the gastric output of acid can be controlled by medical means, it is highly desirable, since a surgical approach, especially one involving pyloroplasty or gastroenterostomy, would interfere with another physiological sphincter of the gastrointestinal tract.

When the patient enters Stage II, with diarrhea less than 2 liters per day on a limited oral intake, intravenous hyperalimentation should be continued for a period of time. When the oral caloric intake begins to exceed 2000 calories per day without accentuating the diarrhea, intravenous support may be gradually reduced. Since appetite tends to be poor during this period. alimentation with an elemental diet through a soft small-bore nasogastric tube may be helpful in the transition to full oral nutrition. When oral nutrition is commenced, carbohydrates and proteins should be started first. Medium-chain triglycerides may also be helpful, but ordinary dietary fat should be eschewed until the diarrhea is well controlled. Small frequent meals are best, prepared to be as appetizing as possible. A balance must be struck between the needs of nutrition and the frequency of bowel movements. Supplemental vitamins and minerals should be continued. A jejunal aspirate should be checked for bacterial overgrowth, since an oral antibiotic may be ehlpful if the small bowel is overgrown with bacteria. In patients who have had limited resection of the ileum (less than 100 cm), cholestyramine may also be helpful.[25] The paradoxical value of cholestyramine, which binds bile salts, may be explained by prevention of the cathartic effect of bile salts on the colon. If the diarrhea is predominantly watery, binding the bile salts with cholestyramine may have an overall benefit, especially when the dietary content of the fat is restricted.

At Stage III, the patient is stable with respect to his diarrhea on a low fat diet. During this stage fat may be added judiciously. Dietary supplements of minerals and vitamins should be continued for life. In addition, the patient should be instructed on a low oxalate diet for life. Viral and other intercurrent illnesses should receive prompt medical attention, since these patients have limited reserves, and episodes of dehydration are common.

Management of these patients is tedious and difficult, but the final result is often very gratifying.

References

Altmann, G. G., and LebBlond, C. P. Factors influencing villus size in the small intestine of adult rats as revealed by transposition of intestinal segments. *Am. J. Anat. 127*: 15, 1970.

Anderson, C. M. Long-term survival with six inches of small intestine. *Br. Med. J. 5432*: 419, 1965.

Bowen, J. C., Paddack, G. L., Bush, J. C., et al. Comparison of the gastric responses to small intestinal resection and bypass in rats. *Surgery 83*: 402–405, 1978.

Bochkov, N. P. Morphological changes in the jejunum and ileum of rats after wide resection of the small intestine. *Bull. Exp. Biol. Med. 47*: 339, 1059.

Buchholtz, T. W., Malamud, D., Ross, J. S., et al. Onset of cell proliferation in the shortened gut; growth after subtotal colectomy. *Surgery 80*: 601–607, 1976.

Clarke, R. M. Control of intestinal epithelial replacement; lack of evidence for a tissue-specific blood-borne factor. *Cell Tissue Kinet. 7*: 241–250, 1974.

Clarke, R. M. Evidence for both luminal and systemic factors in the control of rat intestinal epithelial replacement. *Clin. Sci. Mol. Med. 50*: 139–144, 1976.

Clarke, R. M. "Luminal nutrition" versus "functional work-load" as controllers of mucosal morphology and epithelial replacement in the rat small intestine. *Digestion 15*: 411–42, 1977.

Dobbins, J. W., and Binder, H. J. Importance of the colon in enteric hyperoxaluria. *N. Engl. J. Med. 296*: 298, 1977.

Dowling, R. H., and Booth, C. C. Structural and functional changes following small intestinal resection in the rat. *Clin. Sci. 32*: 139–149, 1967.

Dudrick, S. J, Daly, J. M. Castro, G., et al. Gastrointestinal adaptation following small bowel bypass for obesity. *Ann. Surg. 185*: 642–648, 1977.

Dworkin, L. D., Levine, G. M., Farber, N. et al. Small intestinal mass of the rat is partially determined by indirect effects of intraluminal nutrition. *Gastroenterology 71*: 626–630, 1976.

Feldman, E. J., Dowling, R. H., MacNaughton, J., and Peters, T. J. Effect of oral versus intravenous nutrition on intestinal adaptation after small bowel resection. *Gastroenterology 70*: 712–719, 1976.

Feldman, E. J., Carter, D., and Grossman, M. I. Intestinal adaptation: Evidence for a non-luminal factor which stimulates mucosal growth in dog. *Gastroenterology 74*: 1033, 1978.

Fenyö, G., and Hallberg, D. Intestinal hypertrophy after small intestinal bypass in the rat. *Acta Chir. Scand. 142*: 261–269, 1976.

Fenyö, G., Backman, L., and Hallberg, D. Morphological changes of the small intestine following jejuno-ileal shunt in obese subjects. *Acta. Chir. Scand. 142*: 154–159, 1976.

Fenyö, G., Hallberg, D., Soda, M., et al. Morphological changes in the small intestine following jejuno-ileal shunt in parenterally fed rats. *Scand. J. Gastoenterol. 11*: 635–640, 1976.

Fenyö, G. Morphological changes of the adapting small intestine deprived of gastric, duodenal, biliary and pancreatic secretions in the rat. *Eur. Surg. Res. 9*: 122–130, 1977.

Forrester, J. M. The number of villi in rat's jejunum and ileum: Effect of normal growth, partial enterectomy, and tube feeding. *J. Anat. 111*: 283–291, 1972.

Friedman, H. I., Chandler, J. G., Peck, C. C., et al. Alterations of intestinal structure, fat absorption and body weight after intestinal bypass for morbid obesity. *Surg. Gynecol. Obstet. 146*: 757–767, 1978.

Gleeson, M. H., Cullen, J., and Dowling, R. H. Intestinal structure and function after small bowel bypass in the rat. *Clin. Sci. 43*: 731–742, 1972.

Goss, R. J. Hypertrophy versus hyperplasia. *Science 153*: 1615, 1966.

Hanson, W. R., Osborne, J. W., and Sharp, J. G. Compensation by the residual intestine after intestinal resection in the rat. I. Influence of amount of tissue removed. *Gastro-enterology 73*: 692-700, 1977.

Hanson, W. R., Rijke, R. P. C., Plaisier, H. M., et al. The effect of intestinal resection on Thiry-Vella fistulae of jejunal and ileal origin in the rat: Evidence for a systemic control mechanism of cell renewal. *Cell Tissue Kinet. 10*: 543-555, 1977.

Hoffman, A. F., and Poley, J. R. Role of bile acid malabsorption in pathogenesis of diarrhea and steatorrhea in patients with ileac resection. I. Response to cholestyramine or replacement of dietary long chain triglycerides by MCT. *Gastroenterology 62*: 918, 1972.

Hughes, C., Bates, T., and Dowling, R. H. The trophic effect of cholecystokinin/secretin stimulated pancreatobiliary secretions on dog intestine. *Eur. J. Clin. Invest. 6*: 320, 1976.

Jeejeebhoy, K. N., Zohrab, W. J., Langer, B., et al. Total parenteral nutrition at home for 23 months, without complication, and with good rehabilitation: A study of technical and metabolic features. *Gastroenterology 65*: 811-820, 1973.

Johnson, L. R., Copeland, E. M., Dudrick, S. J., et al. Structural and hormonal alterations in the gastrointestinal tract of parenterally fed rats. *Gastroenterology 68*: 1177-1183, 1975.

Johnson, L. R., Litchtenberger, L. M., Copeland, E. M., et al. Action of gastrin on gastrointestinal structure and function. *Gastroenterology 68*: 1184-1192, 1975.

Keren, D. F., Elliott, H. L., Brown, G. D., et al. Atrophy of villi with hypertrophy and hyperplasia of Paneth cells in isolated (Thiry-Villa) ileal loops in rabbits. *Gastroenterology 68*: 83-93, 1975.

Laplace, J. P. Effect humoral de la résection intestinale chez des porcs en circulation sanguine croisée chronique. *Biol. Gastroenterol. 6*: 359, 1973.

Levine, G. H., and Deren, J. J. Dietary and non-dietary factors mediating hyperplasia of residual gut mucosa after small bowel resection in the rat. *Clin. Res. 22*: 363A, 1974.

Loran, M. R., and Carbone, J. V. The humoral effect of intestinal resection on cellular proliferation and maturation in parabiotic rats. In *Gastrointestinal Radiation Injury*, M. F. Sullivan, ed. Amsterdam: Excerpta Medica Foundation, 1968, pp. 127-141.

Masesa, P. C., and Forrester, J. M. Consequences of partial and subtotal colectomy in the rat. *Gut 18*: 37-44, 1977.

Menge, H., Werner, H., Lorenz-Meyer, H., et al. The nutritive effect of glucose on the structure and function of jejunal self-emptying blind loops in the rat. *Gut 16*: 462-467, 1975.

Nundy, S., Malamud, D., Obertop, H., et al. Onset of cell proliferation in the shortened gut: Colonic hyperplasia after ileal resection. *Gastroenterology 72*: 263-266, 1977.

Nygaard, K. Resection of the small intestine in rats. III. Morphological changes in the intestinal tract. *Acta Chir. Scand. 133*: 233, 1967.

Obertop, H., Nundy, S., Malamud, D., et al. Onset of cell proliferation in the shortened gut. Rapid hyperplasia after jejunal resection. *Gastroenterology 72*: 267-270, 1977.

Osborne, M. P., Frederick, P. L., Sizer, J. S., et al. Mechanism of gastric hypersecretion following massive intestinal resection: Clinical and experimental observations. *Ann. Surg. 164*: 622-634, 1966.

Oscarson, J. E. A., Veen, H. F., Williamson, R. C. N., et al. Compensatory postresectional hyperplasia and starvation atrophy in small bowel: Dissociation from endogenous gastrin levels. *Gastroenterology 72*: 890-895, 1977.

Pullan, J. M. Massive intestinal resection. *Proc.R. Soc. Med. 52*: 31, 1959.

Rijke, R. P., Plaisier, H. M., de Ruitier, H., et al. Influence of experimental bypass on cellular kinetics and maturation of small intestine epithelium in the rat. *Gastroenterology 72*: 896-901, 1977.

Roy, C. C., Laurendeau, G., Doyon, G., et al. The effect of bile and of sodium taurocholate on the epithelial cell dynamics of the rat small intestine. *Proc. Soc. Exp. Bioo. Med. 149*: 1000-1004, 1975.

Spector, M. H., Levine, G. M., and Deren, J. J. Direct and indirect effects of dextrose amino acids on gut mass. *Gastroenterology 72*: 706-180, 1974.

Tilson, M. D., and Wright, H. K. Adaptation of functioning and bypassed segments of ileum during compensatory hypertrophy of the gut. *Surgery 67*: 687, 1970.

Tilson, M. D. Compensatory hypertrophy of the gut in an infant with intestinal atresia. *Am. J. Surg. 123*: 733-734, 1972.

Tilson, M. D., and Wright, H. K. Adaptational changes in the ileum following jejunectomy. In *Regulation of Organ and Tissue Growth*, R. J. Gross, ed. New York: Academic Press, 1972, pp. 257-277.

Tilson, M. D., and Livstone, E. M. Radioautography of heaterotopic autografts of ileal mucosa in rats after partial enterectomy. *Surg. Forum 26*: 393-394, 1975.

Tilson, M. D. Sweeney, T., and Wright, H. K. Compensatory hypertrophy of the ileum after gastroduodenojejunal exclusion. *Arch. Surg. 110*: 309-312, 1975.

Tilson, M. D., and Axtmayer, A. Antral exclusion enhances compensatory hypertrophy of the gut after partial enterectomy. *J. Surg. Res. 20*: 275-279, 1976.

Tilson, M. D., Michaud, J. T., and Livstone, E. M. Early proliferative activity in the left colon of the rat after partial small-bowel resection. *Surg. Forum 27*: 445-446, 1976.

Tompkins, R. K., Waisman, J., Watt, C. M-H., et al. Absence of mucosal atrophy in human small intestine after prolonged isolation. *Gastroenterology 73*: 1406-1409, 1977.

Williamson, R. C. N., Bauer, F. L. R., Ross, J. S., et al. Contributions of bile and of pancreatic juice to cell proliferation in ileal mucosa. *Surgery 83*: 570-576, 1978.

Williamson, R. C. N., Bauer, F. L. R., Ross, J. S., et al. Proximal enterectomy stimulates distal hyperplasia more than bypass or pancreaticobiliary diversion. *Gastroenterology 74*: 16-23, 1978.

Williamson, R. C. N. Intestinal adaptation. I. Structural functional and cytokinetic changes. II. Mechanisms of control. *N. Engl. J. Med. 298*: 1393-1402, 1444-1450, 1978.

Winawer, S. J., Broitman, S. D., Wolochow, A., et al. Successful management of massive small bowel resection based on assessment of absorption defects and nutritional needs. *N. Engl. J. Med. 274*: 72-78, 1966.

Winborn, W. B., Seelig, L. L., Nakayama, H., et al. Hyperplasia of the gastric glands after small bowel resection in the rat. *Gastroenterology 66*: 384-395, 1974.

Wright, H. K., and Tilson, M. D. Changes in structure and function of the small intestine after colectomy. In *Intestinal Adaptation,* R. H. Dowling and F. O. Riecken, eds. New York-Stuttgart: E. K. Schattaner Verlag, 1974, pp. 99-106.

Wright, H. K., and Tilson, M. D. The short gut syndrome. *Curr. Prob. Surg.* Chicago: Year Boodk Medical Publishers, June 1971.

Endoscopy for the Abdominal Surgeon: Indications and Results, Techniques, Complications

PAUL H. SUGARBAKER, M.D.
Surgery Branch
National Cancer Institute
National Institutes of Health
Bethesda, Maryland

Fiberoptic endoscopy is one of the few medical technological advances that has resulted in simultaneous decrease in patient morbidity and mortality as well as cost. In addition, time lost by patients from employment has been minimized by reducing the magnitude of several surgical procedures.

These advances have been made possible by the delivery of high intensity cold light and high resolution images through fiberoptic light bindles. Direct visual inspection of many intra-abdominal organs is now possible, permitting increased accuracy of diagnosis. Photography, biopsy, and excision of many pathologic lesions is now possible. Surgeons, because of their familiarity with gross anatomy, tissue strengths, and electrocautery apparatus, have led the way toward developing fiberoptic instruments to their full potential. In this chapter we explore the indications and results, techniques, and complications of instruments often useful to abdominal surgeons. Throughout the discussion we will emphasize proper techniques, for only with meticulous attention to technical detail can these procedures be repeatedly employed without appreciable morbidity or mortality.

LAPAROSCOPY

Indications and Results

To Assess Operability in Patients with Cancer. Laparoscopy frequently provides information traditionally obtained only by exploratory laparotomy. Laparoscopy enables the abdominal surgeon to *assess operability* without making an abdominal incision; consequently many patients can be spared needless exploratory procedures. Liver metastases plus peritoneal and pelvic tumor implants can be visualized and biopsied to determine the state of intra-abdominal malignant neoplasms. Perhaps, in order to establish operability, all patients who have advanced primary cancer with statistically low cure rates should undergo laparoscopy before proceeding with potentially curative surgical therapy. Such a practice adds only minutes to operative procedures and has a low complication rate. Patients in this category might include those with pulmonary, esophageal, gastric, and pancreatic cancers. Advanced endometrial and rectal cancer patients would also be included. We have not subjected patients with primary colonic or ovarian cancer to preoperative laparoscopy. Colonic cancer (and occasionally gastric cancer) requires resection to prevent intestinal obstruction and bleeding. If possible, ovarian cancer requires an attempt at resection of bulk disease to improve local control and perhaps augment response to subsequent chemotherapy.

Liver Biopsy Under Direct Vision. Few pieces of clinical information change patient management more than the presence or absence of hepatic metastases. The tests used to detect hepatic disease are multiple; they include physical examination, liver function tests, liver scintiscan, ultrasonography, computerized axial tomography, hepatic angiography, percutaneous liver biopsy, liver biopsy under laparoscopic control, and direct examination of the liver at the time of laparotomy. However, all the noninvasive techniques can only provide clues to the presence of liver metastases. Only histologic examination of liver biopsy specimens provides reliable proof of hepatic metastases. Percutaneous liver biopsy can often provide this information in those patients whose livers are extensively involved by tumor; however, the problem in detection of hepatic metastases is not usually difficult with far advanced disease. The clinically relevant problem occurs in those patients with less than 25% of the liver parenchyma replaced by tumor. Blind liver biopsy will show metastatic disease in 10% or fewer of these patients; however, liver biopsy under laparoscopic control gives positive biopsies in 60 to 75% of patients with limited hepatic metastatic disease (Figure 1).

Assessment of Acute and Chronic Abdominal Pain. Approximately 20% of patients who undergo laparotomy for acute abdominal pain are found to have a condition that does not require surgery for its treatment. However, since it is often safer to operate than to risk subsequent perforation or infarction of an intra-abdominal structure (usually the appendix), surgery must be recommended. However, laparoscopy provides an alternative approach to the patient with abdominal pain in whom the diagnosis is in doubt (Figure 2). It can prevent both needless exploratory laparotomy and prolonged periods of clinical observation by quickly and accurately establishing a diagnosis. We reduced diagnostic error from 22 to 4% in a group of patients with acute abdominal pain when preoperative laparoscopy was routinely used. An accurate differentiation of pelvic inflammatory disease, ectopic pregnancy, or appendicitis can usually be made (Figure 2). Length of hospital stay and cost of treatment were reduced when the

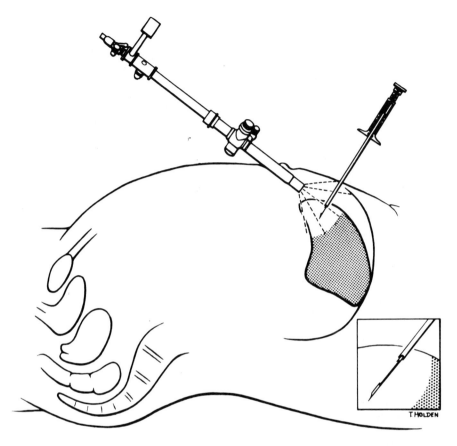

FIG. 1. Liver biopsy under laparoscopic control. (From Sugarbaker, P. H., and Wilson, R. E. *Arch. Surg. 111:* 41, 1976. Reprinted with permission.)

accuracy of diagnosis was increased by preoperative laparoscopy (Sugarbaker et al., 1975).

Laparoscopy is of clinical value in female patients with chronic pelvic pain. An assessment of the severity of adhesions to ovaries and/or Fallopian tubes can be made. A diagnosis of endometriosis can often be made if cystic structures containing dark blood are visualized within the pelvis.

Laparoscopic Tubal Ligation. Gynecologists now routinely use laparoscopy to divide the Fallopian tubes. This method of birth control has proved safe and reliable; however, it is irreversible using currently available techniques.

Other Indications. In patients with possible penetrating abdominal trauma, laparoscopy can be used to determine if the parietal peritoneum was violated. Even with meticulous probing or sinogram, the extent of abdominal penetration

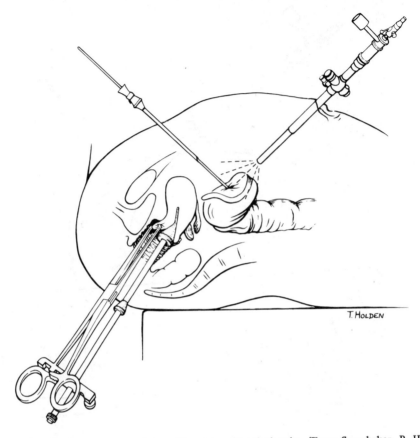

FIG. 2. Laparoscopy in patients with acute abdominal pain. (From Sugarbaker, P. H., Bloom, B. S., and Sanders, J. H. *Lancet 1:* 442, 1975. Reprinted with permission.)

may be difficult to assess. However, the laparoscope views the parietal peritoneum from the inside and can accurately judge if the abdominal cavity was entered. Abdominal masses can be investigated with the laparoscope, although laparotomy is eventually required in a majority of patients. Cholangiography can be performed by entering the gall bladder through the liver; however, cholangiography using an ultrathin (Chiba) needle is usually successful and is a less invasive procedure.

Techniques

All examinations are done in the operating room. With women patients, the buttocks should be 5 cm off the end of the table, with the legs in stirrups. If local anesthesia is planned, intravenous therapy is started, and the patient is heavily sedated with diazepam (Valium), 5 mg and meperidine hydrochloride (Demerol), 50 mg. An umbilical block of 20 ml of 0.5% lidocaine (Xylocaine) hydrochloride is used; 5 ml of lidocaine hydrochloride is also injected just above the peritoneum, inferior to the umbilicus. A second puncture site lateral to the course of the deep epigastric artery may be infiltrated at this time. However, we have found general anesthesia to be more satisfactory when double-puncture technique is being used. If general anesthesia is used, a nasogastric tube should be passed into the stomach to allow escape of air that is often introduced during induction. This will prevent possible gastric perforation as the trochar is introduced. In women, a Cohen-Eder cannula is placed in the uterus and secured with a tenaculum.

A 2-cm incision is made through the skin only at the lower edge of the umbilicus. In extremely obese individuals, it is made directly in the depths of the umbilicus. If a patient has had multiple abdominal incisions with possible diffuse fibrous adhesions, the peritoneum is surgically exposed, and the trochar is introduced under direct vision.

The peritoneum is punctured with a Verres needle through the skin incision, and 2 liters of carbon dioxide is introduced into the abdominal cavity under manometric control. As the carbon dioxide is insufflated, the air pressure noted on the gauge should be below 15 cm of water. It is difficult and usually impossible to determine if an endoscope is within the abdominal cavity before gas infusion allows visualization. Insufflation of subcutaneous tissue in the space of Retzius gives a pressure of 20 to 30 cm of water; pressure within the bowel is about the same. Patients who strain while intubated under general anesthesia may cause much higher pressures to develop. The patients must be relaxed so that one is sure carbon dioxide is going into the free peritoneal cavity. Pressure within venules of the anterior abdominal wall is 16 to 22 cm of water in supine normovolemic persons, and just a few centimeters of water higher within the portal system. Uncontrolled insufflation of gas by syringe or hand pump should not be performed because it exposes patients to a needless risk of air embolism.

The trocar in the sleeve is introduced at an angle of 45° with the abdominal wall. It is passed through the abdominal incision and toward the pouch of Douglas. During penetration, strong traction is applied to the anterior abdominal wall by grasping a fold of skin midway between the umbilicus and the os pubis and pulling upward. As the trocar is removed, a rush of air from the abdominal cavity is noted. The operating peritoneoscope is advanced through the sleeve; a second puncture can now be made in other parts of the abdomen under direct vision.

When the peritoneal cavity is entered, it is visualized by a standard routine starting at the pelvis and proceeding clockwise around the abdominal cavity. A complete exploration is not performed in all patients, especially if local anesthesia is used. A percutaneous needle biopsy of most intra-abdominal organs can be performed under direct vision. Biopsy examinations of less stationary lesions or organs are performed using forceps through the laparoscope.

We have found it useful to tilt the table to examine different abdominal quadrants; reverse Trendelenburg position is used to look into the upper part of the abdomen and Trendelenburg position to look into the pelvis. The spleen is only seen in sharp reverse Trendelenburg position with the patient's right side downward. In women, the entire pelvis is visualized if the uterus is moved inward and upward. Rotation of the uterus to the opposite side of the abdomen may allow improved visualization of a Fallopian tube. All carbon dioxide should be evacuated from the abdomen at the end of the procedure. The skin incision is closed by a single absorbable subcuticular suture.

Complications

The problems encountered following laparoscopy include bleeding and bowel perforation. Bleeding most frequently occurs from a biopsy site. If bleeding develops after a needle biopsy of the liver, hemorrhage into the free peritoneal cavity or into the bile (hemobilia) may occur. This blood loss can be controlled usually by angiography and clot embolization. Bleeding from other more accessible biopsy sites is usually easily controlled by electrocoagulation through the laparoscope. Bleeding that occurs from the anterior abdominal wall as a result of the trochar puncture can be controlled without surgery. A large Foley catheter is inserted into the abdominal cavity through the bleeding puncture wound; the Foley balloon is inflated and traction exerted until bleeding stops.

Bowel perforation rarely occurs as the trochar is being introduced into the abdominal cavity. A more common cause of perforation is full thickness heat necrosis occurring inadvertently as a biopsy or tubal ligation is being performed. Perforations almost always involve small bowel; they are difficult to diagnose, for free air was introduced into the peritoneal cavity by laparoscopy, and symptoms may be delayed in their onset. Surgical repair of a perforation immediately after diagnosis is indicated.

COLONOSCOPY

Indications and Results

Colonoscopic Polypectomy. Colonoscopy can be utilized in the clinical management of multiple diseases of the colon and rectum. Colonoscopy has had its greatest impact by reducing the morbidity, mortality, and cost of medical care by allowing colonic polypectomy without laparotomy. All but the largest and most sessile benign lesions can be removed *in toto*. For some very small lesions excision should not be attempted, for "hot biopsy" can be used to sample and destroy the lesion simultaneously (see below).

Differential Diagnosis of Diverticulitis and Cancer. Not infrequently these two disease states produce similar clinical and radiologic findings. Cancer can be ruled out if the colonoscope can be passed through the entire segment of colon in question and no cancerous lesion is seen. A diagnosis of cancer is made if biopsy or cytologic brushing reveals malignant cells.

Assessment of the Extent and Severity of Inflammatory Bowel Disease. Not infrequently patients who have abdominal pain, blood per rectum, and leuko-cytosis may have inflammatory bowel disease with an entirely normal barium enema. In many of these patients, colonoscopy with blind biopsy of each seg-ment of the colon has revealed inflammatory changes in the mucosa. Also serial colonoscopic examination with biopsy has been useful to follow the response to therapy in patients with colitis.

Evaluation of Suture Lines. Following resection and anastomosis for colon cancer, tumor cells may implant on the suture line and result in recurrent dis-ease. These mucosal recurrences are difficult to diagnose by barium enema and often impossible to visualize by sigmoidoscopy. Colonoscopy and suture line biopsy may confirm local recurrence and lead to curative reresection.

Clarification of Confusing Findings Seen on Barium Enema. The ileocecal valve and midsigmoid areas often are not clearly defined even with the most meticulous radiologic techniques. Barium enema and colonoscopy often comple-ment each other; we have found the barium enema to be the indicated procedure after a careful history, physical examination, rectal examination, and stool test for blood are made. We think the endoscopist should not perform colonoscopy prior to obtaining a barium enema for several reasons: (1) Colonoscopy with biopsy delays barium enema examination by at least ten days. If pathology is seen on colonoscopy, a biopsy should be performed; following biopsy, barium enema should be delayed ten days to allow healing of mucosal and submucosal damage, thus preventing submucosal dissection of barium or perforation. (2) The barium enema tells if diverticuli are present; if they are, special precautions need to be taken so the colonoscope is not moved into a diverticulum and then through the colon wall causing a perforation. (3) The barium enema in identify-ing pathology gives the endoscopist a definite area within the colon to reach and then to inspect and photograph. Sometimes the segment of colon in question by barium enema may look entirely normal by colonoscopy. Success rates in reach-ing lesions known to exist are much better than success rates in reaching un-defined lesion. (4) A barium enema defines the anatomy of the colon so that the endoscopist knows the length and configuration of the bowel. (5) Patients whose barium enema suggests inflammatory bowel disease should have multiple biopsies performed.

Techniques

The most difficult aspect of colonoscopy is the most fundamental maneuver—advancement of the colonoscope tip up into the colon. Experience indicates that a definite sequence of maneuvers repeated in every patient allows most rapid advancement. A barium enema is displayed and is used as a road map. The well-lubricated tip of the colonoscope is introduced into the anus on the index finger, as in performing a rectal examination. Upon insufflation of air, the rectal ampulla appears as a large cavern; its exit can be located using moderate flexion and then rotation of the tip. The sigmoid colon is usually navigable under direct vision until the acute angle at the junction of the sigmoid and descending colon is encountered. Often despite an open lumen ahead, insertion does not advance the tip but merely increases the sigmoid inverted U loop. At this point, 2 to 3 inches of retraction are used to relax but not completely reduce the loop of the sigmoid; $360°$ counterclockwise rotation and reinsertion modify the loop into an alpha configuration, markedly decreasing the acute angle the colon makes with itself at the junction of the sigmoid and descending colon (Figure 3). If the loop of the sigmoid is completely reduced, the colonoscope may merely turn within the lumen of the colon rather than change its configuration. Advancement through an alpha loop causes the tip to slide by into the descending colon. During a slide-by maneuver, insertion should be discontinued if the mucosa blanches or the patient experiences pain. Because the descending colon is fixed to the retroperitoneum, navigation straight to the splenic flexure is usually uncomplicated. After just entering the splenic flexure, the tip of the colonoscope is gently fixed in a mucosal fold, and the reverse alpha maneuver is performed by retraction and $360°$ clockwise rotation. This straightens the sigmoid colon on the colonoscope and lowers the splenic flexure (Figure 3).

The transverse colon usually becomes quite ptotic as the tip of the colonoscope reaches the hepatic flexure. More insertion only elevates splenic and hepatic flexures while depressing further the middle portion of the transverse colon (Figure 3). Rotational elevation of a ptotic transverse colon is accomplished by partial reduction of the U loop and clockwise rotation. This maneuver slides the colon onto the undersurface of the diaphragm, relieves the ptosis, and pushes the tip of the colonoscope down into the ascending colon. Slight, continued clockwise torque upon further insertion moves the tip into the cecum.

Localization of the colonoscope tip can be accomplished with fluoroscopy; however, colonoscopy without fluoroscopy acquires increased versatility, for examinations can then be performed in the operating room, at the patient's bedside, or in the physicians office, replacing the use of the rigid sigmoidoscope. Guidance for locating the tip of the colonoscope is available from the light transmitted through the abdominal wall, the internal appearance of the colon, and certain gross anatomic landmarks.

ALPHA MANEUVER

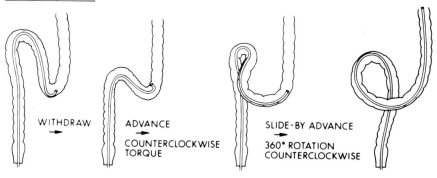

REVERSE ALPHA MANEUVER

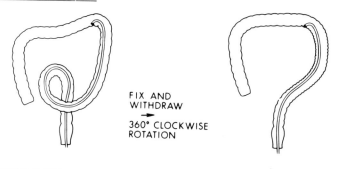

ROTATIONAL ELEVATION TRANSVERSE COLON

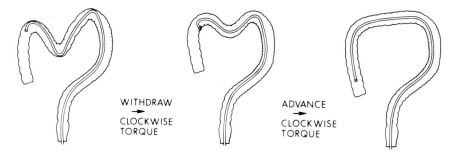

FIG. 3. Maneuvers for colonoscopic advancement. (From Sugarbaker, P. H., Vineyard, G. C., and Peterson, L. M. *Surg. Gynecol. Obstet. 143:* 457, 1976. Reprinted with permission.)

External Localization from Transmitted Light. As the colonoscope is passed from the anus to the ileocecal valve, the transilluminated intracolonic light on the abdominal wall can be located at key check points in a darkened room in most patients. The patient is initially positioned in the right lateral decubitus position. As the colonoscope is passed up into the middle portion of the sigmoid, transmitted light first appears in the left lower quandrant; then the light disappears as the junction of the sigmoid and descending colon is traversed. As the tip of the colonoscope moves up the descending colon, transmitted light appears in the left flank and becomes visible at the tips of the 11th and 12th ribs. The transilluminated light can occasionally be seen moving up and down with respiration when at the splenic flexure. When the light is seen at the level of splenic flexure, the patient is turned onto the back. Light travels across the abdomen at the level of the umbilicus during navigation of the transverse colon and then disappears behind the liver to reappear at McBurney's point when the cecum is entered.

Localization Using Internal Appearance of Colon. Overinsufflation of air may distort characteristic anatomic features. Often the internal appearance is sufficient to localize the tip of the colonoscope. Various portions of the internal anatomy are shown in Figure 4. The rectum is a smooth-walled cavity partially bound by transverse rectal folds, the valves of Houston. The inferior fold lies left and posterior in the patient; the middle fold lies right and anterior; the superior fold lies left and posterior. The middle fold marks the level of the peritoneal reflection. The sigmoid colon is characterized by low-profile, irregular mucosal folds, tubular lumen, and, if the colonoscopic examination is prolonged, forceful peristaltic waves. Acute angulations from pelvic adhesions or from overdistention with air may occur upon insertion, for the mesentery allows great mobility of the sigmoid colon within the abdominal cavity. The transverse colon is characterized by a triangular lumen with prominent, repetitive, draperylike mucosal folds, the interhaustral septums. Deep pockets, the haustra, separate triangular interhaustral septums at regular intervals. In the ascending colon and cecum, the lumen is capacious and circular in outline; the folds between irregular haustra are widely separated and deep. Small mucosal lesions may be especially difficult to locate. The appendicular orifice may be a mere dimple if the lumen of the appendix is scarred, or a shallow diverticulum if a previous appendectomy has been done. When viewed from the ascending colon, the ileocecal valve appears merely as a mound of mucosa projecting from an interhaustral fold. It is often recognized by a fleck of ileal contents within it. In the terminal ileum, the delicate mucosa is arranged in closely spaced folds around the oval lumen. Peristalsis is continuous and makes further advancement of the colonoscope difficult.

Localization Using Gross Anatomic Landmarks. A major landmark may be the obstruction to easy advance encountered at the junction of sigmoid and

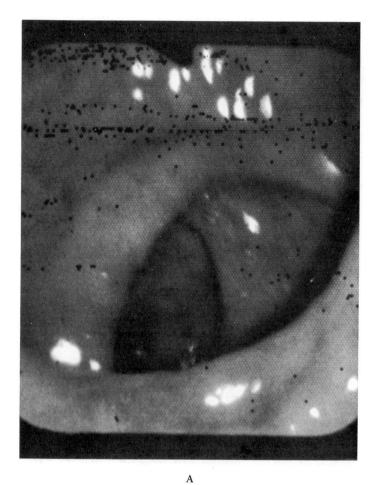

A

FIG. 4. Internal anatomy of the colon. 4A, Rectum. 4B, Sigmoid colon. 4C, Transverse colon. 4D, Ilececal valve. 4E, Appendicial orifice. 4F, Ilioceal valve. (see pages 412–416).

descending colon, which may be navigated using the alpha maneuver. At the splenic flexure, respiratory excursions are seen. With further advancement, motion imparted by cardiac contractions is first noted. A darkened indentation caused by the spleen is frequently seen at the splenic flexure, and a similar darkened area is produced by the liver at the hepatic flexure. Both cardiac and respiratory movements disappear as the instrument enters the hepatic flexure. The transverse colon and cecum are close enough to the abdominal wall to allow easy appreciation of pressure that is applied externally.

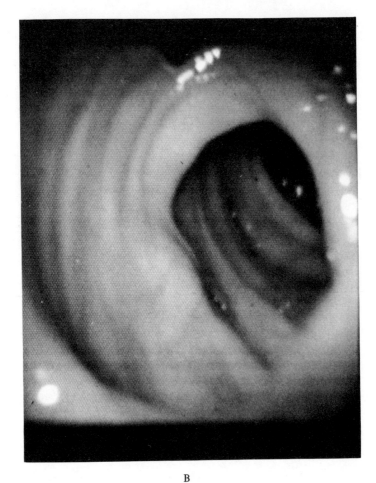

B

FIG. 4. Cont'd.

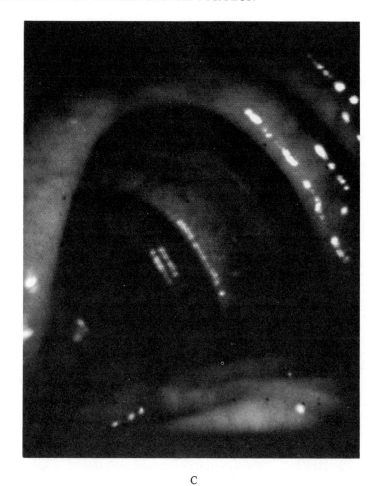

C

FIG. 4. Cont'd.

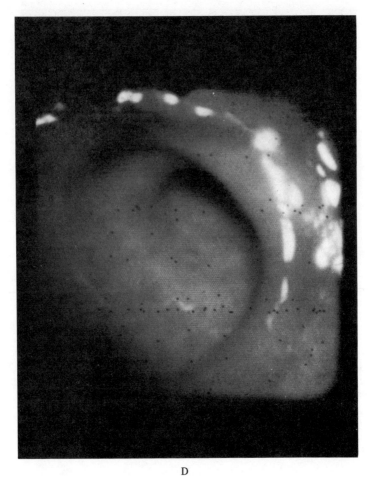

D

FIG. 4. Cont'd.

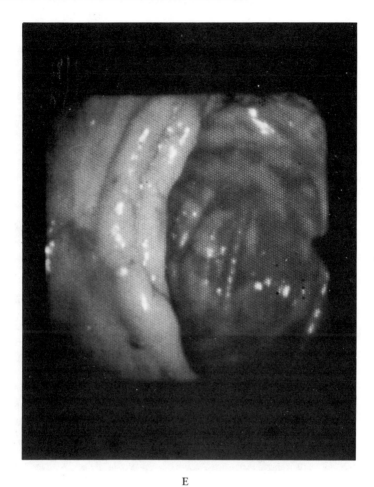

E

FIG. 4. Cont'd.

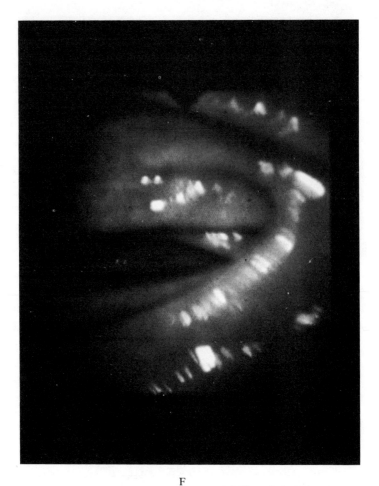

F

FIG. 4. Cont'd.

Once the navigation from anus to cecum is complete, the colonoscope is slowly withdrawn to visualize, biopsy, or remove pathologic findings. Usually, location of lesions seen on barium enema is not difficult; however, certain portions of the colon require special effort for visualization (see Figure 5). In portions of the colon immediately beyond an acute angulation, pathology may often be overlooked.

Biopsy is seldom difficult; problems in passing the biopsy forceps through the biopsy channel do occur unless this channel is kept well cleaned and lubricated. If difficulty arises during a procedure, 10 to 20 cc of mineral oil injected down the biopsy channel will facilitate passing the biopsy forceps.

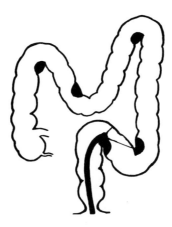

FIG. 5. Trouble spots for colonoscopic visualization. (From Williams, C., and Teague, R. *Gut 14:* 990, 1973. Reprinted with permission.)

Colonoscopic Polypectomy. Few recent technical advances have had an impact on the standard of medical practice like that of colonoscopic polypectomy. Drs. William Wolfe and Hiromi Shinya must be congratulated for developing and popularizing the technique in the United States. The technique is basically a simple one. A wire loop is passed over the head of a polyp, and secured loosely around its stalk. The loop is pulled into its catheter as electrocautery is applied. However, no two polyps are the same, and multiple technical details must be practiced to keep complications at a minimum (see Figure 6).

Complications

Complications resulting from diagnostic colonoscopy have been few, and usually occur in patients with underlying colorectal pathology. Diverticular disease causes problems in that increased intracolonic air pressure can result in a "blow out." Also the orifice of a large diverticulum can be mistaken for the colon lumen and the colonoscope passed into the free peritoneal cavity. These problems are greatly magnified in the patient with diverticular disease on corticosteroid medication. Active ulcerative colitis results in a weak colon wall, making examination and biopsy more hazardous. Active granulomatous colitis does not frequently weaken the bowel wall, but patients experience severe pain if traction is put on the involved segment of bowel. A narrowed segment of bowel caused by adenocarcinoma may be extremely friable, and minimal pressure from the colonoscope tip may result in free perforation. Because narrowed or obstructing lesions present a serious risk if not recognized prior to the colonoscopic examination, barium enema should always be obtained before colonoscopy is performed.

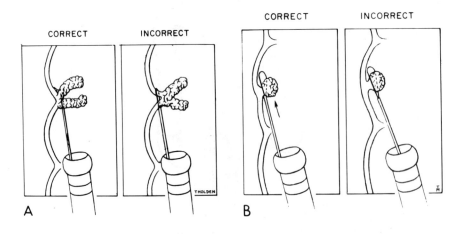

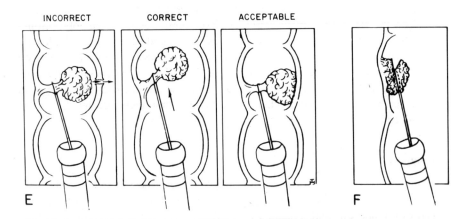

FIG. 6. Techniques of colonoscopic polypectomy (Plates A–G). (A) Sessile multilobed polyps: Sessile multilobed polyps should be excised piecemeal. *En bloc* excision may include bowel wall in the specimen, especially if the polyp occurs on an interhaustral fold. (b) Excision of small polyps: In excising small sessile or small pedunculated polyps the catheter should be advanced to the base of the polyp before beginning to even up on the snare wires. If this is not done the polyp will slip out of the snare as the wires are manipulated to secure the polyp (Shinya manuever). (c) Minimally pedunculated polyps: Many polyps that do not appear pedunculated grossly will on microscopic examination be shown to be completely excised. Small sessile polyps can be gently lifted away from the colon wall by tenting up the mucosa. (d) Polyps with long stalks: Excision of polyps with long stalks at their base incurs unnecessary risk of full thickness heat necrosis of the colon wall. Divi-

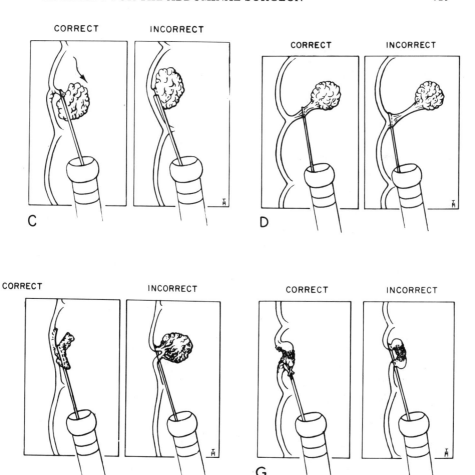

sion of the stalk at its midpoint should always be attempted. (E) Minimizing sparking: Sparking to the bowel wall has caused perforation and should be avoided. The profile of a polyp may be lowered by pushing out on the tightened snare. Or sparking may be avoided if a large portion of opposite colon wall is in contact with the polyp head. (f) Piecemeal excision of sessile polyps: Sessile polyps, if they are to be removed by colonoscopic polypectomy, should be excised piecemeal. Snare excision of a large tissue mass allows the colon wall to be included in the specimen. If the snare wire is slowly tightened while (not before) electrocautery is applied, hemostasis will be better and the colon wall less likely to be puckered into the resected specimen. (g) Carcinoma in sessile polyps: Because of distortion and retraction of tissue surrounding invasive cancer, perforation or bleeding has occurred frequently with excision of carcinomatous polyps. A suspicious sessile lesion should be biopsied before excision is attempted.

The management of colonoscopic complications only rarely requires laparotomy. Bleeding that occurs at the time of polypectomy can be controlled with "hot biopsy" forceps (see Figure 7). This is most easily accomplished if a double channel colonoscope is available. Good exposure of the bleeding point is maintained by sucking blood through the large channel, and passing the hot biopsy forceps through the small channel. Not infrequently bleeding may start three to five days after polypectomy. Early or late after polypectomy, persistent bleeding rarely occurs; but when it does, it is usually controlled by blood replacement and peripheral vasopressin infusion if necessary. If this is unsuccessful, angiography should be used to identify the bleeding point, and the catheter tip positioned near the bleeding vessel. Gelfoam or blood clot can then be used to occlude the bleeding vessel.

Perforations are a more serious problem and require good surgical judgment to prevent a life-endangering situation from occurring. Perforations through a segment of diseased bowel are unlikely to close rapidly; the danger of bacterial contamination of the peritoneal cavity by bowel flora is great, and laparotomy to close the leak is indicated. If the patient has suspected carcinoma, biopsy confirmation on an emergency basis should be obtained, and definitive surgery undertaken. In other situations where a small perforation has occurred through a segment of healthy colon, expectant management is indicated. This can only be recommended if the bowel preparation at the time of endoscopy was excellent. The patient should be placed on nasogastric suction, broad spectrum antibiotics, and bed rest. Daily serial upright chest X-rays should indicate whether intraperitoneal air is increasing or decreasing. Frequent repeat physical examination should reveal if signs of peritoneal irritation are becoming manifest. The patient's temperature and leukocyte count should be monitored. If no signs of continued leak are observed, the patient is continued on all treatments for approximately one week and then gradually progressed back to normal alimentation and activity.

UPPER GASTROINTESTINAL ENDOSCOPY

Indications and Results

Upper gastrointestinal endoscopy is a clinical skill shared by the surgeon with the gastroenterologist; and the endoscopic tasks that surgeons undertake do overlap upon occasion with those of the gastroenterologist. However, the nature of the disease process usually indicates who should manage a particular patient. Usually the gastroenterologist is asked to consult on those patients whose problem requires medical management; he sees radiologically benign-appearing esophageal strictures, uncomplicated hiatus hernias, gastric ulcers appearing

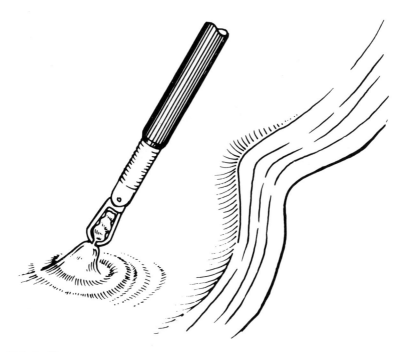

FIG. 7. "Hot biopsy" forceps used to control bleeding point. (After Williams, C. B., *Endoscopy*, 1973).

benign by radiologic examination, duodenal ulcers, and problems in gastrointestinal motility (achalasia) or absorption (sprue). On the other hand, those patients who are likely to need surgical intervention in the near future are directed to the surgeon. His patients with upper gastrointestinal disease include those with esophageal stenosis radiologically appearing malignant, hiatus hernia resistant to conservative management, gastric ulcer radiologically appearing malignant, and duodenal ulcers resistant to conservative management.

Upper gastrointestinal endoscopy is of greatest use to the surgeon in a preoperative setting. Visualization and biopsy of pathologic lesions allows the surgeon better to define the type of operation to be performed and its extent. Endoscopy preoperatively will supply more accurate histopathological diagnosis and allow the pathophysiology of the lesion to be defined better. Many times the gastroenterologist and surgeon will jointly participate in an endoscopic examination.

Esophageal Strictures. Differentiation of esophageal strictures as benign or malignant by biopsy and brush cytology is possible nearly 100% of the time. Benign strictures can be related to reflux (acid or alkaline), infection (monilia), or scar (from ingestion of corrosives). In patients with hiatus hernia, esophageal cancer can be ruled out, the presence of reflux and extent of associated esophagitis evaluated, and the type of mucosa (squamous or columnar as seen with Barrett's ulcer) determined by biopsy.

Gastric Ulcer. Gastric ulcers can be visualized and their appearance evaluated as suggesting a benign (mucosal folds radiating into a flat "punched-out" ulcer) or malignant (mucosal folds terminating before they reach a "shaggy" ulcer with raised edges) process. However, no matter what the gross appearance of the ulcer, multiple biopsies from each quadrant of the ulcer must be taken, followed by brushings from the ulcer crater. If the gross appearance and histopathological examination suggest a benign process, a second endoscopic study after three weeks of conservative management should be performed. If, again, malignancy is not suggested, cancer is highly unlikely, for the accuracy of diagnosis approaches 100% using this plan of management.

A not uncommon problem in differential diagnosis occurrs in patients seen to have remarkably thickened gastric mucosal folds by UGI radiologic examination. These patients may have hypertrophic gastritis, Menetrier's disease, gastric lymphoma, or superficial spreading carcinoma of the stomach. Endoscopy with "macrobiopsy" is the procedure of choice to differentiate these entities definitively (Figure 8).

Upper Gastrointestinal Bleeding. In patients with acute upper gastrointestinal bleeding, endoscopic study of the esophagus, stomach, and duodenum will

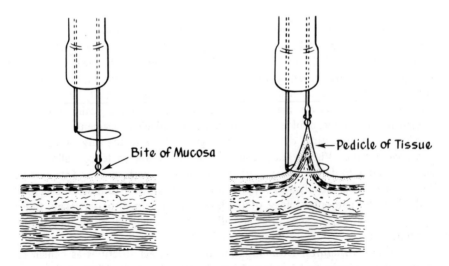

FIG. 8. "Macrobiopsy" of gastric mucosa. (From Martin, T. R., *et al. Gastrointest. Endosc. 23:* 29, 1976. Reprinted with permission.)

afford a correct diagnosis about 90% of the time if the examination is performed within 12 hours of the bleeding episode. Knowledge of the patient's history is helpful but must not be relied on for diagnosis. In about half the patients with esophageal varices, the actual bleeding site is erosive gastritis or peptic ulcer. A Mallory-Weiss tear at the esophago-gastric junction occurs usually without prior symptomatology, but may cause as many as 25% of UGI bleeding episodes.

Surgical Follow-up. UGI endoscopy is useful to the surgeon for follow-up. Malignancy may often first recur at the previous suture line; anastomoses are traditionally difficult to evaluate radiologically because postoperative changes distort the normal anatomy. The size and shape of an anastomatric channel, marginal ulceration, and inflammatory changes can be readily evaluated. One must be cautioned, however, that although endoscopy is sensitive to the presence of recurrent cancer intrinsic to the gut wall, recurrent disease extrinsic to intestinal lumen is difficult or impossible to evaluate. Radiologic examination is more accurate than endoscopic examination in assessing progressive extrinsic distortion of a hollow viscus.

Endoscopic Retrograde Cholangiopancreatography (ERCP). A final UGI endoscopy technique, seldom performed by surgeons but occasionally useful to them in clinical decision making, is ERCP. This procedure may be indicated in patients with jaundice in whom a definite diagnosis cannot be established. Percutaneous transhepatic cholangiography with the Chiba needle may also be helpful in this clinical situation. In patients with pancreatic disease, ERCP preoperatively may help the surgeon plan his procedure. A smooth-walled but dilated duct of Wirsung may suggest that a sphincterotomy is indicated. A "chain of lakes" Wirsung's duct suggests the need for a distal pancreatectomy, filet of pancreatic duct, and Rouxen-Y pancreaticojejunostomy.

Techniques

UGI endoscopy is probably the least technically demanding of the procedures discussed so far. The sedated patient is asked to gargle a local anesthetic agent while seated. Then with the patient in the right lateral decubitus position, the endoscope tip is passed on the forefinger into the pharynx. The patient is asked to swallow to open the cricopharyngeal sphincter and the endoscope passes into the esophagus. The cardioesophageal sphincter is visualized from above and below by retroflexing the endoscope (Figure 9). If the endoscope tip just below the cardioesophageal sphincter is flexed 45° in the plane of the instrument, the greater curvative comes into view. Rotation of the endoscope clockwise scans the anterior surface of the stomach; rotation counterclockwise scans the posterior surface of the stomach. If the endoscope tip is repositioned just below the cardioesophageal sphincter and extended 45° in the plane of the instrument, the lesser curvature is visualized. This is followed to the antrum and then

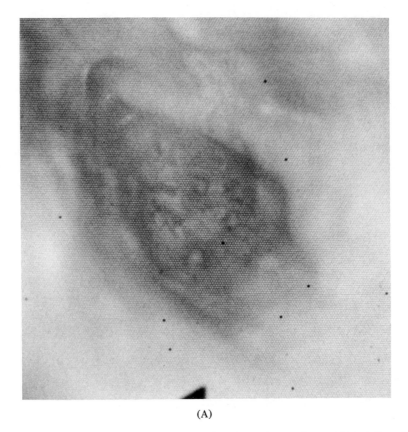

(A)

FIG. 9. Views of the cardioesophageal junction from the esophagus (A) and from the stomach (B).

through the pylorus into the duodenum. Persistent advancement will move the tip to the ligament of Treitz and even beyond.

It should be mentioned that the techniques involved in UGI endoscopy and colonoscopy are entirely different. The esophagus, stomach, and duodenum are structures whose position within the abdominal cavity are fixed; therefore, as the hollow viscus is inflated with air, the endoscope is moved readily ahead under direct vision. Not so with the colon. The sigmoid, the transverse, and often the ascending colon are free to move nearly anywhere within the abdominal cavity; therefore, maneuvers to reduce bowel loops by accumulating collapsed colon on the endoscope are required.

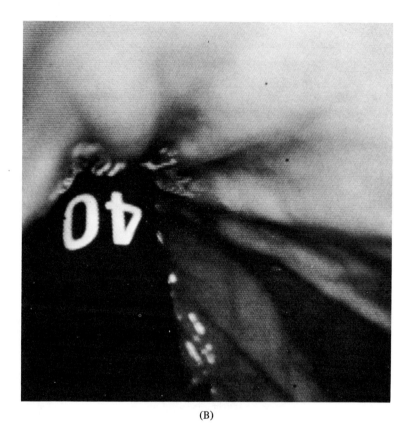

(B)

FIG. 9. (Cont'd)

Complications

The number-one rule for the UCI endoscopist is "Don't push." Perforations are rare, but they do occur—often through a cancer. If this occurs, surgery needs to be performed immediately, and the pathologic lesion resected. If a perforation occurs through normal stomach or through a benign duodenal ulcer, nasogastric suctioning, intravenous antibiotics, and careful observation are usually enough. Perforation of the normal esophagus should be rare but does occur. If the diagnosis is suspected (substernal pain, subcutaneous emphysema in the neck, elevated temperature), pharyngeal suctioning, antibiotics, and careful observation are indicated. Patients may often need surgical drainage; this is done through the neck if the perforation is in the upper mediastinum or through the left chest if it is in the middle or lower third of the esophagus.

References

Colcher, H. Current concepts gastrointestinal endoscopy. *N. Engl. J. Med. 193:* 22, 1975.
Elias, E., Hamlyn, M. B., Jain, S., et al. A randomized trial of percutaneous transhepatic cholangiography with the Chiba needle versus endoscopic retrograde cholangiography for bile duct visualization in jaundice. *Gastroenterology 71:* 429, 1976.
Sugarbaker, P. H., and Wilson, R. E. Using celioscopy to determine stages of intra-abdominal malignant neoplasms. *Arch. Sugr. 111:* 41, 1976.
Sugarbaker, P. H., Bloom, B. S., Sanders, J. H., and Wilson, R. E. Preoperative laparoscopy in diagnosis of acute abdominal pain. *Lancet 1:* 442, 1975.
Sugarbaker, P. H., Vineyard, G. C., Lewicki, A. M., Pinkus, G. S., Warhol, M. J., and Moore, F. D. Colonscopy in the management of diseases of the colon and rectum. *Surg. Gynecol. Obstet. 139:* 341, 1974.

Carcinoma of the Rectum— Can the Sphincter Be Saved?

JOSEPH H. FELLER, M.D.
PETER J. DECKERS, M.D.

Colo-rectal carcinoma is the most frequent gastrointestinal cancer and the second most frequent visceral neoplasm with over 100,000 new cases and over 50,000 deaths reported each year. The surgical procedures available for treatment of colon cancer are well defined, but operations for rectal carcinoma are less standardized. Design of surgical procedures is generally based on such considerations as experience and technical competence of the surgeon, bulk and location of the primary lesion, age and body habitus of the patient, physical properties of the tumor, and accepted methods of dealing with rectal carcinoma in a specific locale.

Furthermore, since Miles described the abdomino perineal resection for rectal carcinoma in 1908, many thousands of these procedures have been performed with what is thought to be a very acceptable morbidity and mortality and low incidences of perineal recurrence. It is, therefore, incumbent on any less frequently utilized method of dealing with rectal carcinoma to demonstrate comparable figures in these areas.

We believe that an adequately conceived cancer operation, which satisfies all criteria regarding en block dissection and still could be performed with preservation of sphincteric function, would certainly represent a considerable advance in the treatment of rectal cancer.

We will, moreover, raise certain other questions regarding the feasibility of performing less than radical cancer surgery in certain highly selected cases of rectal cancer. We intend to question the blind application of the Miles resection to all patients with rectal cancer, regardless of the clinical presentation. Finally, we will demonstrate the necessity for adjuvant radiation therapy in rectal lesions with poor prognosis and draw conclusions regarding its use in conjunction with certain sphincter-saving operations.

The rectum (Figure 1) is a muscular organ that occupies the most posterior part of the pelvis. It is bounded posteriorly by the sacrum, coccyx, anococcygeal body, and superior hemorrhoidal artery, and is bounded anteriorly by the bladder, prostate, and seminal vesicles in the male and by the uterus and adnexa in the female. On each side of the rectum lie the so-called rectal stalks, which are situated at the level of the distal rectum and contain the middle hemorrhoidal artery and vein. The rectum traverses a musculo-aponeurotic diaphragm consisting of the levator ani muscles and puborectalis sling to end in the anal canal, which is bounded by a complex sphincteric system, consisting of an external sphincter with subcutaneous, superficial, and deep portions. The superficial component of the mechanism is made up of the subcutaneous and superficial portions of the external sphincter, while the deep component is formed by the deep external sphincter and the puborectalis. Each puborectalis muscle passes around the anorectal junction to form a sling. At the intersection of the internal and external sphincters and puborectalis sling is the anorectal sling, which, when destroyed, produces incontinence. (See Figures 2 and 3.)

The blood supply to the rectum is by both the inferior mesenteric and internal iliac and course in the fat of the ischi rectal fossa to supply the lower hemorrhoidal vessels. The inferior hemorrhoidal vessels are branches of the internal iliac and course in the fat of the ischial rectal fossa to supply the lower rectum. The extensive collateral circulation around the rectum usually assures adequate vascularity during the performance of low resections. (See Figure 4).

In order to understand the effectiveness of sphincter-preserving procedures, the concept of continence must be understood. Four factors constitute continence according to Bacon:[1]

1. The pressure receptors and afferent reflex arcs that five rise to the sensation of impending defecation.
2. Reflexes that are produced by feces passing over the sensitive anal epithelium.
3. Reservoir function, which may be defined as the ability of the rectum to adapt to increasing bulk of stool, which is dependent on its smooth muscle property, permiting increasing lengths at constant tension until pressure stimulates peristalsis, initiating defecation.

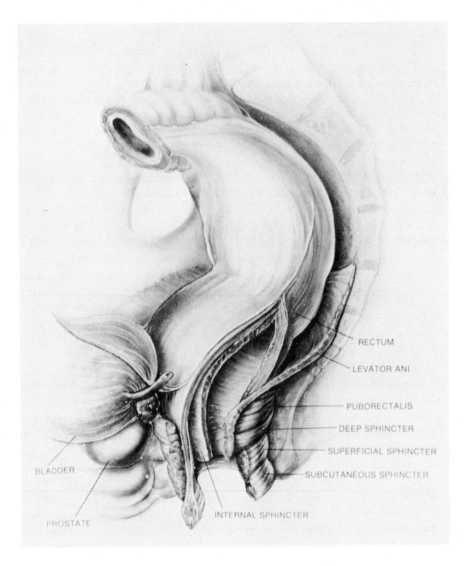

FIG. 1. Anatomy of the rectum, sphincteric apparatus and relationship to the other pelvic organs. (Reproduced from Localio with permission of the publisher.

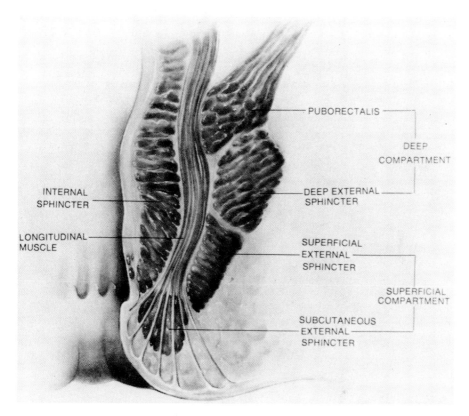

FIG. 2. Anal sphincteric mechanism. (Reproduced from *Localio* with permission of the publisher.

4. Sphincter continence, which is the ability to prevent involuntary evacuation by conscious control of the external sphincter. Continence may be defined as the voluntary control over defecation, whereas defecation is the physical explusion of stool.

This preceding discussion is essential to an understanding of "pull through" procedures, of which there are four major varieties in use today. All involve resection of tumors within the rectum and mobilization of the proximal bowel through the anus, securing it to the rectal stump. Bacon states that after "pull through" operations the urge to defecate is retained, and since continence implies the ability to control defecation by volition, the patient is continent. If the urge to defecate arises, the patient is able to contract the preserved sphincters and inhibit the expulsion of stool. He further states that after "pull through"

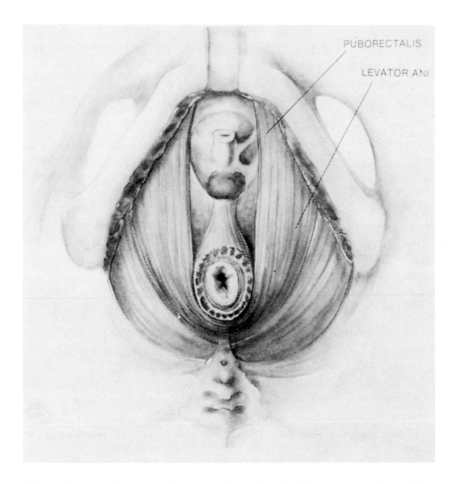

FIG. 3. The pelvic diaphragm. (Reproduced from *Localio* with permission of the publisher)

operations, pressure of the distended colon at the level of the sphincters acts as another stimulus which incites the need to defecate. In this instance again, the patient may react to prevent expulsion of fecal content. The popularity of "pull through" procedures lies in the ability to retain fecal continence—a result of preservation of the anal sphincteric mechanism.

Since tumors of the rectum frequently metastasize by lymphatic channels, an understanding of the lymphatic drainage of the rectum has been thought critical for the design of an appropriate operation. Briefly, there are two extensive anastomotic lymph channels that drain the rectum. The first consists of those lymph structures located in the submucosal and subserosal layers of the bowel

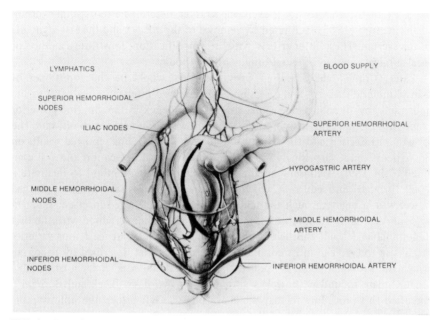

FIG. 4. Lymphatic and vascular supply to the rectum. (Reproduced from *Localio* with permission of the publisher)

wall. These, in turn, drain into extramural lymphatic structures, which, in general, follow the course of the vessels of the anatomic area concerned. Lymphatic channels may also drain into lymph structures in areolar tissue surrounding the longitudinal muscle. These node-bearing areas are located posterior to the rectum above the levator muscles. Nodal drainage occurs, thereafter, along the course of both the superior hemorrhoidal and inferior mesenteric vessels. The chief path of metastatic spread is, therefore, upward from the rectum and pararectal tissues.

Villemin et al.[2] have demonstrated that lymph drainage from rectal tissues above 7 to 8 cm from the anus is essentially upward. Below 7 to 8 cm, on the other hand, drainage may occur in either direction, inferiorly to the middle hemorrhoidal vessels or to the lymph nodes on the lateral pelvic wall.

The anal canal drainage is made up of channels that are located in the ischiorectal space, superior hemorrhoidal areas, and middle hemorrhoidal areas. Drainage from the anal verge may occur to the inguinal nodes.

The first reported amputation of the rectum was described by Lisfranc[3] in 1826. Limited use of this operation was associated with numerous serious complications, and justification for the procedure was questioned. Verneuil[4] (1873) and Kocher[5] (1874) suggested excision of the coccyx to afford better exposure of the area for local excision. Kraske[6] described a transsacral excision of the rectum (1885) facilitated by removal of the coccyx and the last segments of the sacrum. These latter efforts, with little modification, constitute a method of local surgical excision of rectal tumors utilized today.

Later, Cripps[7] described an operation that would be the forerunner of transphincteric surgery of the rectum. This involved inserting a scalpel into the anus; and, by directing the scalpel toward the coccyx in the anterior posterior plane, the rectum and sphincteric mechanism were transected with one cut. The growth was excised and the wound left to granulate. Cripps reported results on 36 patients, and, surprisingly, 23 had regained normal defecation and full continence. In 1892, Maunsell[8] used this sphincter-dividing method to facilitate a "pull through" procedure in which, after the tumor was excised, the proximal bowel was brought through the rectal remnant and anchored in place. Hochenegg[9] of Vienna in the late nineteenth century is generally credited with the first abdominal-anal "pull through" type procedure, of which at least four varieties are in use today. The most common operation was that described by Bacon, in which the proximal colon is "pulled through" a denuded anal canal of variable length.[1] The redundant bowel is amputated in ten days. Black and Botham[10] modified this procedure in that the anal canal was left intact, the union taking place between the cut edge of the anus and the pulled-through specimen. More recently Turnbull and Cuthbertson[11] and Cutait and Figlione[12] modified this, in that the proximal bowel was drawn through the everted anal stump, the union was allowed to occur, and subsequently the excess bowel was amputated at a second stage.

Abdominal transsacral resection as practiced by Localio and Eng[13] is based on the Kraske operation, the abdominal phase of the operation being performed as a low anterior resection with the subsequent anastomosis being performed posteriorly (the sacrum and coccyx being removed).

Cripps[7] in England in 1877 and Balfour[14] in the United States in 1910 were the first to perform anterior resection. This procedure and the classic abdomino perineal resection described by Miles[15] in 1908 are currently the mainstays in the surgeon's armamentarium with respect to rectal cancer.

Several methods of local treatment (which are considered sphincter-preserving procedures) have been described. Crile and Turnbull[16] and Madden and Kandalaft[17] utilized electrocoagulation in the treatment of rectal carcinomas with good results. Recently, Papillon[18] described the use of intracavitary irradiation in the primary treatment of rectal carcinoma. These methods will be described in greater detail subsequently.

It has been noted previously that the lymphatic spread of rectal cancers progresses in an orderly, predictable manner until widespread lymphatic disease is present, at which time some degree of lateral extension may occur. Localio suggests that basic anatomic facts should be considered in procedures applied to rectal cancer and challenges Miles's work. He believes that the original concept of the operation was formulated from autopsy data on patients dying with far advanced and inoperable disease. At this late stage, lateral extension through the levators was noted. Patients with early disease confined to the immediate para-rectal tissues were, by and large, excluded. Localio further cites other studies by McVey[19] in 100 patients with rectal tumors. Forty-seven patients presented with lymph node metastases, and only one patient had involvement below the lower limit of the resection. Similarly, Coller et al.[20] have failed to find metastasis in lateral zones in lesions 3 cm or more above the ano-rectal junction. Citing these and other studies, Localio[13] suggested that only a very small percentage of rectal lesions spread laterally. Guernsey[21] described 42 patients whose rectal cancers were 2 cm or less above the levators, and lateral extension was not present. Gabriel et al.[22] suggested after detailed anatomic studies that lateral and down-ward spread is only seen after wisespread local and advanced disease, not in the early lesion best-suited for sphincter-saving procedures.

Certain other facts must be considered when evaluating the efficacy of various operative procedures. We know that colo-rectal cancer has a decided tendency to spread through the thickness of the bowel wall and only to a lesser degree intramurally. Therefore, the biologic characteristics of this tumor are different from esophageal carcinoma, for instance, in this respect. Only 1 to 2% of well-differentiated lesions spread more than 2 cm from the resection margins, and this figure only increases to 5 to 6% when more undifferentiated varieties are studied.[23]

Numerous authors have demonstrated the effect of increasing Dukes' stages on prognosis. In various series, modified Astler-Coller A lesions carry a 74 to 100% five-year survival. If extension into the muscularis, but not through the bowel wall, occurs, this percentage drops to 64%. If, however, extension is noted into pericolic fat, the five-year survival is between 40 and 60%.

Survival is further adversely effected by the presence of lymph node meta-stases. Such metastases exist in approximately 50% of cases at the time of initial surgery for rectal cancer, and survival is decreased 15 to 30% when lymph node metastases are found.

The location and number of nodes influence survival as well. Copeland et al.[24] found that survival was 27% if one node was involved, but the figure dropped to 9% if more than five nodes were involved. Dukes suggested that if only positive pericolonic nodes were present in the resected specimen, survival was 41%. If, on the other hand, nodes were positive at the highest resection margin, the survival dropped to 14%.

Gunderson and Sosin[25] examined the problem of local recurrence after resection for colo-rectal cancer by reviewing the University of Minnesota re-operative experience. These patients underwent reexploration at varying inter-vals after the initial operation for rectal carcinoma. Seventy-four patients with modified Astler-Coller B_2, C_1, and C_2 lesions had planned single or multiple reoperations. Tumor recurrence was present in 52. Local failure occurred alone or in combination with distal metastasis in 33% of the entire group.

Studies from Portland, Maine[26] demonstrated that groups at highest risk for local recurrence (LR) were those presenting with lesions through the entire thickness of the bowel wall, whether or not nodes were involved (50–65% LR) or uninvolved (35% LR). Interestingly, failure was noted only in 20% when nodes were involved but the lesion was confined to the bowel wall. Gunderson showed essentially the same data.[25] If C_1 lesions were considered in the University of Minnesota series, local failure was 23.5% as opposed to 70% with positive nodes associated with full wall thickness lesions.

The implications of the above findings are discussed in detail in the monograph by Gunderson.[27] It is obvious, however, that local recurrence is a major problem in full thickness lesions with or without positive nodes. Some form of adjuvant therapy is necessary in this regard. Cuthbert Dukes[28] suggests:

> The dissection of operative specimens of rectal cancer has shown that the first glands to receive metastases are almost invariably those lying nearest to the primary tumor. In the case of growths of the lower third and ampulla of the rectum the first metastases are found to the pararectal glands on the same level with or immediately above the primary tumor. The next glands to be affected are the superior hemorrhoidal, which are usually invaded in sequence from below upwards. In an advanced case of cancer of the lower third or ampulla the metastases come to form an unbroken chain extending from the regional group of glands to those situated at the point of ligature of the inferior mesenteric vessels. Occasionally, a case is met with in which a metastasis is present high up in the chain of hemorrhoidal glands though those at a lower level are free from deposits. This may be due to an anomaly whereby some lymphatic trunks bypass glands en route and pass directly upwards to reach the glands in the recto-sigmoid region.
>
> The general direction of lymphatic spread for growths situated in the upper third of the rectum and recto-sigmoid region is also upwards, and it is very rare to find metastases in glands below the primary tumor, though this may occur if the upward spread is blocked. Downward spread of this character has been met with in less than 1% of cases. Evidence of lateral lymphatic spread may sometimes be seen in tumors situated in the lower third of the rectum, but even in these situations it would seem that the upward path is the main highway of lymphatic drainage and is the one most commonly taken by cancerous emboli.

We have not improved on this review. Therefore, certain conclusions may be drawn from the preceding arguments. First, resection margins in rectal cancer could be approximately 3 to 4 cm, since only rarely, even in undifferentiated malignancy, does rectal cancer spread beyond 2 cm from the growing edge of the tumor. Second, lateral extension in early operable carcinoma of the rectum is rare, and, therefore, lateral dissection and ablation of strictures at the level of the levator ani muscles is not always necessary. Third, in tumors above 7 cm, downward spread is not noted, and, therefore, excision of elements cephalad to the lesion suffices. Finally, lymph node metastasis and lateral spread are uncommon with small well-differentiated polypoid lesions. This fact implies that less than radical cancer operations may be applied to these lesions.

In general one may define a spectrum of operations that preserve the innate sphincter musculature of the rectum and thus permit defecation to proceed in the normal fashion with preserved continence and reservoir effect. These procedures (Figure 5) are listed below:

A. Low anterior resection
B. Combined procedures
    1. Abdominal transsacral resection
    2. Abdominal anal "pull through" procedures
C. Local procedures
    1. Electrocoagulation
    2. Contact radiation therapy
    3. Transsphincteric resection
    4. Kraske type operations

In general, the combined procedures and anterior resection are true cancer operations. They satisfy all criteria of an en bloc dissection and excision while preserving normal rectal function. The local procedures, on the other hand, are not true cancer operations. They treat the local problem and do not satisfy the criteria of radicality. The most obvious drawback is the fact that lymph node metastases are not controlled by these procedures. We believe, however, that these local procedures do occupy an important place in the management of rectal carcinoma, and with the application of strict selection criteria may be considered as curative procedures. These concepts will be discussed in the following paragraphs.

Since Miles described the abdomino perineal resection for rectal carcinoma in 1908, many thousands of these procedures have been performed with a steady predictable morbidity, mortality, local recurrence, and five-year survival rate. Miles designed this operation as a result of careful analysis of autopsy material from patients dying with widespread as well as locally recurrent disease. Numerous authors have challenged the concepts delineated by Miles with respect to early rectal cancer and extent of resection. We have demonstrated that lateral spread to the levators was uncommon and is, generally, a late occurrence in

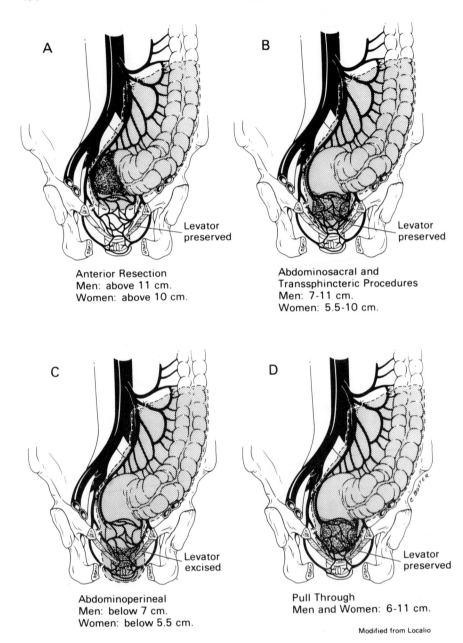

FIG. 5. Extent of resection. A, anterior resection includes superior and middle hemorrhoidal vessels and lymphatics. B, abdominosacral resection extends dissection to the level

patients with advanced rectal carcinoma. Therefore, the combined operations that preserve sphincteric function (i.e., abdominal transsacral excision and abdominal anal "pull through" as well as anterior resection) may be as effective a cancer operation as is the classic Miles resection.

In order to support this hypothesis, one must compare large groups of patients undergoing both abdomino perineal resections and sphincter-preserving combined procedures with respect to operative mortality, morbidity, local recurrence, and five-year survival rates.

Operative mortality of Miles resection has declined in recent years owing to better preoperative and postoperative care, better anesthesia, and surgical techniques. It is now approximately 5 to 10% nationally. Table 1 demonstrates the mortality in various series of various "pull through" procedures. Results are similar in major series.

Stearns[29] reports 8 postoperative deaths in 227 patients undergoing abdomino perineal resection at Memorial Hospital, Kholdin,[30] on the other hand, found that mortality in 824 patients undergoing Miles resection was 12.7% as opposed to a 5.2% mortality in those patients subjected to "pull through" operations. Bacon[1] reported an operative mortality of 3.9% in "pull through" procedures, a 4.1% incidence in anterior resection, and a 2.8% incidence in Miles resections. Therefore, in most major series reviewed operative mortality was similar.

Morbidity (Table 2) is considerable after abdomino perineal resection. Genito-urinary tract complications developed in more than 20% of 305 patients

TABLE 1. Morbidity, Mortality, and Functional Results of "Pull through" Operations for Rectal Cancer

Author	No. Cases	Operative mortality, %	5-Year Survival, %
Bacon (1971)	705	3.4	52.3
Black and Botham (1958)	106	6.8	53
Kholdin (1973)	339	5.2	67.5
Kennedy (1970)	158	4.5	60 (only those with 5-year follow-up)
Stearns (1974)	43	2.3	70

of the levator ani. C, abdominoperineal resection removes, in addition, levator ani, anorectal stump and inferior hemorrhoidal lymphatics. D. Abdominal anal pull through sacrifices superior and middle hemorrhoidal vessels and leaves the levator ani muscle intact. Shaded areas indicate extent of resection. Darker shading indicates zone of tumor. (Modified from *Localio,* reproduced with permission of the publisher.)

TABLE 2. Analysis of Local Recurrence Rates and Surgical Morbidity after
"Pull through" Procedures for Rectal Cancer

Author	No. patients	Local recurrence	Acceptable functional result	Morbidity
Gardner	12	(16%)	83% (10/12)	2/12 (16%)
Grimson	13	(15%)	100% (0/survivors)	3/12 (25%) prolapse or hernia
Kennedy	158	(7%)	90%	74/158 (46%)
Bacon	705	(11%)	99%	28/705 (3.9%) mortality

Morbidity (Table 2) is considerable after abdomin perineal resection. Genito-urinary tract complications developed in more than 20% of 305 patients at the Mayo Clinic.[31] A high rate of importence has been reported after abdomino-perineal resection.[32] On the other hand, Bacon[1] suggested that impotence is not noted after "pull through" procedures unless disection is carried out exten-sively along the iliac vessels. Urinary retention was only noted in three patients in the Bennett et al.[33] series of "pull through" procedures. This complication usually occurs during the postoperative course in most patients undergoing Miles resection. Bacon[1] reported that his most serious complication was intestinal obstruction, which occurred in 6 out of 705 cases. Perhaps the most serious morbidity of the Miles resection is the presence of a permanent colostomy, for which the morbidity in terms of psychologic problems cannot be quantified. Indisputably, therefore, a greater morbidity appears to be associated with ab-domino perineal resections.

The problem of local recurrence (Table 2) after operation has been described previously. Several points merit further discussion. In a comparative series by Bacon[1] in which anterior resection or a "pull through" procedure was per-formed, Bacon noted that this problem occured in 30% of the anterior resection patients and 11.8% of the "pull through" patients. Only 6.3% of these local recurrences were suture line recurrences. Kennedy et al.[34] noted 11 recurrences in 125 patients treated with curative resections and "pull through" procedures.

Gunderson,[25] in the Minnesota reoperative series, noted recurrence alone in 50% of the original 75 patients with Dukes B_2, C_1, and C_2 lesions. Fifty-two were found to have tumor at the second-look procedures. In Gunderson's study 90.5% of the patients had classic abdomino perineal resections, but only 7 pa-tients had sphincter-saving operations. Local recurrence rates, therefore, seem less with "pull through" procedures, but this may be skewed since the majority of cases reviewed come from only one series (Bacon).

In analyzing five-year survival rates (Table 1) of various sphincter-saving operations as opposed to sphincter-ablating procedures, comparable results are found. Five-year survival rates of various "pull through" procedures are noted in Table 1, where 53 to 70% survival rates are documented. Survival rates of patients undergoing Miles resections are comparable in major series.[29,30] In ten major series reviewed by Kholdin,[30] five-year survival rates ranged between 43.4 and 56% for Miles resections, and between 49 and 65.4% for "pull through" procedures, in contrast to rates of 33 and 74% for anterior resections.

The functional aspects of "pull through" or combined sphincter-saving operations must of necessity be compared to assess the worth of the procedure. Function (Table 2) returns rather rapidly in terms of sphincter control and continence after X-ray therapy and fulguration. It is similar with low anterior resections. Mason[35] reported continence and a satisfactory result in all 72 patients treated by either abdominal transsphincteric or local transsphincteric methods. Bacon[1] reports the most favorable results in the literature, and, of 705 patients, only three required a colostomy subsequent to the "pull through" procedures. In his first series of cases, only three wore pads. Other authors report less encouraging but generally acceptable results.[30,32,34] Bennett[33] suggests that only 25% of his patients have bowel function that is indistinguishable from normal, but fully 80% have had acceptable results. After careful analysis of this group, he deemed 90% to exhibit adequate function. Furthermore, Bennett[33] and Kennedy[34] both noted a marked improvement in function with the passage of time. Kennedy examined functional results meticulously and noted that fully 77% demonstrated good results defined as the ability to control defecation, the capability to differentiate between feces and flatus, and the rarety of soiling. This finding coupled with a survival rate of 60% and an operative mortality rate of 4.5% with a local recurrence rate of 9% constitute excellent results comparable in all respects to Miles resection. Kennedy notes, in a word of caution, however, that a high percentage of these lesions were stage B lesions.

Byrne,[36] in 1889, followed by Strauss et al.[37] and Wassink,[38] first utilized electrocoagulation for destruction of rectal tumors. Since this time and especially during the last 15 years, numerous authors have suggested that electrocoagulation be considered as the procedure of choice for rectal carcinoma. Madden and Kandalaft[17] suggested that this technique should be considered the preferred method of dealing with this lesion. They presented a series of 77 patients, of whom 60% were alive from 1 to 17 years postoperatively. The failure rate in the operable group was only 24%. In their inoperable cases, there was a failure rate of 60%. Madden and Kandalaft[17] argue that results with the Miles resection have never yielded greater than 45 to 60% five-year survivals, and the procedure has been associated with a mortality of about 5% and a high morbidity rate—problems notably lacking when electrocoagulation is used appropriately.

Crile and Turnbull[16] compared a series of patients treated by electrocoagulation with those treated by abdomino perineal resection. In their series electrocoagulation was combined with implantation of radon seeds or cobalt teletherapy.

The technique employed by Crile and Turnbull utilizes a low-intensity cutting current, and, with the use of a brass wire loop 1 cm in diameter, the carcinoma is "combed" away until the muscle is encountered. The muscle is heated but not resected if the tumor is distinct from it. The procedure is performed under caudal anesthesia, and the operation lasts between 15 and 45 minutes. No serious complications and no deaths were observed. Other authors have suggested that the procedure should take as long as a classic resection for rectal carcinoma. Madden described three to six fulgurations per patient, and emphasizes that all tumor should be removed in one session.

In the Crile and Turnbull series of coagulation versus resection, five-year survivals were 67% with fulguration and 54% with resection. A strong argument which has been echoed in other papers concerning the effectiveness of local treatment was forwarded by Crile and Turnbull. These authors suggested that in their resected patients only one-third had nodal metastases, and only one-fifth of the patients with nodal metastases were cured by radical surgery. They infer that for resection to produce a cure in one patient, 15 patients would have to undergo surgery—the overall survival, therefore, being increased by only 7%. It must be stated, however, that in most series in the literature fully 50% of patients present with lymph node metastases at operation.

Crile, therefore, demonstrated a 68% five-year survival for the electrocoagulation group as opposed to 54% five-year survival in the resection group. Surprisingly, 93% of patients treated with coagulation who presented with polypoid tumors (probable Dukes A) have lived five years. In the above study none of the patients treated by coagulation developed known abdominal carcinomatosis. It must also be noted that the average age of the patients was five years greater in the electrocoagulation group, and that the average size of the tumors was greater in the resection group. These factors may certainly have influenced survival rates but the data suggest that in selected patients electrocoagulation is an acceptable method of local control and cure. Selection criteria include patients with:

1. Polypoid lesions
2. Well-differentiated lesions
3. Small lesions
4. Lesions easily fully exposed

As has been stated previously, not all rectal tumors are amenable to major surgical resection. Recently, Papillon[18] has described a technique of intracavitary irradiation in a highly selected group of patients. He reported a series of 186 patients who were treated in Lyon, France from 1951 to 1972. Most of these carcinomas were situated in the lower rectum (93% below 10 cm from the anal verge). The techniques used were both contact radiotherapy and interstitial implants.

Of 133 patients available for five-year follow-up, 104 (78%) are alive and disease-free. There were only three local failures, and these underwent subsequent resection. Of the total group of 186 patients, 26 failures (14%) were noted—a figure consistent with other major series. Failures were twice as frequent with ulcerative lesions as opposed to the polypoid variety.

There are advantages noted with this technique. Tolerance is excellent even in the poor-risk patients. There is no need for general anesthesia. Morbidity and mortality are negligible. During intracavitary treatments the time dose fractionation is changed according to the apparent tumor regression. The tolerance of the rectal tissues is good, and only one patient developed a fistula which healed spontaneously. The fibrous reaction that occurs after intracavitary irradiation is supple, and it is easy to detect recurrent carcinoma. Moreover, if local failure does occur, radical surgery may still be applied with cure.

It is emphasized that Papillon states that polypoid, well-differentiated adenocarcinomas are the most suitable for contact radiation therapy. He maintains, however, that limited, fairly confined ulcerative lesions are amenable to this technique.

One may take exception to Papillon's statement that the rate of local control and cure after irradiation is higher than it is after surgical procedures. It is certainly true that five-year survival rates seem to indicate this. However, given the highly selected nature of the patient population, no conclusion may be drawn by comparison with other surgically treated patients who, by and large, had more unfavorable lesions. This criticism aside, our basic premise that, with the use of strict selection criteria, results of radical resections and local therapy are similar, is given added support by the Papillon data.

The role of preoperative and postoperative radiation therapy has been better defined during the last several years. Several large series have demonstrated the inordinately high local failure rate after operations for rectal carcinoma.

The question of adjuvant preoperative or postoperative radiation therapy is vast, and the reader is directed to the detailed comparison by Gunderson.[27] Several points are important to note from the author's analysis. Gunderson suggests the use of a "sandwich technique": a preoperative therapy utilizing portals sufficient to encompass the tumor-bearing area but supplying low doses of radiation is used, and may prevent growth of tumor cells shed at operation and still allow the performance of an anastomosis in an irradiated area. Postoperatively, those patients with lesions associated with a high percentage of local recurrence (i.e., B_2, C_1, and C_2) would receive full doses of radiation therapy to sterilize any tumor-bearing lymphatic areas. (See Table 3 for cancer classification.)

TABLE 3. Modified Astler-Coller Classification for Cancer of the Colon and Rectum

A	Confined to the mucosa with no penetration of the muscularis
B_1	Penetration into the muscularis
B_2	Penetration through the muscularis into the pericolic fat
C_1	Involvement of regional lymph nodes with lesion confined to the bowel wall
C_2	Involvement of the regional lymph nodes with lesion through the bowel wall
D	Distant metastasis

Several large series have documented the benefit of preoperative radiation therapy. A large VA study[39] utilizing 2000 to 2500 rads showed a difference in five-year survivals of 12.4% (28.4 as opposed to 40.8%). Local recurrence decreased, from 47 to 29% in the nonirradiated group as opposed to the irradiated group. The results are more striking in the Oregon series[40] utilizing tumorcidal doses of 5000 to 6000 rads. Only 1 of 50 patients demonstrated local recurrence.

Several large series utilizing postoperative radiation therapy have been published, and these are summarized by Gunderson.[27] All studies show a marked and dramatic reduction in local recurrence. Utilizing data from the University of Florida, University of Chicago, Maine, M. D. Anderson Hospital, and Latter Day Saints Hospital, Gunderson showed that local recurrence rates were: 0% versus 25 to 35% for the B_2 and B_3 lesions; 8% versus 45 to 50% for the C_2 and C_3 lesions.

These results dramatically demonstrate that no longer can one rely on surgery alone in the treatment of rectal carcinoma. The use of a sandwich technique would permit the performance of a low anastomosis (be it anterior resection, abdominal-anal, or abdominal transsacral resection) in an area with a very low radiation injury. If the resected specimen contained a lesion with a known poor prognosis (Dukes B_2, C_1, or C_2), further radiation therapy would be delivered to tumoricidal doses after the anastomosis had healed. Theoretically, low anastomoses or classic "pull through" procedures would be equally as effective. More data and a randomized prospective trial of radiation therapy in association with combined procedures are necessary.

In reviewing results of operations for rectal cancer, we have shown that when large series are considered, results with respect to operative mortality and local recurrence rates are similar for the various procedures. We have shown that morbidity is certainly less with the combined sphincter-saving operations. At least 75 to 80% of patients are content with the functional results achieved with combined sphincter-saving operations. This fact, in association with a low morbidity rate, makes the operation a very viable instrument in the surgeon's armamentarium in rectal cancer.

Several studies have demonstrated the effectiveness of local sphincter-saving proccedures in curing rectal cancer. These procedures, when well-performed with strict selective criteria, yield results comparable to combined sphincter-saving procedures and to abdomino perineal resection.

Finally, we feel that the Miles resection certainly maintains an important place in poor-prognosis lesions less than 6 to 7 cm from the anal verge. We have, however, questioned its blind application to all forms of mid- and high midrectal lesions. We feel that strict selection criteria should be applied when dealing with rectal cancer and that combined and local sphincter-saving procedures should be considered much more frequently when operating for rectal carcinoma.

References

Bacon, H. E. Present status of the pull through sphincter-preserving procedure. *Cancer 28*: 196, July 1971.

Villemin, F., Huard, P., and Montaque, M. Recherches anatomiques sur les lymphatiques du rectum et de l'anus. *Rev. Chir. 63*: 39, 1925.

Lisfranc, J. Memoire sur l'excision de la portie inferieure du rectum devenue carcinomateuse. *Mem. Acad. Med. 3*: 291, 1826.

Verneuil, M. Resection du coccyx pour faciliter la formation d'un anus perineal dans les imperforations du rectum. *Boll. Soc. Clin. 2*: 299, 1873.

Kocher, T. Die exstirpation recti nach vorheriger excision des steissbeins. *Zentralbl. Chir. 1*: 145, 1874.

Kraske, P. Zur exstirpation hochsitzenden mastdarmkrebs. *Verh. Dtsch. Ges. Chir. 14*: 464, 1885.

Cripps, H. *On Disease of the Rectum and Anus* (4th ed.). London: Churchill, 1914.

Maunsell, H. W. A new method of excising the two upper portions of the rectum and the lower segment of the sigmoid flexure of the colon. *Lancet 2*: 473, 1892.

Hochenegg, J. Meine operations serfalge bei rectumcarcinom. *Weiu Klin. Wocheuschr. 13*: 399, 1900.

Black, B. M., and Botham, R. J. Combined abdomino-endorectal resection for lesions of the mid and upper parts of the rectum. *Arch. Surg. 76*: 688, 1958.

Turnbull, R. P., and Cuthbertson, A. Abdomino-rectal pull through for cancer and Hurschprung's disease, delayed posterior colorectal anastomosis. *Clev. Clin. Q. 28*: 109, 1961.

Cutait, D. E., and Figlione, F. J. A new method of colo-rectal anastomosis. *Dis. Colon Rectum 4*: 335, 1961.

Localio, S. Arthur, and Eng, Kenneth. Malignant tumors of the rectum. *Curr. Probl. Surg.* Chicago: Year Book Medical Publishers, Sept. 1975.

Balfour, D. C. A method of anastomosis between sigmoid and rectum. *Am. Surg. 51*: 235, 1910.

Miles, W. E. A method of performing abdominoperineal excision for carcinoma of the rectum and terminal portion of the pelvic colon. *Lancet 2*: 1812, 1908.

Crile, G., Jr., and Turnbull, R. B. The role of electrocoagulation in the treatment of carcinoma of the rectum. *Surg. Gynecol. Obstet. 135*: 391, 1972.

Madden, J. L., and Kandalaft, S. Clinical evaluation of electrocoagulation in the treatment of cancer of the rectum. *Am. J. Surg. 122*: 347, 1971.

Papillon, J. Intracavitary irradiation of early rectal cancer for cure. *Cancer 36*: 696, Aug. Supp., 1975.

McVey, J. R. Involvement of lymph nodes in carcinoma of the rectum. *Ann. Surg. 76*: 755, 1922.

Coller, F. A., Kay, E. B., and MacIntyre, R. S. Regional lymphatic metastasis of carcinoma of the rectum. *Surgery 8*: 294, 1940.

Guernsey, D. R. Carcinoma of the rectum prognosis based on the distance of lesions from, or involvement of, the levator ani muscle, and involvement of the anal sphincters. *Surg. Gynecol. Obstet. 92*: 529, 1951.

Gabriel, W. B., Dukes, C. E., and Bussey, H. J. R. The lymphatic spread in cancer of the rectum. *Br. J. Surg. 23*: 395, 1935.

Black, W. A., and Waugh, J. M. The intramural spread of carcinoma of the descending colon, sigmoid, and rectosigmoid. *Surg. Gynecol. Obstet. 87*: 457, 1948.

Copeland, E. M., Miller, L. D., and Jones, R. S. Prognostic factors in carcinoma of the colon and rectum. *Am. J. Surg. 116*: 875, 1968.

Gunderson, L. L., and Sosin, J. Areas of failure found at reoperation following "curative" surgery for adenocarcinoma of the rectum. *Cancer 34*: 1278, 1974.

Gilbert, S. G. The significant of symptomatic local tumor failure following abdominoperineal resection (quoted in Gunderson). *Int. Cong. Radiol.*, Oct. 1977.

Gunderson, L. L. Combined irradiation and surgery for colo-rectal carcinoma. *Int. Cong. Radiol.*, Brazil, Oct. 1977.

Dukes, C. E. The surgical pathology of rectal cancer. *J. Clin. Pathol. 2*: 95, 1949.

Stearns, M. W., Jr. The choice among anterior resection, the pull through and abdominoperineal resection of the rectum. *Cancer 34*: 969, Sept. Supp., 1974.

Kholdin, S. A. Evaluation of sphincter saving operations for cancer of the rectum and sigmoid. *Am. J. Proctol.*, 464, Dec. 1973.

Judd, E. S., The risk of surgery of the colon. Current trends in hospital mortality rates. *Proc. Staff Meet. Mayo Clin. 36*: 492, Sept. 1961.

Long, D. M., Jr., and Bernstein, W. C. Sexual dysfunction as a complication of abdominoperineal resection in the male. *Dis. Colon Rectum 2*: 540, Nov.–Dec., 1959.

Bennett, R. C., Hughes, E. S. R., and Cuthbertson, A. M. Long term review of function following pull through operations of the rectum. *Br. J. Surg. 59*: 723, Sept. 1972.

Kennedy, J. T., McComish, D., Hughes, E. S. R., and Cuthbertson, A. M. Abdomino-anal pull through resection of the rectum. *Br. J. Surg. 57*: 589, Aug. 1970.

Mason, A. York, Transsphincteric surgery of the rectum. *Prog. Surg. 13*: 66, 1974.

Byrne, J. *Clinical Notes on the Elective Cautery in Uterine Surgery*. New York: William Wood & Co., 1873, p. 68.

Strauss, A. A., Strauss, S. F., Carwford, R. A., and Strauss, H. A. Surgical diathermy of carcinoma of the rectum. Its clinical end results. *J. A. M. A. 104*: 1480, 1935.

Wassink, W. F. The curative treatment of carcinoma recti by means of electrocoagulation and radium. *Arch. Clin. Neurol. 8*: 313, 1956.

Kligerman, M. M., Urdaneta, N., Knowlton, A., Vidone, R., Hartman, P. V., and Vera, R. Preoperative irradiation of rectosigmoid carcinoma including its regional lymph nodes. *Am. J. Roentgerol. Radium Ther. Nucl. Med. 114*: 498, 1972.

Stevens, K. R., and Allen, C. V. Preoperative radiotherapy for adenocarcinoma of the rectosigmoid. *Cancer 37*: 2866, 1976.

Reproductive Endocrinology and Infertility

DR. ARTHUR SHAPIRO, Associate Professor
Division of Reproductive Endocrinology
Dept. of Obstetrics & Gynecology
University of Miami School of Medicine
Miami, Florida

The definition of infertility is the failure to conceive or to carry a pregnancy and deliver a living baby after one year of sexual intercourse. The reason that one year is chosen is that studies have shown that it would take six months for 75% and 12 months for 85% of normal fertile couples to conceive.

Approximately 10% of all marriages are involuntarily childless, which would mean that three to four million couples in the United States are infertile.

The need for physicians to understand and help treat problems of patients with infertility is greater today than it ever was. This is partly due to the change in abortion laws: the availability of babies for adoption has declined dramatically. In addition, there seems to be an increase in the incidence of infertility which may be due to an epidemic outbreak of venereal diseases, in particular gonorrhea, leading to obstructive diseases of the female as well as male genital tract. The use of birth control pills may also give rise to a potential complication of "post pill amenorrhea."

Reproductive endocrinology is rapidly becoming a more and more complex science. Research is continuing to uncover and explain more of the mysteries of contraception and pregnancy. These new findings not only help us to understand and cure problems of infertility, but may define areas that hold promise for future contraception as well.

The incidence of the major causes of infertility may be divided as follows: (1) male factor—30 to 35%; (2) ovulatory problems—20%; (3) obstructive diseases of the female—25%; (4) cervical factor (cervical mucus or cervical incompetence)—10%; (5) uterine factor (adhesions, irregularities, anomalies)—5%. In 10% of couple no etiology can be identified; approximately 30% of couples will have multiple problems.

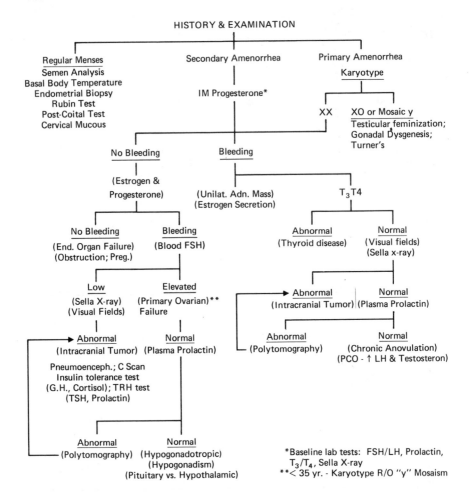

HISTORY & EXAMINATION

Regular Menses
Semen Analysis
Basal Body Temperature
Endometrial Biopsy
Rubin Test
Post-Coital Test
Cervical Mucous

Secondary Amenorrhea

IM Progesterone*

Primary Amenorrhea
Karyotype

XX   XO or Mosaic y
Testicular feminization;
Gonadal Dysgenesis;
Turner's

No Bleeding

(Estrogen &
Progesterone)

Bleeding

(Unilat. Adn. Mass)
(Estrogen Secretion)

T_3T4

No Bleeding   Bleeding
(End. Organ Failure) (Blood FSH)
(Obstruction; Preg.)

Abnormal   Normal
(Thyroid disease) (Visual fields)
                   (Sella x-ray)

Low   Elevated
(Sella X-ray)   (Primary Ovarian)**
(Visual Fields)   Failure

Abnormal   Normal
(Intracranial Tumor) (Plasma Prolactin)

Abnormal   Normal
(Intracranial Tumor) (Plasma Prolactin)

Pneumoenceph.; C Scan
Insulin tolerance test
(G.H., Cortisol); TRH test
(TSH, Prolactin)

Abnormal   Normal
(Polytomography) (Chronic Anovulation)
                  (PCO - ↑ LH & Testosteron)

Abnormal   Normal
(Polytomography) (Hypogonadotropic)
                  (Hypogonadism)
                  (Pituitary vs. Hypothalamic)

*Baseline lab tests: FSH/LH, Prolactin,
T_3/T_4, Sella X-ray
**< 35 yr. - Karyotype R/O "y" Mosaism

BASIC PRINCIPLES OF INFERTILITY INVESTIGATION

The most important aspect of infertility investigation is the doctor–patient relationship. The problem should be defined as it relates to the couple, and it is therefore preferable to have both husband and wife present at least at the initial interview. The couple should be made to understand, in general, the type and purpose of each of the tests that are going to be done, and most important, the amount of time that is usually required for the infertility work-up, which in most cases will range from three to six months. At least two-thirds of the couples can be helped by the appropriate therapeutic measures, which are in turn based on the results of the infertility testing.

DIAGNOSTIC PROCEDURES

The usual diagnostic procedures for infertility include a complete history and physical, CBC, serology, urinalysis, Pap, and rubella titer (consider immunization if a patient shows a negative rubella titer).

The male factor is tested by a semen analysis done by a reliable laboratory, which reports the count given per milliliter, the volume, and the percentage of sperm motile. The percentage of abnormal forms, a description of abnormalities of motility and the presence of immature forms should be noted.

An additional test of the "male" factor is the postcoital or Sims-Huhner test, which is done to evaluate both the woman's cervical mucus in the immediate preovulatory state and the survival of sperm in this mucus.

Ovulation is judged on the basis of a biphasic basal body temperature and endometrial biopsy. The tubal patency is judged by the use of a hysterosalpingogram (carbon dioxide insufflation has been abandoned by most infertility experts on the basis of its limited information and discomfort to the patient), and, in certain cases, endoscopy. These tests are described in detail below.

EVIDENCE OF OVULATION

The simplest test that can establish a presumptive diagnosis of **ovulation is** the use of a basal body temperature chart. The patient charts her temperature upon arising in the morning before getting out of bed or having a cigarette or coffee.

An "ovulatory" temperature pattern should be biphasic, with the temperature rising one or two days after ovulation owing to the increasing amounts of progesterone, which is found only in the luteal (postovulatory) phase of the menstrual cycle.

It has been stated that a woman with regular menstrual periods and a biphasic temperature chart is ovulating and therefore need not be examined further for an ovulation problem. However, we have found that even under these circumstances, an endometrial biopsy should be done. The reason for this is the recent recognition of a diagnosis of "inadequate luteal phase," in which there is inadequate progesterone secretion and therefore delayed maturation of the lining of the uterus in the post-ovulation, luteal state. It is also important to do the endometrial biopsy approximately two to four days *before* menstruation. Second, in order to properly judge the development lining of the uterus and to make proper histologic diagnosis as to whether or not an inadequate luteal phase is present, it is important that the pathologist be familiar with the Noyes, Hertig and Rock "dating" of the endometrium. This is based on the morphologic changes of the glandular epithelium and stroma of the endometrium during the luteal phase with the diagnosis given on the basis of the number of days post ovulation. The patient informs the physician when her **next** period after the biopsy begins, and this date is then corrollated with the date given on the endometrial biopsy report. There should not be a difference of greater than two days between the predicted date of menses by the biopsy report and the actual onset of the next menses. An example of this is the following: The patient undergoes an endometrial biopsy on day 25 of her menstrual cycle. The report of the biopsy reads "consistent with day 18 or four days post ovulation." Her menses then begin three days after the biopsy procedure. There is a seven-day difference between the biopsy report and the onset of the next menses $(18 + 3 - 28 = -7)$, which is therefore consistent with the diagnosis of "inadequate luteal phase." On the other hand, had her menses begun ten days after the biopsy, the report would have been normal. It is therefore important to evaluate the endometrial biopsy in relation to the onset of the *next* menses and for the histologic pattern to be within two days of the cycle.

SEMEN ANALYSIS

The semen analysis should be collected according to the coital history; abstinence before the semen analysis should be the same as the average interval between sexual relations. The specimen is collected in a dry clean jar by masturbation. Contraceptive condoms should not be used for this collection because they are spermicidal. However, there are commercially available plastic "pouches" that have no spermicidal action. Specimens should be examined within two hours after collection, and the following should be noted in the report: (1) liquefaction—which is usually complete in 20 to 30 minutes; (2) volume—normally 2.5 to 4 ml; (3) motility—at room temperature, should be 60 to 70% and demonstrating vigorous *progressive* activity, and at six to eight hours (although this length of time is not routinely done) 25 to 40% should still be showing vigorous progressive activity; (4) the cell count should be at least 20 to 30 million/ml; (5) morphological examination should show greater than 60% normal forms. In addition, the notation of any sperm agglutination or presence of immature sperm cells should be included. The combination of decreased motility, increased abnormal forms, and the presence of immature sperm cells strongly suggests the presence of a varicocele.

THE POSTCOITAL TEST (SIMS-HUHNER TEST)

The purpose of this test is to evaluate the interaction of sperm with the cervical mucus and to evaluate the quality of the cervical mucus itself. The patient is instructed to have intercourse within 10 to 12 hours preceding the exam. The test must be timed within two days of the expected ovulation and therefore may need to be repeated several times during the same cycle. Intercourse should be performed in the normal fashion, and no period of abstinence is necessary. The patient should be warned not to use any douches or lubricants. A nonlubricated speculum is placed in the vagina, and the ectocervix is gently wiped with a clean sponge with care taken not to produce any bleeding. In the presence of unopposed estrogen (without progesterone), the cervical mucus becomes clear, watery, and abundant, and develops stretchability, or spinbarkait of 10 to 15 cm. The microscopic exam may show 0 to 4 white blood cells per high power field, and if any more are present, this will either indicate an "endocervicitis" or that the test has been done at the wrong time of the cycle. The number of sperm should be about 10 to 20 per high power field. In addition, the percentage of good forward progression versus poor progression or immotile sperm should be noted. The mucus is then dried, and a classic "ferning" pattern should develop. The absence of sperm in the presence of good mucus may be due to: (1) azoospermia; (2) retrograde ejaculate; or (3) a problem in coital technique (e.g., use of lubricants) or sexual dysfunction. Immotile sperm may be noted in "hostile" mucus, which may contain an antibody to the sperm antigen. The absence of good mucus may denote a hypoestrogen state, or the presence of progesterone, and most important, may only mean that the test was performed at the wrong time of the cycle.

HYSTEROSALPINGOGRAM

The purpose of this test is to determine uterine or tubal pathology. The test is specially indicated in women with a history of pelvic inflammatory disease or previous pelvic surgery (laparoscopy is also important in these types of situations), suspected uterine malformations, or intrauterine adhesions. A pelvic exam should be done prior to the procedure to rule out any adnexal pathology or infection; the procedure should not be done if the patient is bleeding. Therefore, the best time to perform this procedure is a few days after menstrual bleeding has ceased.

A water-soluble or an oil medium may be used. The advantage of the water-soluble medium is its rapid absorption and is the best medium for identifying uterine abnormalities. The advantage of the oil medium is that the 24-hour film may help to diagnose pelvic adhesions. If any tubal occlusion is diagnosed on the hysterosalpingogram, a laparoscopy then becomes essential prior to any surgical correction.

LAPAROSCOPY

Laparoscopy is indicated in the following conditions: (1) suspicion of endometriosis, pelvic mass, or ectopic pregnancy; (2) pelvic pain of unknown etiology; (3) to confirm the diagnosis of ovarian dysgenesis, absent uterus, or pelvic inflammatory disease; (4) when there is inability to conceive after two or three years of unprotected coitus in the presence of normal fertility testing; (5)

to confirm the diagnosis of fallopian tube occlusion; (6) to diagnose and/or remove an intra-abdominal IUD; (7) an abnormal hysterosalpingogram; (8) tubal sterilization. Before contemplating any tubloplastic procedure, a laparoscopy should be done so that an unnecessary laparotomy is avoided in those conditions where the tubes are irreparably destroyed. Last, laparoscopy should be considered in those patients who failed to conceive after six cycles of appropriate infertility therapy (e.g., fertility drugs or artificial insemination).

THE MALE FACTOR

A careful history should be obtained as to the adequacy of sleep, exercise, and the possible excessive use of alcohol or marijuana. Emotional tension or the possibility of excess or prolonged heat to the scrotom should be ruled out on the basis of history. Urological consultation should be obtained if an abnormal semen analysis is present, and serum FSH—Fullicle Stimulating Hormone, LH—Luteinizing Hormone, thyroid, testosterone and prolactin levels should be obtained in cases of oligo- or azoospermia. Men demonstrating azoospermia with normal tests are required to have a testicular biopsy in order to rule out an obstruction of the distal epididymus or proximal vas deferens. Epididymosotomy can be curative in these particular cases. If low motility and/or an increased number of abnormal and mature forms is detected, a varicocele may be suspected. Varicocelectomy may improve an abnormal semen analysis in 65% of the cases, with an approximately 40 to 50% pregnancy rate. Some investigators have considered ligating the left spermatic vein even in the absence of a varicocele, when these abnormalities are reported on repeated semen analyses. Pharmacological management of oligospermia with fertility drugs has included: human menopausal gonadotropins (Pergonal), clomiphene citrate, or testosterone. The cost of Pergonal is presently $15 an ampule, and requires that the husband be treated for a minimum of 70 days (cycle of sperm) before determining a positive response. This therapy is best reserved for those men with documented gonadotropin insufficiency. Clomiphene citrate is used for its gonadotropin-stimulating ability and has been reported to improve semen analysis in 30% of the cases. The dosage used is 25 to 50 mg per day, and it is not approved for treatment of male infertility. Testosterone therapy has been used for its "rebound" effect on the sperm count. However, in some instances, the suppression of spermatogenesis by testosterone has resulted in persistent azoospermia and for this reason its use has been discouraged.

ARTIFICIAL INSEMINATION

Artificial insemination can be done with the use of a donor (AID) or the husband (AIH). AIH or husband insemination can be used in those cases in which oligospermia, low volume (less than 1 ml), or other abnormalities in the semen analysis are noted. Since the first portion of the ejaculate continas 75% of the total spermatozoa and the motility is usually better in the first than in the second portion, a split ejaculate may be of particular value in those cases of oligospermia secondary to a large volume of semen (greater than 5 ml). AIH may also be considered in cases of poor cervical mucus (see cervical factor).

In cases of severe oligospermia (less than 5 million/ml), azoospermia, or when a significant number of AIH fail to result in conception, consideration should then be given to use of a donor insemination.

ANOVULATION FACTOR

Patients presenting with primary or secondary amenorrhea, oligomenorrhea, or dysfunctional uterine bleeding may all have a common infertility factor-

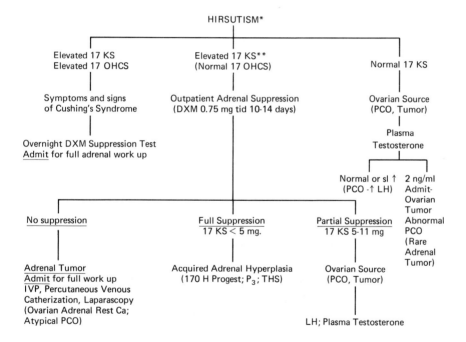

*If Primary Amenorrhea — do Karyotype R/O Incomplete T.F. or Gonadal Dysgenesis

**17 KS > 50 mg/24 hrs. — IVP → will reveal almost all Adrenal Ca
  17 KS > 25 mg/24 hrs. — rarely seen with PCO (75% of PCO or Cushing's have normal 17 KS)

Adapted in part from Speroff et al Clinical Gyn. Endocr. & Infertility, 1973.

PCO — Polycystic Ovaries   17 OHCS — 17 Hydroxysteroids
T.F. — Testicular Feminization   17 KS — 17 Ketosteroids

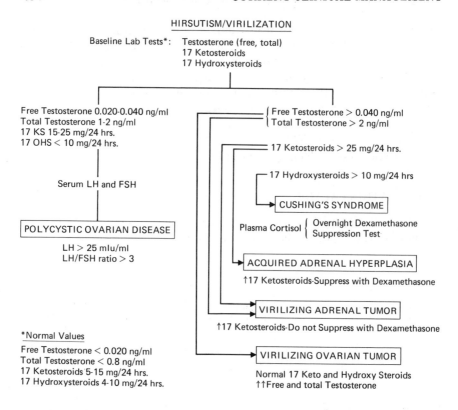

HIRSUTISM/VIRILIZATION

Baseline Lab Tests*: Testosterone (free, total)
17 Ketosteroids
17 Hydroxysteroids

Free Testosterone 0.020-0.040 ng/ml
Total Testosterone 1-2 ng/ml
17 KS 15-25 mg/24 hrs.
17 OHS < 10 mg/24 hrs.

Serum LH and FSH

POLYCYSTIC OVARIAN DISEASE
LH > 25 mIu/ml
LH/FSH ratio > 3

Free Testosterone > 0.040 ng/ml
Total Testosterone > 2 ng/ml

17 Ketosteroids > 25 mg/24 hrs.

17 Hydroxysteroids > 10 mg/24 hrs

CUSHING'S SYNDROME

Plasma Cortisol { Overnight Dexamethasone Suppression Test

ACQUIRED ADRENAL HYPERPLASIA
↑17 Ketosteroids-Suppress with Dexamethasone

VIRILIZING ADRENAL TUMOR
↑17 Ketosteroids-Do not Suppress with Dexamethasone

VIRILIZING OVARIAN TUMOR
Normal 17 Keto and Hydroxy Steroids
↑↑Free and total Testosterone

*Normal Values
Free Testosterone < 0.020 ng/ml
Total Testosterone < 0.8 ng/ml
17 Ketosteroids 5-15 mg/24 hrs.
17 Hydroxysteroids 4-10 mg/24 hrs.

anovulation. A diagnostic approach to the work-up of patients with amenorrhea is shown on the amenorrhea flow sheet. Note that precocious menopause or ovarian dysgenesis would represent cases of absolute sterility, and therefore attempts at ovulation induction should not be done. These patients present with hypoestrogenism and amenorrhea, and elevated serum gonadotropin levels, in particular FSH.

As outlined on the flow sheet, every anovulatory patient should be evaluated with a pituitary polytomogram, serum prolactin, FSH, LH, and thyroid profile. Presence of endogenous estrogen is documented by withdrawal bleeding after 100 mg of progesterone IM. If no bleeding occurs, exogenous estrogens are then administered to demonstrate the presence of a uterus and a responsive endometrium. Patients with amenorrhea due to intrauterine adhesions do *not* bleed in response to exogenous estrogens, i.e. endometrial failure. In the presence of hirsutism, serum testosterone (total and free), urinary 17 ketosteroids and 17 hydroxysteroids, determination may be warranted in differentiating between hirsutism due to androgens of ovarian and adrenal sources. (See "Hirsutism" flow sheet.) If a prolactin-secreting pituitary tumor is noted on a polytomogram,

DISEASE STATE	OBSERVATION	BROMCRYPTINE	SURGERY	
Amenorrhea-Galactorrea (no tumor)	+	+	−	
Amenorreah-Galactorrea and Pregnancy Desired	−	+	−	
Microdenoma (< 1 cm)	+	+*	+	Transphenoidal Microsurgery
Microadenoma and Pregnancy Desired	−	+**	+	
Macroadenoma (> 1 cm)	−	?+*	+	
Macroadenoma with Suprasellar Extension	−	?+*	+	
Macroadenoma (all) and Pregnancy Desired	−	−	+	

*Recent evidence indicates that Bromcryptine Therapy may prevent growth of
and/or shrink Prolactin-Secreting Pituitary Adenomas.
**Careful followup of pregnant patients with Microadenomas is indicated.

FIG. 1. Choices of treatment in the management of anenorrhea-galactorrhea-pituitury adenona.

the patient is best treated with either radiation or transphenoidal surgery. In the latter case, a therapeutic response may be noted in over 50% of patients with the return of ovulatory menstrual cycles, and a normal prolactin level. With radiation therapy, symptoms are slow to regress and may not do so for a number of years. Although these pituitary tumors are slow growing, they may suddenly enlarge, impinging on the optic chiasma and requiring emergency therapy in the form of corticosteroid medication and/or emergency surgery. Therefore, it may be best to treat these tumors before consideration is given to induction of ovulation and pregnancy unless they are less than 1 centimeter in size (see Figure 1).

AMENORRHEA-GALACTORRHEA-HYPERPROLACTINEMIA

Amenorrhea-galactorrhea, an important syndrome related to infertility and ovulation failure, is associated with elevated serum prolactin levels. It is therefore important to obtain prolactin levels in patients with anovulation to rule out pituitary adenoma, a principal cause of elevated prolactin levels. However, clini-

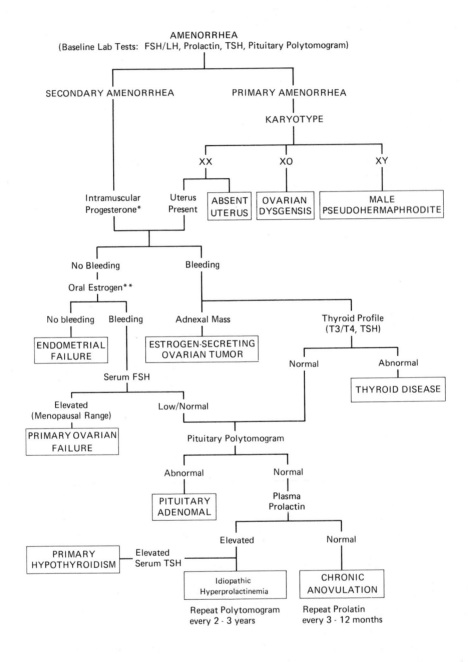

cal galactorrhea may be found in only one-third of the patients with hyperprolactinemia. A prolactin-secreting pituitary adenoma may be found in 30% of patients with hyperprolactinemia. This percentage is higher if the prolactin levels are greater than 100 ng/ml. Primary hypothyroidism should be ruled out, since this may also give rise to amenorrhea, galactorrhea and elevated **in prolactin levels**. If there is no evidence of hypothyroidism or a pituitary adenoma, the syndrome of amenorrhea-hyperprolactinemia may be treated with the use of a new drug, Brom-ergocryptine (sold under the commercial name of Parlodel by Sandoz Pharmaceuticals). The usual dose is 2.5 mg B.I.D. and the side effects are mild nausea and dizziness. The mechanism of action is that of dopamine agonist, which acts on both the hypothalamus and the pituitary to suppress prolactin secretion and to reestablish normal ovulatory cycles. For choices of management for this problem see Figure 1.

OVULATION INDUCTION

When an anovulation woman shows evidence of estrogen secretion (an endometrial biopsy showing proliferative endometrium, cervical mucus showing good spinbarkait and ferning, and withdrawal bleeding following intramuscular injection of progesterone clomiphene citrate is of therapeutic value in inducing

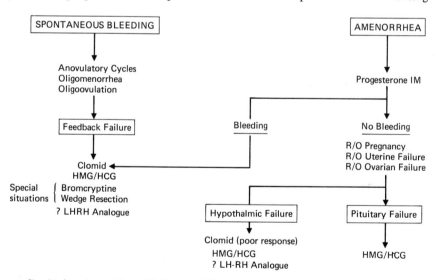

Clomid - (may be combined with Estrogen, HCG, or Dexamethasone, or HMG)
HMG   - Human Menopausal Gonadotropin (Pergonal)

FIG. 2. Ovulation induction.

ovulation. On the other hand, if there is evidence of hypoestrogenism, based on lack of a bleeding response to intramuscular progesterone (and *no* evidence of ovarian failure), the patient may be a candidate for primary treatment with Pergonal. In the future, long-acting luteinizing hormone releasing hormone (LH–RH) may become available, which may be used for ovulation induction in patients with an intact pituitary gland. (A basic approach to ovulation induction therapy is shown on the ovulation induction flow sheet)

CLOMIPHENE CITRATE

This drug is a nonsteroidal weak estrogen that acts as a gonadotropin stimulator. The initial dose is 50 mg daily for 5 days starting **on the fifth day of the cycle,** which may require progesterone therapy for its induction. The biologic activity of Clomiphene is not well understood; but being a weak estrogen, it competes with estrogen binding in the hypothalamus and pituitary. The hypothalamus and pituitary interprets this as an estrogen deficiency state and results in the secretion of increasing amounts of gonadotropins. This in turn stimulates the growth of an ovarian follicle. Ovulation usually occurs four to seven days after the last day of Clomiphene. If ovulation fails to occur, the dosage is increased in subsequent cycles, progressing up to 200 to 250 mg for five days plus HCG (human chorionic gonadotropin) 10,000 IU four to six days after the course of Clomiphene. If this maximum dose is still not effective in inducing ovulation, human menopausal gonadotropin (Pergonal) may then be used. Although Clomiphene will usually yield "ovulation" in 65% of the cases, approximately only half of these patients will conceive. The reason for this discrepancy is not completely clear, but the following should be ruled out: (1) Presence of another infertility factor in the male or female; (2) Inadequate luteal phase as shown by a biopsy done during an "ovulatory" cycle induced by Clomiphene; (3) antiestrogen effect on the cervical mucus in which the cervical mucus fails to develop its characteristically clear, watery appearance in the preovulatory state. This latter side effect can be overcome by the use of oral ethinyl estradiol, starting on the *last* day of Clomiphene therapy in doses ranging from 20 to 150 μg per day for ten days. It is important that the postcoital examination be done *prior* to any Clomiphene treatment in order to document the presence of normal cervical mucus prior to any therapy. The inadequate luteal phase can be corrected by increasing the dose of Climiphene or adding HCG.

Possible side effects of Clomiphene therapy include menopausal-like hot flashes, transient visual disturbance, headache, nausea, and vomiting. The miscarriage rate is approximately 20%, and twinning may occur in 5 to 7% of pregnancies. There is no evidence of any teratogenic effect above that expected for the normal population. If a patient develops ovarian cysts, the drug should be stopped until the ovaries regress to their original size. Patients with polycystic ovaries syndrome, who fail to respond to Clomiphene, may be treated with Pergonal or bilateral wedge resection. However, patients with enlarged ovaries may react to Pergonal with tremendous ovarian stimulation in spite of the proper safety precautions, which we will outline below. On the other hand, bilateral ovarian wedge resection may result in a 15 or 20% incidence of postoperative pelvic adhesions, and the surgery may only temporarily result in ovulatory cycles. In certain patients with polycystic ovarian syndrome, who are Clomiphene failures, continous low dose corticosteroid therapy (e.g., Prednisone 5 to 10 mg nightly) may improve their response to Clomiphene.

PERGONAL

Pergonal is a urinary extract of menopausal women, with each ampule containing 75 mg of FSH and 75 mg of LH. As opposed to Clomiphene, in which case an intact pituitary gland is essential, Pergonal, which is itself a gonadotropin, does not require an intact pituary. The drug is indicated in patients with amenorrhea, especially those who are hypostrogenic and do not have primary ovarian failure. It may also be given to those patients who failed to ovulate with maximal doses of Clomiphene citrate. In addition, patients who failed to conceive after apparent ovulation with Clomiphene citrate may also be considered for Pergonal therapy, although their potential for pregnancy may not be as good. Before proceeding with Pergonal, the patients who failed to conceive on Clomiphene should be reevaluated with a complete infertility workup; laparoscopic examination of the pelvic organs should be considered.

Patients with lack of endogenous estrogen are started on two ampules daily, and those with evidence of endogenous estrogens are started with one ampule a day. The cervix is observed for development of watery, elastic, "ferning" mucus, and estrogen levels are measured in the urine or blood. If estrogen secretion does not increase (i.e., there is a lack of cervical mucus and no rise in urinary or plasma levels after six or seven days of therapy), the dose should be increased by an additional ampule. Intramuscular HCG, 10,000 IU is given when the plasma estradiol reaches 1000 to 1500 pg/ml, or the total urinary estrogen reaches the range of 60 to 120 μg/24 hours. It is therefore important to have the estrogen report within the *same* day so that the therapy can be adjusted on a day to day basis.

It is a prerequisite that the patients receiving Pergonal be examined frequently to ensure that there is no enlargement of the ovaries, and that daily blood or urinary estrogens be measured. If these two criteria cannot be met, the patient should be referred to the appropriate medical facility.

With appropriate selection of patients, Pergonal therapy is highly successful. Over 90% of patients ovulate, and 65% of patients conceive. It is important to remember that the miscarriage rate is approximately 20%, and that the incidence of twins is 25%, and of triplets is 2 to 5%. An ultrasound should be done early in pregnancy to diagnose multiple gestational sacs.

The main complication of Pergonal therapy, apart from multiple gestations, is the ovarian hyperstimulation syndrome. The latter is characterized by tremendous ovarian enlargement (**due to multiple** theca lutein cysts), ascites, hydrothorax and finally hypotension, oliguria, and hypovolemia resulting from "third spacing" of fluid into the peritoneal cavity. This also produces an electrolyte imbalance, in particular hyperkalemia. The ovaries not only enlarge to tremendous size, but may twist or hemorrhage, causing an acute abdomen. The syndrome reaches a peak approximately two weeks post ovulation and subsides within the next few weeks. The hyperstimulation syndrome is usually preventable by checking for ovarian enlargement and monitoring the estrogen levels; if the HCG is withheld, hyperstimulation will not develop.

INADEQUATE LUTEAL PHASE OR CORPUS LUTEAL DEFECT

The inadequate luteal phase may be a cause of infertility or early miscarriage (eight weeks or less). It is diagnosed by an endometrial biopsy taken approximately three to four days before the onset of menstruation. Luteal defects are thought to be due to a deficient follicular development, which in turn causes deficiency of luteal progesterone as demonstrated by depressed serial blood progesterone levels. This has led to one of the first therapeutic approaches, i.e., the use of progesterone medication in the form of IM progesterone injections (12.5 to 25.0 mg per day) or progesterone vaginal suppositories (25 mg bid) during the luteal phase of the cycle. If pregnancy occurs, the therapy is continued for 10 to 12 weeks, at which time placental takeover is assured. Progestagens other than progesterone are best avoided because of there being a possible teratogenic or luteolytic side effects. Other therapeutic approaches to this problem have been to improve the follicular development by using Clomiphene or Pergonal.

CERVICAL FACTOR

Cervical factor is diagnosed on the basis of an abnormal postcoital test, in which a male factor has been ruled out by a normal semen analysis. It may be characterized by the absence of the characteristic preovulatory mucus as described above. In a well-timed preovulatory mucus, the presence of white blood cells indicates endocervicitis. This type of infection may be primarily treated with local antiseptic douching in combination with vaginal antibiotic creams and systemic antibiotics. Should this form of therapy prove unsuccessful, consideration may be given to cryosurgery. When the cervical mucus is decreased or viscous, the patient may be treated with oral ethinyl estradiol starting at about four days prior to ovulation. If the cervical mucus remains inadequate despite estrogen therapy, consideration may be given to the use of artificial insemination (AIH). The presence of a sperm antibody may be suspected on the basis of a normal semen analysis, and a postcoital test in which the quality and quantity of the mucus is adequate, but contains many dead or immotile sperm. This may be documented by an in vitro "penetration test," which microscopically quantitates the migration of the sperm in a capillary tube filled with cervical mucus. This condition is one of the most difficult problems to treat in the field of infertility. Therapy may include the long-term use of a condom, which prevents antigenic exposure. This may be combined with corticosteroid in order further to depress the wife's antibody formation. Lastly, intrauterine insemination has been used in order to overcome this cervical "barrier," although the sperm antibody may still be present higher up in the genital tract. Pregnancy rates are approximately 10 to 15%.

TUBAL FACTOR

The principal causes of problems related to tubal pathology such as tubal obstruction or peritubal adhesions are pelvic inflammatory disease or endometriosis. In addition, owing to the increased rate of divorce and remarriage, there are many patients who are asking for reanastomosis of a previous tubal ligation. A full fertility workup should be obtained preoperatively and laparoscopy should be done in advance, in order to avoid an unnecessary laparotomy in those cases where the tubes are beyond repair. The various types of surgery may involve: (1) salpingolysis, which is the lysis of peritubal adhesions; (2) reanastomosis of tubal obstructions such as those resulting from previous tubal sterilizations; (3) salpingostomy, in which a new distal tubal opening must be re-created (with the fimbria destroyed, the results of this latter operation are poor); (4) tubo-uterine reimplantation or reanastomosis for a cornual obstruction. Success rates may vary from 10 to 75%, depending on the type of procedure done. One important complication of tubal surgery is a 5 to 10% incidence of ectopic pregnancy. The use of an operating microscope has become increasingly popular, although controversy still exists as to whether it is actually required for all tubal surgery. In any case, the highest pregnancy rate can be obtained with the least surgical manipulation of the tube, fine suture material (e.g., 8-0 nylon or vicryl or nylon), preservation of a relatively normal length of the tube, and normal-appearing fimbria. If the operating microscope is not available, magnifying loupes (3-4X) may be equally effective for most cases.

ENDOMETRIOSIS

Endometriosis has been treated in various ways over the years, including conservative surgery with or without pre- and postoperative ovarian suppression with sex steroids. Endometriosis may be suspected on the basis of significant secondary dysmenorrhea or tender nodularities palpated on uterosacral ligaments on pelvic exam. These are best confirmed with laparoscopy. If at the time of laparoscopy, no evidence of tubal obstruction or adhesions are present, and only "power burn" spots of endometriosis are found, the patient is treated with ovarian suppression in the form of constant administration of birth control pills, or a newer steroid called Danazol, for six to nine months. Surgery is indicated with the presence of tubal obstruction and/or peritubal adhesions. Consideration may be given perhaps to a preoperative six-week course of hormonal therapy to shrink very large endometriotic nodules. Postoperatively, if no endometriosis is left behind, the patient is instructed to get pregnant as soon as she is able to resume coitus. When endometriosis has been left behind, a short course of approximately six to eight weeks of birth control pills or Danazol may be used before attempting pregnancy. The more severe the amount of endometriosis, and the longer the postoperative course of hormonal suppression, the less success the patient has in conception, ranging from 25–75%. At the time of surgery, a uterine suspension may be performed in order to prevent the tubes from falling back into the cul de sac and readhering into the peritoneal surface. A presacral neurectomy may be done in those cases with intractable dysmenorrhea.

UTERINE SURGERY

Intrauterine adhesions usually result from a traumatic D and C, and are characterized by a syndrome of amenorrhea or hypomenorrhea, cyclic pelvic pain, and little or no bleeding in response to exogenous estrogens (see amenorrhea flow sheet). The diagnosis is confirmed by hysterosalpingogram, and the treatment is to resect the adhesions. The operative hysteroscope is a suitable instrument for this purpose and results in a 50% pregnancy rate.

Uterine anomalies such as a bicornuate or septate uterus may be related to repeated spontaneous abortions. Uterine reunification procedures are associated with a better than 65% successful pregnancy rate.

Another cause of repeated spontaneous midtrimester abortions amenable to surgery is the incompetent cervix. This can be corrected by a circlage procedure usually done early in the second trimester of pregnancy, confirmed by a diagnostic ultrasound. A permanent suture such as mersile or nylon is used, which may be removed at term, thereby allowing the patient to deliver vaginally.

Further Reading

Behrman and Kistner, eds. *Progress in Infertility* (2nd ed.). Boston: Little, Brown and Co., 1976.

Gold, ed. *Gynecologic Endocrinology* (2nd ed.) New York: Harper and Row, 1975.

Hafez, E. S. E., ed. *Human Semen and Fertility Regulation in Men*. St. Louis: C. V. Mosby, 1976.

Hafez and Evans, eds. *Human Reproduction—Conception and Contraception.* New York: Harper and Row, 1973.

Martini and Besser, eds. *Clinical Neuroendocrinology,* New York: Academic Press, 1977.

Netter, Frank H. *Reproductive System—The CIBA Collection of Medical Illustrations,* Vol. 2, 1965.

Odell and Moyer, eds. *Physiology of Reproduction.* St. Louis: C. V. Mosby, 1971.

Reid, Ryan, and Benirschke, eds. *Principles and Management of Human Reproduction.* Philadelphia: W. B. Saunders, 1972.

Simpson, ed. *Disorders of Sexual Differentiation.* New York: Academic Press, 1976.

Speroff, Glass, and Kase, eds. *Clinical Gynecologic Endocrinology and Infertility.* (2nd ed.). Baltimore: Williams and Wilkins, 1978.

Williams, ed. *Textbook of Endocrinology* (5th ed.) Philadelphia: W. B. Saunders, 1974.

Yen and Jaffe, eds. *Reproductive Endocrinology.* Philadelphia: W. B. Saunders, 1978.

Total Joint Replacement

JOSEPH S. BARR, Jr., M.D.
Assistant Clinical Professor of Orthopaedic Surgery
Harvard Medical School
Assistant Orthopedic Surgeon
Massachusetts General Hospital
Boston, Massachusetts

The reconstructive surgery of major joints has been revolutionized by the introduction of the total joint replacement. Much of the early work was done in England by Sir John Charnley. He conceived the idea of a "low friction" arthroplasty and began by using a Teflon (polytetrafluoroethylene) socket and stainless steel femoral prosthesis for hip replacement. Although laboratory wear studies had been promising, Teflon wore quickly, and the resultant small plastic particles proved toxic, causing wound breakdown and sinus tract formation. Charnley then turned to high-density polyethylene for the hip socket, and this material has proved successful in a variety of joints over the past 15 years (Figure 1). Charnley also pioneered the fixation of prosthesis to bone with the acrylic plastic, polymethylmethacrylate. Methylmethacrylate is a cement; it does not have adhesive properties. It is a brittle material when subjected to torque or bending forces, but has excellent strength when compressed. It is mixed at the operating table from a liquid monomer and powdered polymer, producing a dough after 3 to 5 minutes and then fully polymerizing or setting in 8 to 12 minutes (Figure 2). The reaction is an exothermic one, but the temperature in a large mass does not exceed 100°C., and it can be lowered by the "heat sink" effect of the metal prosthesis, or by irrigating the plastic as it sets.

THE HIP JOINT

Major disability from arthritis of the hip is more common than from the knee, ankle, or other joints. The hip is well suited for total joint replacement because it is a ball-and-socket joint with one center of rotation, and it is inherently quite

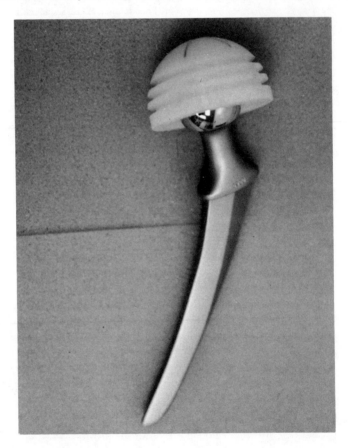

FIG. 1. Total hip replacement in common use. The high-density polyethylene socket has grooves to allow cement fixation and metal wires imbedded to mark its position in an x-ray. The femoral prosthesis is a stainless steel alloy with a highly polished head to avoid scratching of the socket.

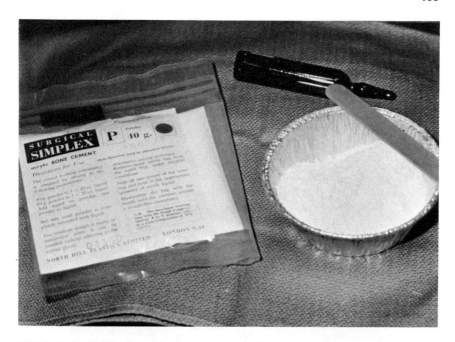

FIG. 2. Polymethylmethacrylate bone cement consisting of liquid monomer (brown vial) and powdered polymer supplied sterile in measured amounts to be mixed at the operating table. At 3-5 minutes after mixing the "dough" in non-sticky and ready to be inserted into the bone.

stable and well protected by thick layers of muscle and subcutaneous tissue. Total hip arthroplasty has become the model and stimulus for the development of replacement techniques for other major joints. Approximately 75,000 total hips are now done in the United States yearly (Figure 3). The quality and reliability of this surgery has been good to excellent in 85 to 90% of patients at five-year follow-up. Pain, which is the major indication for this type of joint surgery, is virtually always relieved. The prosthetic joint provides a good functional range of motion and usually allows the patient to increase his activity. Rehabilitation of the patient following surgery is guided by the surgeon and the physical therapist, and proceeds quite routinely with crutches for about 6 weeks, followed by a cane. Most vigorous patients can discontinue a cane at 12 weeks and are able to walk lengthy distances and resume essentially normal activity. Strenuous activities such as running or jumping are not advisable due to the danger of prosthetic or cement loosening or breakage. Because of this relative activity limitation, the yet-unknown long-term wear characteristics, and the possibility of toxic or carcinogenic properties of wear products, total joints are not routinely advised for patients under the age of 50 years.

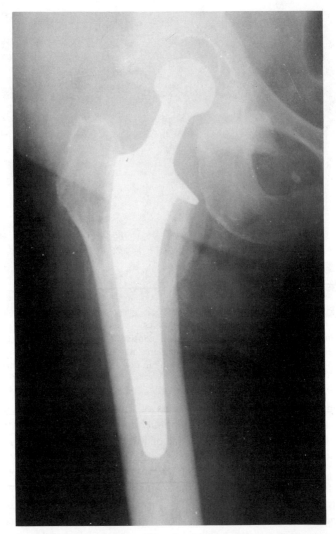

FIG. 3. Total hip replacement. The methylmethacrylate has been made radiopaque with barium and is visable between prosthesis and bone. The greater trochanter was not osteotomized in this instance.

While total hips have been highly successful, a number of problems have occurred, the most important of which will be considered separately.

Sepsis

Deep infection is a true disaster in a total joint, as the volume of foreign inert material puts normal body defense mechanisms at a disadvantage. The same is true with the prosthetic heart valve. The sepsis rate in over 18,000 total hips recorded in the literature has been 1.5%. During total joint surgery, scrupulous attention must be paid to sterile technique; and the use of laminar-flow, sterile-air operating rooms is helpful to decrease air-borne bacterial contamination of the open wound. Interestingly, about half of the infections occur late, as much as several years postsurgery. Late infection following dental procedures or cystoscopy has been documented, and patients with total joints should be cautioned to take a broad spectrum antibiotic (e.g., a cephalosporin) prophylactically before any invasive procedure. Deep sepsis may present as an erythematous, swollen, draining wound, as one would expect with a typical wound infection, or may be subtle and hard to diagnose. X-rays may show loosening of the cement and prosthesis or even dislocation of the hip. Pain may be the only symptom at times. Any painful total joint must be suspected of having a low-grade sepsis, and aspiration of joint fluid with careful aerobic and anaerobic culture technique is mandatory. A persistent elevated sedimentation rate is another clue to deep sepsis.

When deep infection does occur, the joint and methylmethacrylate cement must be removed along with all devitalized tissue and bone. Removal of cement from the femoral medullary canal can be technically difficult, and at times the femur must be "guttered" or opened longitudinally. The end result of this procedure is a pseudoarthrosis (Girdlestone procedure), which is not very stable, may be painful, shortens the leg 2 or more inches, and requires permanent use of crutches or a cane while walking. If the offending organism is not too virulent, and can be controlled with appropriate antibiotics, it is sometimes possible to replace the total joint following the debridement, or after a suitable wait of 6 weeks or more to make sure a dry uninfected wound has been obtained. Intensive parenteral antibiotics for 6 weeks followed by oral antibiotics for an extended period is the commonly used protocol for the replacement of an infected total joint. Buchholz in Germany has pioneered in the use of methylmethacrylate cement impregnated with antibiotics (usually gentamycin) for the replacement of a septic total hip. Gentamycin is heat-stable and leaches slowly out of the cement for many months. Buchholz reports a 75% success rate in this difficult surgery using only antibiotic-impregnated cement after a meticulous debridement. Most surgeons in the United States prefer parenteral antibiotics with antibiotic cement as an adjunct. In the United States currently, the Food and Drug Administration does not allow the sale of a methacrylate-antibiotic combination.

Loosening

This is the most common complication of total hip replacement and is more frequently seen in the femur than the acetabulum. Heavy patients or patients with osteoporosis are particularly subject to this complication. Diagnosis of loosening by X-ray is made by the appearance of a radiolucent zone between the bone and cement, sinking of the prosthesis lower in the femur, cracks in the cement mass, or fatigue fracture of the stem of the prosthesis (Figure 4). Approximately 20% of patients show some radiographic signs of loosening at five-year follow-up, but fortunately most are stable, and not symptomatic or progressive. The rate of operative revision for loosening has been about 2% in most series. Obviously, this rate could increase with longer follow-up and gives pause for thought.

Revision is technically difficult and much more demanding than a primary total hip. It is necessary to remove cement from the medullary canal of the femur in order to insert a long-stem prosthesis. Special high-speed drills and burrs have been developed to remove the cement, but it is difficult to avoid weakening the femur, and perforation of the femoral cortex is frequent. Fracture of the femur is another hazard. In acetabular loosening, metallic mesh can

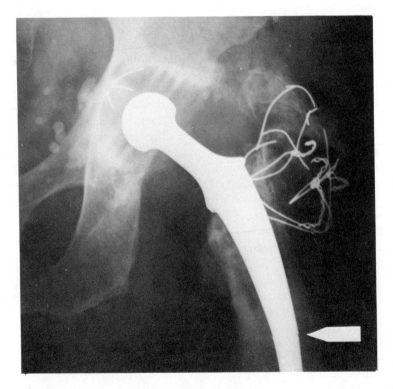

FIG. 4. Failed total hip in an obese patient. Non-union and upwards displacement of the greater trochanter is evident. The cement in the femur is loose and the stem of the prosthesis has fatigued and broken (arrow). Cultures were sterile, although sepsis might well be suspected with this x-ray appearance.

be used to reinforce the cement, and a polyethylene cup with a wide rim can be used to help prevent migration and intrapelvic protrusion. Occasionally, fatigue fracture of the femoral stem has occurred in conjunction with cement failure. Redesign and strengthening of the prosthetic stem should effectively control this problem. Improvement of surgical techniques should provide a better mechanical bond between bone and cement. Bone debris and blood are more effectively removed from the medullary canal of the femur by a pulsatile irrigation system than by ordinary irrigation. The medullary canal of the femur can be plugged with bone or cement distally below the tip of the prosthesis and the cement inserted with a syringe gun apparatus. As the prosthesis is inserted and impacted, the cement will penetrate better into the cancellous bone and form a better mechanical bond.

Dislocation

This occurs in about 1% of total hips, usually within the first few weeks of surgery before a new joint capsule has formed. Closed reduction is usually possible, followed by several weeks of bed rest with the leg abducted to allow the muscles to tighten up. The patients are cautioned to avoid adduction, internal rotation, or excessive (beyond 90%) flexion of the operated hip within the early postoperative period. Occasionally, malposition of the socket is responsible for recurrent dislocation, and revision is necessary.

Heterotopic Ossification

Some degree of this occurs in 20 to 30% of patients. However, only 1 to 2% show a significant decrease in motion. This problem occurs most commonly in mesomorphic males with degenerative arthritis. If loss of function is severe because of ossification about the total hip, removal of this new bone can be carried out when the alkaline phosphatase level is normal and bone scan shows no increased activity. This may take a year or more from the original surgery. If the new bone is disturbed before it is fully mature, it tends to recur even more densely. The biochemical cause of this phenomenon is unknown; it also tends to occur about the joints of patients with spinal cord injuries or severe burns.

Thromboembolism

This problem occurs much more frequently after hip surgery than other operative procedures. In patients who are not given some form of prophylaxis, the rate of thromboembolic disease reaches 50%, and approximately 2% will suffer fatal pulmonary embolism. Newer diagnostic measures including radioactive fibrinogen scanning, cuff plethysmography, phlebography, lung scans, and pul-

monary angiography have helped to define the true incidence of this problem.
More accurate diagnosis also allows for accurate comparison of different forms
of anticoagulant therapy. Effective prevention is given by warfarin, dextran, and
aspirin. Aspirin is most easily administered and best tolerated, but is not as effective in females as in males.

THE KNEE JOINT

The knee joint ranks second to the hip in terms of frequency of replacement,
approximately 30,000 a year being performed in the United States. The technology already discussed for the hip replacement has been adapted to the knee,

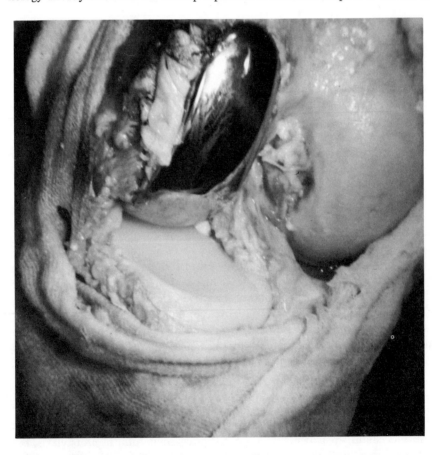

FIG. 5. A unicondylar knee replacement with metallic femoral and polyethylene tibial
components. Here only the lateral side of the knee joint required replacement. Cement is
seen at the edges of the components.

but the knee presents certain problems. Biomechanical studies indicate that while the hip in normal gait is subjected to loads up to 2½ times body weight, the knee during walking or climbing stairs may be loaded to 5 times body weight. The knee is a triaxial joint, being subjected to axial rotation and angular force as well as flexion and extension. Forces at the patello-femoral joint are also very high at times. The knee needs good ligaments for stability and does not have the soft tissue protection that the hip does. Development of total knee prostheses has proceeded along several different lines, and by 1974 at least 300 types were available. Many of them differed only slightly, but one can sense the problems inherent in a satisfactory design.

The first type of total knee was a metal hinge joint developed by Walldius

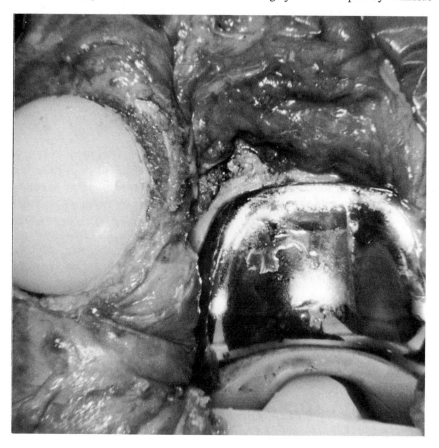

FIG. 6. The metallic component covers the femoral condyles and articulates with a one-piece polyethylene tibial prosthesis. The everted patella is seen to the left and its articulating surface has been covered with a polyethylene button.

in Sweden in the 1950s. Intramedullary stems are fitted into femur and tibia, and are generally cemented into place. Virtually all of these fully constrained prostheses loosen with time, and tissue inflammation from wear particles of the metal is another problem. This type of joint is rarely used now.

The most commonly used total knee prostheses are unconstrained and generally consist of a metallic femoral condylar portion that articulates with a high-density polyethylene component. In addition, the patella may be resurfaced with polyethylene (Figures 5 and 6). These prostheses require stable collateral ligaments. Representative types of the unconstrained prostheses are the Geometric, Duopatellar, or Polycentric.

There is a third general group of semiconstrained knee prostheses. Examples are the Spherocentric and Sheehan knees. They are useful in knees with ligamentous laxity, in severe angular deformity (varus or valgus), and for failure of an unconstrained prosthesis through loosening. This type of prosthesis allows some axial rotation and thus hopefully will provide needed stability while at the same time allowing absorption of the forces that cause loosening of the fully constrained prosthesis.

Success Rates

Unfortunately, knee replacement has not been nearly so successful as that of the hip. Failure rates of 15 to 25% are commonly reported during the first several years after knee replacement. Loosening is the primary cause of failure, and its frequency and severity appear to increase with time. Although the radiographic diagnosis of total hip loosening is common, the majority of hip replacements have remained clinically stable or nonprogressive to date. Thus, loosening is a much greater clinical problem in the knee replacement. Fixation of the tibial component depends mostly on the relatively weak cancellous bone of the upper tibia.

Sepsis in the total knee is an even greater disaster than in the hip. Only rarely can a septic total knee be salvaged. Pseudoarthrosis of the knee is painful and functionally unacceptable. Fusion (arthrodesis) after removal of a septic total knee prosthesis is difficult to achieve, even with compression techniques. The septic total knee often ends tragically in above-knee amputation. Overall, the total knee provides excellent pain relief and improved patient function, but its higher complication rate and poor salvage potential confine its use to older patients in whom no satisfactory alternative (e.g., osteotomy) is available.

OTHER JOINTS

Total joint replacement is possible for the shoulder, elbow, wrist, fingers, and ankle. Experience and follow-up are quite limited in all except finger joints.

Shoulder

Prosthetic designs for this joint generally resurface the glenoid with polyethylene and the humeral head with metal. The normal shoulder has a wide range of motion and depends on the rotator cuff, deltoid, and other supporting muscles for stability. If the rotator cuff is damaged or torn in an arthritic shoulder, total replacement may cure pain but may not be a functional success. Thus, candidates for total shoulder replacement must be selected carefully and may require a rather extended rehabilitation period for the shoulder musculature.

Elbow

Early attempts at replacement were with a hinged (constrained) type of joint (Figure 7). Initially, these produced excellent results, but torque eventually caused the humeral stem to loosen in most. New designs allow for some medial-lateral motion at the hinge to absorb torque, or attempt to resurface the humerus and ulna, allowing some play between the components. Numbers are too small, and follow-up has been insufficient to allow a realistic appraisal at this time.

Wrist

As in the elbow and shoulder, the need for wrist replacement is much less than in the hip and knee. The arthritic wrist can often be well treated by excision of the distal ulna or by arthrodesis. Ball-and-socket replacements are available, (Figure 8), but results are still in a preliminary stage.

Fingers

Much experience has been accumulated with replacement for the metacarpophalangeal and proximal interphalangeal joints. Early hinged metallic joints fatigued and broke with regularity. The most popular prosthesis is the silicone rubber "spacer" for the metacarpophalangeal joints popularized by Swanson. Breakage of these prostheses was a problem at first, but redesign and strengthening have alleviated fatigue and breakage.

Ankle

The adjoining surfaces of distal tibia and talus can be replaced with metal and polyethylene (Figure 9). This is usually done for arthritis that is primary, or traumatic following a fracture. The short-term experience with total ankle replacement has been encouraging, and it appears to be a viable alternative to bracing or arthrodesis in many instances.

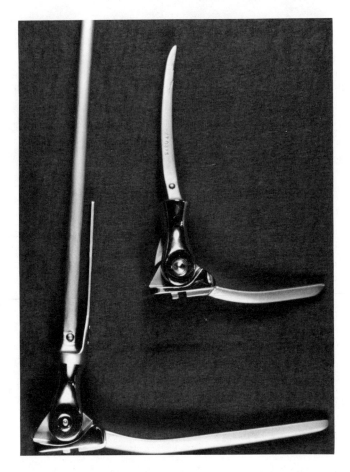

FIG. 7. Hinged elbow replacements. The upper stem is inserted into the humerus, the lower (horizontal) stem into the ulna. The larger prosthesis (at left) has an interior flange to fit outside the humerus and provides better fixation.

FUTURE DEVELOPMENTS

Surface Replacement

A major design change in total hip replacement has been brought about by the efforts of Wagner, Amstutz, and others. The acetabulum is replaced with a thin polyethylene cup while the femoral head is "capped" with a metal shell, and

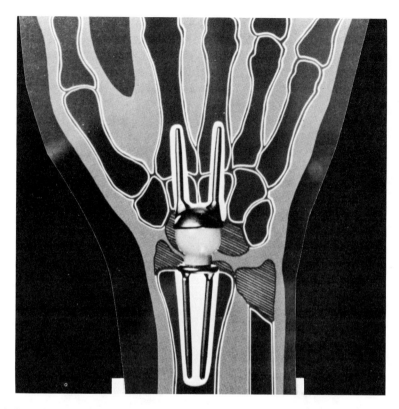

FIG. 8. Ball and socket total wrist replacement shown schematically. Shaded areas of bone are resected during insertion of the prosthesis.

both are cemented in place (Figures 10 and 11). Thus, normal anatomy is more closely preserved, range of motion is improved, and dislocation is less likely to occur. Theoretically, the surface replacement has much to recommend it. Possible disadvantages include weakening of the femoral neck with reamers and later fracture, as well as the danger of damage to the blood supply of the femoral head, which could cause avascular necrosis with pain or settling of the femoral shell.

Hopefully, this method will avoid the loosening seen with prosthetic stems in the femur. Surface replacement seems a more attractive choice for younger patients, as bone stock is conserved and revision to a "conventional" total hip would be possible if the resurfacing failed for reasons other than sepsis. The resurfacing concept has already been used to some extent in the elbow, knee, and ankle, and seems almost certain to be the prototype for the "second generation" of total joints.

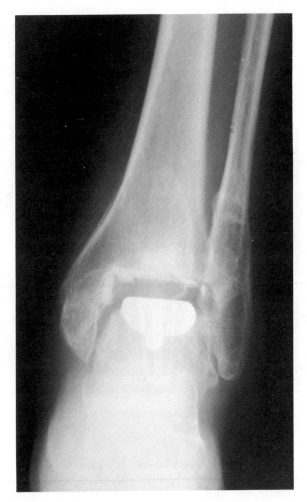

FIG. 9. Total ankle with polyethylene cemented to distal tibia and metal prosthesis for the dome of the talus. Radiopaque cement can be seen in the distal tibia.

Prosthetic Fixation

Loosening has been the most common mode of failure, and various efforts have been made to solve this problem. One promising development is the production of prostheses with stems that have a porous or "sintered" surface. Pores of $100\,\mu$ or greater allow bone ingrowth and, in experimental animals, produce rigid

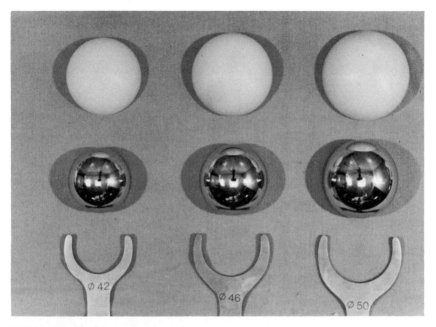

FIG. 10. Surface hip replacement showing various sizes of acetabular cups (top row), femoral shells (middle row), and gauges to measure the femoral head after reaming (bottom row).

fixation in about 6 weeks without the use of cement. Early results with sintered prostheses appear favorable, but some recent data suggest that disuse atrophy of bone may be a problem unless the stress is transferred evenly from prosthesis to bone. Long-term favorable follow-up is necessary before this type of prosthetic design can be put into routine use.

New Materials

Methymethacrylate works quite well, but is too brittle to be an ideal bonding agent between metal and bone. Various additives such as carbon fibers have been tried to strengthen methacrylate. It seems logical to think that a biocompatible and more mechanically satisfactory bonding agent will be found in the future. Prostheses are being fabricated of new alloys (titanium) and other more "exotic" materials such as ceramic, boron, and so on, will probably find clinical application in the near future.

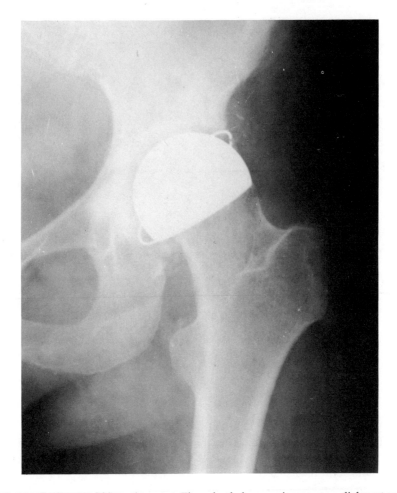

FIG. 11. Surface total hip replacement. The polyethylene cup is seen as a radiolucent zone outside the metal sheel covering the head of the femur.

SUMMARY

The first 15 years of total joint replacement have been most stimulating to orthopedic surgeons and beneficial to patients. The total hip provides freedom from pain and increased function in a reliable manner. Results are not quite as reliable and optimistic for the knee and other major joints at present, but are steadily improving with better prosthetic design and fixation. While a "perfect" joint may be unattainable, cooperation between the fields of surgery, biomechanics, and engineering seem certain to improve the quality and reliability of total joint replacement in years to come.

Bibliography

Beckenbaugh, R. D., et al. Review and analysis of silicone-rubber metacarpophalangeal implants. *J. Bone Jt. Surg. 58A*:483, 1976.

Charnley, John. *Acrylic Cement in Orthopaedic Surgery*. Baltimore: Williams and Wilkins, 1970.

Sonstegard, D. A., et al. The surgical replacement of the human knee joint. *Sci. Am. 238*: 44–51, 1978.

Walker, P. S. *Human Joints and Their Artificial Replacements*. Springfield, Illinois: Charles C. Thomas, 1978.

Reconstructive Microsurgery

JAMES W. MAY, Jr., M.D.
Chief of Hand Surgical Services
Division of Plastic Surgery
Massachusetts General Hospital
Assistant Professor of Surgery
Harvard Medical School

It is a curious commentary on the passivity of the reconstructive surgeon, toiling with staged ischemic pedicle tissues for wound closure, when the solution to one stage free tissue transfer lay simply in the micro application of his surgical art.

Reconstructive microsurgery is reconstructive surgery performed under various degrees of magnification. This magnification makes the application of accepted Halstedian principles possible on a micro level. Surgical techniques under magnification are applicable to virtually any field of surgery and have recently seen great use and expansion in the fields of ophthamology, ear, nose, and throat surgery, gynecology, urology, and cardiac surgery. In this chapter reconstructive microsurgery will be reviewed.

HISTORY

In 1960 Jacobson and Swarez successfully demonstrated patent repair of 1-mm arteries and veins under the operating microscope, utilizing meticulous surgical techniques. These techniques required micro instrumentation and suture material appropriately scaled to the repair of 1-mm structures.

In 1962 Malt replanted the arm of a 12-year-old boy with macrosurgical technique but established human replantation as a possibility. In the early 1960s, Kleinert and his group in Louisville, Kentucky were perfecting vascular techniques for revascularization of partially severed digits. In 1965 using microvascular technique, Komatsu and Tamaii performed the first replantation of a human digit, the thumb.[1] In 1976 Cohen reported a case of human penis replantation.

Sidenberg in 1959 reconstructed a cervical esophageal defect by the use of a free micro vascularized loop of jejunum. The bowel was revascularized in the neck by micro technique connecting the vessels of the bowel with recipient vessels in the neck region. This marked a major milestone in elective reconstructive clinical microsurgery.

In 1972 Millesi and Berger[2] reported upon results of peripheral nerve repair using the intrafascicular graft and the operating microscope. Here the "no tension and meticulous fascicular alignment concept" of peripheral nerve repair was endorsed.

Thoughts of free skin transfer in elective reconstructive surgery were begun by Gibson in 1957, who suggested that possibly flaps of skin could be transferred by connecting nutrient vessels to vessels of the recipient area. With this thought, Buncke, the father of contemporary reconstructive microsurgery, began to pursue the concept in the experimental animal. Impressed with the report of a near-successful free flap transfer in 1969 by Buncke, Daniel, working in Australia, performed the first successful human free flap transfer in 1973.[3]

Since this operation literally hundred of free flaps and segments of tissue have been transferred in the human from one area to another for the purpose of reconstruction. Since 1965 literally thousands of digits and portions of extremities have been replanted with the use of microsurgery. Both in the area of extremity reconstruction and in the area of general reconstructive surgery, the use of the operating microscope is beginning to take its proper place. Microsurgery can enhance some previously available techniques, and it can replace others which are no longer effective.

PRINCIPLES AND TECHNIQUES

In most reconstructive microsurgical procedures, the actual time required to repair the micro structures is small when compared to the overall time needed to

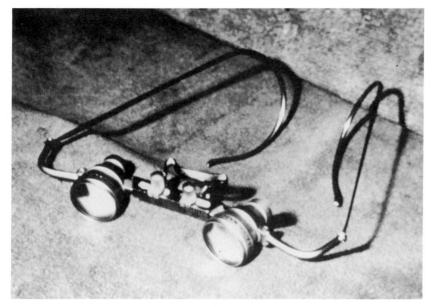

a

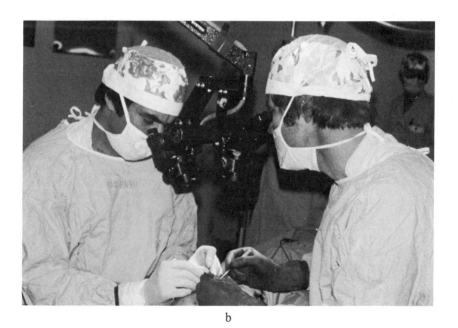

b

FIG. 1. (A) Loups used in clinical micro dissection. (B) operating diploscope. (C) 10–0 nylon suture tied around a human hair (photograph courtesy of Dr. Robert Acland). (D) Micro instruments.

481

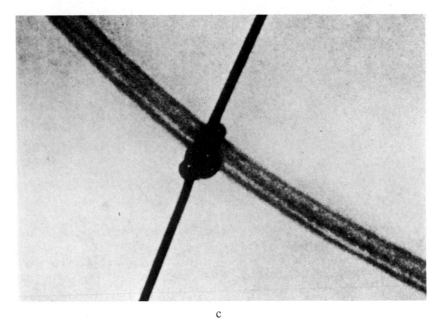

c

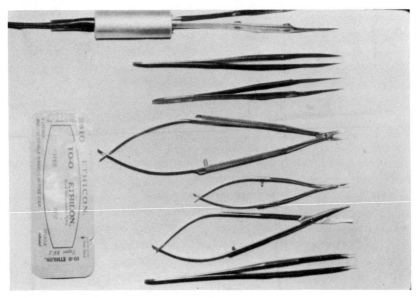

d

FIG. 1. (continued)

set the stage for the repair. Nonetheless, the micro repair itself requires special techniques, instrumentation, and magnification. In a microsurgical case much of the dissection can be done under 2 to 4 power loups (Figure 1A). The vascular and nerve repairs are best done under the operating diploscope (Figure 1B), which can zoom from 5 to 40 power. The same field can be viewed by the surgeon and the assistant. Special fine nylon (10-0) is used (Figure 1C) with very fine needles. The instrument list also includes (Figure 1D) micro needle holders, scissors, and jeweler's forceps plus a micro bipolar coagulator to provide specific hemostasis in tiny blood vessels.

The basic technique of microvascular repair involves the same Halstedian principles as macrovascular repair. Specifically, the blood vessel is dissected freely with a minimum of trauma (Figure 2A). The vessel is then freshened and

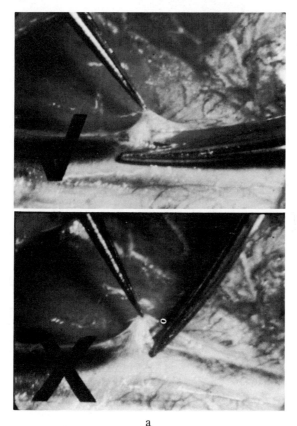

a

FIG. 2. (A) Trauma-free dissection (photograph courtesy of Dr. Robert Acland). (B) 1-mm vessel in micro clamp (photograph courtesy of Dr. Robert Acland). (C) Appropriate alignment for anchoring sutures in microvascular repair. (D) Micro clamp rotation (photograph courtesy of Dr. Robert Acland).

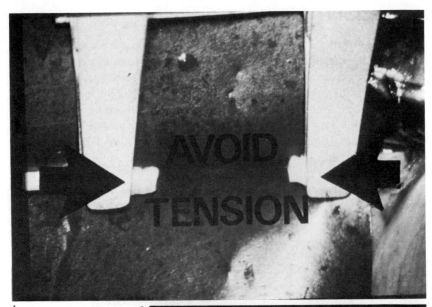

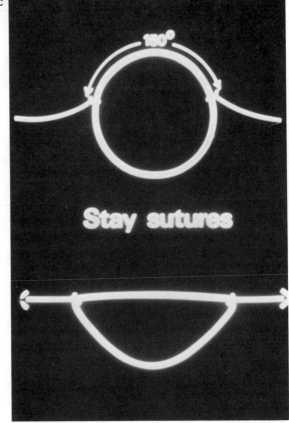

FIG. 2. (continued)

prepared for repair by inclusion in a microvascular clamp (Figure 2B). Micro sutures are then placed at 150 degrees in opposing sides of the vessel to support the anterior wall in such a way that the posterior wall falls away from the anterior wall (Figure 2C). Finally the anastomosis is completed after the anterior row of interrupted sutures is finished by turning the micro clamp over and completing the posterior row (Figure 2D). After the entire circumference is complete using approximately ten sutures per 1-mm vessel, the clamps are removed and blood flow is reestablished.

Micro neural repair involves essentially the appreciation that tension-free fascicular alignment with contained axons will provide the most encouraging environment for axonal regeneration across a nerve division interface. Under the operating microscope, the recognition of damaged nerve endings has been greatly improved as the traumatized nerve or neuroma can be meticulously dissected from normal nerve tissue. The defect or loss of nerve tissue can then be assessed. In the judgment of the surgeon if the gap between two nerve ends which are to be repaired is extensive, then a nerve graft must be used. In small peripheral nerves, the nerves may be repaired by placing the 10-0 nylon sutures only

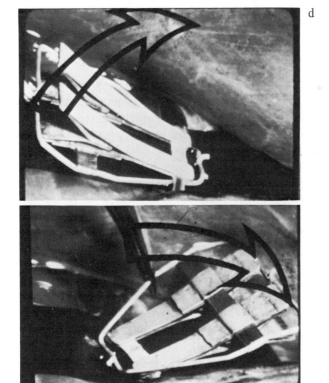

d

FIG. 2. (continued)

through the epineurium. However, in major trunk nerves, it may provide better fascicular alignment in selected cases to place the sutures actually through the perineurium surrounding each fascicle and thus repair each fascicle or fascicular group one to the other. Although the merits of one technique over the other in clinical microsurgery are still controversial, it is nonetheless clear that the use of the operating microscope improves one's view of normal and damaged nerve tissue and enhances one's ability to align fascicular content no matter which technique is used.

CLINICAL APPLICATION

Revascularization

Before 1960 blood vessels smaller than 1 mm in diameter were considered beyond the level of surgical manipulation. Presently, however, digits that have sustained significant injury but have not been totally amputated may be revascularized either to allow survival or to allow an improved level of perfusion which subsequently may improve the level of function.

When an injury has been sustained, the decision must be made by the treating physician as to whether the injured part has enough circulation to remain viable, or whether it does not. If the decision is no, then the injured part should be cooled until a time when revascularization surgery can be done if appropriate. If the decision is yes, then no cooling is necessary.

Case Report.   A 20-year-old male presented with a thumb injury (Figure 3A) that was sustained with a large broken drinking bottle. The thumb flexor tendon and both digital neurovascular bundles were cut. Pulse volume recordings showed no pulsatile flow to the digit, and the digit remained white. A revascularization procedure was carried out after tendon repair was completed. The princeps pollicis artery was sharply lacerated, and therefore little of the vessel needed debridement. The vessel was sutured together employing standard microvascular technique with interrupted 10-0 nylon sutures (Figure 3B). Both nerves were repaired under the operating microscope with interrupted 10-0 nylon epineural sutures. Postoperatively pulsatile flow (Figure 3C) was returned to the thumb, as was its clinical pink color. Six months postoperatively the 2 point discrimination was less than 1 cm, and acceptable flexion and extension were demonstrated (Figure 3D, E).

Replantation Surgery

Replantation means to plant again or anew. For something to be planted again, therefore, it must be completely amputated. Patients with incomplete amputations may be candidates for revascularization, whereas patients with complete amputations are candidates for replantation. The complexities of replantation

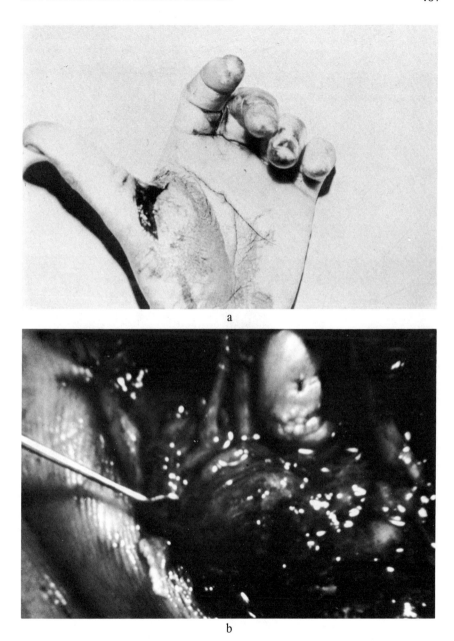

FIG. 3. (A) Devascularized thumb following sharp-glass volar injury. (B) Repair of princeps pollicis artery, both volar digital nerves, and flexor pollicis longus tendon. Case done with Dr. B. Cohen. (C) Pulse volume recording following revascularization. (D, E) Range of motion of injured thumb six months postoperatively.

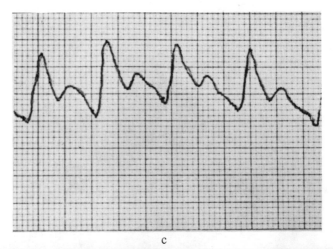

c

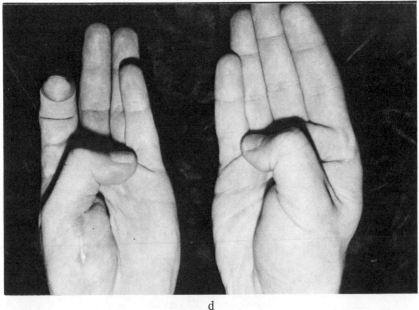

d

FIG. 3. (continued)

are vast and involve different considerations at each different level of digital, palm, hand, forearm, and arm amputation. For optimal results replantation as a clinical service is best practiced by a team of reconstructive surgeons acquainted with micro techniques and experienced in acute care of the injured hand.

When a patient has sustained an amputation injury, the part to be replanted should be cleansed and stored in a sterile dressing. The dressing should then be

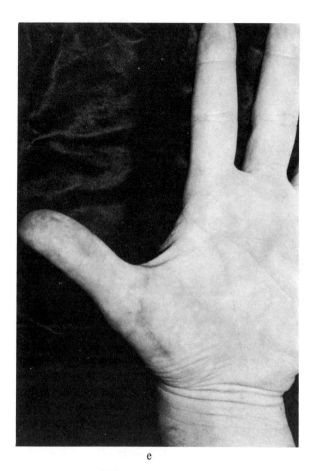

e

FIG. 3. (continued)

placed inside a plastic bag, and the bag should be placed in a water–ice interface. This lowers the metabolic rate of the amputated part and greatly extends the ischemia time that the part may tolerate before replantation. Upon the patient's arrival at the replantation center, many factors should be reviewed and assessed before the decision to proceed with replantation surgery (Table 1). If replantation in the judgment of the experienced hand microsurgeon would give the patient a better chance for a functional extremity than stump closure with or without a prosthesis, then replantation should be considered. If physical examination of the total patient and the amputated part are consistent with replantation as a possibility, then, with the patient's desires, replantation should be attempted.

A detailed knowledge of hand functional anatomy will avoid converting a

TABLE 1. Factors to Be Reviewed and Assessed Prior to Replantation Surgery

History
1. Nature of injury
2. Desire for replantation
3. Vocation and avocational interest
4. Age
5. Chronic disease
6. Handedness

Exam
1. Associated injuries
2. Anatomy of injured part
3. Level of amputation
4. Method of part preservation

TABLE 2. Sequential Steps* in Replantation Surgery

1. Structure identification in stump and amputated part
2. Bone fixation
3. Extensor and flexor tendon repair
4. Dorsal vein and volar artery repair
5. Nerve repair
6. Wound closure

*Some maneuvers are slightly modified, depending on the level of injury.

technical microvascular triumph into a clinically useless disaster. The replantation team is organized in such a way that two surgeons can start vessel identification in the amputated part while two other surgeons are operating on the proximal stump. The general steps or stages in extremity replantation as outlined in Table 2 are carried out. Each of these steps should be done with meticulous technique as though it were the only part of the operation. To allow this, the replantation team needs at least four surgeons available so that no two surgeons are working at the same time for extended periods of time.

Case Report. A 21-year-old female presented several hours after amputating the radial side of her hand through the proximal area of no man's land of the middle, index, and thumb digits. Replantation was carried out in stages that required 14 hours of surgery (Figure 4A). Six months post replantation, the patient had sensation in her digital tips and had acceptable extension and flexion (Figure 4B, C). One year following replantation the patient had 2 point discrimination of less than 1 cm in all digits with sudomotor activity present.

With replantation procedures of this type, if a length of diseased or damaged vessel is appreciated, this gap can be bridged by use of micro vein grafts usually harvested from the volar surface of the forearm or dorsum of the foot.

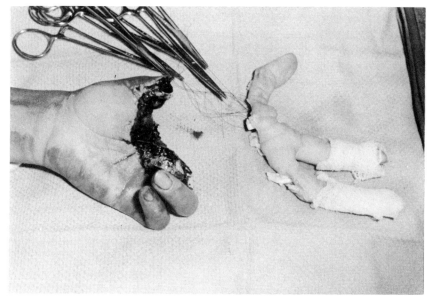

a

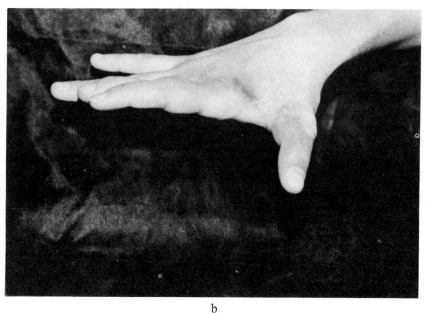

b

FIG. 4. (A) Amputation in 21-year-old female of thumb, index finger, and middle finger through proximal no man's land. Case done with Dr. H. Rosen. (B, C) Range of motion of replanted part six months postoperatively.

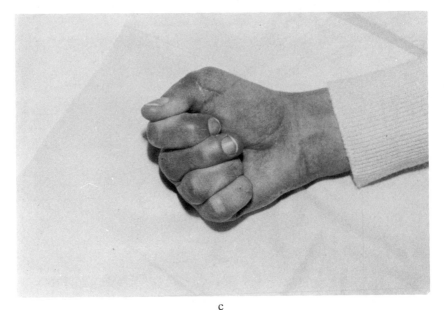

c

FIG. 4. (continued)

In general, as replantation procedures have become more common, the incidence of replantation viability has increased (Table 3), with several replantation centers recording survival rates of better than 90%.

As confidence with microvascular repairs has increased, clearly the pendulum has swung toward improvement in functional results. This improvement will come in part as a manifestation of meticulous anatomic repair during replantation.

With the proper goals in mind, the vast majority of replantation patients will have functional results following successful replantation far superior to what they would have had with simple stump closure or prosthesis use.

Free Tissue Transfer

Free tissue transfer refers to the movement of a mass of tissue based on its isolated vasculature from one area of the body to another where it is revascularized through vascular repair in the recipient area. In the human body most potential free tissue transfers are suppled by vessels smaller than 3 mm in diameter, and therefore require the use of microvascular and microneural techniques for safe transfer.

Basically free tissue transfers are classified as in Table 4. From this review one can see that single free tissue transfers are those tissues of the body that are moved from one area to another to fulfill a single overall purpose. Compound

TABLE 3. Massachusetts General Hospital Upper Extremity Replantation,
July 1, 1976-January 1, 1978 (18 Months)

Patients	Replantations	Unit survival
27	36	35
	Unit survival percentage	
	97%	

A replantation unit is defined as a separate portion of amputated tissue that requires the repair of at least one artery and one vein for survival.

TABLE 4. Classification of Human Free Tissue Transfer

I. Single free tissue transfer
  A. Free flap
    1. Free cutaneous flap—skin and subcutaneous tissue with direct cutaneous vessels
    2. Free myocutaneous flap—skin, subcutaneous tissue supplied by vessels from underlying muscle with axial vessels in the nonfunctional muscle
  B. Free bone transfer
  C. Free muscle transfer
  D. Free nerve transfer
  E. Free bowel transfer (stomach, small bowel, large bowel)
  F. Free omental transfer
II. Compound free tissue transfer*—multipurpose tissues moved to solve more than one problem
  A. Free osteocutaneous transfer
  B. Free myocutaneous transfer
  C. Free neurovascular flap
  D. Free toe-to-hand transfer

*Many additional combinations are possible.

free tissue transfers, however, are made of more than one type of functional tissue and thus can fulfill the multipurpose roles of their included tissues.

For any method of reconstructive surgery to achieve acceptance, the method must have a high incidence of success and must provide the patient with lower morbidity and a superior reconstructive result. In experienced hands, free tissue transfer operations are as safe as standard methods of reconstructive surgery and in most cases provide the patient with less overall morbidity and an excellent finished product. In some difficult reconstructive situations, a free tissue transfer may make possible that which was previously "nonreconstructable."

In any free tissue transfer type of reconstructive surgery, there are several basic steps which must be accurately conceived, meticulously planned and carried out, and appropriately managed postoperatively: (1) accurate assessment of other more standard methods of reconstruction, through adequate overall surgical experience; (2) appreciation of the defect to be reconstructed with extrapolation of appropriate donor site qualities to match the requirements of the recipient site; (3) identification of recipient and donor vessels that are healthy and can be manipulated in the microsurgery realm (greater than .75 mm in diameter); (4) confident evaluation that the tissue to be transferred is safely supported by the donor vasculature; (5) transfer of that donor tissue to the recipient area following meticulous vascular dissection; (6) accurate microvascular anastomoses; (7) astute postoperative management with early recognition of vascular problems and immediate revision when necessary.

With increasing appreciation of the axial blood supply to many component tissues of the body, many free tissue transfers are now available that require microsurgical technique for their reliable transfer. Skin flaps from donor sites that are supported by axial artery and venous supply in the skin include the scalp, forehead, deltopectoral flap, groin flap, dorsalis pedis flap, and upper arm flap.

With the realization that loose skin in the body is supplied by perforators from the underlying muscle, many potential free flap donor sites have now become available as the axial blood supply that enters the muscle can be harvested with muscle and overlying skin and can be transferred to recipient areas with microvascular repairs. This anatomic realization, however, has decreased the number of free tissue transfers necessary, since many myocutaneous flaps can be simply rotated from an adequate local area into the defect.

For large bony defects where standard nonvascularized bone grafts would have a high incidence of failure, the vascularized fibula has answered many problems. Here the fibula is isolated with a cuff of muscle, and the peroneal vessels can be transferred to any appropriate recipient area.

In certain areas where bone and large amounts of skin are necessary, the compound osteocutaneous groin flap has been useful in supplying not only a large surface of skin but also up to 10 cm of anterior iliac crest for bony primary reconstruction. Although the blood supply to this segment of bone may not be as good as the free fibular transfer, nonetheless with healthy overlying skin, this composite transfer has been useful in its dual role of bone reconstruction and skin coverage.

Case Report. A 13-year-old male was admitted to the Massachusetts General Hospital in January of 1978 following a snow mobile accident in which he amputated his left leg. Original physical examination revealed a lower leg that was avulsed by skin level 1 inch below the tibial plateau and by bony level some 4 inches below the tibial plateau (Figure 5A). Ten inches of neurovascular struc-

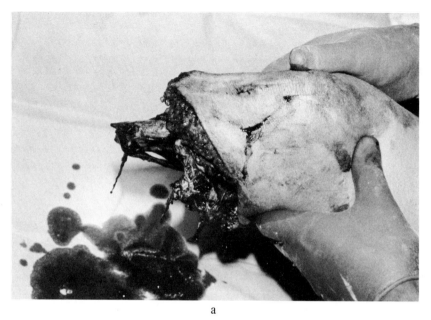

a

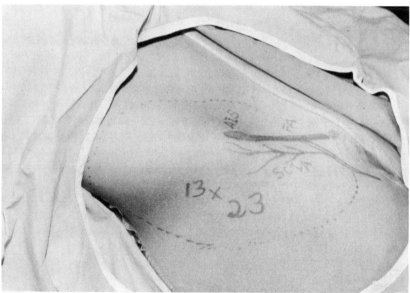

b

FIG. 5. (A) A 13-year-old male with lower leg snow mobile amputation with 10 inches of avulsed nerve from the midthigh region. (B) 23 by 13 cm groin flap. Case done with Dr. M. Donelan. (C) Three months postoperatively with full flap survival.

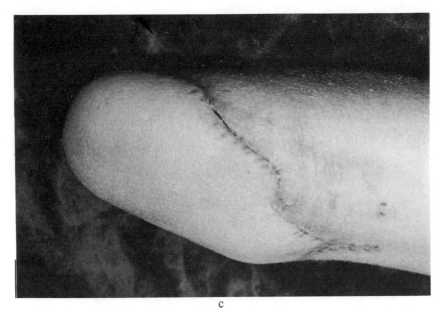

c

FIG. 5. (continued)

ture remained with the leg, and under the operating microscope severe avulsion was noted. For this reason replantation of the lower extremity did not appear to be in the patient's best interest.

To avoid an above-the-knee amputation, and to preserve the full remaining length of the tibia below the knee, a free groin flap was elected for coverage.

Preoperative arteriography revealed geniculate branches in the recipient area and a superficial circumflex iliac artery trunk in the groin donor area.

Twelve days after admission to the hospital after wound debridement and dressings, a 23 by 13 cm groin flap (Figure 5B) was transferred by microvascular technique to the left lower leg amputation site. The donor site of the free flap was closed primarily. The flap survived in full (Figure 5C).

The patient was discharged from the hospital on the twelfth postoperative day and began wearing a lower extremity prosthesis six weeks postoperatively.

Now eight months postoperatively, the patient is ambulating fully on his resurfaced stump and has no evidence of flap breakdown.

Case Report. A 25-year-old female was involved in a rifle accident in August of 1976, in which an open severe shattering fracture of the distal left tibia, fibula, and talus were incurred. Initial treatment involved open debridement with Hoffman apparatus extremity stabilization, and split thickness skin graft coverage.

Because of nonunion of her tibial fracture in January of 1977, a posterior iliac wing bone graft was done. However, in July of 1977 nonunion persisted, and a second bone graft procedure was carried out. Despite these two bone-grafting procedures, nonunion continued to be present, and pain continued to plague the patient with ambulation (Figure 6A). Ambulation was not possible without crutches.

Because of unstable skin, poor circulation, and nonunion following two bone graft procedures, the patient was thought to be a candidate for composite free tissue transfer including groin flap skin with underlying anterior iliac wing. It was hoped that this combination would not only provide better skin cover for the unstable skin grafted area but in addition would improve circulation to the soft tissues and provide a vascularized bone graft.

In late February 1978, a right composite groin flap with iliac wing was transferred to the left lower tibial position. A 10-cm length of iliac wing bone graft was harvested with the flap (Figure 6B), and this was slotted into the tibial defect. At the time of harvest, fluoroscene was injected systemically into the patient, and fluoroscene was seen to be coming from the cut edge of the iliac wing transferred with the flap. This was presumptive evidence that the bone circulation at least to some degree was being supplied by perforating periosteal vessels originating through the superficial circumflex iliac system. Following microvascular arterial and venous anastomoses, the flap became pink, and the procedure was terminated.

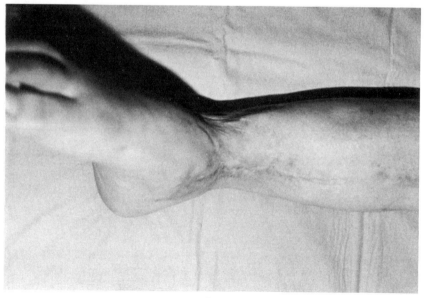

a

FIG. 6. (A) Painful lower extremity with unstable skin graft coverage. (B) Iliac wing bone graft with flap. (C) Living flap, three weeks postoperatively.

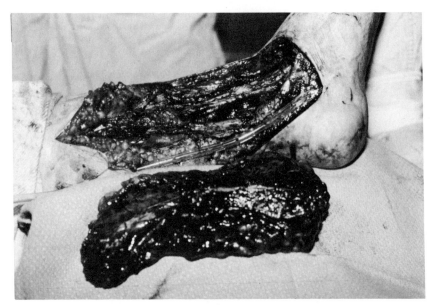

b

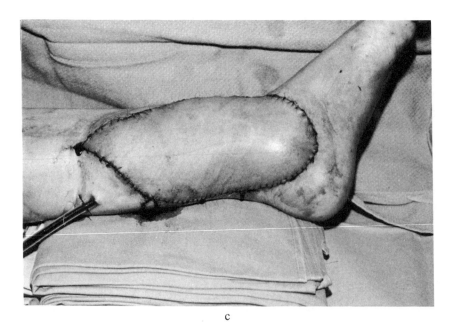

c

FIG. 6. (continued)

Three weeks postoperatively the transfer had survived completely (Figure 6C), but a bone scan was performed that did not show significant uptake in the iliac wing. The interpretation of this finding is unclear at this point. Four months postoperatively the bone graft itself looks unchanged, although there is no significant evidence of callous formation at the distal end of the bone graft. The patient is pain-free and is ambulating without crutches in a tibial plateau weight-bearing splint. She has returned to work and is on her feet eight hours a day.

The neurovascular free flap from the foot first web has allowed skin coverage in hand reconstruction with a potential for innervation by harvesting nerves of the hand.[4] The free intestinal transfer has provided an excellent conduit for esophageal replacement in cases where no other solution may be possible. Free muscle transfer from the pectoralis or gracilis muscles has been done with limited success but offers great promise in improvement in conditions such as Volkmann's ischemic contracture and certain facial paralyses. The vascularized nerve transfer using the radial artery, vena comitantes, and radial nerve as a transfer unit has been shown to be effective, although the use for this particular type of transfer must compete favorably with free nonvascularized nerve grafts before wide acceptance will be seen. Vascularized free omental transfers can allow wound coverage that will support a skin graft. This form of transfer is very flexible.

The free toe-to-hand transfer is an excellent example of the compound free tissue transfer concept.[5] Here in selected cases, the thumb or other digits can be replaced with toes in a single procedure with all component tissues which are necessary for functional use in the hand.

Case Report. A 20-year-old male injured his right hand severely in a jeep accident in July of 1976, and following an established clostridial gas gangrene infection in the right hand was transferred to the Massachusetts General Hospital. Subsequent debridement of the thumb, index, and middle fingers was necessary in addition to a large surface of the palm of the hand (Figure 7A).

Because of a paucity of transferable local digits, in January of 1978 a toe-to-hand transfer was completed (Figure 7B) with primary repair of the deep perineal nerve to the superficial radial nerve and bilateral plantar digital nerves of the toe to thumb branches of the median nerve. The flexor hallucis longus was repaired to the flexor pollicis longus tendon. The dorsalis pedis artery of the toe was repaired to the dorsal radial artery of the hand, and the dorsal toe vein was connected to the cephalic vein of the wrist.

Postoperatively all tissue primarily survived, although delayed healing was seen in the toe donor site, which ultimately required revision.

Now seven months postoperatively, the patient has protective and light touch sensibility to the tip of the thumb. There is 45 degrees active range of motion of

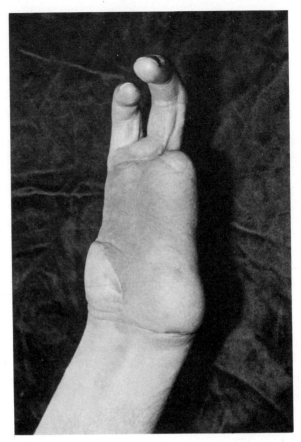

a

FIG. 7. (A) Hand following debridement of all necrotic tissues with groin flap coverage to the palm. (B) Free transfer of the great toe to the hand. Case done with Dr. R. J. Smith. (C, D) Range of motion of thumb mobility at the CM joint seven months postoperatively. An adductor transfer is planned for the thumb to augment motor power in the previously injured intrinsic muscles to the thumb.

the interphalangeal joint of the thumb, and the thumb is being used effectively (Figure 7C, D). There are no ambulation abnormalities, and the patient has continued to be a jogger.

Free tissue transfers in general are considered whenever a more standard method of reconstruction either has little chance to be successful or would be extremely time-consuming with multiple stages. In addition, free tissue transfers are frequently called upon when more standard methods of reconstruction have failed.

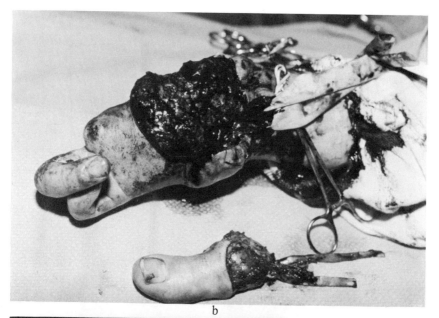

b

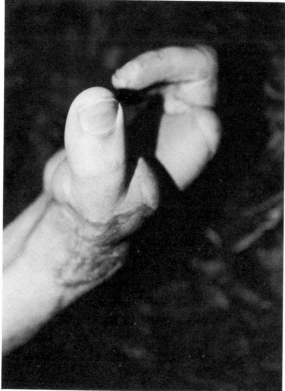

c   **FIG. 7.** (continued)

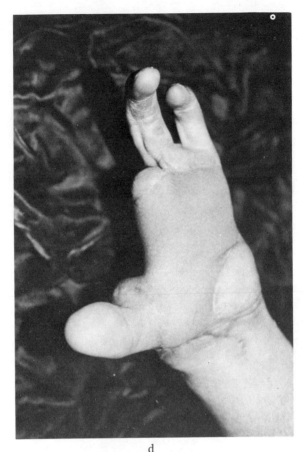

d

FIG. 7. (continued)

Advantages of Free Tissue Transfer.   When compared to conventional reconstructive techniques, free tissue transfers offer many advantages (Table 5).
Although the disadvantages are few, they are formidable and include extensive
preoperative preparation, extensive microvascular technical surgical experience,
and tedious long operations with an all-or-none outcome.

TABLE 5.   Advantages of Free Tissue Transfer in Reconstructive Surgery

1. Less patient morbidity and hospitalization
2. Fewer staged procedures
3. Less overall operation time
4. Problem solution where no solution may have existed

Reconstruction microsurgery is a new surgical frontier with application as broad as the surgeon's imagination.

References

Komatsu, S., Tamai, S., et al. Successful replantation of a completely cut-off thumb case report. *Plast. Reconstr. Surg. 42*: 374–377, 1968.

Millesi, H., and Berger, S. The interfascicular nerve graft. *J. Bone J. Surg. 54A*: 727, 1972.

Daniel, R. K., and Taylor, G. I. Distant transfer of an island flap by microvascular anastomoses. *Plast. Reconstr. Surg. 52*: 111, 1973.

May, J. W., Jr., Chait, L. S., et al. Free neurovascular flap from the first web of the foot in hand reconstruction. *J. Hand Surg. 2:5*: 387–393, 1977.

May, J. W., Jr., and Daniel, R. K. Great toe to hand free tissue transfer. *Clin. Orthop. Relat. Res. 133*: 140–153, 1978.

Musculotaneous Flaps in Reconstructive Surgery

J. WILLIAM FUTRELL, M.D.
Professor of Surgery (Plastic Surgery)
Chairman Division of Plastic Surgery
Univ. of Pittsburgh Medical Center
Department of Surgery (Plastic Surgery)
University of Pittsburgh Medical Center
Pittsburgh, Pennsylvania

A fundamental principle of reconstructive surgery consists of replacement of missing parts with autologous tissue and thereby execution of this principle requires the ability to move healthy, vascularized integument from one area of the body to another. The development of the concept of myocutaneous flap surgery has permitted the achievement of this objective with a minimum of uncertainty. As is the case with many clinical procedures thought to be of modern innovation, however, the recent "discovery" underlying this concept (i.e., that in addition to direct cutaneous blood flow the skin receives a significant portion of its blood supply from underlying muscle) was more a reawakening of past knowledge than a modern revelation. Nontheless, that recognition diminishes in no way the vast importance and indeed fundamental percipience of this imminently useful clinical technique, which in the last two years has virtually revolutionized much of reconstructive surgery.

In past years the lack of enthusiasm and oftentimes begrudging acceptance of many reconstructive techniques by even the medical community was explainable primarily on the basis that customarily numerous operative procedures were required in order to obtain the availability of even modest amounts of distantly transferred tissue for reconstructive purposes. This was due to the diminution in cutaneous blood flow and often ultimate tissue necrosis when a poorly vascularized skin flap was elevated from its bed and rotated into a new position. Even in generally successful cases many people remained critical of the concept of reconstructive surgery because of the long, tedious, and expensive multiple operations often required. Primarily because of the dedication of numerous post-World War I and II pioneer reconstructive surgeons, the premise that restorative surgery is a worthy goal was finally established, and now, along with the development of microsurgery, the evolution of the clinical principles involved in myocutaneous flap surgery has demonstrated that most of these procedures can be done safely as one-stage operations, with consistent reliability, often in conjunction with primary ablative surgery and with excellent long-term results.

DEFINITION OF SKIN AND MYOCUTANEOUS FLAPS

As used in medical terms a flap refers to a piece of tissue partially severed from its place of origin but maintaining a source of blood supply. A skin flap is a composite of the skin and subcutaneous tissue that can be transferred from a donor to a recipient site with its blood supply preserved through cutaneous vessels. Similarly, a myocutaneous flap (Gk. *mys,* L. *cutis;* a hybrid shortened word from musculocutaneous, L. *musculus* and Gk. *cutis*) refers to a compound skin and muscle flap in which the underlying muscle is retained with the skin flap as a primary source of blood supply. Either type of flap can be used in standard rotation fashion, in which case the base of the tissue remains stationary providing the source of blood supply, while the partly severed portion of the flap is rotated through an arc into a new position. When blood flow through the tissue is sufficient, an "island" flap can be created, in which situation a portion of the skin or skin and muscle is completely divided from the body, except for its arterial and venous communication through a dominant vascular pedicle. Likewise, both types of tissue can be transferred as "free" flaps, in which situation the donor site blood supply to the flap is completely severed, and following transplantation of the tissue to a new anatomic site the flap vessels are immediately reanastomosed with new recipient site vessels. The concept of "delay" of a flap refers to the clinical technique of sequentially severing the blood supply to the flap margins in an effort to augment blood flow from the base vessels and thereby improve perfusion when the flap is eventually rotated. This often requires multiple operative procedures. With regard to myocutaneous flaps, the "axis" of rotation (or "rotation point") of the flap is the point of entry of its dominant vascular pedicle into the muscle, and this point determines the mobility of the flap; the "arc" of the flap refers to the dimension that the cutaneous tip of the flap circumscribes. The muscle portion of the flap, therefore, acts as the "carrier" of the skin or cutaneous segment of the myocutaneous flap providing the skin blood supply.

BLOOD SUPPLY TO SKIN AND MUSCLE

The vascular supply of the skin can derive from any of three sources: (1) segmental or major vessels arising from the aorta; (2) perforating vessels from underlying muscle; or (3) direct cutaneous vessels. Skin flaps nourished predominantly by cutaneous vessels can be classified as "random" if no specific anatomically recognizable arteriovenous system exists, or as "axial" if the flap contains at least one artery and vein extending from the base along the flap dimensions. Clinical examples of axial cutaneous flaps are the deltopectoral flap nourished by perforating vessels from the internal mammary artery and vein, and the groin flap usually supplied by the superficial circumflex iliac vessels. Reliable surviving length of axial pattern flaps is considerably enhanced over that of random pattern flaps. Unfulfilled optimism held that the eventual demonstration of numerous specific cutaneous axial vessels would ultimately be achieved, making transfer of multiple anatomic axial pattern flaps possible. Extensive animal and cadaver experimentation, however, has identified only a limited number of such axial flaps, stimulating the recent renewed interest in delineating cutaneous blood supply from the second vascular source, namely, perforating vessels through the underlying musculature. This search has resulted in the demonstration that there are multiple available myocutaneous flaps which due to their excellent blood flow can be elevated and transferred in one operation without prior "delay" procedures.

SEGMENTAL VERSUS DOMINANT PEDICLE
BLOOD FLOW

Many muscles have a segmental blood supply via numerous perforating vessels, whereas those most useful in myocutaneous flaps have a single "dominant" vascular pedicle. When a dominant pedicle does exist, the portion of the muscle that is directly supplied and its immediately overlying skin can be raised as a myocutaneous flap without previous delay and with little detectable change in the blood supply of the cutaneous portion. This is true even when the cutaneous "island" is completely circumscribed and attached only by adherence to its carrier muscle. When the cutaneous segment of a myocutaneous flap extends beyond its nourishing muscle, that portion of the tissue is less well vascularized and may depend upon peripheral cutaneous blood flow in addition to the muscle perforator vessels. This additional skin can often be carried primarily as part of a myocutaneous flap receiving adequate perfusion through the muscle vessels. When a large portion of such "random" skin is carried, however, a preliminary "delay" procedure is recommended even in myocutaneous flaps.

HISTORY OF MYOCUTANEOUS FLAPS

The credit for the modern reintroduction of the clinical usefulness of the myocutaneous flap principle must go to McCraw.[5,6] He and his associates including Dibbell,[5,6] Carraway,[6] and the Emory University group of Mathes,[4] Vascondez,[1,3,4] and Jurkiewicz[1] have defined the vascular territories and extended the applications of numerous muscle and myocutaneous flaps. Significant recent contributions have continued from the Atlanta group, including those from Bostwick,[1] Nahai,[3,4] and Hill.[3]

In historical terms, Manchot, in 1889, suggested that virtually all of the skin vascular supply was via specific arterialized cutaneous vessels. The vascular territories so created were shown to be anatomically sharply delineated, although it has subsequently been found that few such territories are supplied directly by existing longitudinal cutaneous vessels; rather, the predominant blood supply is from perforating vessels through the underlying muscle. Cole was among the first, in 1918, to describe clinical use of a musculocutaneous flap when he used portions of the sternocleidomastoid muscle and cervicle skin to resurface wounds of the oral mucous membrane and nose. Owens, in 1955, and subsequently Bakamjian, in 1963, pioneered further the use of the compound sternomastoid myocutaneous flap for reconstruction of massive facial defects after radical ablative cancer surgery. In addition these surgeons designed flaps in which supraclavicular skin was also carried as random tissue by the sternocleidomastoid muscle and used to repair defects of the cheek and palate. Houston and McConchie, in 1968, utilized blood supply through the pectoralis major muscle to transfer a compound chest wall flap. Taking advantage of the same principle, DesPrez, Kiehn, and Eckstein, in 1971, were able to close large meningomyelocele defects by use of composite skin-muscle flaps based posteriorly on the latissimus dorsi muscles. In 1972, Orticochea demonstrated the feasibility of using the gracilis compound skin-muscle flap for phallus reconstruction. This initial use of the gracilis myocutaneous flap was performed in several stages, although the same flap was subsequently elevated primarily and immediately inset as a cross leg flap.

Each of these clinical applications recognized the principle of a certain cutaneous dependence on the vasculature of the underlying muscle. It remained, however, for McCraw and associates to build upon these observations and demonstrate in an extended experience of animal and clinical studies the fact that the cutaneous portion of a compound skin-muscle flap will survive as a "primary island" when completely separated from any cutaneous attachments and maintained only as the integral skin-muscle unit perfused by a single muscle vascular pedicle. Clinical definition of multiple independent myocutaneous vascular territories has subsequently been delineated. Use of the myocutaneous flap principle to develop methods of free tissue transfer in microsurgery, including vascular and neural reanastomoses, has further extended the clinical application of these observations.

CLINICAL DEFINITION OF MYOCUTANEOUS
VASCULAR TERRITORIES

A myocutaneous vascular territory refers to the anatomic area of skin and muscle tissue supplied by a perforating muscular vessel. Space limitations prohibit the discussion of more than a few of these territories, although among the muscles providing significant cutaneous blood flow are the sternocleidomastoid, trapezius, latissimus dorsi, rectus abdominis, gracilis, rectus femoris, biceps femoris, gastrocnemius, tensor fascia lata, and platysma. To intelligently select a myocutaneous flap for clinical use, the surgeon must know the vascular territory of the principal vessels and also the anatomic location of the dominant pedicle which will determine the rotation point axis of the flap. Additional surgical considerations include the need for understanding regarding the functional expendability of the carrier muscle, the desirability (or not) of muscle bulk in the reconstruction site, and the cutaneous and muscular innervation of the tissue. Ultimate cutaneous sensibility in myocutaneous flap transfers is variable, although occasionally maintenance of protective sensation can be achieved when some cutaneous nerve supply is preserved. Likewise, some degree of muscle atrophy will occur with muscle denervation or when the origin and/or insertion of a muscle is released.

CLINICAL PREDICTION OF VIABILITY
OF A MYOCUTANEOUS FLAP

Whenever vascular perfusion of a flap is questionable, it is important to determine the viability of the most distal portion of the tissue immediately at the time of surgical transfer. Probably the best currently available method to do this with predictable reproducibility is by intravenously administering 10 ml of 10% fluorescein and then after 20 minutes observing the questionable tissue for fluorescence under ultraviolet light. In simple terms, visual fluorescence indicates vascular perfusion that is adequate for tissue survival, as characterized by a

bright, confluent chartreuse color. Nonfluorescence, indicated by a blue appearance under ultraviolet light, indicates lack of good perfusion and suggests that
the tissue will probably be lost. If fluorescence is identified to the distal margin
of the cutaneous portion of a myocutaneous flap, ultimate survival is highly
predictable. Conversely, if no staining is apparent, ischemia with eventual
necrosis is likely such that if adequate tissue is available, the flap should be
appropriately tailored to the distal margin of fluorescence at the time of the
primary operative procedure. This maneuver results in significantly improved
safety and outcome of the operation, besides its being economically beneficial over simply waiting for eventual tissue slough and demarcation during
hospitalization.

ADVANTAGES AND DISADVANTAGES
OF MYOCUTANEOUS FLAPS

Among the significant potential advantages of the use of myocutaneous flaps
are: (1) proven clinical reliability with improved blood supply over most skin
flaps; (2) a single-stage surgical procedure allowing primary tailoring and inset of
the flap at the initial operation; (3) added bulk to the flap by inclusion of
muscle as well as skin; (4) minimal donor site deformity due to frequent use of
primary closure without concern of vascular compromise of flap; and (5) large
vessel size and pedicle length, often allowing use of tissue as a free flap. Potential
disadvantages include: (1) excess bulk when transferred to an area requiring only
a thin portion of tissue; (2) loss of intended function of the carrier muscle; and
(3) lack of long-term evaluation of results due to recent reintroduction of the
technique.

CLINICAL APPLICATION OF SELECTED
MYOCUTANEOUS FLAPS

Latissimus Dorsi Myocutaneous Flap

Because of the large expanse of this muscle and its dominant blood supply off
the thoraco-dorsal vascular trunk, the latissimus dorsi muscle provides the
carrier for one of the most durable and versatile myocutaneous flaps. The muscle
itself is one of the largest "flat" muscles in the body and extends from the lower
6 thoracic vertebrae and the thoraco lumbar fascia to the iliac crest. The thoraco-
dorsal nerve (C6, 7, & 8) is the sole nerve supply, and the anterior two-thirds of
the muscle is supplied by the thoraco-dorsal artery and vein. An independent
myocutaneous vascular territory representing the anterior 12 cm of the muscle
can be raised reliably without delay. The posterior 6 cm of the muscle is sup-

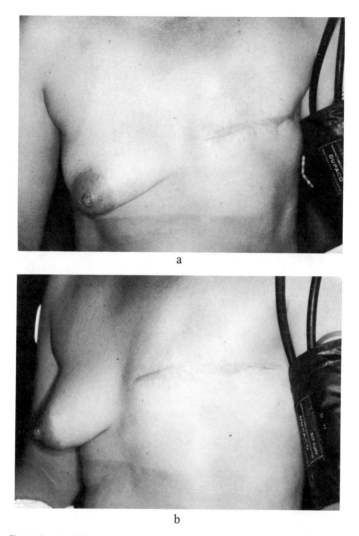

FIG. 1. Frontal and oblique view of patient six months following left complete mastectomy for carcinoma of breast.

plied by perforator vessels arising approximately 8 cm from the posterior midline. If inclusion of this additional skin is needed on the flap, preliminary division of the perforator vessels in a delay procedure can be recommended, although the author has personally employed latissimus dorsi myocutaneous flap measuring as much as 35 cm × 25 cm with complete survival and without previous delay. Technical elevation of the flap is performed by making an incision 3 to 5 cm in front of the anterior border of the muscle and elevation of the

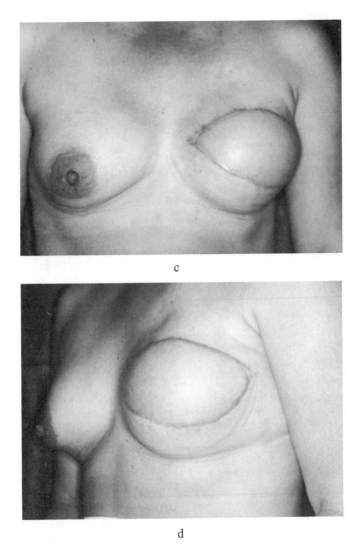

c

d

FIG. 1. (continued)   Same patient following reconstruction of left breast using a latissimus dorsi myocutaneous flap and subcutaneous mastectomy and immediate reconstruction of the right breast.

latissimus dorsi from the underlying serratus anterior muscle. Care is taken to avoid injury to the long thoracic nerve. On the undersurface of the latissimus muscle and approximately 10 cm below the axillary apex, the thoraco-dorsal neurovascular pedicle is identified and protected. The inferior skin incision is then made and the muscle divided from its origin on the iliac crest. The extent of posterior skin extension will be determined by the need for tissue in the

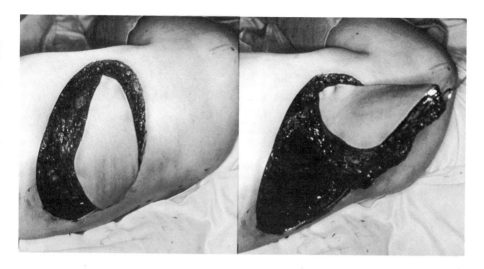

FIG. 2 and 3. Intraoperative views of creation of "skin island" receiving blood supply from thoracodorsal vessles via the latissimus dorsi muscle. 92/2 posterior views of skin incision and elevation of latissimus dorsi muscle.

reconstructive procedure and by the desire for primary closure of the donor site. The flap can reliably be used as a completely circumscribed "island" allowing 180° rotation. A distinct advantage of this flap is that the vascular pedicle arises high in the axilla, providing a rotation point that allows easy coverage of the entire upper half of the anterior chest wall. Use of the flap in breast reconstruction and chest wall replacement after cancer surgery has proved highly effective. Due to the large vessel size and pedicle length, this tissue also provides an excellent "free" flap when a large amount of tissue transfer is required. The flap can also be advanced posteriorly for use in closure of meningomyeloceles by dividing the posterior perforator vessels. Adequate posterior advancement requires incision of the deep fascia in front of the anterior border of the latissimus muscle, although it is rarely necessary to incise the anterior skin.

Tensor Fascia Lata Myocutaneous Flap

One of the most unlikely muscles has actually provided one of the most remarkable myocutaneous flaps. The tensor fascia lata muscle is an accessory flexor and medial rotator of the thigh, and originates from the anterior portion of the outer iliac crest and iliac spine. The nerve supply is through a branch of the superior gluteal nerve with fibers from L. 4,5, and S 1. The consistent blood supply to the tensor fascia lata is the transverse branch of the lateral femoral cutaneous artery as it passes between the vastus lateralis and the rectus femoris muscles.

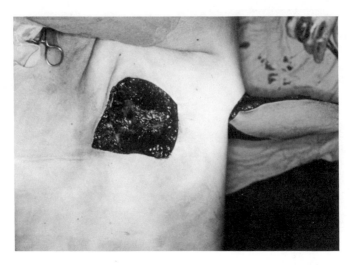

FIG. 4. Patient prone with left mastectomy defect recreated. Latissimus dorsi myocutaneous flap elevated to left.

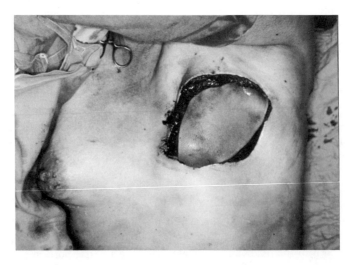

FIG. 5. Latissimus dorsi myocutaneous flap "tunneled" beneath left axillary skin and into place over left breast implant. Subcutaneous mastectomy and implant placement completed on right.

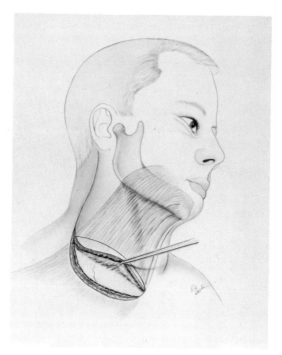

FIG. 6. Development of cervical myocutaneous flap based on platysma muscle. Skin "island" incised and inferior portion of platysma muscle divided.

Venous drainage is via paired venae comitants of this vessel. The vascular pedicle enters the muscle approximately 6 cm distal to the anterior iliac crest with branches superiorly and inferiorly providing a large myocutaneous vascular territory. Clinical elevation of the tensor fascia lata myocutaneous flap usually commences inferiorly along the desired cutaneous margins with isolation and protection of the vascular pedicle by subfascial elevation of the muscle. Flap dimensions of 15 cm X 20 cm are predictably achievable. Clinical use of this flap has involved medial rotation over the inguinal area and posterior rotation over the gluteal and ischial regions for closure of decubitus ulcers. The extreme length and relatively large size of the vascular pedicle also encourages the use of this tissue as a free myocutaneous flap.

Platysma Myocutaneous Flap

Unlike most other muscles supporting a myocutaneous flap, the platysma has no large dominant blood supply. But presumably because of its intimate cutaneous attachments (as demonstrated in phylogenetically lower species where it

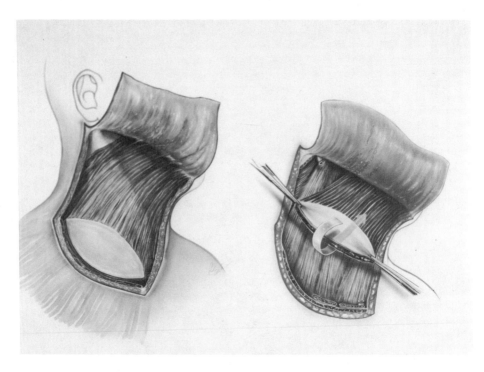

FIG. 7. Superior cervical skin elevated and following neck dissection platysma myocutaneous flap prepared for rotation into oral cavity defect.

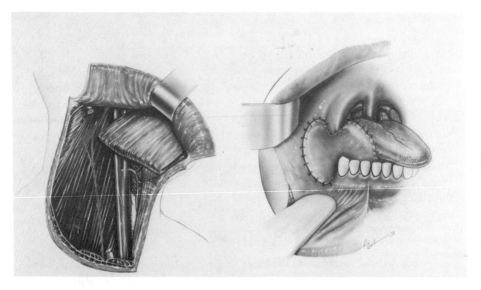

FIG. 8. Platysma myocutaneous flap rotated superiorly and sutured into oral cavity infection defect.

514

functions as a skin motion muscle; e.g., twitching of the hide in domestic animals to divert insects), blood supply through the platysma muscle to the overlying skin is extremely reliable. Muscle blood supply is predominately from cephalad through tributaries of the facial artery and vein, while innervation of the platysma is from the cervical branch of the facial nerve (Cranial N 7). Clinical application of the platysma myocutaneous flap has been demonstrated by the author[2] by isolation of a cutaneous island of cervical skin nourished by vascular communications from the underlying platysma muscle and use of the flap as a one-stage procedure for primary intraoral reconstruction following ablative cancer surgery. Technical elevation of the flap is begun by marking an island skin ellipse on the neck and making the lower cervical incision along the inferior ellipse margin through both skin and platysma muscle. The superior incision of the ellipse is then made through only skin, which isolates the cutaneous skin island based on the platysma muscle which is still attached cephalad. Following reflection of the upper neck skin, the flap can be rotated cephalad and a radical neck dissection performed. The skin island of the platysma myocutaneous flap can then be rotated into the mouth to replace resected tissue. Primary closure of the cervical defect and one-stage total reconstruction of the oral cavity is reliably achievable.

CONCLUDING REMARKS

The availability of a reliable, single-stage reconstructive method to provide large volumes of healthy vascularized tissue has recently been afforded through clinical use of myocutaneous flaps. Recent practical application of the old observation that a significant portion of the skin blood supply is from underlying muscle has virtually revolutionized much of reconstructive surgery. Although long-term evaluation of results and clinical determination of the appropriate uses of each flap must await further experience, even now it is apparent that this technique makes many previous reconstructive flap procedures obsolete.

References

Bostwick, J., Vasconez, L. O., and Jurkiewicz, M. J. Breast reconstruction after a radical mastectomy. *Plast. Reconstr. Surg. 61*: 682, 1978.

Futrell, J. W., Johns, M., Edgerton, M. T., et al. Platysma myocutaneous flap for intraoral reconstruction. *Am. J. Surg.,* Oct. 1978.

Hill, H. L., Nahai, F., and Vasconez, L. O. The tensor fascia lata myocutaneous free flap. *Plast. Reconstr. Surg., 61*: 517, 1978.

Mathes, S. J., Nahai, F., and Vasconez, L. O. Myocutaneous free flap transfer: Anatomical and experimental considerations. *Plast. Reconstr. Surg. 62*: 162, 1978.

McCraw, J. B., Dibbell, D. G., and Carraway, J. H. Clinical definition of independent myocutaneous vascular territories. *Plast. Reconstr. Surg. 60*: 212, 1977.

McCraw, J. B., Dibbell, D. G., and Carraway, J. H. Clinical definition of independent myocutaneous vascular territories. *Plast. Reconstr. Surg. 60*: 341, 1977.

Breast Reconstruction

WALTER R. MULLIN, M.D., P.A.

This chapter is designed to familiarize the reader with what is presently available for women who have been unfortunate enough to require breast reconstruction. The different surgical techniques currently available to accomplish reconstruction, insight into what the patient experiences, and also realistic results will be discussed. Of these, the most difficult area to cover will be the emotional and philosophical parameters of this topic.

Generally, a plastic surgeon sees patients for breast reconstruction from one of several variable sources. The optimal patient is one who has been sent by a doctor familiar with the possibilities of reconstruction. The patient is sent after it is felt that she is reasonably free of persistent tumor and she is able to comprehend the preoperative explanation of the procedure and possible complications.

It seems that the reason most physicians have been reluctant to encourage reconstruction of breast lost to carcinoma is that they somehow feel that the reconstruction will decrease the patient's longevity, namely, hide a recurrence or alter host resistance to persistent or de novo carcinoma. It is the obligation of every treating physician to gain as much information as he can regarding these topics so that it may be validly related to each individual patient in a way that she may make an intelligent decision.

Several thoughts come to mind with respect to the above:

1. Some authors have written that there is very early dissemination of breast carcinoma even with very small lesions.[1] This thought carried further leads some to believe there is a substantial likelihood that there is incurable disease present. If one strongly adheres to this dismal outlook, then one could argue for immediate reconstruction to allow the patient maxium benefit of her remaining time.

2. Another point relative to the idea of concealing recurrent or persistent carcinoma is directed toward the question of where recurrent or persistent disease would have to be located if it were to be concealed. Obviously, it would have to be on the chest wall behind the implant, and this location carries a very poor prognosis as compared to skin or scar line recurrence. It seems logical that a patient destined to have this problem might be in a better situation if a silastic implant had previously been placed below this predetermined site of recurrence in the scar, therefore physically preventing direct extension into the chest wall during the critical time of detection, biopsy, and definitive surgery for such recurrences.

3. The topic of altering host resistance and possibly inciting "dormant tumor cells" is covered elsewhere and is not within the scope of this chapter. One must evaluate the evidence for or against this in advising a patient to have reconstruction.

4. The basic question arises of how long should one postpone reconstruction so that most of the recurrences can be detected. I doubt if this question will ever be answered satisfactorily in such a way that every physician involved feels comfortable in dealing with this problem.

We, as physicians, are interested in prolonging life of the best quality possible. The difference between individual patients in how they handle the loss of a breast and the overwhelming idea that they have a potentially gruesome and fatal disease is phenomenal.[2-4] It is very important to gain a feeling as soon as one can as to where each individual patient fits in this spectrum. Some patients seem truly not to care if they lose a breast, and they do very well postoperatively with or without an external prosthesis. They go about their daily routine with an "as if it never happened" attitude. More and more, however, we are seeing patients who have received their "medical education" through the medium of popular magazines and television. Sadly, often just enough information is retained to confuse the patient, and they respond to the loss or potential loss of a breast drastically. We should not be impatient with their questions and demands for a more thorough explanation. They are often the more educated medical consumers, and want to know if the reasons for surgery are valid and based on reliable studies. This attitude is good for the overall progress of this branch of plastic surgery. Presently, our best information is that 85% of patients who do develop recurrent disease have it detected within the first two years.[5] This information is helpful in deciding when reconstruction is to be initiated in each individual based on the patient's philosophies and desires.

Leaving aside the philosophical aspects of breast reconstruction, let us progress to the technical features. The amount of skin that remains and the status of the pectoralis muscle and the major features that dictate the type of procedure that will be offered to the patient. Other factors that are important are: history of radiation, general health, status of pathology report, motivation, family support, and location of local and distant scars. We should pause here to reemphasize the importance of the word "offer," for this first evaluation conference is so important. The patient must be made to realize what the surgery entails and what her alternatives are. Many patients feel they have only to come into the hospital for one relatively simple operation, and they will have a breast. However, in patients who do not have adequate skin coverage, this is not possible, and they must be given a clear understanding of what the more involved methods of reconstruction entail.

The following outline of surgical techniques describes the ones currently in use for reconstruction.

A. First, a patient who has an adequate skin envelope remaining after her surgery is the best candidate for reconstruction. If the pectoralis major is intact and the nipple has been banked,[6-8] all the better. A very reasonable breast can be made by simply introducing an appropriately sized silastic implant beneath the skin or skin and pectoralis major if possible. Time, usually three to four months, is allowed for the reconstructed breast mound to settle and stabilize. Since the opposite breast is at a greater risk of developing carcinoma,[9-12] and sometimes it is large or ptotic, then a subcutaneous mastectomy with implant replacement is in order to afford better symmetry and also an improved sense of security for the patient with respect to possible development of carcinoma in her remaining breast.

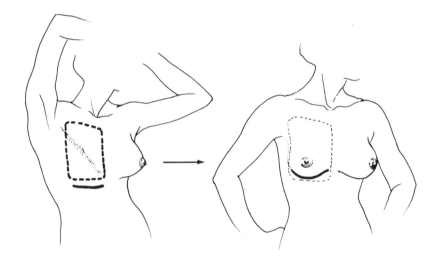

After a radical or modified radical mastectomy in a patient who has been left with infraclavicular flatness and an inadequate amount of skin that can not safely retain an implant without severe risk of skin breakdown due to tension, skin and subcutaneous tissue must be brought in from elsewhere. There are a number of ways this can be done. In general, use is made of one of the most practical principles of plastic surgery, namely, to evaluate what is missing as compared to the ideal normal, then use the most optimal area of excess to provide the needed material to reconstruct the defect.[13]

B. One way this skin is brought into the desired area is to use the excess skin and subcutaneous fat in the area of the lateral chest wall,[14] going posteriorly toward the subscapular area. This flap is delayed, elevated, and then turned into position, and allowed to pick up blood supply and settle. Next, an implant is placed, and the edges of the flap are tailored to mimic a natural breast. Once the

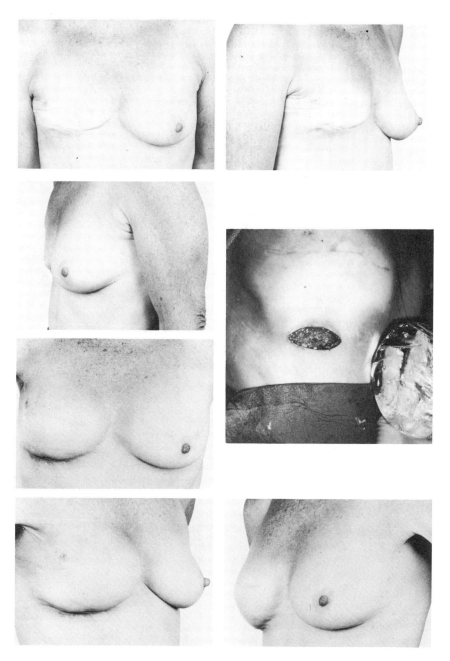

FIG. 1. Utilization of adequate remaining skin. An incision is made, and adequate skin is elevated for an implant to be placed to provide volume for the breast mound. Adequate cover is a must, for if too much tension is placed on the overlying skin, then breakdown and loss of the implant will result.

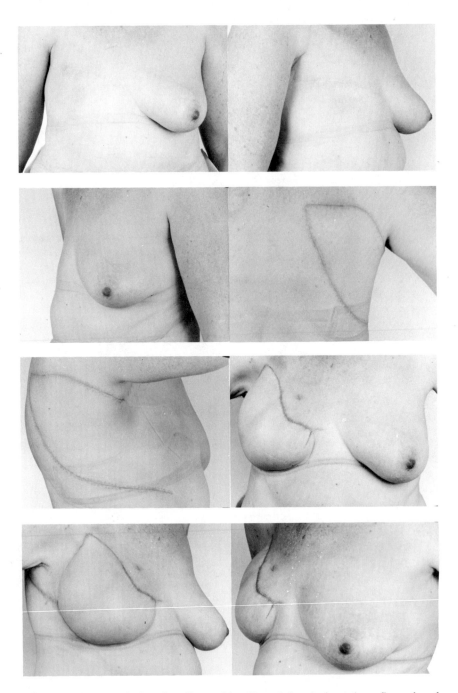

FIG. 2. Medially based chest flap. Excess skin of lateral chest is elevated as a flap and used to provide the needed cover for the implant.

mount is formed and settled, then the same procedure of managing the opposite breast is considered as outlined earlier.

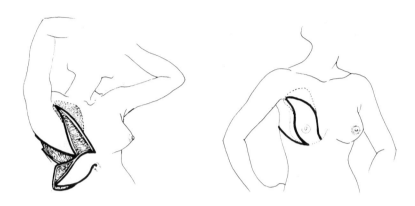

C. Use may also be made of a flap with the base laterally so that the scar of the donor area is not in an area that would be exposed by a low-back dress or a bathing suit. This flap provides a nice cupping contour of the inferior aspect of the breast.[15]

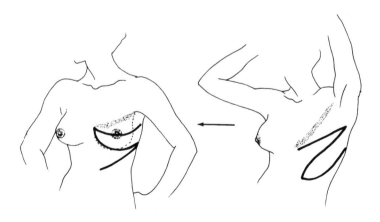

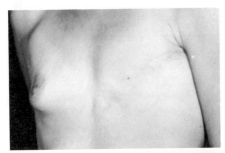

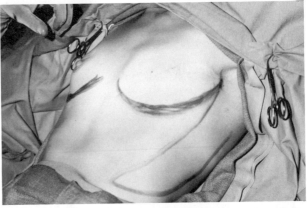

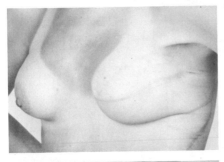

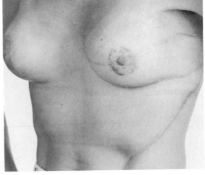

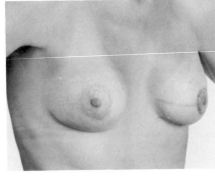

FIG. 3. Lateral-based chest flap.

D. In some women who have very large breasts and in whom one feels the risk of using opposite breast tissue[8-12] in the reconstruction is warranted, a flap taken from that large breast may be used for cover. Also in patients with a large breast, this may be a "life boat procedure"[13] if the flap from the chest is lost at any time during its transfer to the desired position.

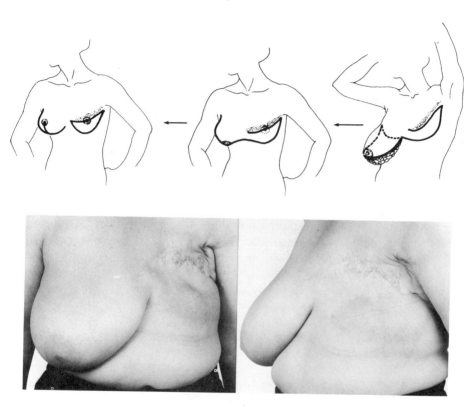

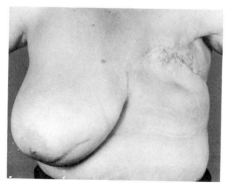

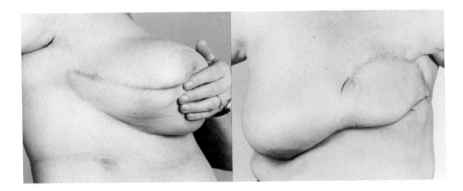

FIG. 4. Opposite breast flap. Use is made of a very large breast to provide flap cover for the deficient side. This case is obviously not completed but is well on its way to providing nice cover for the implant. Once the flap is stable, then the other breast will be reduced to match the reconstructed breast.

E. Advantage may also be taken of the fact that many patients in the age group of this disease have an excess of abdominal skin, which they will donate to "their cause" with great enthusiasm.[16] Most often this method is reserved for patients who have very tight, scarred or skin-grafted chest wall defects and ample abdominal tissue, or are unwilling to accept the donor area scars of the lateral chest area. Care must be made in selecting these patients, for certain locations of old abdominal surgical incisions may make this method a poor choice. There are

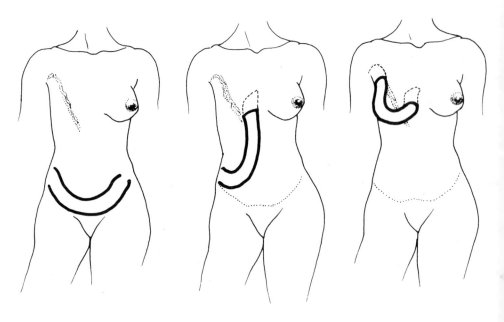

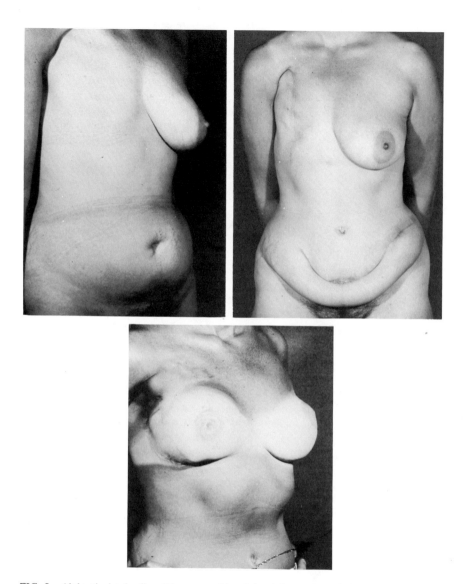

FIG. 5. Abdominal tube flap. The excess skin of the abdomen is used that would normally be discarded in the typical adbominoplasty. The tube is brought up in stages and inset artistically for the desired effect.

multiple stages involved in this procedure, but the end result is most rewarding as the donor area scars are in the most desirable location possible. Seldom is it possible in the field of reconstructive plastic surgery for one to be able to take so much tissue from an area for reconstruction and still benefit the donor area. Once again, the reconstruction of the nipple areolar complex and management of the remaining breast must be dealt with on an individual basis.

F. Another method for reconstruction is the use of a composite myocutaneous flap, utilizing the latissimus dorsi muscle and overlying skin.[17] This is a very good flap and has the advantage of reducing the number of stages required by the above flaps. The drawback however, is, the scar over the latissimus border and the defect caused by the loss of the amount of latissimus required to move the needed tissue.

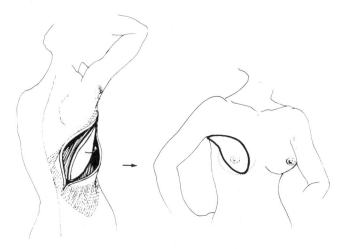

FIG. 6. Latissimus dorsi flap. The desired amount of skin, subcutaneous tissue, and muscle is elevated and repositioned in the desired position to provide bulk and cover for the implant.

G. Another method of getting the required tissue into the appropriate position is by use of microsurgical transfer of a free flap.[18] This requires a surgeon who is proficient in microsurgical techniques. The donor area is often not optmal, but if the flap is successful, it does provide the needed cover in a short period of time.

H. Omentum[17,19,20] has been used successfully to provide a vascular bed upon which a skin graft may be placed, both over a silastic prosthesis. Omentum with grafting also provides cover for chest wall defects that are sometimes seen after radical excision of tumor involving the chest wall, or for radiation necrosis of the area.

There are more elaborate methods in the literature such as large abdominal flaps or use of the buttocks tissue carried on the wrist, but the cost to the donor area is excessive.

One can see that moving tissue into the tight area resulting from certain mastectomies can be required regardless of the method chosen. The patient

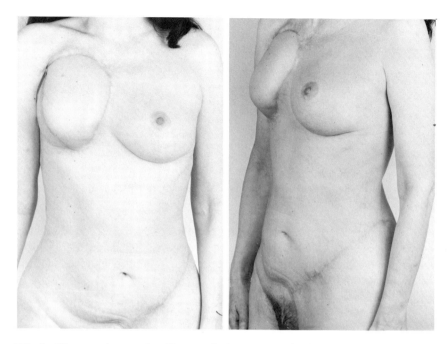

FIG. 7. Microvascular transfer. Photograph demonstrates the amount of cover tissue that can be brought into position with this technique. This flap will need to be adjusted to provide a more natural contour.

should be made to understand at the beginning that the common complications of infection, hematoma, loss of tissue secondary to inadequate blood supply and problems with the implants, such as capsular contracture, do occur. The extent to which this effects the final result is greatly variable.[21]

The subject of reconstructing the nipple-areolar complex has been saved for the end of the list of surgical techniques, for it is the "icing on the cake." The breast mound that has been constructed should be stable and not in need of revisions at this point. If the uninvolved breast is about the same size as the reconstructed breast, then the location of the nipple-areolar complex is made to match. If the nipple has been banked on the groin[6-8] (and this should only be done under very careful pathologic control, i.e., tumor-free at base of nipple), then it can simply be transferred up into position. This affords the simplest and usually the best cosmetic result. However, since those ducts that would be involved exit in the nipple and not the areola, an outer "donut" of areolar perimeter skin might be considered for reconstructive use in patients who have a very wide areola. (See Figure 11.)

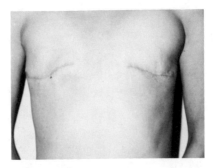

FIG. 8. Banked nipples. Patient lost both breasts secondary to *injections* of silicone.

If the nipple was not saved, then any of a number of sharing procedures may be used. The areolar skin is thin and grafts do very well placed on a de-epithelized receptor site of appropriate diameter and position. The techniques are outlined below:

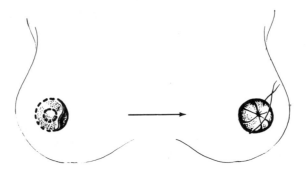

FIG. 9. Total area split graft. Split graft taken from normal side and used to construct the needed nipple areolar complex. This technique is useful in women with a small-diameter nipple areola complex.[22,23] A drum dermatome should be used.

The use of distant tissue to reconstruct the nipple is often less desirable because it does not follow the principle of using like tissue for reconstruction.[13] In the past, a graft from the labia was used to imitate areolar skin, but the result was often too dark.[24,25] A better color match is obtained in some patients by using the very high inner thigh skin for areolar grafts.[26] In most surgeons' hands, the use of tattooing has been unsatisfactory because of its lack of texture and color match.

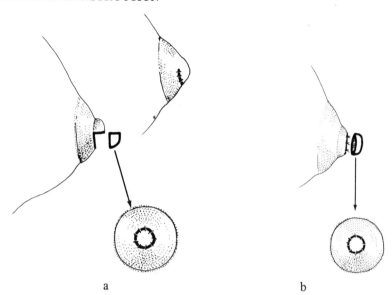

a   b

FIG. 10. Nipple projection. Composite grafts of the normal nipple may be obtained by one of the two methods outlined with minimal defect to the donor area.[17] Method "A" is used most often.

Another excellent method of reconstructing a very realistic nipple-areolar complex is obtained by utilizing the ear.[28]

As one can see from reflecting on the surgical gymnastics required to provide adequate cover for reconstruction, one might logically ask if perhaps there might be a better location for the ablative surgical scars that would result in less waste of uninvolved tissue. As in all surgical endeavors, each case should be evaluated on its own merits and individualized. If there are skin changes or if the lesion is close to the overlying skin, this area must be included with the specimen. However, in cases where the lesion is small or far removed from the overlying skin, one should ask himself if using the typical fusiform excision to include all the breast skin possible is of real established benefit to the patient. A very adequate mastectomy and axillary node dissection after removal of the pectoralis minor and leaving thin skin flaps can be easily accomplished through the incisions outlined in Figures 14–16.

In summary, this chapter has aimed at familiarizing the reader with what is currently available for patients wishing breast reconstruction. It should be re-emphasized that treating the disease is *the* top priority and that the patient should be given every chance to live out the rest of her days free of persistent or recurrent disease. Breast reconstruction is focused on the quality of life of those days in between initial treatment and the patient's demise, regardless of

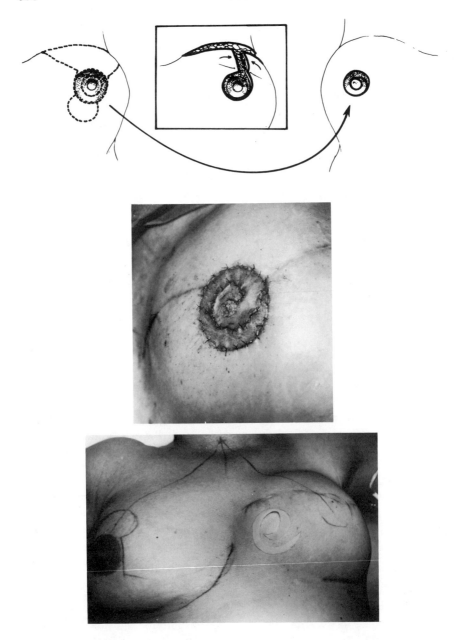

FIG. 11. Use of excess full thickness areola strip. In patients who have a large-diameter areola, the thin outer edge may be taken as a full thickness strip and coiled into position on the de-epithelized receptor site.[14,27]

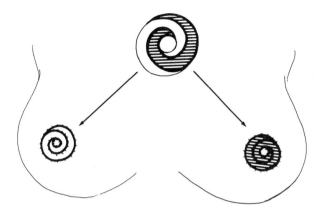

FIG. 12. Conjoined spirals method. This technique, the details of which are carefully outlined in Cronin's article,[14] reduces one large areola to two smaller ones with similar scar patterns.

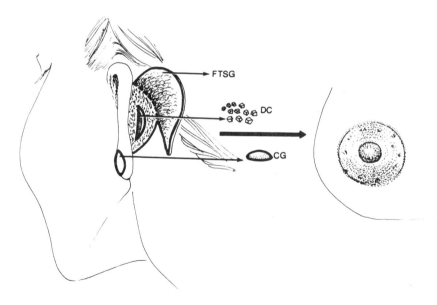

FIG. 13. Nipple areola reconstruction from auricular components. The pink areola is reconstructed from a full thickness graft from the postauricular skin. Nipple projection is constructed from a composite graft of earlobe. The glands of Montgomery are simulated with diced cartilege. Attention to careful detail pays off and can give a very rewarding result.

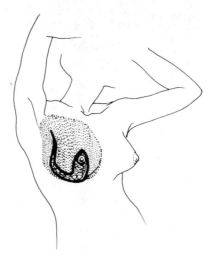

FIG. 14. Surgical approach to position scars for ideal reconstruction. Opening a breast via this approach allows exposure of the breast gland and axilla while preserving the needed skin cover. The nipple may be removed totally, or if frozen section clears the base, the nipple may be banked.

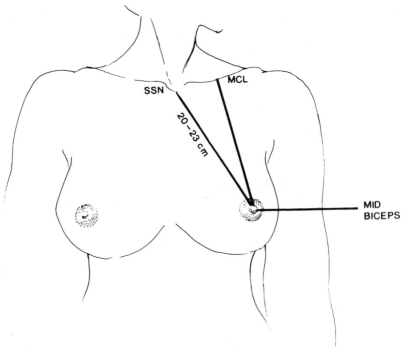

FIG. 15. Ideal nipple location. This diagram gives coordinates that are used to locate the ideal nipple location. It would help to locate the upper end of the apex above the nipple in Figure 14, if the involved breast were ptotic.[29]

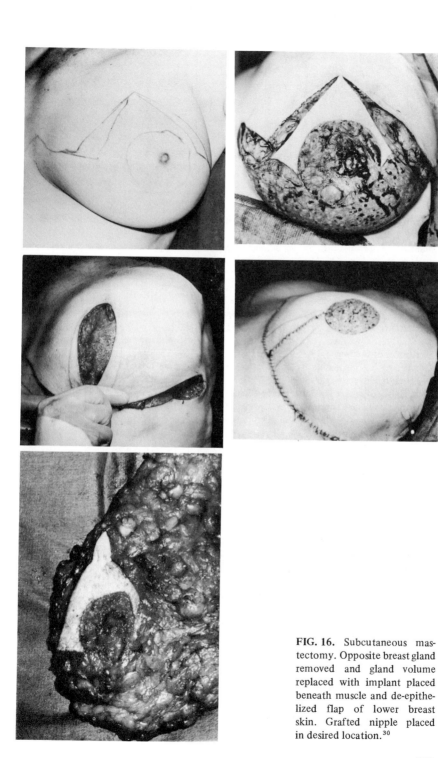

FIG. 16. Subcutaneous mastectomy. Opposite breast gland removed and gland volume replaced with implant placed beneath muscle and de-epithelized flap of lower breast skin. Grafted nipple placed in desired location.[30]

the cause. We must be able to give the patient a clear understanding of what can be realistically expected from breast reconstruction.

References

Foulds, L. Experimental study of the course and regulation of tumor growth. *Ann. R. Coll. Surg. 4:* 2: 93–101, August 1951.

Women's Attitude Regarding Breast Cancer: Summary conducted for The American Cancer Society. The Gallop Organization, Inc., 53 Bank Street, Princeton, New Jersey.

Adsett, G. A. Emotional reaction to disfigurement from cancer therapy. *Canad. Med. Assoc. J. 89:* 385, 1963.

Renneker, R., and Cutler, M. Psychological problems of adjustment to cancer of the breast. *J. A. M. A. 148:* 383, 1952.

Ketchum, A. Personal communication, 1978.

Millard, D. R., Jr., Devine, J., and Warren, W. D. Breast reconstruction: A plea for saving the uninvolved nipple. *A. J. Surg. 122:* 763, 1971.

Allison, A. B., and Howarth, M. D. Carcinoma in a nipple preserved by heterotropic auto-implantation. *N. Engl. J. Med. 298:* 20: 1132, 1978.

Parry, R. B., Cochran, T. C., and Wolfort, F. C. When is there nipple involvement in carcinoma of the breast. *Plast. Reconstr. Surg. 59:* 535–537, 1977.

Kilgore, A. R. Incidence of carcinoma in the second breast after radical removal of one breast for carcinoma. *J. A. M. A. 77:* 354–457, 1921.

Pack, G. T. Argument for Bilateral Mastectomy. *Plast. Reconstr. Surg. 29:* 929, 1951.

Urban, J. A. Bilateral breast cancer. *Cancer 24:* 1310, 1969.

Robbins, L. F., and Berg, J. W. Bilateral primary breast cancer. *Cancer 17:* 1501, 1964.

Gilles, H. D., and Millard, D. R., Jr.: *Principles and Art of Plastic Surgery,* vol. 1. Boston: Little, Brown and Co., 1951, pp. 48–54.

Cronin, T. D., Upton J., and McDonough, J. M. Reconstruction of the breast after mastectomy. *Plast. Reconstr. Surg. 59:* 1, 1977.

Millard, D. R., Jr. Aesthetic aspects of reconstructive surgery. *Ann. Plast. Surg.,* in press.

Millard, D. R., Jr. Breast reconstruction after radical mastectomy. *Plast. Reconstr. Surg. 58:* 283, 1976.

Bostwick, J., Vasconez, L. D., and Jerkiewitz, M. J. Breast reconstruction after radical mastectomy. *Plast. Reconstr. Surg. 61:* 682, 1978.

Seratin, D., Georgiude, N., and Given, K. Transfer of free flaps to proide well-vascularized, thin cover for breast reconstructions after radical mastectomy. *Plast. Reconstr. Surg. 62:* 517, 1978.

Arnold, P. G., Hartrampf, L. R., and Jerkiewiez, M. J. One stage reconstruction of the breast using the transposed greater omentum. *Plast. Reconstr. Surg. 57:* 520, 1976.

Das, S. K. The size of the human omentum and methods of lengthening it for transplantation. *Br. J. Plast. Surg. 29:* 170–174, 1976.

Bouview, B. Problems in breast reconstruction. *Med. J. Aust. 1:* 937, 1977.

Millard, D. R., Jr. Nipple and areola reconstruction by split-skin graft from the normal side. *Plast. Reconstr. Surg. 50:* 350, 1972.

Obi, L. J., cited by Millard, D. R., Jr. Breast reconstruction after a radical mastectomy. *Plast. Reconstr. Surg. 58:* 283–291, 1976.

Adams, W. M. Labial transplants for correction of loss of nipple. *Plast. Reconstr. Surg. 4:* 295, 1949.

Thale, H. B. Follow-up on labial transplant for nipple loss. *Plast. Reconstr. Surg. 8*: 471, 1951.

Broadbent, T. R., Woolf, R. M., and Metz, P. S. Restoring the mammary areola by a skin graft from the upper inner thigh. *Br. J. Plast. Surg. 30*: 220-222, 1977.

Wexler, M. R., and O'Neal, R. M. Areolar shaving to reconstruct the absent nipple. *Plast. Reconstr. Surg. 51*: 176, 1973.

Brent, B., and Bostwick, J. Nipple areola reconstruction with auricular tissue. *Plast. Reconstr. Surg. 60*: 353, 1977.

Spira, M. Subcutaneous mastectomy in large ptotic breast. *Plast. Reconstr. Surg. 59*: 200, 1977.

Parsons, R. W., Burton, F. C., and Shaw, R. C. The versatile mammaplasty pattern of Wise. *Plast. Reconstr. Surg. 55*: 1-4, 1975.

Bone Marrow Transplantation

ROBERTSON PARKMAN, M.D.
FRED S. ROSEN, M.D.
Harvard University Medical School, and Children's Hospital Medical Center, Boston, Massachusetts.

Bone marrow transplantation is effective therapy for individuals with severe combined immune deficiency,[1-3] severe aplastic anemia,[4-8] the Wiskott-Aldrich syndrome,[9-11] and Kostmann's syndrome. Allogeneic bone marrow transplantation is also effective but still experimental therapy for relapsed acute and chronic leukemia (acute lymphoblastic leukemia, acute myelogenous leukemia, chronic myelogenous leukemia in blast crisis).[12-15]

Crucial to the understanding of successful transplantation is an understanding of the marrow populations involved. The infused donor bone marrow contains both hematopoietic and lymphoid stem cells. Although both stem cell populations are derived from a common totipotential stem cell, there is no evidence that there is any interchange between them in postnatal life. Thus, recipient engraftment can be achieved by either the lymphoid stem cells or the hematopoietic stem cells or both. Table 1 shows the marrow composition of individuals with the various disease for which bone marrow transplantation has been attempted. Children with severe combined immune deficiency have normal hematopoietic cells but abnormal or absent lymphoid stem cells. Conversely, individuals with severe aplastic anemia have absent hematopoietic stem cells and normal lymphoid stem cells. Individuals with genetically determined disorders such as the Wiskott-Aldrich syndrome and Kostmann's syndrome have normal numbers of dysfunctional stem cells.

TABLE 1. Preparation for Allogeneic Bone Marrow Transplantation

| Disease | STEM CELLS PRESENT | | Preparation | Result |
	Lymphoid	Hematopoietic		
Severe combined immune deficiency	–	+	None	Lymphoid graft
Severe aplastic anemia	+	–	None	No graft
			CTX	Lymphoid and hematopoietic grafts
Acute leukemia	+	+	None	No graft
			CTX ± other drugs	Irreproducible lymphoid and hematopoietic grafts
			TBI ± CTX	Lymphoid and hematopoietic grafts
Wiskott-Aldrich	+	+	CTX	T-Lymphoid graft
			TBI + ATS	Lymphoid and hematopoeitic grafts
Granulocyte dysfunction	+	+	CTX ± other drugs	No graft
			TBI + ATS	Lymphoid and hematopoietic grafts

The immune system is of crucial importance in engraftment because immunity of the recipient will permit the rejection of all allogeneic donor marrow cells. Therefore, a marrow transplant from a sibling who is HLA-A, –B, –C, and –D identical[16] [major histocompatibility region (MHR) identical] will not engraft because of the immunocompetence of the recipient. Adequate immunosuppression of the recipient's immune system is a necessary prerequisite for successful transplantation in all recipients with normal immunity. The interrelationship of the immune system and the stem cell composition of the recipient marrow in various diseases will now be considered separately.

1. *Severe Combined Immune Deficiency (SCID)*. In this disorder, the affected children are missing normal lymphoid function and have normal hematopoietic function. Therefore, they have an inability to reject foreign grafts and consequently require no immunosuppression of their immune suppression to permit allogeneic marrow engraftment. After bone marrow transplantation, usually with a dose of 50 million cells/kg intravenously,[3] engraftment of only the lymphoid stem cells occurs. Approximately two weeks after transplantation, the presence of donor lymphoid cells peripherally can be detected. No decrease in recipient marrow cellularity is detectable prior to transplantation. Only donor lymphoid stem cells engraft; there is no engraftment of donor hematopoietic stem cells, presumably because of the presence of normal numbers of recipient hematopoietic stem cells. These observations in children with SCID has led to the concept that engraftment is achieved only by those stem cells for which there is "space in the marrow" (i.e., a physiological absence). When there has been a difference in ABO blood group or in red cell enzymes [adenosine deaminase deficiency (ADA)], no evidence for engraftment of donor erythroid elements has been detected.[3]

2. *Aplastic Anemia (AA)*. In AA, there is an absence of hematopoietic stem cells, but normal lymphoid stem cells and immunocompetence are present. Because of the normal immunocompetency, after the infusion of MHR compatible donor marrow no hematopoietic engraftment will occur because the infused marrow cells will be rejected by the recipient's immunocompetent lymphocytes. Therefore, immunosuppression of the recipient's immune system is required for successful hematopoietic engraftment. The immunosuppression required is dependent upon whether the recipient is sensitized to the donor or not. Nonsensitized individuals can be immunosuppressed with cyclophosphamide alone, whereas individuals who are sensitized may require multiagent immunosuppression.[17,18] With the reduction or abolition of the recipient's immune system including the lymphoid stem cells, engraftment of both donor hematopoietic and lymphoid stem cells can be achieved. Therefore, recipients of allogeneic transplants for AA have both lymphoid and hematopoietic function of donor origin.

3. *Wiskott-Aldrich Syndrome (WAS)*. The WAS is a genetically determined

X-linked disorder in which affected males demonstrate abnormal cellular immunity, decreased antibody production to carbohydrate antigens, decreased platelet production, abnormal platelet function, and eczema.[11] These individuals have normal numbers of circulating lymphocytes and normal numbers of bone marrow megakaryocytes with decreased circulating platelets. When such individuals have been prepared for transplantation with cyclophosphamide (CTX) alone, establishment of only donor T-lymphocyte function has been achieved.[9,10] Recipient B-cell function has continued. It is not clear whether the donor T-cells are the progeny of T-cells that differentiated in the donor which are living out their normal life span in the recipient, or whether donor lymphoid stem cells engraft in the recipient and differentiate under the influence of the recipient's thymus. However, no hematopoietic engraftment has been achieved in these children. Although cyclophosphamide reduces the number of hematopoietic stem cells producing peripheral pancytopenia, all circulating hematopoietic elements have returned to normal levels by one month and have been of recipient origin.

The difficulty in the treatment of genetically determined bone marrow disorders is that the disease is produced not by the absence of hematopoietic stem cells but by the presence of dysfunctional cells which have normal self-renewal capacity. Agents such as cyclophosphamide, ara-C, 6-thioguanine, and so on, that have been used as pretransplant preparation do not have significant anti-hematopoietic stem cell activity and therefore do not reduce the number of recipient hematopoietic stem cells to a level where donor engraftment can occur. Various agents have been shown in canine and rodent models to be effective anti-hematopoietic stem cell agents, including total body irradiation (TBI), the nitrosoureas, and dimethyl myleran. For this reason, we have prepared patients with WAS for transplantation with a combination of TBI and rabbit anti-human thymocyte serum (ATS).[11] TBI is an effective antihematopoietic stem cell agent and has some immunosuppressive capacity. ATS has both immunosuppressant and anti-stem cell activity. Three children with WAS have been successfully transplantated after preparation with ATS and TBI, demonstrating that the combination has adequate immunosuppressive and anti-hematopoietic stem cell activity to permit complete donor engraftment.

4. *Kostmann's Syndrome.* Kostmann's syndrome is a genetically determined disorder in which affected individuals have normal numbers of bone marrow myeloid precursors that because of an undefined defect do not mature into circulating granulocytes. The combination of ATS and TBI has permitted adequate immunosuppression, the successful elimination of the abnormal hematopoietic stem cells, and the engraftment of normal histocompatible marrow, establishing both donor hematopoietic and lymphoid function.

SUMMARY

The transplantation of human marrow may achieve lymphoid and/or hematopoietic engraftment. In individuals without lymphoid stem cells, allogeneic lymphoid engraftment can be achieved without immunosuppression or evidence of hematopoietic engraftment, a result suggesting that only those marrow elements for which there is physiological space will achieve engraftment. In diseases characterized by an absence of the hematopoietic stem cells but normal immunocompetence, no engraftment after transplantation will be achieved without immunosuppression because of the immune rejection of the infused marrow. The abolition of recipient immunity is necessary before the successful transplantation of individuals with absent hematopoietic stem cells is achieved. Immunosuppression in such patients can be achieved with drugs alone, resulting in the engraftment of both lymphoid and hematopoietic stem cells. In diseases characterized by the presence of dysfunctional hematopoietic or lymphoid stem cells, chemical immunosuppression alone is not sufficient to obtain both hematopoietic and lymphoid engraftment, since immunosuppressive agents have poor anti-hematopoietic stem cell activity. The addition of agents like TBI must be utilized to eradicate the dysfunctional hematopoietic stem cells. The combination of TBI and ATS generates the requisite immunosuppressive and anti-hematopoietic stem cell activity necessary for the successful engraftment of allogeneic lymphoid and hematopoietic stem cells in individuals with genetically determined dysfunctional stem cells.

References

Gatti, R. A., Meuwissen, H. J., et al. Immunological reconstitution of sex-linked lymphopenic immunological deficiency. *Lancet 2*: 1366, 1968.

Dekoning, J., Van Bekkum, D. W., et al. Transplantation of bone marrow cells and fetal thymus in an infant with lymphopenic immunological deficiency. *Lancet 1*: 1223, 1969.

Parkman, R., Gelfand, E. W., et al. Severe combined immunodeficiency and adenosine deaminase deficiency. *N. Engl. J. Med. 292*: 714, 1975.

Thomas, E. D., Storb, R., et al. Bone marrow transplantation. *N. Engl. J. Med 292*: 832–843, 895–902, 1975.

Thomas, E. D., Buckner, C. D., et al. Aplastic anemia treated by marrow transplantation. *Lancet 1*: 284–289, 1972.

Storb, R., Thomas, E. D., et al. Allogeneic marrow grafting for treatment of aplastic anemia: A follow-up on long-term survivors. *Blood 48*: 485–490, 1976.

Camitta, B. M., Rappeport, J. M., et al. Selection of patients for bone marrow transplantation in severe aplastic anemia. *Blood 45*: 355–363, 1975.

UCLA Bone Marrow Transplant Team. Bone marrow transplantation in severe aplastic anemia. *Lancet 2*: 921–923, 1976.

Bach, F. H., Albertini, R. J., et al. Bone-marrow transplantation in a patient with the Wiskott-Aldrich syndrome. Lancet 2: 1364–1366, 1968.

August, C. S., Hathaway, W. E., et al. Improved platelet function following bone marrow transplantation in an infant with the Wiskott-Aldrich syndrome. *J. Pediatr. 82:* 58-64, 1973.

Parkman, R., Rappeport, J. et al. Complete correction of the Wiskott-Aldrich syndrome by allogeneic bone-marrow transplantation. *N. Engl. J. Med. 298:* 921-927, 1978.

Thomas, E. D., Buckner, C. D., et al. One hundred patients with acute leukemia treated by chemotherapy, total body irradiation, and allogeneic marrow transplantation. *Blood 49:* 511-533, 1977.

Gale, R. P., Feig, S., et al. Bone marrow transplantation in acute leukemia using intensive chemoradiotherapy (SCARI-UCLA). *Transplant. Proc. 8:* 611-616, 1976.

Santos, G. W., Sensenbrenner, L. L., et al. HL-A identical marrow transplants in aplastic anemia, acute leukemia, and lymphosarcoma employing cyclophosphamide. *Transplant. Proc. 8:* 607-610, 1976.

Graw, R. G., Jr., Yankee, R. A., et al. Bone marrow transplantation from HL-A matched donors to patients with acute leukemia. *Transplantation 14:* 79-90, 1972.

Amos, D. B., Batchelor, R., et al. Nomenclature for factors of the HLA system. *Cell. Immunol. 21:* 382-385, 1976.

Parkman, R., Rappeport, J., et al. Successful use of multiagent immunosuppression in the bone marrow transplantation of sensitized patients. *Blood, 52:* 1163-1169, 1978.

Storb, R., Floersheim, G. L., et al. Effect of prior blood transfusions on marrow grafts: Abrogation of sensitization by procarbazine and antithymocyte serum. *J. Immunol. 12:* 1508-1516, 1974.

Status of Transplantation of Human Organs

ROBERT J. CORRY, M.D.
JOHN C. WEST, M.D.
Department of Surgery
University of Iowa
College of Medicine
Iowa City, Iowa

Although prolongation of life by replacement of a diseased organ with a normal organ had been considered just after the turn of this century, it has been only within the last two decades that organ transplantation has been realized in practice. In spite of the fact that many mechanical artificial organs are meeting with increasing success, including portable (wearable) dialysis units, artificial limbs, and even artificial hearts, it is obvious that healthy living tissue is the ideal substitute for damaged organs.

It is now firmly established that the most important factor governing survival of an organ transplanted from one individual to another is the degree of genetic or "immunogenetic" disparity between the donor and the recipient. For example, transfer of a kidney from a healthy individual to his identical twin brother whose own kidneys have inexorably failed, should result in the recipient's living a normal and full life. However, transplantation of a kidney from an unrelated cadaver donor who has been healthy prior to sustaining irreversible brain injury, has a little better than a 50% chance of succeeding for more than one year. Nonidentical sibling and parent donors are in between these two extremes in terms of graft success. Although the surgical procedure of transplantation of any primarily vascularized organ must be carried out with precise technique, the major problems are concerned with preventing and controlling the rejection process and dealing with complex complications that may arise as a result of nonspecific immunosuppression.

We are now getting closer to a more satisfactory solution of the problem of rejection, and even at the present time a completely workable approach to its control has been worked out with renal transplantation and with cardiac and liver transplantation in a few select centers. From all we have learned in the recent past, there are strong reasons for expecting that a combination of partial prevention and complete control of the rejection process can be worked out that will move clinical surgery more in the direction of supplementing bodily functions by adding rather than removing something.

REJECTION

Rejection is the primary cause of failure of a transplanted organ. The recirculating small lymphocytes are able to recognize the foreign target cell through specific surface receptors, leading to membrane changes responsible for cytotoxic destruction. The lymphocyte, and most particularly the T-cell lymphocyte (thymus-dependent), has come to be known as the "killer cell." Rejection can occur on a cellular basis, or can result from a humoral B-cell (bone marrow-dependent) factor.

Hyperacute rejection is a phenomenon that occurs within minutes or hours after transplantation as a result of a preformed cytotoxic antibody directed against foreign antigens of the grafted tissue. Cytotoxic antibodies develop as a normal response to transfusion of whole blood (white blood cells) or a previous transplant. Fortunately, the phenomenon of hyperacute rejection rarely occurs, since pretransplantation cross matches, testing the patient's serum with donor lymphocytes, is an automatic procedure immediately prior to organ transplantation. A positive lymphocytotoxic cross match precludes this disaster.

Acute rejection occurs between five days and three weeks following transplantation and is a cell-mediated hypersensitivity type of rejection involving the

T-lymphocytes. In most cases, this reaction can be successfully treated with the use of high dose steroid hormones administered for a few days to the recipient. However, even after total reversal of the rejection process, second, third, and even fourth episodes of cellular rejection may occur. Usually, with each attack of this "army of lymphocytes" some permanent destruction of grafted tissue occurs. Fortunately, there is usually a long interval between these rejection reactions.

Late rejection or *chronic rejection* may occur after several years in a slow but inexorable manner. This type of tissue destruction occurs as a result of the binding of immunoglobulins and complement on the vascular endothelium, producing a secondary endothelial proliferation and consequent obliteration of the lumens of small blood vessels. Cardiac transplant surgeons have recently had some success in dealing with this problem by the administration of aspirin, dipyridamole, and a lipid-free diet. Steroid hormones in high doses are totally ineffective in reversing chronic rejection.

Although there are killer T-cells and cytotoxic antibodies elaborated by B-cells on the one hand, it is well established that there are suppressor cells and enhancing antibodies on the other. Therefore, the successful long-term normally functioning transplanted organ has entered a state of equilibrium with the recipient in which the appropriate balance has been achieved. This balance between the factors leading to destruction and those producing enhancement and suppression of rejection occurs in those few cases in which grafted organs from unrelated individuals have functioned without any evidence of rejection for many years. In these ideal cases, recipient unresponsiveness has developed.

HISTOCOMPATIBILITY TYPING

Since survival of grafted tissue transferred from one individual to another of the same species depends to a large extent on genetic differences between donor and host, efforts have been made in clinical organ transplantation to achieve the best possible tissue match. Rules of tissue transfer were defined and histocompatibility testing in man was initiated by Dausett's description of the first HLA antigen (1954) and further delineated with his description of the HLA complex in 1958. Further refinements came from Amos's study of varying techniques for identifying leukocyte antigens, VanRood's confirmation of the same in 1965, and finally, at the Turin International Workshop on Histocompatibility, Ceppellini's proof that the highly polymorphic leukocyte antigens were controlled by a region on the sixth pair of chromosomes, now called the MHC (major histocompatibility complex) locus. The genetic region on the sixth pair of autosomal chromosomes (MHC or HLA) is further subdivided into four specific regions and designated by the letters A, B, C, and D (Table 1).

TABLE 1.   Genetic regions for histocompatibility typing

MHC or HLA	Major histocompatibility complex, region of the chromosome encompassing the whole complex of closely linked genes.
A, B, C, D	The locus symbols: where HLA–A corresponds to the first segregating serologically defined series, previously called LA.
HLA–B	Corresponds to the second segregating series, previously termed four.
HLA–C	Corresponds to the AJ or third locus.
HLA–D	Corresponds to the locus of genes related to mixed lymphocyte reactions, previously termed LD-1.

Early methods pioneering the detection of these leukocyte antigens involved microscopic agglutination procedures. Wolford first developed a lymphocytotoxicity test, which was further perfected by Terasaki and his colleagues. Lymphocytes from the individual recipient to be typed are isolated from peripheral blood, one lambda of antiserum known to detect HLA antigens is added, and the mixture is incubated for 30 to 60 minutes. Complement is added from fresh rabbit serum, and, after incubation, a vital dye is added, and the percentage of dead to live cells determined. In determining the HLA type of a specific individual, approximately 60 to 80 antisera known to detect specific antigens are required. This rather complex procedure is carried out on each cadaver donor. Recipients and their families have been tissue-typed previously so that a genotypic analysis can be determined.

If a living related donor is not available, the best possible matched cadaver kidney is used. Histocompatibility testing procedures on cadaver donors and their families can be accomplished within four to five hours, and two appropriately matched recipients can be selected. Donor kidneys matched for a haplotype with the recipients have been selected in our own institution in about 50 cases (Figure 1).

Nationwide and even worldwide sharing systems are developing which permit the best possible matched recipients to be selected. Accordingly, the kidneys are then sent to the appropriate transplantation center by commercial or private airplane, usually within a few hours after their removal. Either simple cold storage or pulsatile perfusion of kidneys has been used to preserve the organs. The two methods of storage have proved to be equally satisfactory.

IMMUNOSUPPRESSION

Despite advances in histocompatibility testing procedures, and attempts to match donors with recipients, the administration of immunosuppressive agents to recipients of transplanted organs is necessary except possibly in an identical twin donor-recipient combination. Rejection remains the chief cause of graft loss, and circumventing this inexorable process is a major goal. Prednisone and azathioprine were initially used independently, but upon recognition of their pharmacological synergism, the two drugs were combined. This drug combination remains the cornerstone upon which successful transplantation of organs rests. Although antilymphocyte globulin (ALG) has been shown to be highly effective in prolonging graft survival in rodents and other experimental animals, its promise in humans has not yet fully materialized. Recent reports, presented by Levey in Boston and Thomas at the Medical College of Virginia, have been encouraging in terms of the ability of xeno-specific antisera produced in rabbits to delay rejection. Results in controlled studies using other preparations of ALG, however, have not yet been as encouraging as was originally anticipated. Recent data presented by Calne at the Seventh International Congress of the Transplantation Society in Rome suggests that Cyclosporin A, a fungal metabolyte, known to inhibit humoral immunity and to suppress cell-mediated immunity while exerting only mild myelotoxicity, might represent a major breakthrough. Although only in the early experimental stages, total lymphoid irradiation (TLI) followed by donor bone marrow injection may have promise in the future. Renewed interest in thoracic duct drainage to deplete lymphocytes has occurred and is being investigated in Denver by Starzl.

Evidence was presented in 1973 by Terasaki and Opelz that blood transfusions administered to recipients prior to the kidney transplantation lead to an

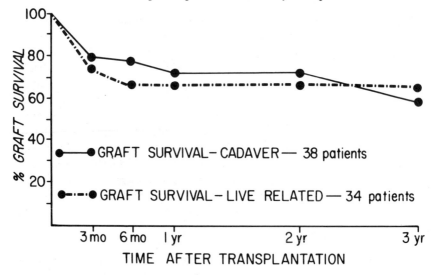

FIG. 1. Actuarial survival curves of single haplotype living related grafts compared to single haplotype matched cadaver grafts. Note that survivals of both types of transplants are equal.

improved graft survival. Investigators in numerous other centers since then have presented unequivocal evidence that patients who have received blood transfusions actually have a better graft survival rate than those who have never been transfused at all. Our own group has shown in a large series that patients transfused only on the day of the transplant procedure have the same improved graft survival as those patients transfused before transplantation. Both groups have a substantially better graft survival rate than those patients who have received no blood transfusions at all (Figure 2).

Since most immunosuppressive agents are relatively nonspecific, the partial immune paralysis that ensues inevitably leads to a higher infection rate. For example, infections with opportunistic organisms as well as bacterial and viral agents are not uncommon in recipients of transplanted organs. The transplantation team must become expert in diagnosing and treating a variety of infections, and when potentially fatal infections occur, immunosuppressive drugs should be stopped immediately, and steroid hormones should be reduced to a maintenance level. Fevers should be evaluated aggressively to determine the source of infection. Close cooperation with infecious disease services and clinical microbiological laboratories are of vital importance.

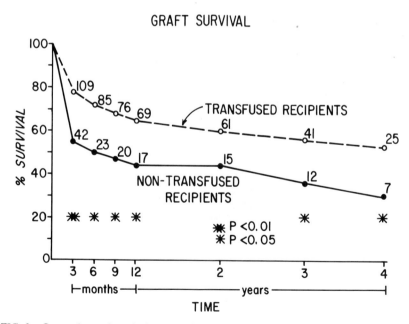

FIG. 2. Comparison of survival curves of transplants in recipients who have received blood transfusions with those who have not been transfused. Note the beneficial effect on graft survival of blood transfusions.

RENAL TRANSPLANTATION

More than 25,000 renal transplants have been performed throughout the world in the last two decades. In 1958, Murray and his colleagues performed the first successful transplant from an identical twin donor. In 1963, Starzl reported the first series of transplanted patients using combined azathioprine and prednisone for immunosuppression. The major indications for transplantation of the kidney are a variety of end-stage renal diseases, including such disorders as glomerulone-

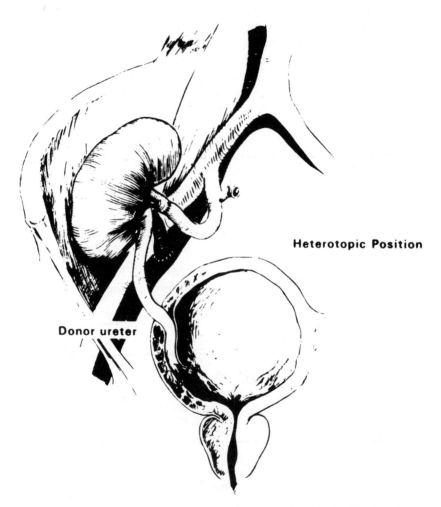

Heterotopic Position

Donor ureter

FIG. 3. Diagrammatic illustration of a kidney transplant placed in the iliac fossa. Ureter is joined to the bladder mucosa beneath the submucosal tunnel to prevent reflux. Alternate method of ureteral anastomosis is pyeloureterostomy.

phritis, pyelonephritis, polycystic renal disease, medullary cystic disease, hereditary nephritis, and other systemic disorders such as systemic lupus erythematosus, juvenile onset diabetes mellitus, hypertension, scleroderma, and a host of congenital bladder neck and urethra malformations that have lead to chronic renal failure.

More than 60,000 Americans reach end-stage renal failure per year and would die unless treated by hemodialysis or renal transplantation. Results of transplantation reported by the larger well-known centers indicate that overall *graft* survival rates from cadaver donors has been somewhere in the range of 60%, from HLA identical sibling donors, 90%, and from nonidentical sibling or parent donors, 75%. Patient survival rates should be at least 90%. Better results from cadaver transplants have been shown to occur when haplotype matched cadaver donors are used, and when patients have received prior blood transfusions.

Since 1973, patients with end-stage renal disease have been classified as Medicare patients. Thus, the enormous financial burdens of chronic dialysis and renal transplantation have been eased considerably for the patient.

LIVER TRANSPLANTATION

Following Starzl's first orthotopic liver transplant in man in 1963, more than 300 patients have undergone this procedure throughout the world. Patients with

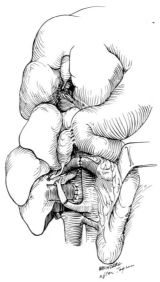

FIG. 4. Heterotopic liver transplant. Most successful liver transplants are in the orthotopic position. This technique has been used in a few cases in which the patient's own liver has not been removed. Note that the portal circulation is directed into the liver.

end-stage liver disease, which includes those patients with biliary atresia, chronic hepatitis, the Bud Chiari syndrome, and, in some circumstances, primary hepatic malignancy, are candidates for hepatic replacement. At the present time, two major centers of hepatic transplantation have developed, Denver (Starzl) and Cambridge, England (Calne). Starzl has performed over 100 hepatic replacements, and in his last series of 30 patients, between August 1976 and December 1977, has reported a one-year survival of 50%. Donor livers are flushed with chilled Collins' solution and can be stored for 12 hours prior to transplantation. Complications that arise following hepatic replacement have usually been concerned with the method of biliary tract drainage. The Denver group has used two methods of biliary drainage: choledochocholedochostomy with a T-tube stent and cholecystenterostomy through a Roux-en-Y limb. The Cambridge group also has reported improved survival within the last couple of years.

CARDIAC TRANSPLANTATION

Progress in heart transplantation has probably been the most impressive of any primarily vascularized organ since Christian Barnard's first successful orthotopic cardiac transplant in man in 1967. Over 400 human heart transplants have been performed in the world, and approximately 100 of these patients are surviving. Major progress in the field has been made by Shumway's group at Stanford. Cave's description of transvenous biopsy of the endomyocardium in 1973 lead to a remarkable facilitation in the diagnosis and treatment of cardiac allograft rejection. Cave's technique, together with electrocardiographic voltage changes, remains the mainstay for the diagnosis of rejection. In 1968, the Stanford group reported a 22% one-year survival rate, which at the present time has been increased to around 60%, a figure that is at least comparable to renal allograft survival rates in major centers. Unfortunately, complete rejection of the heart allograft usually results in death of the recipient unless another cardiac transplant can be performed.

Contraindications for orthotopic cardiac transplantation include *severe pulmonary hypertension* with a high fixed pulmonary vascular resistance in which the donor right ventricle is not capable of carrying out the work load placed upon it because of insufficient hypertrophy, *ongoing infection* in the recipient, juvenile onset *diabetes mellitus,* and a *positive lymphocytotoxic cross match.*

More recently, Barnard has introduced another major breakthrough in the field, the heterotopic or auxiliary heart transplant. Between November of 1974 and 1978, 20 heterotopic heart transplants have been performed by Barnard's group. At present, there is a 58% one-year graft survival. There are several distinct advantages of this "piggyback" heart transplantation procedure, in which the heart is placed essentially adjacent to the recipient's own heart in the mediastinum and right chest. First, patients with severe pulmonary hypertension can be transplanted, since the patient's own right ventricle has become hyper-trophied and is equipped to overcome the increased pulmonary vascular resis-tance. Second, the recipient can better tolerate severe rejection episodes in that the patient's own heart can usually take over temporarily. Third, the "piggy-back" heart can be replaced with another transplant with more time to spare, should rejection be complete.

Progress in heart transplantation has been of such magnitude that additional programs in this country are cautiously developing in centers that have had successful renal transplantation programs where facilities for such programs have already been in operation, including histocompatibility typing, immunological monitoring, infectious disease groups experienced in handling problems of infections, and experienced transplantation and cardiac surgeons.

PANCREATIC TRANSPLANTATION

Around 50 pancreatic transplants have been attempted with only four long-term survivors. Although an enormous amount of research has been carried out in perfecting techniques of islet cell transplantation, complete amelioration of the

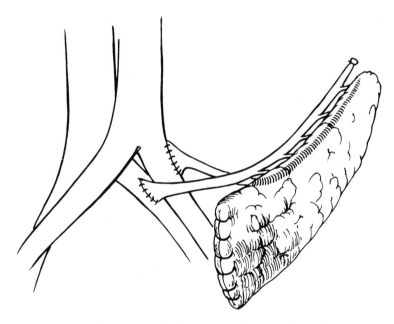

FIG. 5. Illustration of a partial heterotopic pancreatic transplant. Blood supply of the distal half of the pancreas is based on the splenic artery and vein. In this case, the transected pancreas is sutured. Drainage of the pancreatic duct into the ureter or a Roux-en-Y limb would be preferable.

diabetic state using this procedure has not yet been accomplished. Apparently, rejection of the islet cells occurs in a fairly vigorous fashion. Therefore, renewed interest has developed in whole organ transplantation of the pancreas. Some success has been achieved in Lyon, France, in which the tail of the pancreas is transplanted based on the splenic artery and vein. A major obstacle in this technique has concerned the most appropriate method of draining the pancreatic juice. Methods of handling this problem have been the subject of research in larger animals, and include injection of the entire ductal system with Neoprene, a rubberized synthetic that essentially fills the large and small exocrine ducts, free drainage of pancreatic juice into the peritoneal cavity, and diversion by means of a duct-ureter anastomosis or Roux-en-Y drainage to the small intestine.

Probably the most ideal recipients are those patients who have received successful renal transplants and have not rejected their kidneys over a period of several months to years.

SUMMARY

The therapeutic value of transplantation of organs is obvious, particularly when compared to the alternatives. In no other area is there such an intense cooperation between clinicians and basic scientists as exists in transplantation biology. As more clearly defined methods of specifically altering recipient responsiveness to foreign tissue antigens are worked out, a fully satisfactory solution to the problem of the rejection response will be inevitable.

References

Proceedings of the Sixth International Congress of the Transplantation Society. *Transplant. Proc. 9*, No. 1. New York: Grune & Stratton, 1977.
Najarian, J. S., and Simmons, R. L., eds. *Transplantation*. Philadelphia: Lea & Febiger, 1972.
Russell, P. S., and Monaco, A. P., eds. *The Biology of Tissue Transplantation*. Boston: Little, Brown and Co., 1965.
Calne, R., ed. *Immunological Aspects of Transplantation Surgery*. New York: John Wiley and Sons, 1973.

Maintenance of Life by Blood Replacement: Modern Treatment for Hemophilia

MARTIN J. INWOOD, B.Sc., M.D. F.R.C.P. (C).
Associate Professor
Department of Medicine
Faculty of Medicine.
The University of Western Ontario
London, Ontario, Canada

Transfusion of various components of the blood is the most frequent transplantation procedure performed in the current practice of medicine. Transfusion is a transplantation process because the majority of the cells transfused, particularly the red cells, are viable, and in the circulation for a finite period of time. The components of the blood that may be transfused include:

1. Cellular elements—erythrocytes (red cells), leucocytes (white cells), and platelets
2. Plasma
3. Fractionated components of plasma

The modern principle of blood transfusion is to give the appropriate blood component the patient has an absence or deficiency of, rather than transfuse blood directly from a suitable donor. Using this approach of component therapy, one blood donation may be fractionated into in excess of seven different components, which, in turn, can be used to treat numerous patients, each missing a different blood component.

Historical Perspective on Blood Transfusion Therapy

The transfusion of blood from one person or animal to another was first recorded in the middle of the seventeenth century, but the deaths caused by inappropriate apparatus and blood incompatibility caused it to fall rapidly into disrepute. Blundell, a British surgeon, rekindled enthusiasm by designing apparatus to successfully transfuse women dying of postpartum hemorrhage. Subsequently, the major problem of the donor blood clotting prior to or during transfusion was solved by the successive modifications of defibrinated blood, paraffin-wax-coated apparatus, and the most important discovery, in 1917, of sodium citrate as a nontoxic blood anticoagulant. This final discovery, made possible for the first time the storage of refrigerated blood for elective and emergency transfusion. The advantage of such a system was first demonstrated on a large scale during the Spanish Civil War, thus laying the foundations for modern transfusion practice.

The problems of interdonor incompatibility were largely solved by the discovery of the ABO blood group system by Landsteiner in 1901. Prior to that time transfusions of human blood were complicated by serious reactions which often caused death rather than therapeutic benefit to the patient. Landsteiner demonstrated that each ABO group had an antithetical naturally occurring antibody. Table 1 shows the four ABO blood groups, with their corresponding antibodies and the choice of ABO compatible blood. It can be appreciated that if a group A individual is transfused with group B blood, the recipient's naturally occurring Anti-B will react with the group B donor cells, causing them to hemolyze or be destroyed in the blood stream. This destruction of donor cells will not only negate the benefit of the transfusion, but often causes death of the recipient. Landsteiner's simple but important observation has led to the further demonstration of 16 major blood group systems, with an almost infinite number of subgroups. Thus, although the prospective donor blood has the same ABO type as the recipient (patient), careful cross matching of the two bloods is required prior to transfusion, in order to assure that compatibility exists between all the other blood group systems.

TABLE 1. The ABO Blood System

Red cell group	Plasma antibody	ABO compatible donors
A	Anti-B	A and O
B	Anti-A	B and O
AB	Nil	A, B, and O
O	Anti-A	O only
	Anti-B	

Blood Donation

Modern transfusion practice encourages two methods of blood donation:

Whole Blood Donation. Approximately 420 ml of blood can be removed from a normal healthy adult at two- to three-month intervals without adverse donor reaction. Suitable anticoagulants allow storage of the blood at 4°C for up to 28 days prior to transfusion. At the expiry date the red cells have to be discarded because of their lack of viability in the recipient's circulation. However, the plasma can be either used as whole plasma or broken down into a variety of fractions, all with approximately five years of storage life.

Plasmapheresis. If plasma, leucocytes, or platelets are required, the donor can donate up to 500 ml of plasma, along with these cells, at weekly intervals, provided there is no red cell loss. These three components are quickly produced by the body, as opposed to the red cell mass, which takes one month or more to replace. The platelets and leucocytes require immediate transfusion, but the plasma can be used either as whole plasma or as fractions. The great advantage of this plasma is that it is collected and fractionated or stored in a fresh state, thus allowing for preservation of clotting factors, which, in stored plasma, have deteriorated to a large extent. As will be seen, this is used to great advantage in the treatment of hemophilia, and other disorders of blood coagulation.

Transfusion of Blood

Early techniques had encouraged the direct donation of blood from donor to recipient to avoid clotting. Although this had the added advantage of giving absolutely fresh blood to the patient, it required having a suitable donor available, and this is extremely difficult because of the complexities of providing group-compatible blood.

The vast majority of blood is now collected using either whole blood or plasma collected into plastic bags. Thus, an array of suitable groups of blood is always on hand in the blood bank ready for an emergency—the situation for which blood is most often used. Transfusion is accomplished by attaching a plastic administration set, which has a visible drip chamber for adjusting the rate of transfusion, a filter to remove small blood clots or cell aggregates, and a coupler enabling it to be attached to a needle or catheter placed within the vein of the recipient. Five hundred milliliters of blood is routinely given over a period of 4 hours, but in an emergency situation, it can be transfused in under 10 minutes, using suitable pressure infusors.

Occasionally it may be necessary to replace the patient's total blood volume with donor blood. This replacement, rather than a simple addition, is used to remove all the patient's red cells or a noxious substance in the circulating plasma. An example of the need for such a procedure would be in the "rhesus baby," where the infant's cells are being destroyed by a substance in its plasma. In such circumstances, exchange transfusion not only corrects the anemia, but can prevent brain damage, which often accompanies the untreated condition.

Risk Factors in Blood Transfusions

Blood incompatibility has already been described as a potential cause of death to the recipient. Other reactions can occur which must be considered when assessing the overall risk of transfusing an individual. Such risks include:

Transfer of Infectious Agents. Viral hepatitis is a serious complication. Fortunately testing for contamination of donor blood with these viruses is rapidly advancing, and is approaching the sophistication of syphilis testing, which is mandatory in blood transfusion. Malaria, cytomegalovirus, and many different forms of bacteria can all be transmitted by donor blood, and in the absence of suitable screening testing, careful donor selection is necessary.

Transfusion Reactions. If careful blood transfusion practice is used, the fatal hemolytic reaction can be largely avoided. Thus the majority of such reactions are usually allergic or febrile (fever-producing) reactions that, although common, rarely cause more than transitory discomfort for the patient. Rarely, delayed reactions occur in which the donor blood is gradually destroyed. Routine assessment of the patient's post-transfusion blood level will alert the physician and patient to this complication.

Cardiovascular Reactions. Increasing the blood volume of healthy individuals can usually be done without complication. However, if patients with weakened hearts and/or lungs are transfused, the change in volume can cause serious complications, which often result in the lungs becoming overloaded with fluid, or the heart failing because of the increased work load placed on it. Careful monitoring of the patient and the use of blood concentrates as in the therapy of hemophilia avoids such complications.

Clinical Use of Blood Transfusions

Reference to Table 2 shows there are seven main blood components, each of which has a specific transfusion function. Thus, not only may one blood donation provide essential therapy for seven individuals with different blood defects, but, more appropriately, each individual receives only the fraction he requires, thus avoiding reactions from the other unwanted components in the event whole blood was transfused. Red cells can only be stored for 28 days, leucocytes and platelet viability is counted in hours rather than days, whereas the plasma fractions can be stored indefinitely if freeze-dried. Thus, component therapy

TABLE 2. Blood Components Obtained from a Whole Blood Donation

---

Cellular components
Packed red cells
Leucocyte concentrate
Platelet concentrate

Plasma components
*Fresh whole plasma
Albumen
Gamma-globulin
Clotting factor concentrates

---

*Starting material for the production of all the other plasma components.

represents an ultimate in utility and conservation of a vital life-sustaining material, which cannot be artificially manufactured.

Packed Red Cells. This fraction is used for individuals with a deficiency of red cells due to anemia (lack of production) rather than blood loss. The former patients require just red cells, while the latter group require both red cells and other components (e.g. whole blood).

White Cells (Leucocyte) Concentrates. This fraction contains many of the cells required by the body to fight infections and be involved in inflammatory reactions. Patients with a white cell deficiency often contract life-threatening infections which require such transfusions along with appropriate antibiotic therapy.

Platelet Concentrates. These cell participate in the process of blood coagulation, and thus the prevention of hemorrhage from the blood vessels. A wide variety of conditions will cause a platelet deficiency and bleeding from many different sites of the body. A platelet transfusion will provide a dramatic cessation of bleeding in such situations, and is analagous to the use of clotting factors in hemophilia.

Plasma. This is the liquid carrier for the above cellular components of the blood. It contains a wide variety of materials, many of which can be further concentrated as demonstrated with the use of plasma fractions. Whole plasma is mainly used for the restoration of volume in patients who have lost large amounts of fluid (plasma), rather than the cellular portions of the blood. If it is not replaced, the blood becomes increasingly viscid, the cardiovascular system has a great deal of difficulty circulating it through the body organs, and the patient's blood pressure falls. In a fresh state, plasma is often used to provide coagulation factors for conditions other than hemophilia.

Albumen. This is the major protein of blood (approximately 5g/dl) and is of major importance in maintaining both essential nutrition and balanced fluid mechanics in the body. It is often used in shock to maintain blood pressure.

Gamma-globulin. This is the protein fraction of blood containing antibodies that protect the individual from infectious diseases. People deficient in this fraction often succumb, either early in life because of a congenital absence, or as the result of an acquired deficiency. Replacement of the missing gamma-globulin confers temporary protection. Furthermore, it can be used for prophylaxis by administering it to an individual who has been exposed for the first time to an infectious agent for which he has no immunity (e.g., has not formed antibodies to the agent).

Coagulation Factor Concentrates. The following section relates the use of these components to hemophilia. However, there are other coagulation factor deficiencies, rarer than hemophilia, which can be treated with specific concentrates. An example would be afibrinogenemia, a deficiency of fibrinogen which causes continued precipitous bleeding in deficient individuals. Fibrinogen, a major clotting factor, is fractionated and can be given in the same manner as the hemophilia concentrates, thus allowing individuals to live a relatively normal existence. Fibrinogen concentrate was also used up to comparatively recent times for the treatment of obstetrical bleeding, but because of the high incidence of hepatitis in such fractions, its use has now been reserved for individuals with congenital deficiencies.

HEMOPHILIA–MAINTENANCE OF LIFE BY BLOOD TRANSFUSIONS

Definition of Hemophilia

Hemophilia is a hereditary deficiency of a blood clotting factor which can be replaced by the transfusion of the appropriate clotting factor from a human blood donation. This broad definition of hemophilia is currently used by the majority of national voluntary societies representing hemophiliacs throughout the world.[1] Hemophilia is a relatively rare condition, the most common type being classical hemophilia, with an incidence of approximately 1.4 individuals per 10,000 live male births. The three major forms of hemophilia are:

1. Factor 8 deficiency–classical hemophilia or AHF deficiency
2. Factor 9 deficiency–Christmas disease or PTC deficiency
3. VonWillebrand's disease–Vascular or Pseudo-hemophila

All three conditions are characterized as follows:

1. There is a well defined hereditary transmission of the defect, which in the first two is sex-linked in that only the males usually exhibit clinical signs of the defect.
2. The defect is temporarily corrected by the transfusion of the appropriate blood clotting factor into the individual.
3. Spontaneous hemorrhage not related to trauma can occur into any part or organ of the body, with the greatest danger being seen in occult bleeding, that is, bleeding that cannot be seen and occurs into the body spaces (e.g., joints, abdomen, cranium, etc.).
4. Precipitous bleeding occurs if trauma or surgery is performed on the affected individual.
5. If the hemophiliac is not treated with blood products, there is a marked decrease in both quality of life and life span.

Evolution of Hemophilia Treatment

Hemophilia was first officially recorded in 1000 B.C., and because of its frightening and curious bleeding symptoms, it has been referred to in a wide variety of literature since that time.[2] Even though the condition was a scientific enigma until recent times, the early observers were quick to appreciate its hereditary pattern. Most of the affected males died very early in life, as the result of either usually innocuous procedures or trauma (e.g., circumcision), events that were accompanied by unexpected or uncontrollable hemorrhage. If they did survive to adulthood, progressive joint hemorrhages caused crippling and reduced them to being bedridden. A wide variety of treatments were evolved on an empiric basis, and included extracts of spider webs, snake venom and milk, injection of calcium, horseblood, and vaccines; and finally a wide variety of appliances were designed to protect the hemophiliac from incurring hemorrhages. All of these proved singularly ineffective in either preventing or treating hemophiliac bleeding, and indeed, in many instances, caused exacerbation of fresh bleeding.

Nevertheless, as knowledge of the blood coagulation mechanism improved, it became obvious that the blood of hemophiliacs lacked a clotting factor which was present in nonbleeding (i.e., normal) individuals. Furthermore, transfusion of whole blood or plasma was able to staunch the hemorrhage. Unfortunately, this fact was not immediately exploited because the effect of the transfusion was only temporary, owing to the small amount of clotting factor that could be transfused in this manner. If excessive whole blood transfusions were given, the hemophiliac's heart and lungs failed because of the excessive amounts of red cells transferred into his blood system. These obstacles were enhanced because the hemophiliac more often bleeds internally rather than externally, making it difficult to assess the effectiveness of such transfusions.

The major advance came when a specific clotting factor was found to be missing in a hemophiliac, and this factor was appropriately called antihemophiliac globulin or factor (AHF). A specific blood fraction was isolated from fresh plasma that allowed for the concentration of the fraction from 10 to 20 pints of blood into a volume of 30 to 40 ml. Thus, an individual who had no AHF, by receiving such an injection intravenously, had his level of AHF restored to normal, thus either preventing further hemorrhage or treating existing hemorrhage. Unfortunately, this satisfactory and comforting state of affairs did not last long.

It soon became apparent that hemophiliacs with the same bleeding problems and inheritance pattern as AHF-deficient individuals did not respond to AHF concentrates. In 1950 this therapeutic impasse was found to be a deficiency of another blood clotting factor, then called Christmas factor. The choice of name did not relate to the season in which the discovery took place, but was the name of the patient, Stephen Christmas, a young Canadian hemophiliac living in

Stratford, Ontario. The presence of this second form of hemophilia was quickly compounded by the demonstration that VonWillebrand's disease (VWD), which had been described in the early twentieth century as pseudo-hemophilia, was indeed closely related to AHF-deficient or classical hemophilia. Originally it had been thought to be a defect of the blood vessels, which, coupled with a different inheritance pattern to the other two forms of hemophilia, thus constituted a completely distinct entity. However, when a deficiency of AHF was also found in VWD, it became apparent that the two conditions did have a similar molecular defect, which current research is exploiting. Thus, what was thought originally to be a single condition, was found to have three major forms, each of which required specific blood factor therapy and which have now been found to have further significant subgroups.

The complexity of the biological defect in hemophilia was further complicated by the need for therapy using specific and separate blood plasma fractions in adequate quantity. Although the administration of normal fresh plasma replaced each of the missing blood clotting factors, for reasons previously stated, the level of clotting factor required in the hemophiliac's circulation to stop or prevent bleeding could not be attained using such a product. Furthermore, owing to the relatively short survival of the transfused clotting factors (varies from 4 hours for the VWD factor to 18 hours for Christmas factor), repeated infusions were necessary to maintain the level of transfused factor and prevent recurrence of the hemorrhage. The demands being made on the blood donor to provide the raw material and the apparatus necessary to produce the fractions, now constitute a formidable obstacle to successful therapy of the hemophiliac. Nevertheless, in those countries where it is possible to sustain the manufacture or use of such products, the life style and life span of the hemophiliac have been radically altered.

Fractionation of plasma is a demanding task that requires a large eligible blood donor pool, a high level of technological sophistication, a large financial investment in manufacturing plant, and careful quality control of the finished product. Since it is a relatively new science, the expertise and experience is not easily come by, while there are relatively few voluntary or commercial organizations that can sustain the donor demand and capital investment. Fortunately for the majority of hemophiliacs (AHF and VWD deficiencies), a relatively simple process was discovered by Pool and Shannon in 1964[3] that enabled the production of Factor 8 or AHF concentrate using conventional apparatus and existing technology. Fresh plasma is snap-frozen at -70°C, and upon subsequent controlled thawing, the AHF precipitates to the bottom of the bag, allowing for relatively easy removal from the supernatant AHF-depleted plasma. Thus any conventional blood transfusion service can provide a therapeutically useful concentrate for the treatment of the day-to-day emergencies facing severely affected hemophiliacs. Since this fortuitous discovery, not only have AHF- and VWD-deficient hemophiliacs greatly benefited, but this progress has been reinforced by the development of more sophisticated cryoprecipitated freeze-dried concentrates and methods of administration.

Blood Clotting Concentrates Currently Available to the Hemophiliac

It is accepted that whole blood is inappropriate and unsatisfactory for the treatment of hemophilia unless red cells are also being lost as the result of hemorrhage. Fresh frozen plasma is used in special circumstances for mildly affected individuals and children. For the severely affected hemophiliac (level of factor is zero or less than 1% of normal), the following concentrates represent their current lifeline to maintain health, body function, and normal life span, provided that suitable diagnostic and treatment facilities exist.

AHF Deficiency (Factor 8 or Classical Hemophilia). Frozen Concentrates (Cryoprecipitate). The Pool and Shannon cryo- or cold-precipitated material concentates approximately 250 units of AHF found in a pint (420 ml) of fresh blood into 25 ml containing 80 to 120 units of AHF. This represents a recovery efficiency of 50 to 65% in a concentrate of approximately ten times concentrating efficiency. The advantages of relatively simple production and small volume are offset by the need to constantly freeze the concentrate at -30°C or lower, variability of the factor concentration from one donor to the next, the need to pool up to 20 bags of cryoprecipitate to obtain sufficient material for a simple transfusion, and finally the difficulty in transporting the material unless it is stored in dry ice. Nevertheless, it is a prime source of material for many hemophiliacs, and is often the starting material for more complex and sophisticated dried concentrates.

Dried Concentrates. This process increased the efficiency of concentration by another factor of ten as compared to the cryoprecipitate, but reduces the efficiency of extraction of AHF from whole plasma to approximately 30 to 40%. Therefore, the volume of 250 ml of cryoprecipitate can be reduced to approximately 20 to 30 ml using this type of concentrate, with the obvious advantages of increased speed of infusion and greater increase in circulating level of AHF in the hemophiliac. The freeze-drying process enables easy transportation (no freezer required); rapid reconstitution by dissolving in small amounts of sterile water; and knowledge of the exact amount of AHF in each vial, as opposed to the approximate amount assumed in each cryoprecipitated unit. Its main disadvantage is a reflection of the current axiom that the more concentrated the final form of clotting concentrate, the less efficiency there is in extracting all the available AHF from the starting plasma. This is an important logistical and technological consideration because of the limit to the global supply of fresh frozen plasma. To the seriously affected hemophiliac it represents an ultimate in therapy at this time, and the benefit to human life always tends justifiably to overwhelm technocratic and logistical arguments. Nevertheless, it represents a source of great concern to those voluntary and commercial organizations responsible for obtaining the ever increasing supplies of fresh frozen plasma required for this process.

Christmas Deficiency (Factor 9 or PTC). The great advantage for individuals with this form of hemophilia is that the concentrates can be made from discarded stored plasma (obtained from whole blood from which the red cells have been removed because of lack of viability) or indeed fresh plasma from which AHF has been first removed. This dual source of supply combined with the fact that only 10 to 15% of hemophiliacs have this deficiency, means that their supply of concentrate is relatively abundant as compared to the problems for the AHF- or VWD-deficient hemophiliacs. The freeze-dried Christmas factor concentrates have the same advantages as the AHF concentrates, although there are probably more side reactions associated with them, particularly an increased incidence of viral hepatitis and thrombosis.

VWD Deficiency. Curiously, although there is a deficiency of AHF in this form of hemophilia, AHF dried concentrates currently do not uniformly give satisfactory therapeutic results in such individuals. It is now evident that in this form of hemophilia another factor is also missing, namely the VWD factor, as well as the AHF factor. During the manufacture of the refined freeze-dried AHF concentrate, the VWD factor probably becomes either denatured or discarded. Therefore, cryoprecipitated frozen AHF and fresh plasma are the mainstays of therapy. Fortunately, severely affected VWD-deficient hemophiliacs are even rarer than Christmas deficiencies, so that they place no great demands on material, which is already in relatively short supply for AHF-deficient hemophiliacs.

Principles and Practice of Replacement
Therapy in Hemophilia

Principles. The treatment of bleeding in hemophilia is necessary. If it is left untreated, deaths or crippling results. The main principle of therapy must be either prompt recognition and immediate transfusion, or the prevention of bleeding using prophylactic or maintenance infusions of the appropriate clotting factor.

The waiting for onset of bleeding symptoms requires an unusually close and trusting relationship between the physician and the hemophiliac. Encouragement of the hemophiliac to recognize early bleeding can only be done if he can expect prompt medical and transfusion therapy. If the initial symptoms of pain, tenderness, or slight loss of function are disregarded, the more serious and easily recognized complications naturally follow. This changes a minor hemorrhage requiring a single transfusion into a major catastrophe requiring multiple transfusions, prolonged hospitalization, and chronic disability. A common example is in the progression of joint hemorrhages. Initially, the hemophiliac experiences a vague discomfort in the joint—if left untreated the affected joint can be transformed within three to four hours into a swollen, excruciatingly painful, immobile joint, incapable of weight support or function. Recovery from such a hemarthroses (blood into the joint cavity) is prolonged, with loss of muscle mass and function and deterioration of the joint surfaces. This, along with prolonged pain, immobility, and helplessness, can have a profound effect on a young man who is completely normal except for a deficiency of one clotting factor. The need to recognize and treat early has changed the usual dominant attitude of physician over patient who has little or no knowledge of his illness, to the cooperation of physician and patient through a mutual process of education, experience, and need to avoid complications in this lifelong disorder.[4]

Prophylaxis implies the prevention of hemorrhage rather than allowing a spontaneous hemorrhage to begin and then start emergency treatment. It embodies the principle used in most chronic disorders (e.g., diabetes, heart disease, etc.), where medication is given on a regular schedule to avoid complications of the disorder. Such a principle appears well suited for the therapy of hemophiliacs because hemorrhages, even if quickly treated, contribute to a steady deterioration of body function and life span. Unfortunately, the effect of chronic (continuous) infusion of clotting concentrates into the bloodstream is still unknown. It is evident that hemophiliacs who receive regular infusions of clotting concentrate can have disorders of the liver, spleen, and kidneys, with increased blood pressure, jaundice, formation of inhibitors, and other complications. Whether these complications are directly the result of the transfusions has yet to be fully determined. Nevertheless, it is also well known that lifesaving drugs can, in themselves, cause death-dealing reactions (e.g., penicillin causing anaphylactic shock). This, compounded by the relatively precarious supply of AHF, has not popularized this method of therapy. It is estimated that the average severely affected adult hemophiliac would require the equivalent of 800 whole blood donors or 400 plasmapheresis donations to satisfy a minimal annual prophylactic program. This is not beyond the realm of possibility, but would certainly demand absolute efficiency from world transfusion services. Recognition of the efficacy of prophylaxis is seen in young hemophiliacs who are given a transfusion before participating in energetic (not body contact) sports, or if they are experiencing a bleeding crisis (repetitive spontaneous bleeding for no apparent reason).

Practice.   Up to comparatively recent times the hemophiliac spent a considerable portion of his life attending hospitals in order to receive therapy for emergent hemorrhages, either as an in- or an outpatient. This involved lengthy journeys during inclement weather, at all hours of the day and night, with the hemophiliac exposed to constant anxiety and pain. The effect on relatives and friends would often be traumatic, with a breakdown in family relationships and retardation of normal social development in the young hemophiliac. The hemophiliac was at the mercy of the hospital emergency department, which was attuned to dramatic emergencies rather than the transfusion of an individual without obvious symptoms. Needless to say, any delay in therapy could then transform the hemorrhage into a life-threatening situation. The anxiety that such a system precipitated in a hemophiliac is well documented.[5] It caused members of the medical team to reevaluate therapy for such individuals in the hope of finding a more flexible system.

The analogy of hemophilia to diabetes has already been made. The two conditions share many similarities; each is a lifelong condition, with no apparent cure available, and requires repeated injections of material to replace a missing or defective substance. If the condition is left untreated, life-threatening complications occur with shortening of life span. Diabetics had already shown that, with proper preparation, education, and availability of appropriate therapeutic materials, they could care for themselves within their home and social environment, provided their progress was supervised. Home or self infusion, which has now become an accepted method of care for such individuals, has been translated to the hemophiliac.

Self or Home Infusion.   Injection of material intravenously has usually been associated with illicit drug use. Therefore, the idea of a normal-looking individual doing this posed a very real psychological barrier to the hemophiliac and his family. This, coupled with the almost automatic reflex to attend the hospital in time of need, prevented such an idea from gaining prompt acceptance. Nevertheless, the 1960s saw a combination of enlightened physicians and compliant hemophiliacs embark on individual programs. In the last five years, the procedure has gained widespread approval, now that it has a demonstrated cost benefit and social and medical acceptance.

Current programs emphasize careful screening of severely affected hemophiliacs who are emotionally and educationally capable of assimilating the large amount of knowledge required to perform the procedure successfully. This is not quite as difficult as it sounds, in that many of these individuals routinely receive up to one hundred transfusions a year, and they quickly learn all the intricacies of the procedure by a process of painful repetition.

A bleeding episode in a hemophiliac on a self-infusion program would typically evolve as follows. As soon as it became evident that hemorrhage was oc-

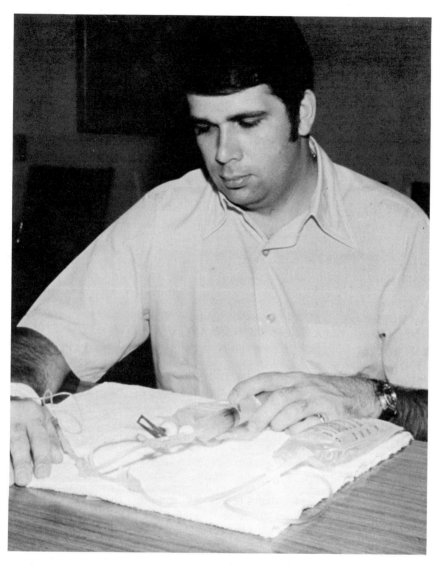

FIG. 1. Currently this represents the ultimate in hemophilia therapy. The hemophiliac is administering his own transfusion within the home environment, using a blood concentrate that is freeze-dried, thus allowing him complete independence and mobility from the hospital.

curring, the hemophiliac would immediately prepare the factor concentrate in an injectable form. Cryoprecipitate would take longer to prepare than dried concentrate, and would probably limit where the procedure could be performed. Dried concentrate means the hemophiliac can inject at home, school, or work, or during a wilderness trip, provided a reliable helper or friend is available. The venepuncture is performed using exactly the same equipment and technique a physician would use. This, again, is simpler than it sounds; the illicit drug user can perform the same maneuver under far more adverse conditions and using the crudest of apparatus. The hemophiliac usually has the best knowledge of where the most accessible veins are, owing to the many hundreds of venepunctures he has had in his lifetime. Injection of the material is performed using either a syringe (see Figure 1) or gravity-fed apparatus, and takes only 20 to 30 minutes if freeze-dried material is used. The hemophiliac can return to his previous activity with little interruption or disability. A number of very real or potential complications can occur, but if the hemophiliac has been carefully trained and has a procedure manual and instant communication with a medical team, it is a medically safe procedure. The author is not aware of a fatal accident occurring during self infusion if the above precautions have been observed.

THE FUTURE TREATMENT OF HEMOPHILIA

Cryoprecipitate has been compared to a thick biological soup, while the freeze-dried concentrates are considered the biological consommé or bouillon soups. Certainly, each clotting concentrate contains substances not required by the hemophiliac to correct his coagulation defect, and which could be responsible for some of the complications of existing therapy. Four alternative approaches appear feasible at this time, which could modify therapy as we currently use it.

Improved Concentrates

Advances in cellulose gel, column technology, and other fractionation methods are producing more refined fractions. However, they still have to be proved therapeutically effective, and have an effective recovery ratio. Animal sources of clotting factors such as bovine and porcine plasma can produce therapeutically effective material, but interspecies allergic reactions prevent their being used on a repetitive schedule in the same hemophiliac. Modification of this animal plasma will, it is hoped, remove the proteins causing such reactions but preserve the clotting activity. Another interesting development is the use of concentrates containing activated clotting factors that bypass those portions of the clotting mechanism where AHF and Christmas factor operate. These experimental concentrates are currently being used in hemophiliacs who have developed antibodies to transfused human AHF, and have enabled such hemophiliacs to have successful surgical procedures, even though their AHF has remained zero both during and after surgery.

Chemical Triggers

AHF and Christmas factor deficient individuals have defective rather than a total absence of biological clotting molecules. Using in vitro and in vivo techniques, the AHF level of mild rather than severe hemophiliacs has been boosted using various amino acid substances. DDAVP, an artificially synthesized posterior pituitary hormone, has such an ability, and again has enabled surgery to be performed in the absence of AHF concentrate infusion.

Prolongation of Concentrate Effectiveness

All the clotting factors have relatively short biological half lives. Extending the effective half life decreases the frequency of infusions, conserves already precious human clotting concentrate, and reduces the possibility of reactions or side effects to the hemophiliac. Such a principle has been successfully accomplished in rabbits by blocking or interrupting the efficiency of their reticuloendothelial system, thus decreasing the catabolism of the transfused factors. It has yet to be attempted in the human.

Tissue Transplants

Various body organs are known to synthesize AHF. A decade ago the spleen was considered the major organ of synthesis. Hemophiliac dogs had normal spleen transplants to provide AHF. Unfortunately, such transplants did not succeed over a sustained time period, and the procedure fell into disrepute. Recently vascular endothelium has been shown to synthesize AHF, and consideration is now being given to either producing exogenous AHF via tissue culture of endothelial cells, or transplanting such tissue into a suitable body cavity in a hemophiliac.

CONCLUSION

Regardless of what approach is finally successful, current therapy for the hemophiliac demonstrates the effectiveness of blood component therapy, and in particular the blood clotting concentrates. It enables normal-looking people (hemophiliacs) to retain normal function and lead relatively normal lives. It provides the hemophiliac the opportunity to be a self-sustaining member of the community. Above all it demonstrates that the gift of life from a blood donor is a palpable truth when one is a hemophiliac.

References

Inwood, M. J. Blood coagulation and hemophilia. In *Canadian Hemophilia Handbook*. Hamilton: Canadian Hemophilia Society, 1976.

Ingram, G. I. C. The history of haemophilia. *J. Clin. Pathol. 29*: 3–13, 1976.

Pool, J. G., and Shannon, A. E. Production of high potency concentrates of anti-hemophilic globulin in a closed bag system. *N. Engl. J. Med. 273*: 1443–1446, 1965.

Inwood, M. J. Hemophilia—Why concern yourself? *U. W. O. Med. J. 47*: 3–4, 1976.

Massie, Robert, and Massie, Suzanne. *Journey*. New York: Alfred E. Knopf Inc., 1975.

Total Parenteral Nutrition: Techniques and Indications

JOHN M. DALY, M.D.
Assistant Professor of Surgery
Departments of Surgery
The University of Texas Medical School
at Houston
The University of Texas System Cancer Center
M. D. Anderson Hospital and Tumor Institute

STANLEY J. DUDRICK, M.D.
Professor and Chairman
Department of Surgery
The University of Texas Medical School
at Houston

EDWARD M. COPELAND III, M.D.
Professor of Surgery
The University of Texas Medical School
at Houston and
The University of Texas System Cancer Center
M. D. Anderson Hospital and Tumor Institute

Total parenteral nutrition (TPN) may be defined as the provision of adequate essential nutrients via the intravascular route to maintain metabolic homeostasis and anabolism. The concept of TPN was made practical in 1968 by Dudrick and

Rhoads, who demonstrated clinically and experimentally that intravenous administration of hypertonic dextrose, amino acids, minerals, and vitamins promoted normal growth and development in infants and puppies and maintained positive nitrogen balance in malnourished, hospitalized adults. Since that time, numerous laboratory experiments and clinical studies have documented the beneficial effects of TPN in a wide variety of diseases that produce a severe catabolic response. Now, with the availability of total parenteral nutrition, the nutritional needs of patients should no longer be neglected in the clinical practice of medicine.

The hypertonic nutrient solution most commonly used for total parenteral feeding consists of approximately 20 to 25% dextrose, 4 to 5% crystalline amino acids or protein hydrolysates, 1 to 3% minerals and the fat- and water-soluble vitamins (Table 1). Each unit of base solution provides approximately 5.25 to 6.0 g of nitrogen and 900 to 1000 calories in 1100 ml of water. Such solutions can be prepared in bulk by a manufacturing pharmacist from commercially available stock products or as individual units by a physician, pharmacist, nurse, or technician using TPN kits. Regardless of who makes the solution, meticulous aseptic mixing under a laminar air flow hood is the vital first line of defense against bacterial contamination. Suitable quantities of electrolytes and vitamins must be added to the base solution, and the usual additions to each unit of base solution are listed in Table 1. While it is possible to illustrate a "standard" IVH solution, the specific water, electrolyte, calorie, and nitrogen requirements of each patient must be individualized so that avoidable metabolic derangements do not occur during the course of therapy.[2]

In formulating a TPN mixture for the average adult patient who has no significant cardiovascular, hepatic, or renal dysfunction or metabolic abnormality, 40 to 50 mEq of sodium (as the chloride, acetate, bicarbonate, or lactate salt) and 30 to 40 mEq of potassium (as the chloride, acetate, bicarbonate, or acid phosphate salt) are usually added to each liter or unit of base solution. Potassium, phosphorus, and magnesium administration are often reduced or omitted in patients with compromised renal function. Some crystalline amino acid solutions are commercially available as the chloride or hydrochloride salt, and a significant risk of hyperchloremic metabolic acidosis exists if sodium and potassium requirements are satisfied solely by the addition of the chloride salt to these solutions. Other crystalline amino acid solutions contain most or all of the amino acids as acetate salts, and the addition of sodium and potassium as the chloride salt is necessary to prevent hypochloremia. There are now several different amino acid preparations commercially available with varying electrolyte content, and the physician must be familiar with the exact composition of these mixtures before adding the electrolytes necessary for patient homeostasis. The exact nutritional and electrolyte requirements of each individual patient must be thoroughly appreciated if iatrogenic metabolic complications are to be prevented.

TABLE 1. Composition of Standard Hyperalimentation Solutions for Adults

	Stock solution method: 350 ml 50% dextrose plus 750 ml 5% protein hydrolysate in 5% dextrose	Kit method: 500 ml 8.5% crystalline amino acids plus 500 ml 50% dextrose
Volume	1100 ml	1000 ml
Calories	1000 kcal	1000 kcal
Dextrose	212 g	250 g
Hydrolysates	37 g	
Amino acids		42.5 g
Nitrogen	5.25 g	6.25 g

Additions to each unit of base solution (average adult):
Sodium (chloride and/or acetate, lactate, bicarbonate)		40–50 mEq
Potassium (acetate, lactate, chloride, acid phosphate)		30–40 mEq
Magnesium (sulfate)		8–15 mEq
Phosphate (potassium acid salt)		12–18 mEq

Additions to only one unit daily:
Vitamin A	5000–10,000	U.S.P. units
Vitamin D	500–1,000	U.S.P. units
Vitamin E	2.5–5.0	I.U.
Vitamin C	250–500	mg
Thiamine	25–50	mg
Riboflavin	5–10	mg
Pyridoxine	7.5–15	mg
Niacin	50–100	mg
Pantothenic acid	12.5–25	mg
Calcium (gluconate)	4.8–9.6	mEq

Optional additions to daily nutrient regimen:
Vitamin K	0.5–1.0	mg	
Vitamin B_{12}	10–30	μg	
Folic acid	0.5–1.0	mg	Alternatively may be given
Iron	2.0–3.0	mg	IM in appropriate daily or
Zinc	1.0–2.0	mg	weekly dosages

Total parenteral nutrition, in contrast to isotonic dextrose therapy, can result in significant hypophosphatemia when solutions deficient in phosphate are used. Symptomatic hypophosphatemia is identified by malaise, lethargy, peripheral and perioral paresthesias, tremors, and dysarthria, which may progress to mental obtundity, respiratory disorders, coma, and death. Phosphorus is an intracellular anion essential in promoting protein synthesis. Hypophosphatemia does not occur as a result of increased urinary losses of phosphorus, but develops secondary to "trapping" of the phosphorus in newly synthesized protein. Under ordinary circumstances, phosphorus should be added to each unit of base solution as potassium or sodium acid phosphate in doses of 15 to 30 mEq per liter, but in severely malnourished patients 30 to 50 mEq per liter may be necessary.

Magnesium and calcium also participate in the anabolic process along with nitrogen, phosphorus, and potassium. The deletion of any one of these elements will inhibit the establishment of anabolism. In adults, 4 to 5 mEq of calcium (as the gluconate or gluconate-heptonate salt) are added to *one* unit of nutrient solution per day. Calcium should always be added to parenteral feeding regimens of infants and children to provide 3 to 4 mEq/kg body weight/day (Table 2). In the average adult, approximately 24 mEq of magnesium (magnesium sulfate) is required per day. The severely malnourished patient treated with TPN has the greatest risk of developing disease states secondary to deficiencies of the aforementioned elements. Total body deficits in these elements may not be identified in the serum profile until TPN has begun. Hypophosphatemia may exist, for example, and the serum calcium may be normal. If the concentration of phosphorus infused is increased without increasing the infusion of calcium, severe hypocalcemia may result. Calcium and phosphorus exist in the serum as if controlled by a constant solubility coefficient; if the infused concentration of one element is increased, consideration should be given to increasing the other.

One ampoule of a mixture containing fat-soluble and water-soluble vitamins suitable for parenteral administration (MVI)* is added to only one unit of the nutrient solution daily. Because each ampoule contains the vitamins in adequate therapeutic dosages, it is not necessary or advisable to administer more than one ampoule per day. Vitamin B_{12}, vitamin K, and folic acid should be given in appropriate doses separately, since these compounds are currently unavailable in parenteral vitamin preparations. These vitamins can either be added to any one bottle of solution daily, or alternatively may be given intramuscularly in cal-

TABLE 2. Composition of Pediatric Total Parenteral Nutrient Solutions

	Daily intake
Nitrogen source	2.5 g/kg
Dextrose	25–30 g/kg
Sodium chloride	3–4 mEq/kg
Potassium acid phosphate	2–3 mEq/kg
Calcium gluconate 10%	0.5 mEq/kg
Magnesium sulfate 50%	0.25 mEq/kg
Multiple vitamin injection*	1 ml
Vitamin B_{12}	50 µg
Vitamin K	250–500 µg
Folic acid	50–75 µg

*MVI (USV Corporation, Tuckahoe, N.Y.).

*Multivitamin injection (USV Corporation, Tuckahoe, N.Y.).

culated weekly doses. Trace elements, such as cobalt, copper, iodine, manganese, and zinc, are present as contaminants in most parenteral solutions and are not added routinely to the nutritional regimen. Trace elements may be required in newborn infants, severely debilitated adult patients, and patients with inflammatory bowel diseases or short-gut syndrome on long-term "home" total parenteral nutrition.

Clinical management guidelines for *safe* total parenteral nutrition include accurate measurements of the patient's temperature, pulse and respiratory rate, and blood pressure at least every 4 hours, fractional urine sugar and acetone concentrations at least every 6 hours, fluid balance at least every 8 hours, and daily body weight. Serum electrolyte concentrations, blood urea nitrogen, and blood glucose levels should be determined at least daily until stable, and every 2 or 3 days thereafter. Serum calcium, phosphorus, magnesium, albumin, bilirubin, SGOT, and alkaline phosphatase should be measured weekly. To avoid osmotic diuresis, the nutrient solution is maintained at a rate that will not allow the quantitative urinary glucose to exceed 2 g/100 ml (greater than 3+ nitroprusside reaction) or the blood glucose to exceed 200 mg%. In patients with diabetes mellitus or persistent excessive glycosuria, crystalline insulin is added to the intravenous infusion in dosages of 5 to 60 units/1000 calories to achieve the desired effect on the blood sugar concentration. Frequent, accurate measurements of blood and urine glucose must be obtained, since insulin requirements can vary abruptly as the patient's condition changes. In the occasional patient with hyperglycemia despite exogenous insulin (usually due to hypercatabolism secondary to sepsis), a decrease in the infusion rate of the solution for several days will allow control of blood glucose levels while attempts to treat the source of the severe hypercatabolism are made (drainage of abscesses, etc.).

TECHNIQUE

Total parenteral nutritional solutions are hyperosmolar (1800–2400 mOsm) and must be delivered to the circulatory system through a large-diameter, high-flow blood vessel, preferably the superior vena cava. The hypertonic nutrient solutions can be infused through an indwelling polyvinyl, silastic, or Teflon catheter directed into the superior vena cava via the percutaneous catheterization of the subclavian vein or the internal or external jugular veins. The subclavian vein is preferred because of the ease in maintaining a sterile, occlusive dressing on the anterior chest wall; moreover, TPN infusion through this vessel has been the safest and most effective technique for long-term infusion of total parenteral nutrient solutions in adults and in infants weighing more than 10 pounds. Either subclavian vein may be used safely unless a specific contraindication exists, such as the presence of ipsilateral giant emphysematous bullae, previous radical neck dissection, clavicular fracture, or radiation therapy through a lower neck portal. Successful percutaneous subclavian venous catheterization requires a thorough knowledge of thoracic and cervical anatomy and familiarity with established techniques. Before the procedure, accurate assessment of the patient's apprehensions and competent reassurance are very important. The patient is entitled to a careful, clear explanation of the steps in the procedure and their rationale. The equipment for a central venous catheterization should be readily available to reduce delay and enhance efficiency.

Before percutaneous subclavian venous catheterization is attempted, the patient should be placed in the Trendelenburg position. Hydrostatic dilation of the subclavian vein will occur, providing a larger target for the needle and increasing central venous pressure so that the risk of air embolization during the procedure is minimized. A rolled sheet is placed longitudinally under the thoracic spine and between the scapulae. With the patient's shoulders depressed, the subclavian vein becomes more accessible.

The skin over the clavicle, shoulder, neck, and upper chest is shaved widely and cleansed with ether, acetone, or other organic solvent to remove skin oil. The same area is then prepared with povidone-iodine solution and is draped with sterile towels. Local anesthetic (1% lidocaine or procaine) is infiltrated into the skin, subcutaneous tissues, and periosteum at the inferior border of the midpoint of the clavicle. Three minutes later, a 2-inch long, 14-gauge needle attached to a 3-ml syringe is inserted through the skin wheal and advanced beneath the inferior margin of the clavicle in a horizontal (coronal) plane. The needle tip is aimed for the anterior margin of the trachea at the level of the suprasternal notch. As the needle is advanced beneath the clavicle, a slight negative pressure applied through the syringe will indicate the accuracy of the venopuncture by a flashback of blood. The bevel of the needle should be down and should be

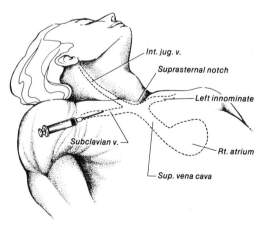

FIG. 1.

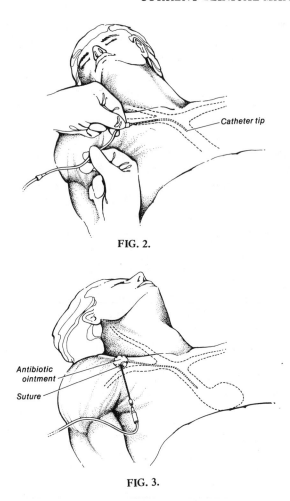

FIG. 2.

FIG. 3.

advanced a few millimeters beyond the point at which blood first appears in the syringe to ensure the placement of the entire bevel tip inside the lumen of the vein. The patient is asked to perform a Valsalva maneuver to minimize the risk of air embolism. The syringe is removed carefully while the needle is still held firmly in place with a hemostat. An 8-inch long, 16-gauge radiopaque catheter is introduced through the needle and threaded its full length into the vein. If any difficulty is encountered during advancement of the catheter through the needle, the needle and catheter must be withdrawn carefully as a unit, and another attempt at venopuncture may be made. The catheter must never be withdrawn through the needle after the tip has passed beyond the end of the needle because transection and embolization of the catheter can result from this maneuver.

When the catheter has been advanced its full length, it is attached to a solution of isotonic saline or glucose by sterile intravenous administration tubing and is flushed immediately with the isotonic fluid to minimize any intralumenal clotting. The needle and catheter are then withdrawn so that at least 3 cm of the catheter is visible, and the catheter is sutured in place just lateral to the skin puncture site. Accurate position within the venous system can be ensured by lowering the solution bottle below the level of the patient and observing a free back-flow of blood into the delivery tubing. A broad spectrum antimicrobial ointment such as povidone-iodine is applied over the puncture site, and an occlusive, sterile gauze dressing is fixed to the skin with tincture of benzoin and adhesive tape. The intravenous administration tubing is looped over the top of the dressing and secured again with adhesive tape to guard against accidental catheter dislodgement.

Conscientious adherence to this technique should ensure successful central venous catheterization. However, if air is aspirated into the syringe during needle advancement, entry of the needle tip into lung parenchyma is suggested, and the needle should be withdrawn. If the needle–syringe connection is airtight and not the source of the air leak, the patient should be observed for signs of respiratory distress, and a portable chest roentgenogram should be obtained immediately. If, during insertion, bright red blood fills the syringe and moves the plunger of the syringe outward, the needle has probably entered the subclavian artery; the procedure should be terminated, and pressure should be applied over the artery for a minimum of 5 minutes.

After the subclavian venous catheter has been properly inserted and secured and before infusion of the hypertonic nutrient solution is begun, a chest roentgenogram must be obtained to verify the position of the catheter tip within the midportion of the superior vena cava.

In infants weighing less than 10 pounds, percutaneous subclavian puncture can be dangerous and difficult. Long-term central venous catheterization in such patients is achieved more safely by inserting the catheter under direct vision via a cut-down over the external or internal jugular vein.

Meticulous care and aseptic maintenance of the catheter and delivery tubing are just as important in preventing bacterial contamination as is proper catheter insertion. Every 2 or 3 days, the dressing over the puncture wound site is removed and the administration tubing is changed. Using aseptic technique and sterile gloves, the nurse or physician cleanses the skin around the catheter exit skin-site with ether or acetone, and reprepares the skin with povidone-iodine. Antimicrobial or antiseptic ointment is again applied around the catheter, and the sterile occlusive dressing is replaced. In order to minimize the risk of catheter-related infection, blood should not be drawn via the catheter, nor should the catheter be used for central venous pressure monitoring, bolus medication injection, or blood constituent administration.

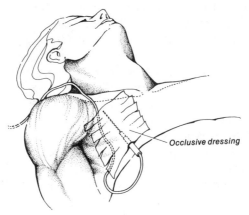

FIG. 4.

INDICATIONS

Ingestion, digestion, and absorption of food may be compromised by a variety of pathologic processes. The option to bypass a malfunctioning gastrointestinal tract and provide nutrients intravenously for as long as necessary allows the physician to "rest" the bowel until normal or maximal bowel function is obtained. The basic clinical indications for the use of total parenteral nutrition are for supportive therapy and primary treatment of patients who *cannot eat, will not eat, should not eat,* or *cannot eat enough.* Patients with specific metabolic needs due to renal, cardiac, and hepatic failure constitute another category in which the application of total parenteral nutrition has proved beneficial.

As shown in Table 3, a variety of pathologic conditions make adequate enteral intake *impossible, inadvisable, improbable,* and/or *hazardous.*[4]

TABLE 3

TOTAL PARENTERAL NUTRITION SHOULD BE USED WHEN GASTROINTESTINAL TRACT FUNCTION IS:

Impossible	Improbable

1. Alimentary-tract obstruction or ileus
    a. Oropharynx–neoplasm
    b. Esophagus–achalasia, neoplasm, stricture
    c. Stomach–benign or malignant ulcer or neoplasm, postoperative atony, gastroschisis
	1. Malnourished geriatric patients
	2. Chronic starvation–marasmus, kwashiorkor
	3. Anorexia nervosa
	4. Hyperemesis gravidarum
	5. Chronic relapsing pancreatitis
	6. Recurrent regional enteritis

TABLE 3 continued

Impossible	Improbable
d. Duodenum—ulcer, neoplasm, veil, atresia, duplication, choledochal cyst, annular pancreas, carcinoma of the head of the pancreas, superior mesenteric artery syndrome	7. Chronic granulomatous or ulcerative colitis
e. Small intestine—atresia, intussusception, neoplasm, polyp, regional enteritis, adhesions, bands, veils, gallstone ileus, foreign body, malrotation	8. Radiation effects
	9. Chemotherapy effects
	10. Short-gut syndrome—after maximal adaptation
	11. Myocardial insufficiency
	12. Chronic respiratory-tract disease
f. Colon—diverticulitis, volvulus, neoplasm, ulcerative colitis, granulomatous colitis	13. Moderate catabolism—burns, trauma, multiple operations

2. Acute hemorrhagic pancreatitis
3. Short-gut syndrome—2 months post-operatively
4. Radiation effects—entire GI tract
5. Chemotherapy effects—entire GI tract
6. Infectious gastroenteritis—cholera, salmonellosis, shigellosis
7. Intraabdominal abscess and/or peritonitis
8. Wound dehiscence
9. Protein-losing gastroenteropathy—sprue, Menetrier's disease
10. Massive catabolism—major burns, multiple trauma
11. Other congenital anomalies—omphalocele, diaphragmatic hernia

Inadvisable	Hazardous
1. Enterocutaneous and enteroenteral fistulas	1. Cerebrovascular accident
2. Renal failure—acute or chronic	2. Mental obtundity
3. Reversible liver failure	3. Reversible coma
4. Partial intestinal obstruction	4. Tetanus
5. Acute pancreatitis	5. Laryngeal incompetence
6. Acute regional enteritis	6. Tracheoesophageal fistula
7. Acute granulomatous or ulcerative colitis	7. Toxic megacolon
8. Chronic respirator dependence	
9. Severe alkaline reflux gastritis	
10. Severe cachexia	
11. Malabsorption syndromes	
12. Extreme prematurity	
13. Failure to thrive	
14. Intractable diarrhea	

In adults, neoplastic and/or inflammatory conditions that gradually produce obstruction of the alimentary tract often cause a progressive and insidious form of malnutrition which is characterized by weight loss, muscle weakness, lassitude, decreased serum protein and immunoglobulin levels, and depressed immunocompetence. Every patient who is to undergo a surgical procedure for an obstructing lesion of the alimentary tract should be given serious consideration as a candidate for *preoperative* parenteral feeding. By use of parenteral nutrition preoperatively in malnourished patients, the incidence of postoperative complications can be reduced because the patient can better tolerate the debilitating effects of the catabolic response to the stress of the operative procedure.

While *complete* gastrointestinal tract obstruction is usually treated best by immediate operation, *partial* intestinal obstruction as a result of inflammatory conditions, such as regional enteritis, granulomatous colitis, ulcerative colitis, or diverticulitis, can often be resolved by treatment with bowel rest and intravenous nutritional repletion. Operation should not be delayed when the clinical condition of the patient suggests imminent danger. However, every opportunity should be taken to improve the nutritional status of malnourished patients prior to definitive surgical therapy.

Total parenteral nutrition and bowel rest are particularly applicable in patients with inflammatory bowel disease. In a series of 52 patients with regional enteritis and granulomatous colitis treated with total parenteral nutrition, 79% of the patients had a favorable nutritional response, and within an average of 36 days of TPN 54% of the patients were able to resume a low-residue, oral diet without exacerbation of their gastrointestinal disease. Most of these patients had been treated initially with corticosteroids, immunosuppressive drugs, and sulfa-containing compounds without remission. Bowel rest and adequate intravenous nutrition reduced intestinal inflammation and edema and often relieved intestinal obstruction if significant fibrosis had not occurred. Thirteen patients required operations for complications of their primary disease such as intestinal obstruction, intra-abdominal abscess, and chronic enterocutaneous fistulas.

Gastrointestinal fistulas developing in patients with inflammatory bowel disease have previously been associated with morbidity and mortality rates as high as 30 to 60%. Inanition from sepsis and malnutrition was the usual cause of death. In a recent series of 62 patients with 78 gastrointestinal fistulas treated with total parenteral nutrition and bowel rest, the overall mortality was only 6.45% and the *spontaneous* fistula closure rate was 70.5%. Successful operative closure of 21.8% of the fistulas produced an overall fistula closure rate of 92.3%. The average period of time between the initiation of TPN and the spontaneous closure of a fistula was 34.9 days.[5]

Complete bowel rest is an important therapeutic measure in the management of acute pancreatitis because the exocrine pancreas is not stimulated to excrete proteolytic and lipolytic digestive enzymes when the bowel remains empty.

However, the application of bowel rest as a therapeutic measure was impossible until TPN was developed.

Extensive loss of the small intestine secondary to resection because of mesenteric infarction, extensive inflammatory bowel disease, multiple gastrointestinal fistulas, or retroperitoneal tumors may be incompatible with life because the remaining absorptive surface is not large enough to assimilate adequate quantities of enterally ingested nutrients. Total parenteral nutrition in the early postoperative period after massive small bowel resection maintains optimal nutritional status, and fluid losses from diarrhea are minimized, since gastrointestinal secretions are not stimulated by oral food ingestion. Oral feeding can be reinstituted after 3 to 6 weeks and slowly increased as tolerated. Chemically defined diets that require little intraluminal digestion before absorption are helpful when treating short bowel syndromes, but the physician must remember that these oral mixtures are hypertonic and can be hazardous if not used properly. Maximum bowel adaptation may not occur for as long as 2 years after the initial operation, and parenteral nutritional support may be required on an outpatient basis to provide essential nutrients for successful recovery or residual bowel function.

Intravenous nutritional therapy is particularly applicable in the clinical management of cancer patients, since the events associated with cancer growth and treatment often result in weight loss, depressed immunologic function, poor wound healing, and malabsorption. The exact mechanism whereby malignant tumors alter host nutritional status is not understood precisely, but several factors including anorexia, gastrointestinal tract dysfunction, and therapeutic intervention with surgery, radiotherapy, and chemotherapy are responsible. In a

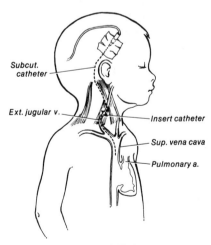

FIG. 5.

group of 175 cancer patients who received chemotherapy, gastrointestinal symptoms of nausea, vomiting, and diarrhea were reduced and/or better tolerated when TPN was used. During an average period of 22.8 days, the average weight gain in these patients was 5.6 pounds, and catheter-related sepsis occurred in only 1.4% of patients. Nutritional repletion of the malnourished cancer patient has also been shown to restore delayed cutaneous hypersensitivity reactions to normal, improve wound healing, reduce septic episodes during treatment, and possibly increase tumor response to chemotherapy.[3] Cachexia should no longer be a contraindication to appropriate cancer therapy, since nutritional repletion via the gastrointestinal tract can be supplemented or replaced by parenteral nutrition.

Total parenteral nutrition can support normal growth and development in infants with congenital anomalies or extreme prematurity who are unable to ingest and absorb adequate quantities of protein and calories. Infants with complex congenital anomalies have little "nutritional reserve" and tolerate semistarvation and perioperative catabolism poorly. Total parenteral nutrition has been lifesaving when extensive operative resection or reconstruction of the gastrointestinal tract has been necessary during the neonatal period. Infants with congenital anomalies such as (1) tracheo-esophageal fistula, (2) small bowel atresia, (3) gastroschisis, (4) omphalocele, and (5) imperforate anus have been supported successfully with TPN during the pre- and postoperative periods.

Acute renal failure in patients who have undergone major operative procedures or severe septic episodes usually is associated with a 50 to 80% mortality rate. Special solutions containing essential L-amino acid mixtures have been formulated to provide sufficient biochemical substrates to promote anabolism while recycling available nitrogen from endogenous urea (Table 4). Use of total parenteral nutrition in patients with acute renal failure has improved the survival rate and shortened the duration of the renal failure.

TABLE 4. Composition of Intravenous Renal Failure Solution

Essential amino acids*	g/100 ml	Solution formulation	
L-Isoleucine	0.56	750–1000 ml 50–70% dextrose	
L-Leucine	0.88	plus	
L-Lysine	1.54	100–250 m. L-amino acids	
L-Methionine	0.88	plus	
L-Phenylalanine	0.88	appropriate electrolytes and vitamins	
L-Threonine	0.40	Volume	850–1250 ml
L-Tryptophan	0.20	Calories	1500–2500 kcal
L-Valine	0.65	Dextrose	375–500 gm
Total	5.1 g	Nitrogen	1–1.5 gm

*Nephramine[TM]

CONCLUSION

Current techniques of total parenteral nutrition are safe and efficacious in patients with a variety of diseases. With increasing knowledge of the exact nutritional requirements during various disease states, precise formulations of nutrient mixtures are now being prepared to provide optimum nutrition and restore metabolic homeostasis. The recognition of protein–calorie malnutrition, however, is essential if patients are to benefit from preventive or corrective nutritional therapy. The nutritional needs of patients should not be neglected in the clinical practice of medicine.

References

Daly, J. M., Ziegler, G., and Dudrick, S. J. Central venous catheterization–Sites and complications. *Am. J. Nurs.* 75: 820–826, 1975.

Duke, J. H., and Dudrick, S. J. Parenteral feeding. In *Manual of Surgical Nutrition,* by the Committee on Pre- and Postoperative Care, American College of Surgeons, W. F. Ballinger, Chair. Philadelphia: W. B. Saunders Co., 1975, pp. 285–317.

Copeland, E. M., and Dudrick, S. J. Nutritional aspects of cancer. In *Current Problems in Cancer,* vol. 1, no. 3, R. C. Hickey, ed. Chicago: Year Book Medical Publishers, Inc., September 1976, pp. 3–61.

Dudrick, S. J., and Long, J. M. Applications and hazards of intravenous hyperalimentation. *Ann. Rev. Med. 28:* 517–528, 1977.

MacFadyen, B. V., Copeland, E. M., and Dudrick, S. J. Application of nutrition to clinical specialties–Surgery. In *Nutritional Support of Medical Practice,* H. A. Schneider, ed. New York: Harper and Row, 1977, pp. 485–500.

Intestinal Obstruction: New Concepts for Fluid and Albumin Replacement

ABELARDO ARANGO, M.D., F.A.C.S.
Clinical Assistant Professor of Surgery
Staff Surgeon V.A. Hospital
Miami, Florida

According to traditional concepts, the fluid resuscitation of patients with advanced intestinal obstruction should include the liberal administration of colloid-containing solutions. In theory this practice appears well founded in

Starling's hypothesis: An increase in serum oncotic pressure would favor absorption of fluid from the interstitial space, through the capillary membrane into the vascular compartment. The fluid reabsorbed would then be held in the circulation, preventing edema and increasing blood volume and urine output. By the same token, a fluid replacement devoid of oncotically active substances could theoretically increase fluid losses and edema because of the reduction in oncotic pressure resulting from the dilution of serum proteins.

The above explanation, however, implies the presence of an anatomically and physiologically intact capillary membrane. It is well known that injuries such as shock, sepsis, and hypoxia result in marked damage to the endothelial membrane, and therefore interference with the normal Starling's mechanism. It is conceivable that in advanced intestinal obstruction, similar capillary damage may occur in the inflamed peritoneum and involved bowel, especially when there is impaired venous and lymphatic return. If such is the case, proteins administered in the resuscitation of these patients may leak from the vascular into the interstitial space, altering the normal oncotic gradients and paradoxically enhancing fluid losses. Experimentally, Rowe and Arango[1] compared the physiologic effects of fluid resuscitation in intestinal obstruction when using an electrolyte or an electrolyte-plus-colloid solution. In their study 20 piglets with 36 hours of untreated intestinal obstruction were resuscitated with either normal saline or 5% albumin in normal saline. Intestinal obstruction was produced by ligating and dividing the jejunum 90 cm from the ligament of Treitz and then volvulizing the distal 30 cm of this obstructed bowel. The results of the experiment are summarized in Tables 1–4, which basically demonstrate that after the 36 hours of untreated obstruction, body weight fell 13%; all animals had proximal bowel distention, edema of the obstructed intestinal wall, and generalized dehydration. Albumin infusion was effective in raising serum oncotic pressure with a pronounced elevation to 45 cm H_2O, whereas the animals infused with a similar volume of colloid-free normal saline solution had a fall in colloid oncotic pressure to 21 cm H_2O (Table 1).

Taking into consideration Starling's law, one might predict that the elevated colloid oncotic pressure in the animals resuscitated with albumin solution would result in fluid shift from the obstructed intestinal segment and surrounding injured peritoneum into the vascular space, leading to a reduction of bowel edema and lower fluid losses into the peritoneal cavity and intestinal lumen. In contrast, the saline-treated animals, because of the low oncotic pressure, would have increased edema and peritoneal and bowel fluid losses. In both sets of animals, the obstructed bowel became markedly edematous, and there was no difference in the water content of the bowel wall between the treatment groups (Table 2). There was, however, a striking difference between the two groups in the volume and composition of fluid that accumulated in the peritoneal cavity. Animals

TABLE 1. Blood and Serum Changes

	SALINE GROUP			ALBUMIN GROUP		
	Basal	After 36 hr obstruction	After 3 hr resuscitation	Basal	After 36 hr obstruction	After 3 hr resuscitation
Hemoglobin (g/100 mg)	8.0 ± 1.7	9.1 ± 2.8	7.6 ± 2.3	8.3 ± 1.7	9.2 ± 2.2	5.6 ± 1.1
Hematocrit (%)	25.0 ± 5.5	27.3 ± 8.1	22.8 ± 6.8	26.3 ± 5.5	27.9 ± 6.0	16.8 ± 3.3
Sodium (mEq/liter)	141.4 ± 7.3	146.7 ± 12.0	141.7 ± 5.7	148.8 ± 8.3	147.1 ± 7.0	153.1 ± 6.8
Potassium (mEq/liter)	3.50 ± 0.52	4.66 ± 1.33	3.61 ± 0.68	3.64 ± 0.30	4.08 ± 1.0	3.08 ± 1.0
BUN (mg/100 ml)	12.1 ± 4.5	61.8 ± 26.5	52.2 ± 19.9	11.0 ± 4.6	58.8 ± 15.4	54.6 ± 18.1
Osmolality (mOsm/kg)	284.8 ± 11.1	318.6 ± 13.0	315.2 ± 8.1	291.2 ± 5.8	326.9 ± 12.2	315.8 ± 9.4
pH	7.409 ± 0.047	7.328 ± 0.110	7.305 ± 0.070	7.373 ± 0.065	7.367 ± 0.062	7.340 ± 0.087
pCO_2 (mm Hg)	37.3 ± 2.6	31.7 ± 9.6	37.8 ± 6.3	37.5 ± 6.3	32.3 ± 5.0	42.9 ± 4.5
Base excess (mEq/liter)	−1.0 ± 2.9	−7.9 ± 9.9	−7.4 ± 2.6	−3.1 ± 4.5	−6.0 ± 5.2	−2.4 ± 6.3
PO_2 (mm Hg)	80.4 ± 12.7	99.2 ± 14.4	88.4 ± 12.0	74.4 ± 10.2	95.2 ± 15.4	72.1 ± 13.8
Total serum protein (g/100 ml)	5.75 ± 0.49	7.84 ± 1.01	4.68 ± 0.39	5.83 ± 0.37	8.13 ± 0.65	7.2 ± 0.26
Colloid osmotic pressure (cm H_2O)	27.6 ± 6.1	41.2 ± 6.5	20.7 ± 2.7	27.9 ± 4.7	39.5 ± 4.9	45.4 ± 3.2

TABLE 2. Changes in Proximal Bowel Fluid

	SALINE GROUP		ALBUMIN GROUP	
	After 36 hr obstruction	After 3 hr resuscitation	After 36 hr obstruction	After 3 hr resuscitation
Sodium (mEq/liter)	152.9 ± 12.4	143.6 ± 15.7	161.6 ± 19.2	103.8 ± 10.5
Potassium (mEq/liter)	8.59 ± 3.16	8.32 ± 2.24	7.94 ± 1.22	8.68 ± 3.4
Osmolality (mOsm/kg)	330.6 ± 14.8	323.2 ± 13.7	349.3 ± 19.3	334 ± 47.8
Specific gravity	1.013 ± 0.005	1.011 ± 0.003	1.012 ± 0.002	1.012 ± 0.004

infused with albumin solution had a significantly greater volume of peritoneal fluid containing a high protein concentration (Table 3).

These findings suggest that with colloid infusion, in spite of the resulting high serum colloid oncotic pressure, there is increased loss of fluid and protein from the vascular spaces of the damaged tissue into the surrounding areas. The key factor may be the integrity of the capillary membrane in the injured tissue—the obstructed bowel. If there is capillary injury, when albumin-containing solutions are infused, albumin molecules may leak out through the damaged capillary membrane. As more protein accumulates outside the capillary, an oncotic gradient may be set up that favors increased fluid loss from the vascular space.

Resuscitation with albumin solutions produced opposite effects in skeletal muscle remote from the site of the obstructed bowel. After protein infusion, the water content of the already severely dehydrated skeletal muscle continued to fall; muscle dehydration increased. In contrast, animals resuscitated with saline solution showed rehydration of skeletal muscle; water content returned toward normal (Table 4). These results imply that in undamaged tissues such as skeletal muscle, the capillary membrane may still be intact and functional once Starling's law is operational. As colloid oncotic pressure increases as a result of albumin infusion, fluid is drawn into the vascular space and intensifies the existing tissue dehydration. The differences in carcass weight and hematocrit and hemoglobin tend to support this concept. The lower carcass weight of the albumin-resuscitated animals implies that they developed more generalized tissue dehydration than the saline-treated piglets. The greater fall in hematocrit and hemoglobin in the albumin-treated group suggest hemodilution and increased plasma volume, partially on the basis of poor mobilization of the fluid into the dehydrated tissues.

During resuscitation, urine output was significantly lower in animals receiving albumin in saline solutions than in those infused with colloid-free saline solution (Table 5). This was in spite of greater hemodilution in the albumin group, which suggests a larger blood volume, and the minimal difference between groups in

TABLE 3. Changes in Peritoneal Fluid

Measurement	SALINE GROUP			ALBUMIN GROUP		
	Basal	After 36 hr obstruction	After 3 hr resuscitation	Basal	After 36 hr obstruction	After 3 hr resuscitation
Sodium (mEq/liter)	138.0 ± 6.2	144.7 ± 7.6	154.8 ± 11.8	145.7 ± 11.1	144.1 ± 6.4	152.5 ± 8.7
Potassium (mEq/liter)	4.84 ± 0.89	5.89 ± 1.58	4.74 ± 0.71	4.90 ± 0.64	6.39 ± 1.28	4.26 ± 1.17
Osmolality (omOsm/kg)						
Specific gravity	1.018	1.035	1.024	1.019	1.033	1.035
Total protein (g/100 ml)	2.54	6.86	3.48	2.58	5.96	6.34

583

TABLE 4. Change in Tissue Water, %

	SALINE GROUP			ALBUMIN GROUP		
Tissue	Basal	After 6 hr obstruction	After 3 hr resuscitation	Basal	After 6 hr obstruction	After 3 hr resuscitation
Proximal bowel	81.4 ± 0.15	82.6 ± 0.27	85.3 ± 0.18	81.3 ± 0.15	82.6 ± 1.8	85.6 ± 0.3
Distal bowel	81.3 ± 0.15	80.3 ± 0.18	83.1 ± 0.16	81.5 ± 0.23	80.1 ± 2.1	84.2 ± 0.13
Skeletal muscle	80.0 ± 0.17	77.8 ± 0.21	79.3 ± 0.18	80.6 ± 0.31	78.2 ± 0.32	77.0 ± 0.21

TABLE 5. Changes in Urine

Measurement	SALINE GROUP			ALBUMIN GROUP		
	Basal	After 36 hr obstruction	After 3 hr resuscitation	Basal	After 36 hr obstruction	After 3 hr resuscitation
Sodium (mEq/liter)	6.8 ± 6.1	24.7 ± 4.9	58.3 ± 18.6	11.3 ± 12.7	21.7 ± 7.9	48.9 ± 24.8
Potassium (mEq/liter)	37.6 ± 19.2	88.7 ± 36.5	35.7 ± 24.9	49.5 ± 26.0	96.4 ± 17.1	53.2 ± 16.2
Osmolality (mOsm/kg)	521 ± 210.5	568.7 ± 278.5	475 ± 190.2	437.3 ± 114.3	511.5 ± 113.9	416.3 ± 85.2
Specific gravity	1.023 ± 0.006	1.029 ± 0.003	1.018 ± 0.008	1.018 ± 0.005	1.025 ± 0.002	1.022 ± 0.006

pulse rate and blood pressure. Two mechanisms may be responsible for the difference in urine output. First, at the systemic level, the tissue dehydration which is persistent and even more marked in the albumin-treated animals will act as a potent stimulus to the osmoreceptors to release antidiuretic hormone. Second, at the local kidney level, the elevated serum oncotic pressure results in lower glomerular filtration rate and, therefore, decreased urine output.

The results of this experiment suggest than in intestinal obstruction there may be extensive capillary membrane damage in the area of primary pathology, colloid infusion leaks of the vascular space, and increased fluid losses. In contrast, in undamaged areas, remote from the area of primary disease, fluid is drawn from the tissue through a normal-functioning capillary membrane, potentiating the local tissue dehydration. But, how do these findings apply to the clinical situation? In a series of 15 patients with nonstrangulated intestinal obstructions, we found that at admission the colloid oncotic pressure, as calculated by the Goldberg refractmeter,[2] was elevated to an average of 42.3 cm H_2O. After fluid resuscitation with electrolyte solution alone, and at the time the patient was considered clinically rehydrated, with adequate urine output and ready for the surgical procedure, the colloid oncotic pressure was 31.8 cm H_2O, a level compatible with a perfectly normal Starling's equilibrium. This finding agrees with Peters's report[3] that massive quantities of nonprotein fluid are needed before serum oncotic pressure falls to a significant degree.

An additional argument against the indiscriminate use of colloid-containing solutions in the resuscitation of intestinal obstruction is pointed out by Shires and co-workers,[4] who emphasized that colloid-containing solutions do not rapidly diffuse into the intestinal space to correct interstitial fluid deficits, whereas electrolyte solutions quickly equilibrate between vascular and interstitial spaces. Moreover, Marty[5] pointed out that infused albumin escapes through the capillary at a rate of 5% per hour in the normal adult, and, once interstitial protein concentration increases, the clearance of albumin by the lymphatics decreases, resulting in the accumulation of albumin in the interstitial space, altering the oncotic gradient, and leading to increased interstitial edema and organ dysfunction.

References

Rowe, M. I., and Arango, A. Colloids versus crystalloids resuscitation in experimental bowel obstruction. *J. Pediat., Surg. 11*: 635–643, 1976.

Rowe, M. I., Lankau, C., and Newmark, S. Clinical evaluation of methods to monitor colloid oncotic pressure in the surgical treatment of children. *Surg. Gynecol. Obstet. 139*: 889–893, 1974.

Peters, R. M. Is fluid overload the culprit in acute respiratory distress syndrome? In *Shock in Low and High Flow States*. B. K. Forscher, R. C. Lillehei, and S. S. Stubbs, eds. Amsterdam: Excerpta Medica, 1972, p. 219.

Shires, G. T., Carrico, C. S., and Canizaro, P. C. *Shock's Major Problems in Clinical Surgery,* vol. XIII. Philadelphia: W. B. Saunders Co., 1973, pp. 15–41.

Marty, A. T. Hyperoncotic albumins therapy. *Surg. Gynecol. Obstet. 139*: 105–107, 1974.

"Dengue Fever"—Review

J. SZEPS, M.D., F.R.C.S.(C), F.A.C.S.
Chatham, Ontario, Canada

Until quite recently dengue fever was a disease only vaguely remembered by practicing physicians in North America and Europe.

With the sporadic cases occurring in the Carribean with increased frequency, as well as recent epidemics in the Carribean area, together with increasing numbers of people traveling to and from those areas, more and more cases of dengue have been diagnosed in Canada and the United States. The U.S. Public Health Center for Disease Control in Atlanta reported that the epidemic of dengue in the Carribean had led to 58 confirmed cases in the United States as of the end of February 1978. The public health authorities in Canada do not yet have the corresponding numbers for this country. This author, convalescing himself from the effects of dengue at the time of this writing, is aware of at least four cases in his area. All these patients spent some time in Haiti prior to the development of the symptoms. The serological studies on these cases are pending, while the author's case has already been confirmed by viral studies.

The Center for Disease Control in Atlanta reported that the cases of dengue in the United States were imported from Barbados, Jamaica, Cuba, Puerto Rico, and the Netherlands Antilles. Cases were also imported from Thailand to Hawaii and from the Philippines and Tahiti into California. Puerto Rico reported 284 cases between January 1 and February 22, 1978.

Dengue, also known as "break-bone fever" or "dandy fever," is an acute febrile disease characterized by a sudden onset, with headache, fever and prostration, joint and muscle pain, and leucopenia. It is caused by a specific filterable virus (arbo virus). Three types of this virus have been isolated. The type I virus was apparently responsible for major epidemics in Jamaica, Antigua, the Bahamas, Bermuda, Cuba, the Dominican Republic, Grand Turk, Granada, Guyana, Haiti, Saint Martin, Surinam, Trinidad, and the U.S. Virgin Islands.

The vector of the disease is a mosquito. The *Aedes aegypti* is apparently responsible for the cases in the most endemic areas, though the *Aedes albopictus* has also been shown to carry the virus. The mosquito becomes infected if it bites the human during the first three days of illness. The virus then takes 8 to 11 days to incubate in the mosquito before it can again be transferred to man. Thereafter the mosquito remains infected for its life. The virus is injected into the skin while the mosquito prepares to feed. The incubation period in the human, after the mosquito bite, is 4 to 10 days. The virus spreads throughout the tissues, but it has particular affinity for the parenchymatous tissues and the lining of the capillaries. The symptoms are produced by the viral toxins.

The acute stage comes suddenly with chills and high fever. It is often associated with excruciating pain in the joints, epigastric region, and orbital region. There is rapid pulse and frequently extreme prostration. The above symptoms may last for four to seven days; on the other hand, they may be very short and quite insipid. Characteristically there is a sudden drop of temperature afterward, profuse sweating, loose stools, and some nosebleeds. The patient usually feels much better at this stage, although he is still weak. Unfortunately in about two-thirds of cases there is recurrence after an interval of 5 to 14 days. The initial symptoms may recur with increased frequency. The patient may break out with a scarlatiniform rash, which lasts for two or three days, and is followed by itching and desquamation. During the progress of the disease there is marked reduction in the neutrophil white corpuscles.

The convalescence is slow and its length unrelated to the severity of the original insult. The recovery period may take many months, with evidence of lassitude, nervousness and irritability, insomnia, and slow pulse; vague or even severe rheumaticlike pains are not uncommon.

It should again be emphasized that the disease may be so mild as to produce only very minimal symptoms and may pass unnoticed. In spite of the fact that the disease is temporarily completely incapacitating, it is almost never fatal. Recovery confers considerable immunity to the homologous strain of the virus. The diagnosis is made on clinical findings, although it may be confirmed by the specific serological tests now available. During the acute stage there is marked leucopenia; the granulocytes may drop to 20 to 40% of total count. There may be some oliguria and albuminuria. The differential diagnosis includes sandfly fever, yellow fever, typhus fever, Rocky Mountin spotted fever, malaria, Weil's disease, relapsing fever, measles, and scarlet fever.

There is no specific therapy, the treatment being purely symptomatic and supportive.

The disease was first accurately described by Benjamin Rush in 1780 during an epidemic outbreak in Philadelphia, Pennsylvania. The causative organism was first demonstrated by P. M. Ashburn and C. F. Craig in 1907 in the Philippine Islands.

Of special interest are the ocular manifestations of dengue fever. Occasionally edema of the lid, with conjunctival injection, lacrimation, and photophobia occur. Ocular and retrobulbar pain accentuated by ocular movements, particularly at the beginning of the disease, is not uncommon. Dacryoadenitis has been mentioned, and keratitis, which may take either punctate or disciform form as well as be dendritic in type, has been described. There have been reports of iritis and even metastatic ophthalmitis as well as retinal and vitreous hemorrhages. An accommodative paresis has been recorded as well as other ocular motor palsies, particularly manifesting themselves from the ninth to the fifteenth day. The seventh nerve may also be affected.

The preventive measures are in the same as in any insect-carried diseases. Screening of suspected as well as diagnosed cases, especially during the first three days of the illness, is important. The unaffected population should also be protected from mosquito bites (by any of the available methods).

Bibliography

Ashburn, P. M., and Craig, C. F. Experimental investigations regarding the aetiology of dengue fever. *Philippine J. Sci. 2*: 93–152, 1907.

Duke-Elder, Sir Stewart. *System of Ophthalmology, viii:* 372–373; *ix:* 313; *x:* 274; *xii:* 700; *xiii:* 608; *xv:* 42. 1976.

Sabin, A. B. Recent Advances in our knowledge of dengue and sandfly fever. *Am. J. Trop. Med. 4*: 198–207, 1954.

Simmons, J. S., St. John, J. H. and Reynolds, F. H. K. Studies of Dengue. *Philippine J. Sci. 44*: 1–251, 1931.

Tropical Parasitology

PROFESSOR L. N. JOHRI, D.Sc.
University of Delhi
Delhi, India

A considerable number of tropical parasites are helminth forms. These organisms live inside the body of men and other animals. The digestive system of these parasites is consequently poorly developed or is altogether missing. These worms possess flattened ribbonlike bodies as in the tapeworm or a cylindrical structure as with the round worm. These parasites have two hosts, a primary host in which they develop into adults and a secondary host in which they pass through some of the early stages of their life cycle.

The plan of construction of the body in these parasites provides maximum spacing facilities for the reproductive organs while considerably reducing other systems in order to produce the largest number of eggs to ensure an easy propagation of their species. Formerly parasites were localized to different parts of the world constituting definite "endemic regions," but today we observe that barriers are shattered; boundaries are dissolved because of free mixing and intercommunication, with easy and quick transport between the most remote parts of the earth resulting in the delivery of unwanted gifts to other doors!

THE PORK TAPEWORM (*TAENIA SOLIUM*)

The adult pork tapeworm is a ribbonlike flat worm found in the intestine of pork-eating people. It may grow to a length of 15 to 18 feet. The body is composed of a large number of segments (800 to 900). The head is about the size of a pinhead, bearing a double row of hooklets with which the worm attaches to the wall of the intestine. The posterior segments, called "gravid segments," contain a large number of eggs. These segments get detached from the worm and are expelled passively along with the feces. The life cycle of the worm is completed in two hosts. The final host is man, harboring the adult worm. The intermediate host is a pig, possessing the larval forms. The pig must eat food contaminated with human feces along with the gravid segments. The eggs find easy access to the intestine of pig. The eggs liberate small embryos that finally reach the muscles and develop into circular vesicles possessing a head, popularly known as bladder worm. The head is deeply penetrated in between the muscle fibers. Pork infected with these vesicles is known as "measly pork." When a person eats improperly cooked measly pork, the head is released from the pork muscle fibers and sticks to the inner lining of the person's intestine where it grows gradually to be a fully developed adult. *Geographical distribution* is worldwide. Conditions have improved owing to strict inspection and hygenic control of pork, in many pork-eating countries.

Prophylaxis. Individual caution is required to avoid eating improperly cooked pork, and adequate pork inspection at the slaughter house is mandatory.

Pathogenicity. Stomach pain with gastrointestinal disturbances and anemia are the usual complaints of the infected persons.

THE BEEF TAPEWORM (*TAENIA SAGINATA*)

This parasite resembles the pork tapeworm. It is longer and differs in absence of hooklets from its head. The life cycle is the same as described for the pork tapeworm. In this case the intermediate host is cattle (cow or buffalo). Human beings suffer the infection by eating undercooked beef.

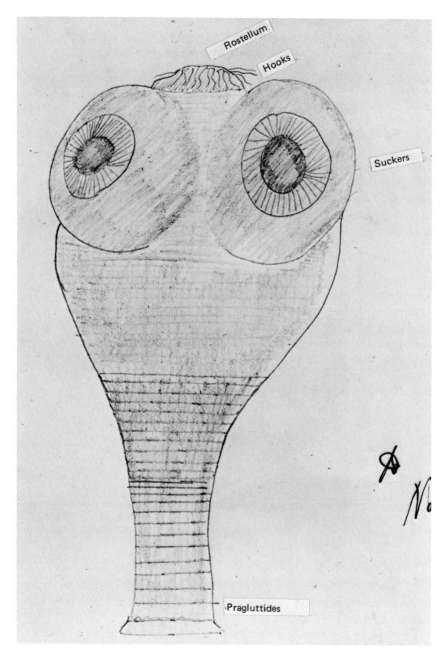

FIG. 1. Scolex of taenia solium. (Illustration courtesy of Prof. Stacey B. Day. Drawn from a high powered microscopic study by Dr. Day in 1945.)

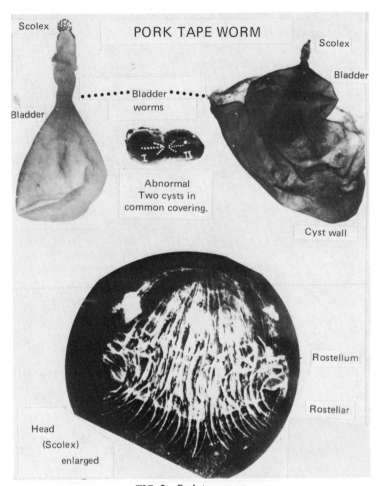

FIG. 2. Pork tapeworm.

Geographical Distribution. It is of world wide occurrence. It is fairly common in countries where beef is consumed as food, especially if adequate meat inspection facilities are not available.

Prophylaxis and Pathogenicity. These parasites require the same caution and care as noted for the pork tapeworm.

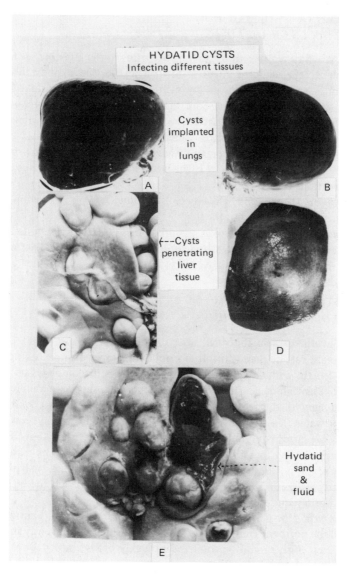

FIG. 3. Hydatic cysts. A and B: cysts implanted in lungs. C, D and E: Cysts in liver tissue. E. Further details in the cyst.

THE DWARF TAPEWORM OF DOG
(*ECHINOCOCCUS GRANULOSUS*)

The adult is a tiny worm 3 to 6 mm long occurring in the intestine of the dog in large numbers. The eggs are infective to man, cattle, sheep, and other herbivorous animals and are swallowed by man through food and drink. The eggs hatch into minute embryos that bore their way through blood vessels, finally reaching the liver and lungs and later invading other organs where they develop into vesiclelike structures popularly called "hydatid cysts." Hydatid cysts develop in size depending on the organ invaded, the diameter varying proportionately (1-2 inches to basketball size). The larval form is most dangerous and even may be fatal to man.

Geographical Distribution. Occurence is worldwide. Man is a victim because of his intimate association with the dog.

Prophylaxis. Hygienic control is essential. It is essential for adults and children to keep dogs at a distance, and thorough washing of hands before eating should be matter of habit.

THE BROAD FISH TAPEWORM
(*DIPHYLLOBOTHRIUM LATUM*)

The adult worm lives in the small intestine of man; it is also reported in fish-eating animals, cat, dog, and fox. It is a ribbonlike tapeworm measuring 8 to 10 meters in length, containing 3000 to 4000 segments. It completes its lifecycle in three different animals. The terminal segments enclosing large number of eggs are shed along with the fecal matter. The eggs are dropped in water and must be eaten by a water flea (cyclops), giving rise first to larval forms. The water flea along with the larval form must be eaten by a fresh-water fish. The second larval form develops in fish muscles. The infected fish in finally eaten by man. The infective larvae are not destroyed by ordinary salting or smoking, or if the fish is insufficiently cooked. The larvae, therefore, successfully reach the intestine of man. The worm requires 6 to 8 weeks to attain maturity.

Geographical Distribution. It is common in Central Europe, Central Africa, Japan, and the northern United States, and was also reported recently in India.

Prophylaxis. Fish should be cooked thoroughly before eating. Dogs and cats should not be fed on offals of fish.

Pathogenicity. It provokes gastrointestinal disturbances and anemia.

THE BLOOD FLUKE (*SCHISTOMA HAEMATOBIUM*)

This worm lives in the blood vessels of man, particularly in the veins of the urinary tract. The male is 7 to 25 mm long and lodges safely in the body of the female (15 to 25 mm long) on its ventral side. The female discharges the eggs into the blood. The eggs gradually find their way into the urinary bladder and escape along with the urine. The eggs penetrate the soft parts of the snail (small-shelled animals in ponds and rivers). Later they develop into larvae, which are released into the water. Infection results when human beings swim, bathe, or wade in such water. Young larval forms very quickly burrow through the skin and gradually reach the blood vessels where they develop into adult males and females.

Geographical Distribution. It occurs in the Mediterranean region, Madagascar, Southwest Asia, Egypt, Africa (tropical and southern), South America, the West Indies, the Philippines, and Celebes, and is also reported in India.

Prophylaxis. Prevention of pollution of water with human excreta is the primary item of concern. It is most important to avoid swimming, bathing, wading, or washing in infected water. Destruction of the snail vector at the government level by appropriate sanitary ordinances should be mandatory.

THE DWARF TAPEWORM OF MAN
(*HYMENELEPIS NANA*)

This worm is commonly available from the intestine of man; also a slightly different form occurs in the intestine of rat. It measures 10 to 53 mm in length. No intermediate host is required to complete its life cycle. Development is continued in the infected host.

Infection first occurs through the ingestion of food contaminated with the eggs of the worm (from the fecal matter of an infected man or rat). Later auto-infection increases the number of parasites in the intestine of the individual.

Geographical Distribution. It is cosmopolitan, being fairly common in the South in the United States, different parts of Europe, Asia, and the Pacific islands.

Prophylaxis. Good personal hygiene must be very carefully observed. Crowded living conditions should be avoided.

THE GUINEA WORM (SERPENT WORM OR DRAGON WORM) (*DRACUNUCULUS MEDINENSIS*)

These worms live under the skin of legs, arms, and back of man. The female measures 12 to 30 mm in length, while the male is much smaller. The life cycle is completed by two hosts. Man is the primary host, while the water flea is the secondary host. Water fleas containing the infective larvae are swallowed by men with *raw* drinking water. The young forms (larvae) are set free in the intestine; later they pierce the intestinal wall and reach the lower surface of the skin, especially of the lower body extremities where the skin is liable to come into

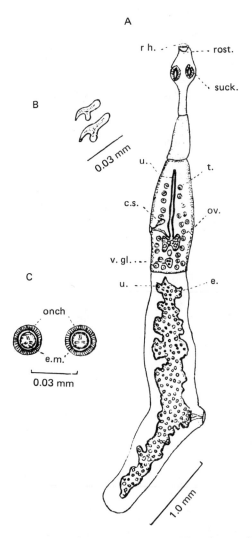

FIG. 4. Dwarf tapeworm of dog. A. Complete worm. B. Hooklets—large and small. C. Eggs.

contact with water, and there they give rise to ulcers. The gravid females migrate to those parts of the skin liable to come in contact with water, particularly the legs of washer men and water carriers. Upon rupture of the ulcer, the young forms are discharged into the water, and water fleas are easily reinfected.

   Geographical Distribution. It is found in India, Burma, Arabia, Persia, Turkestan, Africa (East, West, and Central), the West Indies, and South America.

Prophylaxis. The best way advisable is to break the link of waterflea–man–waterflea. Control pollution of drinking water. Careful filtering and boiling of drinking water is most essential.

Pathogenic Effects. Female worms produce toxic substances, causing allergic manifestations.

THE ROUND WORM (*ASCARIS LUMBRICOIDES*)

This is a cylindrical worm living in the intestine of man. The males grow to 25 cm in length. The females are longer, growing to 40 cm. The male is further distinguished by the possession of a curved tail. Normally they are evacuated along with the feces, but under rare conditions they reach the stomach and are vomited out. The worm passes its life cycle only in man. The eggs are swallowed with food, drink, or raw vegetables. Tiny young forms released from the eggs are drained by blood capillaries, and reach the lungs, trachea, and esophagus. Finally they enter the digestive tract where they grow into male and female worms.

Geographical Distribution. Distribution is worldwide, occurring chiefly in the tropics. People suffer because of unhygienic habits. Children are the first victims.

Prophylaxis. There are three essentials: proper disposal of human feces, education of children in proper hygiene, and care and proper treatment of infected persons.

Pathogenecity. Young forms in the lungs cause serious coughing, fever, and pneumonia. Toxic action is responsible for some physical manifestations. Adult forms rob man of nourishment from the intestine.

THE FILARIA WORM (*WUCHEREIRIA BANCROFTI*)

Adult worms are available in the lymphatic vessels of man only, being long and hairlike (round worm type). The male measures 2 to 4 mm in length, while the female is 7 to 10 mm long. Females lay eggs containing well-developed embryos into the blood. Man is the principal host harboring the adult worms. Embryos (microfilariae) are transmitted to female mosquitoes (*Culex*-type) during their blood meal. They possess a sheath and undergo further development within a fortnight. While the infective mosquito bites the human being, these microgerms are primarily deposited under the skin. Later they migrate to other regions (inguinal, scrotal, and abdominal), and grow to the adult form. Fertilized females keep on producing microfilariae, swarming in the peripheral blood vessels of the patient. The disease is popularly called "elephantiasis." It results in enormous enlargement of the organ affected (foot, arm, scrotum, breast, or vagina). The skin in these parts gets hardened, tough, and fissured. Urine indicates an abnormal condition, showing a milk-white coloration.

Pathogenecity. Morbid changes are produced in the patient by the infection.

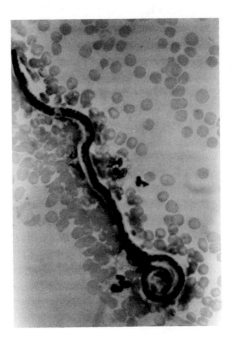

FIG. 5. Peripheral blood smear demonstrating *Wucheria Bancrofti*. Courtesy Drs. Randall D. Bloomfield and Jorge R. Suarez, The Brooklyn Hospital, New York.

THE HOOK WORM (*ANCYLOSTOMA DUODENALE*)

The hook worm is also known as "Old World hook worm." It resides in the small intestine of man. The male worm is nearly 8 mm in length, while the female worm is a little longer. It attaches to the lumen of the intestine, causing hemorrhage and wounds. It resides in the small intestine but does not absorb the digesting food at all. It bites the intestinal wall and sucks blood, resulting in extensive damage to the intestine with profuse bleeding. The excretory waste of these worms cause a general physical *shiftlessness*. Many people throughout the world move bare-footed or with open shoes. In this way the larvae get an excellent opportunity to stick to the skin; once they bore their way inside the body, they are easily carried by blood vessels to the lungs and the trachea. At this stage they are coughed up and maybe swallowed, finally reaching the intestine and alimentary tract.

Geographical Distribution. It is widely distributed in all tropical and subtropical countries.

Prophylaxis. Special attention should be given to treatment of infected persons, prevention of soil pollution with proper control of sewage disposal, and proper use of boots.

Pathogenicity. The worms cause severe anemic conditions.

THE PINWORM OR SEATWORM
(*ENTEROBIUS VERMICULARIS*)

These are very small cylindrical worms. The male grows to 4 mm in length, while the female attains a length up to 12 mm. They live in the cecum or vermiform appendix of man. Mature females wander down the rectum and even work their way out of the anus; this is most convenient for them to do when the patient retires to bed at night and the rectal muscles become relaxed. The worms become fairly active owing to aeration. The patient becomes alarmed and puts the fingers near the anus, contaminating the nails with the eggs. These eggs, which are of very small size (5-60 μ) are heavily embedded in the perianal skin, are swallowed by that same individual and reach the intestine. Another person or other members of the house are infected through food, or linen, or even via a shared bed. In the case of a female patient the worms enter the vagina, causing inflammation and irritation.

Geographical Distribution. The distribution is cosmopolitan, with these worms found all over the world.

Pathogenesis. Irritation is caused by fully grown female pinworms. Inflamation and uneasiness are developed in the human female genital tract as and when worms invade the area.

References

Brumpt, E. *Precis de parasitologies.* (5th ed.). Paris, 1936).

Chaterjee, K. D. *Parasitology.* Calcutta: Sree Saraswaty Press Ltd., 1970, pp. 1–226.

Faust, E. C. *Human Helminthology.* Philadelphia, 1929.

Wradle, R. A., and McLeod, J. A. *The Zoology of Tape Worms.* Minneapolis, 1951.

Yamaguti, S. *Systema Helminthum,* Vols. I and II. London: Interscience Publishers Ltd., 1959.

Hygiene in the Tropics

PROFESSOR J. N. JOHRI
Garhwal University
Srinagar, U.P. India

The tropics include those portions of the earth's surface that lie between the tropics of Cancer and Capricorn, 23½° north and south of the equator respectively. In the present context, however, it would be more useful to include in "tropics" all such regions of the world that show a typical tropical climate irrespective of geographical location.

Contrary to common belief, tropical climates are not very hot. The temperature rarely exceeds 35°C and often ranges between 26 and 32°C. The main feature of the tropical climate is the remarkable uniformity of temperature over a 24-hour period as well as throughout the year. The seasons are, therefore, classified not on the basis of temperature but according to rainfall, which is usually heavy and, in some parts, virtually incessant. As a consequence, humidity is very high almost throughout the year and, coupled with remarkably uniform high temperature, creates an oppressive hot-house atmosphere that is highly conducive to growth of vegetation and lower forms of animal life such as insects in general, and flies and mosquitoes in particular. This generalized description of the tropical climate obviously does not apply to the tropical deserts (between 20 and 30° north and south of the equator) where rainfall and humidity are negligible and diurnal fluctuations in temperature are considerable.

By a curious coincidence, a vast majority of the countries that lie in the tropical belt are poor and densely populated, their inhabitants are undernourished, and civic amenities are poorly developed or, in places, nonexistent. Consequently, many of the problems of health and hygiene in the tropics are due more to *socioeconomic* conditions than to geographical factors. Lack of safe and sufficient drinking water, inefficient sanitary systems, primitive methods of disposal of industrial, agricultural, and sewage wastes, and inadequate medical care, especially in rural reas, have often resulted in massive epidemics of diseases which should otherwise be preventable. Many of the diseases that were once prevalent in Europe and America, have now been virtually eradicated everywhere except in tropical countries where some have now become endemic. With concerted effort involving international cooperation, many of the tropical diseases can be abolished. This is best demonstrated with smallpox, which has now been totally eradicated.

Tropical diseases can be divided into four principal categories. The first comprises diseases that originate as a direct consequence of the hot-humid tropical climate. The second category includes diseases that are transmitted by the bite of insects (malaria, filaria, dengue, yaws, yellow fever), which form the single largest and the most important category of tropical illnesses.

In the third category are diseases whose causative organisms are spread by consumption of unwashed fruits and/or uncooked/improperly cooked vegetables, or by contact with bodily discharges of infected persons. Lastly, there are nutritional diseases like beriberi or general malnutrition, which may occur at any place in the world but are more prevalent in tropical regions.

DIRECT EFFECTS OF TROPICAL CLIMATE ON THE HUMAN BODY

The effects of heat on the human body are influenced by two factors, first, the ability of the body to produce sweat, and second, the ability of the atmosphere to evaporate it. While the severe effects of heat such as heat strokes and heat exhaustion are uncommon in the tropics, milder effects are frequently encountered and are primarily due to excessive production of sweat and the inability of the humid atmosphere to evaporate it.

It is generally accepted that a person doing moderate physical work in the tropics may lose up to 10 liters of water and nearly 28 g salt per day in sweat and urine. These losses may result, over a period of time, in crmaps, giddiness, and severe dehydration. Provision of ample supplies of potable water and intake of about 30 g salt per day are a *sine qua non* for survival in the tropics. Adequate rest and sleep and avoiding overexertion, especially in the sun, are also important. Perhaps the most effective defense against the tropical climate is a daily bath with fresh cool water. A dirty skin, covered with residual products of evaporated sweat, invites bacterial growth, skin eruptions, and prickly heat, which, by mechanically constricting or blocking the sweat pores, interfere with efficient sweating. Clothing should be light, loose, and preferably made of non-synthetic fibers such as cotton. Moderation in food intake, qualitative and quantitative, is advisable. Easily digestible protein-rich food with plently of fresh fruits and vegetables is recommended. Excessive consumption of alcohol and high-calorie items such as fats and carbohydrates raises the internal heat and compounds the ill effects of climate.

While physical effects of heat and humidity are important hazards in the tropics, they pale into insignificance in comparison with the formidable array of diseases that occur exclusively, or almost so, in tropical countries with hot climates, both wet and dry.

INSECT-BORNE DISEASES

The most important of the tropical diseases is *malaria*. It is caused by infection with protozoan parasites of the genus *Plasmodium* transmitted by the bite of infected anopheline mosquitoes and characterized clinically by recurrent paroxysms of chills, fever, and sweating. In man, malaria is produced by four specific parasites which do not infect lower animals. Every year, about a quarter of all adults in Africa and every tenth person in India suffer from malaria, and every year nearly one million children die of the disease.

In addition to malaria, mosquitoes act as vectors for a number of other tropical diseases which are nearly as deadly as malaria, though less widespread. *Yellow fever,* a virulent virus disease, is carried by the mosquito *Aedes aegypti.* This disease has been eradicated from the United States, but a reservoir of yellow fever virus persists in the wild animals of Central and South America.

Another viral disease transmitted by the bites of certain mosquitoes is *dengue.* Appropriately called "break-bone fever," dengue is marked by severe pain in bones and joints, skin eruptions, and rapid high fever.

Another very common insect-borne disease is *elephantiasis* or *filariasis,* which starts by blockage of lymph channels by threadlike worms (*Filaria:* nematodes) conveyed to man by the bite of mosquitoes. The disease is charactized by persistent and chronic swelling of the arms, legs, or scrotum, until they assume gigantic proportions. In Central Africa, there is a species of *Filaria,* carried by the mango fly, that particularly attacks the eye. This disease is called *loa-loa.*

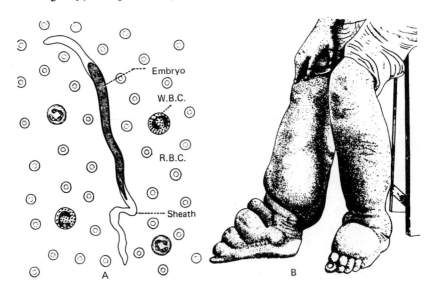

FIG. 1. A. Blood film with embryo. B. Elephantiasis of legs and hands.

Sleeping sickness or *trypanosomiasis* is a tropical disease spread by the bite of the tsetse fly, which transmits the causative organism, a protozoan, into the blood of man. After a long latent period, which may last up to three years, the patient may suffer from periodic high temperature, swelling of spleen and lymph glands, and edema of the legs. The next stage of the disease is marked by tremors, a vacant expression, and slow speech. In the final stages the patient becomes sluggish and sleeps or dozes during the day. A condition like the African sleeping sickness also occurs in tropical America, where it is called *Chagas disease.*

Plague, a bacillary disease, is now restricted to Asia though at one time it was equally prevalent in Europe. The plague bacilli are carried by the bite of rat fleas, but once people get infected, spread may occur by droplet infection such as coughing and sneezing. The disease runs a rapid, severe, and often fatal course. It begins with fever and chills and is soon followed by headache, vomiting and prostration. Bleeding into the lungs or under the skin and enlargement and rupture of glands, especially in the groin, armpits, and neck, are common symptoms.

Asiatic or Indian *cholera* is endemic to the Far East and is almost absent in the Western hemisphere. The primary source of infection is the blood discharge from infected victims which may be spread by flies or carried by raw food and water. Thirst, vomiting, pain, abdominal cramps, and diarrhea leading to severe dehydration and prostration are important symptoms.

Dysentery is a form of diarrhea marked by frequent loose movements and the presence of blood and mucus in the stools. Of the two types of dysentery, *Amoebic* and *bacillary,* the former is confined largely to tropical countries and is caused by a parasitic protozoan (*Entamoeba histolytica*) which is introduced into the human body with contaminated water and uncooked or improperly washed fruits and vegetables. In chronic cases, abcesses may develop in the liver, lungs, or brain, which may lead to *serious complications.*

Conditions of poverty that exist in many of the tropical countries often lead to diseases that are nutritional in origin. *Tropical sprue,* characterized by frequent, soapy stools, sore mouth, raw tongue, weakness, loss of weight and anemia, is often suspected to be due to nutritional causes, although the basic cause is the inability of the stomach and intestine to absorb fats and carbohydrates. Similarly, *beriberi* is a deficiency disease caused by lack of vitamin B_1, which is quite prevalent in regions where people live on diets of polished rice or where the food is cooked in such a way that the heat destroys the vitamins. It is also a disease of alcoholics in which inflammation of the stomach interferes with absorption of vitamins.

Among the most troublesome diseases of the tropics are those caused by parasitic worms. For instance *ancylostomiasis,* an infestation of the small intestine of man by the blood-sucking round worm of the genus *Ancylostoma,* occurs in practically all tropical countries. Man is the sole reservoir of this parasite and is, therefore, himself a source of infection. From the infected host, the eggs of the worm pass out along with stools, and if they reach moist soil, they hatch into hooked larvae (young forms) within about 24 hours. They enter man's body through the skin, especially of the foot, and drain through the blood vessels, finally reaching the stomach and intestine.

Another round worm, *Ascaris lumbricoides,* is worldwide in distribution but is most common in the tropics and subtropics. Infestation of man is due to ingestion of the eggs carried by infected raw vegetables, other eatables, and drinks that are contaminated with human fecal matter. Normally the worm robs the host's food and causes alarming symptoms to man.

Other worm infestations are either too local or too universal (tapeworms) in occurrence and thus need not be described here.

Since many of the insect vectors lay their eggs in standing and stagnant waters or in human and animal excreta, cleanliness of the immediate surroundings is an important prophylactic measure. Uncovered drains and ditches, pools, and puddles should be regularly sprayed with oils or insecticides. Important breeding sites, often overlooked, are overhead storage tanks, room coolers, and air conditioners. It is important to drain out the water completely from these resources.

Unfortunately, man has no natural immunity against the organisms of diarrhea and dysentery, especially when more than one strain of these organisms are present in a certain locality. While water itself is a relatively unimportant carrier of such organisms, it might carry cysts of *Entamoeba* and the eggs of helminth parasites. This necessitates very careful filtration and chlorination of the water at the government level. Human excreta should never be used as manure in fields where vegetables are grown.

Every year there are massive epidemics in several tropical areas whose cause can be traced directly to infection of drinking water. It is therefore essential to avoid such accidents by drinking *boiled and filtered water.*

The practice of defecation in open fields, by the roadside, is very prevalent in the tropics. It is due to the absence of public latrines. The government should take sanitary measures to discourage such practices.

HYGIENE FOR THE TRAVELER

Tourists to tropical countries must realize that conditions in which the natives can remain healthy and disease-free may not be equally healthful for a stranger. Overexertion, lack of adequate rest, and poor sleep predispose a traveler to disease. Similarly a wise traveler should never overindulge in food and drink. A most important precaution is not to drink water from unknown or doubtful sources. It is best to use water treated with purification tablets or by adding 2 to 4 drops of bleach solution per quart of water. It is most advisable to drink boiled or aerated water or freshly prepared tea and coffee. Another needed precaution is to avoid food from open unhygienic stalls. It is also essential not to eat salads, cut fruits, raw berries, or fruits and vegetables that cannot be peeled.

Travelers to most tropical countries are required to take great precautions against a number of communicable diseases. It is very important that travelers safeguard their own health.

References

International Conference on Environmental Pollution. New Dehli, India, June 1978.

Manual of Hygiene for the Armed Forces. Simla: Government of India Press, 1953.

Schifferes, J. J. *The Family Medical Encyclopedia.* 1959.

The State of the World Environment. The 1978 report of the Executive Director of the United Nations. Environment Programme, 1978.

Today's Health Guide. A manual of health information and guidance for the American family. American Medical Association, 1965.

Cryobiology and the Storage of Mammalian Embryos

BRIAN W. W. GROUT
KEITH C. SHORT
Department of Biology
North East London Polytechnic
London, England

The freezing and subsequent storage of biological material at ultra-low temperatures, achieved using liquified gases, has become a valuable tool in developmental biology and the conservation of genetic resources. It is believed that a high degree of genetic stability can be ensured during storage at these reduced temperatures and that all developmental processes are totally inhibited. If suitable material can be frozen and stored successfully, e.g., mammalian embryos, then the technique could be used to store material for the subsequent direct propagation of specific genetic stocks, which would be of benefit to future production and breeding programs.

Despite the problems of freezing and thawing tissues while maintaining viability, there are two other major criteria that a low-temperature storage system must satisfy. The first is relative ease of maintenance of the material under optimal storage conditions, and the second, and perhaps more important, is the guarantee of strict genetic stability over prolonged storage periods. It is believed that these criteria can be met by storage of the tissues in liquid nitrogen (-196°C), which is readily available, is easy to produce, and presents no particular handling problems. Maintenance of a storage system would be limited to ensuring a sufficient level of liquid nitrogen in the storage vessels to maintain the tissues at the temperature of the nitrogen (or very close to it).

At the temperature of liquid nitrogen, normal cellular chemical reactions do not occur, energy levels being too low to allow sufficient molecular motion to complete the reactions. Water exists either in a crystalline or a glassy state, and not as a liquid, and has such a high viscosity ($> 10^{13}$ poises) that rates of diffusion are insignificant over time spans measured at least as hundreds of years. The majority of chemical changes in the tissue are therefore effectively prevented, and so alterations within stored material with time are minimized.

Unfortunately, that is not to say that biological material successfully cooled to -196°C is in a state of suspended animation. Certain types of chemical reaction can occur at these temperatures, such as the formation of free radicals and macromolecular damage due to ionizing radiations. The only real threat to genetic stability of stored material comes from such reactions, especially those that could damage the DNA molecules. Any such damage that does occur wil necessarily be cumulative, as enzymic repair mechanisms are totally prevented at these low temperatures. The practical limit to the storage life of any particular material held at ultra-low temperatures will be reached, therefore, when such damage acculates to an unacceptable level. For certain mammalian cell lines it has been calculated that less than 1% of the spontaneous mutation rate at physiological temperatures is due to background radiation, and so the mutation rate at -196°C should be appreciably lower than at higher temperatures. While there are, as yet, few quantitative data on genetic stability at ultra-low temperatures for higher organisms, recent work by Ashwood-Smith and Grant had indicated that to reach the D_{10} level (where D_{10} is the radiation dose producing 10% survival in the population) a frozen cell culture would have to be exposed to background radiation for some 32,000 years. Assuming no repair at physiological temperatures, it would take 8,800 years to reach this level. There is also some evidence that dimethyl sulfoxide (DMSO), one of the widely used cryoprotectants usually essential for successful freeze preservation, may aid the reduction in the rate of cumulative radiation damage.

It is apparent, therefore, that the infinite storage of biological material at ultra-low temperatures is not yet feasible, although attempts at shielding may further reduce the radiation problems. Radiation resulting from isotopic disintegrations within the storage vessel cannot, however, be eliminated. In practical terms the extended storage of material over decades, even centuries, without significant alterations does, however, seem possible. The problems of genetic alteration can be minimized by setting a realistic storage period, say every 30 years, at the end of which the material is thawed and recharacterized, and fresh samples are taken for a further cycle of storage at ultra-low temperatures.

A second major worry arises if less than 100% survival is achieved after thawing. Unless clonal material is being used, it is always possible that some sort of selection is being imposed on the material, and the resulting progeny must be carefully checked using characters appropriate to the particular situation. One of the challenges that workers in this field face is the improvement of technique to routinely achieve close to 100% survival so that the possibilities of selection are eliminated. A further advantage gained by storage of material at ultra-low temperatures is that internationald transport without the fear of deterioration is possible. Also material could be held in the frozen state while donor organisms were checked to comply with disease and quarantine regulations.

The discovery by Polge and co-workers that spermatazoa could be stored in the frozen state, using glycerol as a cryoprotectant, led to the systematic "banking" of such material and the subsequent flexibility and improvements in animal, especially cattle, breeding. Extensions of this work to human spermatazoa has led to frozen-stored spermatazoa being used for artificial insemination as a way of circumventing clinical barriers to conception in certain cases.

Considerable further advantages to animal breeding could be achieved using techniques of embryo transplantation, which have been used, to date, to introduce new animal breeds to different countries and to multiply rapidly valuable genetic stocks. The major advantage of the technique is that the entire genome from the desired cross lies in the embryo and can be transplanted to a recipient at any geographical location; also a recipient of completely unknown genetic background could be used as a "foster mother." The potential of this technique could be greatly enhanced if there were no limitation to the time that elapsed between obtaining the embryo and its subsequent implantation. If the embryos can be stored for long periods with maintained genetic stability, then this enhancement can be achieved (Polge, 1977).

It is believed that cryopreservation can allow this prolonged storage of a viable embryo in many instances, and that more research will continue to increase the number of species to which it is applicable.

The limitations to the technique are:

1. The ability to freeze the embryo
2. Maintenance of high levels of survival
3. Maintenance of genetic stability
4. Success of the transplanting technique

Much of the early work that led to the successful freezing of mammalian embryos was, in fact, carried out with unfertilized eggs. Notable early experiments carried out with unfertilized rabbit eggs and with glycerol as a cryoprotectant showed that a high percentage (69%) of the eggs could survive storage in a supercooled state at -15°C for 3 days, if 15% v/v glycerol as a cryoprotectant was both added and removed in a stepwise manner. Cooling of these eggs to -79°C at a rate of 1°C min^{-1} reduced viability to 1% after rapid thawing. Further experiments continuing with the use of glycerol as a cryoprotectant demonstrated the survival of rat oocytes slowly cooled to both -79°C and -196°C, the temperature of liquid nitrogen. (Polge, 1977). The transplanting of similarly treated mouse ovarian tissue into previously sterilised mice demonstrated the success and practical implications of the cryopreservative techniques, since normal offspring could be reared from the recipient mothers. The successful freeze preservation of mouse embryos was reported by Whittingham et al. in 1972, in a series of experiments that attempted to assess the contribution of suspending medium and cryoprotectants, cooling rate, and warming rate on the subsequent survival after storage in liquid nitrogen.

Embryos were removed from mice that had been induced to superovulate and were suspended in modified Dulbecco's phosphate-buffered salt solution (PBS medium). The embryos were collected at the one-, two-, and eight-cell states and as blastocysts, and were suspended in 0.1 ml of PBS medium at 0°C, with 0.1 ml of 2 M glycerol or dimethyl sulfoxide added as a cryoprotectant. The embryos were transferred to a bath at c. -4.0°C and seeded with ice. The samples were cooled at rates ranging from 0.3°C min^{-1} to 40°C min^{-1} and warmed at rates from 25°C min^{-1} to 4°C min^{-1}.

The embryos that were intact after thawing were cultured by Brinster's method in small droplets of culture medium at 37°C. Survival was determined as the percentage of recovered embryos that developed into blastocysts. These experiments indicated that for optimal survival the cooling rate had to be lower than 2°C min^{-1}, a rate that had been previously predicted from thermodynamic and kinetic calculations (Mazur, 1963 and 1966). A major factor in lethal freezing injury is the formation of intracellular ice, and a way of preventing this is to cool the cells at a rate sufficiently slow to allow most of the freezable water to come out of the cell during cooling. For the mouse embryos (approx. 70 μm diameter) the theoretical optimal cooling rate would be in the region of 10°C min^{-1}. Survival rates approaching 70% have been achieved with both eight- and two-celled embryos.

These experiments also clearly demonstrated the value of slow warming rates, whereas in more recent studies it has been shown that such warming rates are not generally applicable.

The results indicated that there was a viable potential for such cryopreservative techniques, and subsequently both rat and rabbit embryos have been frozen.

Cow and sheep embryos have also been successfully frozen, making a valuable practical contribution to the conservation of genetic stock of these major agricultural species. Pig embryos have proved to be particularly recalcitrant with respect to freezing, with none surviving cooling below $0°C$, and are at the center of much current research into cryopreservation of embryos.

It is hoped that this overview of work in mammalian embryo freezing has pointed out the major problems that have to be overcome if the successful freezing of the embryos of any species is to be achieved. Difficulties may relate to choice and optimal concentration of cryoprotectant, rates of cooling and warming, embryo size, and indeed other unknown factors that appear to be species-specific. If high levels of survival can be achieved for frozen embryos of laboratory and agricultural animals, then the establishment of gene banks for the maintenance of specific lines and as an aid to the improvement of genetic stocks can become a reality.

Similarly, the storage of human embryos in liquid nitrogen prior to implanting in the mother could be a valuable clinical tool in the solution of problems of infertility in certain situations, e.g., tubal occlusion, oligaspermia, and autoimmunity (Edwards and Steptoe, 1977). In such cases the patients are unlikely to become pregnant unless an oocyte is fertilized in vitro, and the fertilized oocyte is cultured to a suitable stage for implanting in the uterus. Assuming that the implantation was performed at an appropriate time in the hormonal cycle such that the uterus was receptive, then the embryo could develop to full term. In practice, however, the success of these implants is low, for the embryo has to be returned to the mother in the same hormonal cycle as it was collected since it cannot be sustained in culture for prolonged periods. In hormonal terms this particular cycle is some way from natural, as the patient will have been treated with human menopausal gonadotropin (HMG) and human chorionic gonadotropin (HCG) to stimulate follicular growth and ovulation. Despite such problems of implantation, full-term pregnancy and delivery of a normal, healthy child have been demonstrated (Steptoe and Edwards, 1978).

The enormous potential of cryopreservative techniques as an aid to this valuable clinical procedure becomes apparent. If embryos could be stored for prolonged periods, they could be implanted at the appropriate time in a "natural" hormonal cycle of choice, and not in the HMG/HCG modified one. Further, several embryos could be stored from a single batch of collected oocytes so that the chances of achieving a successful implantation without further hormonal treatment and oocyte collection would be greatly increased. A number of pregnancies could also be achieved from such a single batch of stored embryos. The ideal human material for cryopreservation would be the morula/early blastocyst, which would be in the uterus in a normal pregnancy. If such material were successfully recovered after thawing then, providing implantation was at a suitable hormonal period, a high chance of success could be expected.

The value of the cryopreservation of embryos for conservation and breeding of laboratory and agricultural animals has been clearly demonstrated, and an important potential for medical practice highlighted. Although many experimental and ethical questions remain to be answered, this potential should not be ignored.

References

Ashwood-Smith, M. J., and Grant, E. Genetic stability in cellular systems stored in the frozen state. *CIBA Symp. 52*: 251–271, 1977.

Edwards, R. G., and Steptoe, P. C. The relevance of the frozen storage of human embryos. *CIBA Symp. 52*: 235–250, 1977.

Mazur, P. Kinetics of water loss from cells at sub-zero temperatures and the likelihood of intracellular freezing. *J. Gen. Physiol. 47:* 347–369, 1963.

Mazur, P. Physical and chemical basis of injury in a single-celled micro-organism subjected to freezing and thawing. In Cryobiology, ed. H. T. Meryman, Academic Press, London and New York, 214–315, 1966.

Polge, C. The freezing of mammalian embryos: Perspectives and possibilities. *CIBA Symp. 52:* 3–20, 1977.

Steptoe, P. C. and Edwards, R. G. Birth after the reimplantation of a human embryo. *Lancet ii:,* 366, 1978.

Whittingham, D. G., Leibo, S. P., and Mazur, P. Survival of mouse embryos frozen to –196°C and –269°C. *Science (Wash. D.C.) 178*: 411–414, 1972.

INDEX